Workbook for

Mosby's

Paramedic Textbook

Fourth Edition

Workbook for

Mosby's
Paramedic Textbook

Fourth Edition

Kim D. McKenna, MEd RN, CEN, EMT-P
Director of Education
St. Charles County Ambulance District
St. Peters, Missouri

Adjunct Professor
Lindenwood University
St. Charles, Missouri

Mick J. Sanders, MSA, EMT-P
EMS Training Specialist
St. Charles, Missouri

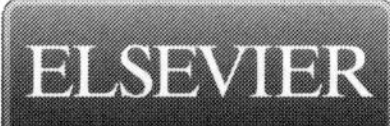

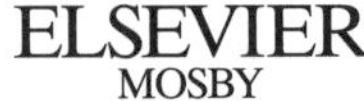
MOSBY

3251 Riverport Lane
St. Louis, Missouri 63043

WORKBOOK FOR MOSBY'S PARAMEDIC TEXTBOOK, EDITION 4   ISBN: 978-0-323-07278-6

Acquisitions Editor: Laura Bayless
Developmental Editor: Mary Jo Adams
Publishing Services Manager: Julie Eddy
Project Manager: Richard Barber/Kiruthiga Kasthuriswamy

Printed in the United States

Last digit is the print number: 9   8   7   6   5   4   3   2   1

Working together to grow
libraries in developing countries

www.elsevier.com | www.bookaid.org | www.sabre.org

ELSEVIER   BOOK AID International   Sabre Foundation

About the Authors

Kim D. McKenna, MEd RN CEN, EMT-P, is the director of education for the St. Charles County Ambulance District located in the metropolitan St. Louis, Missouri, area. There she is primary instructor for the paramedic program and program director for the district's emergency medical technician programs and leads a training staff that provides education for district paramedics and for firefighters and emergency personnel within St. Charles County. Kim has been teaching in EMS for over 25 years. She formerly worked as an emergency and intensive care nurse and served as chief medical officer for the Florissant Valley Fire Protection District for 6 years. Kim was the EMR Project Level Leader for the National EMS Education Standards project and is currently a Board of Director for the National Association of EMS Educators.

Mick J. Sanders, EMT-P, MSA, received his paramedic training in 1978 from St. Louis University Hospitals. He earned a Bachelor of Science degree and a Master of Science degree from Lindenwood University in St. Charles, Missouri. He has worked in various health care systems as a field paramedic, emergency department paramedic, and EMS instructor. For 12 years, Mr. Sanders served as training specialist with the Bureau of Emergency Medical Services, Missouri Department of Health, where he oversaw EMT and paramedic training and licensure in St. Louis city and the surrounding metropolitan areas.

Preface

The *Workbook to Accompany Mosby's Paramedic Textbook,* fourth edition, has been written to enhance paramedic student's understanding and retention of the material presented in the textbook. This has been accomplished using a variety of questions designed to encourage the various levels of learning necessary in this field from recall and memorization to application and analysis of concepts. Some of the features of this workbook include the following:

- A special section on studying and test-taking skills so that good habits can begin early in the program
- A format that follows *Mosby's Paramedic Textbook,* fourth edition, chapter by chapter, with answers referenced to the appropriate objective
- Objectives and Summaries from the textbook chapters to refresh key information
- Wrap It Up sections in each chapter that offer an additional opportunity to use learning in context
- Matching questions that reinforce key terms or content within the chapters
- Extensive use of case study–based questions to help visualize the real-life application of information
- Self-assessment sections that offer the opportunity to review material using multiple-choice questions, a testing format often used by instructors for examinations
- Complete rationales for all answers that ensures understanding of material
- A programmed review of basic math skills that precedes the drug dose calculation section
- Illustrations for student identification of anatomy, patient management techniques, and special equipment
- Paramedic career opportunities section that introduces some of the choices in the paramedic profession

Electrocardiogram and drug flashcards at the end of the book can be removed for easy reference and study purposes. Flashcards are completed by the students and are keyed to questions in the workbook. The electrocardiogram flashcards show actual patient rhythms, and the drug flashcards are based on patient care scenarios.

Before completing each chapter of the workbook, you should read the accompanying chapter in *Mosby's Paramedic Textbook,* fourth edition, and review the learning objectives. When you encounter areas of difficulty while completing the questions, reread the text and attempt the questions again. We hope that this workbook, when used effectively, will facilitate mastery of the complex knowledge necessary to become a paramedic. Enjoy!

# Acknowledgments

This workbook, of course, would never have been possible without the terrific manuscript of *Mosby's Paramedic Textbook,* fourth edition, written by Mick J. Sanders. His commitment to excellence is reflected throughout the text, and his encouragement and suggestions made the completion of the workbook possible.

Thanks to Catherine Parvensky, who wrote the original studying and test-taking tips and the paramedic career opportunities sections of the workbook.

For the original patient electrocardiogram strips, I am indebted to the to my former colleagues at St. John's Mercy Medical Center. A debt of gratitude goes to Gary Denton of Acute Coronary Syndrome Consultants, Inc., and to Wolff Medical Publishing, Inc. for many of the 12-lead electrocardiogram tracings included in the text.

To all of my paramedic students, past and present, I sincerely appreciate all that you have taught me and your suggestions for the content of this workbook.

And to the fellow paramedics and EMTs with whom I work in the field, thanks for showing me where the textbook ends and reality begins.

I am also grateful to the reviewers of this and past editons: Joyce Forsman-Capuzzi, CEN, CPN, CTRN, CCRN, CPEN, SANE-A, EMT-P; John DeArmond, NREMT-P; Jeff DeGraffenreid; Johnson County Medical Action Emergency Medical Services, Olathe, Kansas; Janet Fitts, RN, EMT-P; Bob Nixon, BA, EMT-P; Deborah Petty, BS, CICP, EMT-P I/C; and Monroe Yancie, NREMT-P for their suggestions and fresh ideas.

Thanks to the staff at Elsevier, especially Laura Bayless, who worked so diligently to make this project happen; to Rich Barber whose attention to detail is evident throughout the text; and to Joy Knobbe in marketing, who cheered us all on. We are forever grateful.

Kim D. McKenna
Mick J. Sanders

How to Study for Success in EMS

By Kim McKenna
JEMS Online
Wednesday, February 27, 2008

"Hope is not a strategy."—attributed to General Custer

When it comes to preparing for EMS quizzes, mid-term, final, and registration examinations, no truer words were ever spoken. To ensure success in the EMS classroom, students must plan their study time, use specific study strategies, and have the right motivation. Unfortunately, many students come to EMS classes lacking good skills in this area.

GENERAL STUDY SKILLS

How often have you heard (or said), "I don't understand why I failed that exam. I spent 20 hours studying." Putting in a sufficient amount of time for study is important, but it isn't enough. Students must study with purpose. Reading the written text on the page isn't adequate. You need to engage your senses so the information will "stick" in your brain.

When students study effectively, they study for meaning. To really understand information, you must change it so you comprehend it and it means something to you. Some examples of ways to understand specific information include comparing it to something, coming up with other examples of it, saying what causes it, and determining what an EMT needs to do with it.

There is no "one size fits all" when it comes to studying. Each learner and topic is unique and may require a different approach for success. Try several strategies until you find one that works for you and for the material you're studying.

HIGHLIGHTING AND UNDERLINING

Marking content can be somewhat helpful the first time you read through material. The goal of highlighting is to identify only the most important content in the section you're reading. As a rule, you shouldn't highlight more than 10% of the content. If you're highlighting more, you probably haven't analyzed the content well enough to pick out the most important material.

MARGIN NOTES

Pencil notes in the margin to call out significant thoughts or words. Try to write down different words than those in the chapter; doing this requires you to rephrase and reframe the material. This shows that you understand it.

MAKE STUDY NOTES OR STUDY CARDS

When you make study notes or study cards, it forces you to first pick out important content and then rewrite it. This engages several senses and involves more of your brain. The more of your brain you can involve, the more new memory connections you'll form.

CATEGORIZE THE MATERIAL

Make tables of information to compare and contrast material from a chapter. For example, make a table listing the sympathetic and parasympathetic nervous system and list how each affects the organs. By comparing groups of content, you'll see how they are alike and how they differ. This is a great way to explore a topic and really get to know it.

Mind maps, concept maps, algorithms, and drawings all require you to reorder the material and "see" it in a different way. To prepare these visual aids effectively requires you understand it thoroughly.

ORGANIZE STUDY GROUPS WITH PURPOSE

Quizzing one another and discussing material can be very helpful. Effective study groups come together prepared to study (not to copy each other's homework) with a specific purpose and a time limit. If you fail to properly use study groups, you will waste valuable study time.

Just as students learn differently, each student will study differently. The bottom line is that the earlier a student learns to study effectively for their learning style, the better chance he or she has for success in the EMS classroom and beyond.

x

How to Prepare for the Big One

By Kim McKenna
JEMS Online
Monday, May 12, 2008

For most EMS students, the exam with the highest stakes is the final registration examination, and for most EMS students in the United States, that means the National Registry of EMTs (NREMT) computer adaptive test.

For this exam—as for any test—the key to success is to know and to understand the material. Period. But you can take certain steps to prepare for this "mother" of all exams.

Review the materials provided on the NREMT website. This will give you specific information related to the test.

Practice taking tests in a similar format. Instructors can deliver tests that will only allow you to see one question at a time. These tests often also have a running timer clock on the screen. Adapting to these seemingly small things can help to diminish unnecessary anxiety the day of the test. Tests available for a fee can help to predict your success on the registry examination and help you target weak areas so you can focus your study time.

The NREMT exams cover airway, medical/OB, trauma, cardiovascular, and operations. Pediatrics is integrated throughout each section. Prepare for all sections of the test. Failing to study for the operations section so you can spend extra time studying for the cardiovascular section could be a critical error.

Make your first attempt your best. Taking the test "just so you can see how you do" is never a sound strategy. The test will be different each time, and the personal cost in terms of time, money, and anxiety will be greater with each subsequent attempt.

Keep your eye on the prize: Remind yourself why this is important to you. Your motivation will be critical to ensure adequate preparation.

Develop a study plan: A schedule allows you to devote sufficient time to prepare. Cramming is *not* effective. Divide your time into manageable blocks so you can study properly. Set goals and include "rewards," such as exercise, if you meet your goal.

Identify effective study strategies: These will vary depending on whether the material requires memorization, application, or problem solving. Study skills vary by student.

Focus on understanding: The licensure exam has many questions that require you to apply your knowledge or to solve problems. You must understand what you're doing, why you're doing it, when to do it, and how to do it. In addition, you must understand the pathophysiology behind each sign, symptom, and intervention.

Monitor your study effectiveness: At the end of each section, ask yourself, "Did I really get it?" If the answer is no, you may be in the wrong place to study or you might be using the wrong strategy. Just because you've spent time studying doesn't mean you know the material. Don't waste your time; study effectively!

Control the environment: Get enough sleep the night before the exam. Take the test at the time of day when you know you'll be at your best. Take care of your physical needs before the exam. Eat a small meal and go to the restroom before testing. You don't want to be distracted by little things.

During the test: Treat each question as if it's the last. Don't rush. Read each word in the stem (introduction) of the question carefully. Professionally written examinations avoid using unnecessary words. If a word is in the question, it's there for a reason. For example, the patient's age is often an important clue. Difficulty breathing in a 6-month-old patient has very different causes than in a 72-year-old patient. Pay careful attention to words that can modify the meaning or priority of the answers. Words such as "best," "first," or "most important" can help you distinguish between two or three choices (distractors) that look correct but aren't so you can pick the "best" answer.
Try to read the question (stem) first to see if you can think of the answer before you read the distractors. If none of the answer choices presented in the question match the one that you thought of or if you have no idea what the answer is, go back and reread the question. Break the problem (stem) into small pieces and be sure you understand what the question is' asking. For example, when you carefully reread, you may notice that you missed the fact that your patient's heart rate was very slow. That could be the clue you need to solve the problem! If you carefully reread the question and still can't pick out the right answer, try to rule out answers that you know for sure are wrong. This may at least increase your odds of getting the question right.

Don't forget the priorities of care when you choose an answer. If two answers one that involves treating the airway and the other breathing are attractive, the former may be correct if the question asks you to choose the intervention that you should perform *first*. That said, don't just blindly choose answers that include the airway. Answer the specific question being asked.

For many EMTs, AEMTs, and paramedics, the registry examination is the final stop on the journey to a new career. Current research shows factors related to your EMS program, your instructors, and your field and clinical experience play critical roles in your success on the final exam. However, you play the final—and most important—role in preparing for this test. Give it the attention it deserves. Your future depends on it.

How to Prepare for the Big One

# Paramedic Career Opportunities

Since its inception in 1967, emergency medical services (EMS) has developed into a sophisticated profession with various levels of care that result in improved care of sick and injured patients. With the evolution of EMS have come career opportunities for emergency medical technicians, paramedics, nurses, and physicians. Although specific job opportunities depend on geographical locations, in general, opportunities for prehospital emergency responders have emerged from volunteer to paid career positions. For a certified paramedic, many options are available.

OTHER AREAS OF INTEREST

Aside from traditional prehospital roles, some paramedics have taken on expanded duties. Some hospitals in the United States employ paramedics in the emergency department. Others hire them as patient care technicians, pathology assistants, intravenous team members, phlebotomists, and suture technicians.

Some hospitals also have urgent care centers in which paramedics have an expanded function. These facilities offer treatment for minor illnesses or injuries, physical examinations, and health screenings. They often are located within industrial settings, universities, and stand-alone buildings not part of hospitals.

Finally, paramedics who pursue advanced education can find additional opportunities. Many colleges and universities offer credit hours toward an associate or bachelor's degree for any individual with a paramedic certification. Some paramedics return to school for advanced training as nurses, physician's assistants, or medical doctors.

POSITION

A *field paramedic* requires current state licensure or certification as a paramedic. Some states and organizations also require National Registry certification.

A *paramedic supervisor* or *captain* usually requires substantial experience as a field provider and supervisory experience. Many departments awards point in the promotional process to paramedics who have college degrees.

A *flight paramedic* usually requires substantial experience as a field paramedic and the ability to work under pressure. Additional certifications or training may be required by the individual service.

An *interhospital transport medic* requires certification/licensure as a paramedic. Additional specialized training may be required or provided by the employer.

An *EMS administrator,* in addition to paramedic certification or licensure, often requires advanced degrees in EMS, business, or health care administration.

An *EMS educator* usually requires paramedic certification and experience as an instructor. Specialized training in education to meet the minimum requirements set forth by each state usually is needed. New paramedic program directors must have a minimum of a bachelor degree. Advanced-degree certification often is desired for high-level training programs. Attaining other instructor credentials such as the Nationally Certified EMS Educator (NCEE) is also desirable.

DESCRIPTION

Many paramedics enjoy the day-to-day operations of a field provider, administering emergency care to sick and injured patients. Roles and responsibilities of paramedics undoubtedly will grow as the emergency department extends into the community through advanced life support personnel.

An advanced life support supervisor is usually an experienced paramedic with administrative or management skills. Responsibilities for this position generally include recruitment, scheduling, monitoring quality, discipline, and supervision of emergency care personnel.

Flight paramedics use their knowledge and skills to care for patients who require air medical evacuation and rapid transport to hospitals. A flight crew usually is composed of a pilot, a flight paramedic, and a flight nurse. Some organizations hire paramedics to assist with the interhospital, intercontinental, or international transfer of patients requiring monitored transportation. Responsibilities for this position generally include monitoring of patients during transport and initiation of emergency care when necessary. Additional training for specialty skills often is necessary in this role to meet the needs of high-risk infants, children, and other patients who are critically ill or injured.

Experienced paramedics with backgrounds in management can act in administrative capacities within various organizations. Although advanced training often is necessary, administrative positions in hospitals, government emergency services organizations, and independent companies are possibilities.

Many colleges and universities offer programs in EMS, including paramedic certification programs, associate's degrees, bachelor's degrees, and even master's degrees. Paramedics with experience in education can obtain positions as instructors for such programs.

xiii

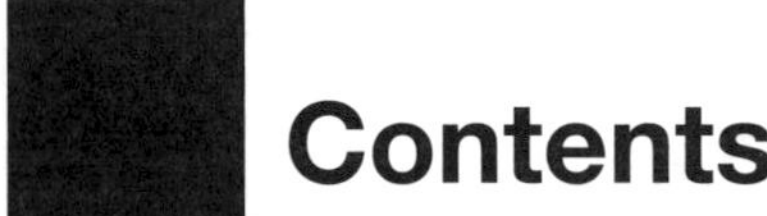

Contents

1

EMS Systems: Roles, Responsibilities, and Professionalism

READING ASSIGNMENT

Chapter 1, pages 1-23, in *Mosby's Paramedic Textbook*, ed. 4.

OBJECTIVES

Upon completion of this chapter, the paramedic student will be able to do the following:

1. Outline key historical events that influenced the development of emergency medical services (EMS) systems.
2. Identify the key elements necessary for effective EMS systems operations.
3. Outline the five components of the EMS Education Agenda for the Future: A Systems Approach.
4. Describe the benefits of continuing education.
5. Differentiate among training and roles and responsibilities of the four nationally recognized levels of EMS licensure/certification: Emergency Medical Responder, Emergency Medical Technician, Advanced Emergency Medical Technician, and Paramedic.
6. List the benefits of membership in professional EMS organizations.
7. Differentiate among professionalism and professional licensure, certification, registration, and credentialing.
8. List characteristics of the professional paramedic.
9. Describe the paramedic's role in patient care situations as defined by the U.S. Department of Transportation.
10. Describe the benefits of each component of offline (indirect) and online (direct) medical direction.
11. Outline the role and components of an effective, continuous quality improvement program.
12. Recognize EMS activities that pose a high risk for patients.
13. Describe actions the paramedic may take to reduce the chance of errors related to patient care.

SUMMARY

- The roots of prehospital emergency care may date back to the military.
- In the early twentieth century through the mid-1960s, prehospital care in the United States was provided in a few ways. Care was provided mostly by urban hospital-based systems. These systems later developed into municipal services. Care also was provided by funeral directors and volunteers who were not trained in these services.
- The operations of an effective EMS system include citizen activation, dispatch, prehospital care, hospital care, and rehabilitation.
- Each level of EMS personnel has its own distinct roles and duties. These roles include telecommunicators (dispatchers), emergency medical responders, EMTs, Advanced EMTs, and Paramedics. These levels combine to make an effective prehospital EMS system.
- Many professional groups and organizations help to set the standards of EMS. These groups exist at the national, state, regional, and local levels. The groups take part in development, education, and implementation. Being active in such a group helps to promote the status of the paramedic.
- Continuing education is crucial. It provides a way for all health care personnel to maintain basic technical and professional skills.
- *Professionalism* refers to the way in which a person conducts him- or herself. It also refers to how one follows the standards of conduct and performance established by the profession.
- The roles and duties of the paramedic can be divided into two categories. These groups are *primary* and *additional* duties.
- The two types of medical direction are online (direct) and offline (indirect) medical direction. Both are equally important. They help to ensure that the components of quality medical care are in place in an EMS system.
- A continuous quality improvement (CQI) program identifies and attempts to resolve problems in areas such as medical direction, financing, training, communication, prehospital management and transportation, interfacility transfer, receiving facilities, specialty care units, dispatch, public information and education, audit and quality assurance, disaster planning, and mutual aid.
- Patient safety should be a high priority during every call. Errors that may cause injury or illness often involve handoffs, communication issues, medication issues, airway issues, lifting or moving patients, ambulance crashes, and immobilization.

1. While working late, a 56-year-old man develops chest pain. The man is alone in his office when the chest pain increases, and he falls to the floor, having a cardiac arrest.

   Identify the missing components of the EMS system in Fig. 1-1 that are necessary to effectively resuscitate this victim and return him to a productive role in society.

   a. ____

   b. ____

   c. ____

   d. ____

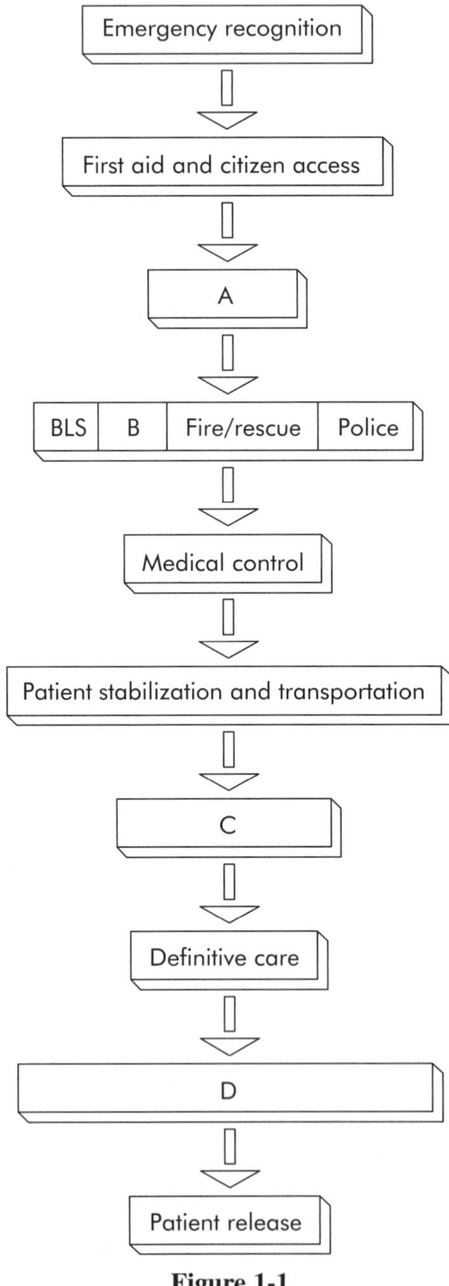

Figure 1-1

Chapter 1 **EMS Systems: Roles, Responsibilities, and Professionalism**

After attending a continuing education lecture on advances in trauma care, you report to work for your 12-hour shift. You carefully check out your vehicle for equipment and mechanical readiness for a call and then head to the company fitness room to exercise. Just as you finish your workout, the tones sound. You are dispatched to a nursing home for a person with "difficulty breathing." The street alarm is activated, and as you pull out, you carefully glance to ensure that traffic has come to a stop before proceeding onto the busy roadway in front of your station. When you arrive at the nursing home, you obtain a rapid history from the nursing home staff and begin your assessment of the 87-year-old patient. She is in obvious respiratory distress, and you recognize the need for rapid interventions to prevent further deterioration of her condition. Your partner gives oxygen and then applies continuous positive airway pressure (CPAP) and prepares to insert an intravenous (IV) line as you contact online medical direction. You briefly describe your patient's condition and request orders for nitroglycerin. The physician advisor agrees with your treatment plan. As soon as your partner secures the IV line, you administer the drug, carefully checking for allergies and appropriate dosing before giving it. A repeat assessment of the patient in 5 minutes shows some improvement. You continue plans to transfer her into the ambulance. The nursing home staff tells you she should be transported to the city hospital. This is consistent with your medical protocols, so you agree. As you depart, another evaluation demonstrates even more improvement. On arrival at the hospital, you give a report and transfer care of the patient to the nursing staff and then complete your patient report. You ask the physician about another drug that you had considered requesting, but she agrees that in this patient's circumstance, the treatment plan you had chosen was appropriate. Back at base, you restock the vehicle with the drugs and equipment used on the call. Then you head down to the classroom to help teach the 8 PM community cardiopulmonary resuscitation (CPR) class.

2. List 10 primary responsibilities of the paramedic that were demonstrated in this simulated call.

a. ____

b. ____

c. ____

d. ____

e. ____

f. ____

g. ____

h. ____

i. ____

j. ____

3. List two additional responsibilities of the paramedic that were demonstrated in this scenario.

a. ____

b. ____

Match the historical role in EMS in column I with the appropriate person or event in column II. Use each answer only once.

Column I

4. _______ First use of helicopter for medical evacuation during an armed conflict.

5. _______ Demonstrated the value of mouth-to-mouth ventilation

6. _______ Twentieth century battlefield ambulance corps developed

7. _______ Dr. Eugene Nagel trains firefighters as paramedics.

8. _______ Earliest American battlefield ambulance corps

9. _______ Clara Barton performs battlefield emergency medical care and brings this organization to the United States

10. _______ Jean Larry transports wounded in a covered cart

11. _______ Fixed-wing medical transports were developed in this conflict.

Column II

a. American Red Cross
b. US Civil War
c. Korean conflict
d. Miami, 1967
e. Napoleonic Wars
f. Peter Safar, MD, 1958
g. World War I
h. World War II
i. Vietnam conflict

Match the description in column I with the appropriate licensure and certification level in column II. Use each answer only once.

Column I

12. _______ Trained in basic life support, including defibrillation

13. _______ Trained in all aspects of basic and advanced life support

14. _______ Trained in all aspects of basic life support and IV therapy

Column II

a. EMT (EMT-B)
b. AEMT (EMT-I)
c. Paramedic (EMT-P)
d. Emergency Medical Responder (First Responder)

Match the activity in column I with the appropriate term in column II. You may use each term more than once.

Column I

15. _______ Education and training of EMS personnel

16. _______ Personnel selection for employment

17. _______ Appropriate equipment choice selection

18. _______ Clinical protocol guidance and direction

19. _______ Clinical problem resolution

20. _______ Interface among EMS systems

21. _______ Advocacy within medical community

22. _______ Online communication with physicians and EMS

23. _______ Patient care report reviews

24. _______ Establish standards of care

25. _______ Serve as resource experts

26. _______ Introduction of new information

Column II

a. Continuing education
b. Continuous quality improvement
c. Medical direction
d. Professional associations

27. Give at least one specific example of patient harm that could occur because of an error that could be caused in the field related to each of the following high-risk activities.

Activity	Cause of Error	Patient Harm
a. Handoffs		
b. Communication issues		
c. Poor sterile technique		
d. Airway issues		
e. Dropping patients		
f. Ambulance crashes		

28. List two specific actions you could take to reduce the chance of error in the following situations.

   a. Giving report at the hospital

   ____

   b. Administering medication

   ____

   c. Choosing the proper airway device

   ____

STUDENT SELF-ASSESSMENT

29. Which federal law enabled creation of the U.S. Department of Transportation and the National Highway Traffic Safety Administration and provided funding for EMS?
   a. Accidental Death and Disability Act
   b. Consolidated Omnibus Reconciliation Act
   c. Emergency Medical Services Systems Act
   d. Highway Safety Act

30. Which component is at the center of the EMS system?
   a. Disaster planning
   b. Consumers
   c. Intensive care units
   d. Paramedic training

31. Which component of the EMS Education Agenda for the future is designed primarily to protect the public?
   a. EMS certification
   b. EMS Program Accreditation
   c. National EMS Core Content.
   d. National EMS Education Standards

 Chapter **1** **EMS Systems: Roles, Responsibilities, and Professionalism**

32. Which of the following describes the manner in which a paramedic follows the practice, guidelines, and ethical considerations of prehospital emergency care?
  a. Certification
  b. Licensure
  c. Professionalism
  d. Registration

33. Which of the following is within the role of the paramedic as defined by the U.S. Department of Transportation?
  a. Dispatching public safety agencies to emergency calls
  b. Coordinating collection of outstanding patient bills
  c. Diagnosing and prescribing medication therapy
  d. Making sure the ambulance is adequately stocked

34. The EMS physician medical director is responsible for which of the following?
  a. Ensuring maintenance of ambulances and equipment
  b. Monitoring the quality of EMS care
  c. Negotiating staff salary and benefit disputes
  d. Providing patient care in the field on advanced life support units

35. A man who claims to be an emergency department physician is attempting to direct care in an inappropriate manner on a cardiac arrest call. You should do which of the following?
  a. Contact online medical direction for instructions
  b. Follow his orders because he has appropriate credentials
  c. Ignore him and carry on as you see appropriate
  d. Immediately ask the police to arrest him

36. Which of the following demonstrates a prospective method of a continuous quality improvement model?
  a. Continuing education programs
  b. Listening to audio tapes of EMS reports
  c. Observation of prehospital care by the medical director
  d. Reviewing prehospital patient care records

37. Which error prevention strategy involves asking yourself, "Am I doing the right thing?"
  a. After-action review
  b. Reflection bias
  c. Reflection in action
  d Questioning assumptions

38. Which is an example of an environmental method to reduce the risk of medication error?
  a. Applying colored tape to distinguish between look-alike medicines
  b. Requiring the dose be repeated three times before administration
  c. Having your partner double check the dose calculation
  d. Using a pocket reference source to verify correct administration

39. Which of the following activities represents the highest risk activity on an EMS call?
  a. Administering medication
  b. Inserting an advanced airway
  c. Lifting and moving a patient
  d. Responding lights and sirens

Your rural EMS service responds to a call for a vehicle accident with possible rescue. Your ambulance arrives on the scene first, and you provide the scene size-up on the radio for the incoming units: "4017 on the scene, two vehicles involved, major damage, investigating." A bystander shouts to you that he called 9-1-1 on his cell phone and that there is a guy "hurt real bad" in one of the cars. You and your EMT partner split up, going to separate cars to triage the injured. Major damage to the car prevents access through the doors, so you break a window to gain access. The driver, an unrestrained teenage boy, has trauma to the head. He is taking agonal gasps and has a rapid radial pulse. You shout to your partner that you have a critical patient and immediately call dispatch to send a helicopter and a second ambulance. As you begin to manage the patient's airway and to ventilate him, the rescue pumper arrives. Your partner tells you that there are two patients in the second car: a woman with minor lacerations and her 9-year-old daughter, who has significant cervical spine tenderness and is hysterical. The second ambulance crew arrives, and you tell them that extrication is needed. You direct the paramedic on the rescue pumper to manage the two patients in the second car while you and your partner care for your critically injured patient as extrication efforts proceed. Your patient has apparent head, chest, and abdominal injuries. Dispatch notifies you that the helicopter has a 2-minute estimated time of arrival (ETA). Police have blocked the highway for safety and are assisting with the landing zone. Moments before the helicopter lands, rescue crews remove the car door, and you perform rapid extrication. You carefully move the patient to the spine board, secure him, and move him to your ambulance. With your partner's assistance, you intubate the patient using inline spinal immobilization. Then, as your partner ventilates the patient, you initiate an IV line while firefighters assist with monitoring and assessment of vital signs. The air medical crew arrives. You give them a rapid, thorough report and direct them to take the patient to the closest level I trauma center. The rescue pumper paramedic reports that the two patients from the second vehicle are being transported by ground past the local hospital to the trauma center. You quickly clean your rig and return in service to the station to write your patient care report.

1. What role did citizens play in this call?

2. What steps did dispatch take to coordinate the activities in this call?

3. What role, if any, did medical direction play in this call?

4. Why was the use of the helicopter indicated in this situation when the other two patients were taken by ground to the same facility?
   a. The male patient needed intubation.
   b. The ETA of the second ambulance was delayed.
   c. Prolonged extrication was needed.
   d. Multiple trauma patients were involved.

5. Why were the patients taken to the trauma center rather than a closer hospital?
   a. Definitive care is rapidly available for trauma patients at a trauma center.
   b. Mileage charges are greater to a more distant hospital.
   c. Helicopters transport only to trauma centers.
   d. Local hospitals have poorer quality of care.

          Chapter **1** **EMS Systems: Roles, Responsibilities, and Professionalism**

6. Why were you performing the advanced skills on this call rather than your partner?
   a. The attending paramedic always performs the skills.
   b. The first person reaching the patient performs invasive skills.
   c. Your partner is an EMT, and these skills exceed his license in many states.
   d. The most experienced crew member is designated to perform skills.

7. Rank the attributes of the professional paramedic that you think would be most important on this call from 1 to 11, with 1 the most important and 11 the least important.

   __________ Integrity   __________ Empathy
   __________ Self-motivation   __________ Appearance and personal hygiene
   __________ Self-confidence   __________ Communication
   __________ Time management   __________ Teamwork and diplomacy
   __________ Respect   __________ Patient advocacy
   __________ Careful delivery of service

8. Would your rankings from the question above change for the following situations? If you answer yes, indicate how they would change.

   a. A 75-year-old patient who is despondent over the loss of his wife is threatening to kill himself. Yes/No

   ____

   ____

   b. A 27-year-old woman has just miscarried a 20-week pregnancy; this is her sixth miscarriage in 2 years. Yes/No

   ____

   ____

   c. A 54-year-old patient in the mayor's chambers has chest pain, and electrocardiogram (ECG) readings suggest a heart attack. He does not want to be transported to the hospital. Yes/No

   ____

   ____

9. Place a ✓ beside the roles/responsibilities of the paramedic used on this call.

   __________ Preparation   __________ Response
   __________ Scene assessment   __________ Patient assessment
   __________ Recognition of injury or illness   __________ Patient management
   __________ Appropriate patient disposition   __________ Patient transfer
   __________ Documentation   __________ Returning to service

REVIEW QUESTIONS

1. a. Dispatcher; b. Advanced life support; c. Hospital delivery; d. Patient rehabilitation and education
(Objective 2)

2. a. Physical preparation for the job (exercise program)
b. Having appropriate equipment and supplies
c. Responding to the scene in a safe manner
d. Performing a quick patient assessment to determine priorities for care
e. Contacting medical direction for assistance with the care plan
f. Managing the emergency in the appropriate manner
g. Stabilizing the patient in the field
h. Providing transport by the appropriate means to the correct facility
i. Reporting to the staff regarding the patient's condition on arrival
j. Replacing equipment and debriefing the call
(Objective 7)

3. a. Advocating citizens' role in the EMS system by teaching community programs such as CPR
b. Continuing personal professional development by attending continuing education programs
(Objective 7)

4. c

5. f

6. g

7. d

8. b

9. a

10. e

11. h
(Questions 4–11: Objective 1)

12. a or d

13. c

14. b
(Questions 12–14: Objective 3)

15. a, b, c, d

16. c

17. a, b, c

18. b, c, d

19. a, b, c, d

20. c, d

21. c, d

22. b, c

23. b, c

24. b, c, d

25. c, d

26. a, c, d
(Questions 15–26: Objectives 4, 5, 8, 9)

27. a. Handoffs: Paramedic fails to tell hospital patient is allergic to a drug: Patient has anaphylactic reaction.
b. Communication issues: Paramedic hears an order for 10 mg of a drug when physician said 1 mg; paramedic fails to repeat back order: Patient receives an overdose and stops breathing.
c. Poor sterile technique: Paramedic fails to use sterile technique when suctioning the trachea: Patient develops pneumonia.
d. Airway issues: Paramedic takes too long on intubation attempts: Patient experiences hypoxic brain injury.
e. Dropping patients: Paramedic leaves stretcher in a full upright position with bariatric patient; stretcher falls to the side: Patient sustains fractures.
f. Ambulance crashes: Paramedic fails to stop at an intersection and collides with a vehicle: Patient and paramedic's partner sustain severe head and spine injuries.
(Objective 12) (Note: there are many possible correct answers to this question).

28. a. Giving report at the hospital: use a standard report format such as "I Pass the Baton"; listening attentively to the other person's questions; preparing to repeat the report more than once.
b. Administering medication: Use the standard "rights" of medication administration; say the drug and dose out loud; repeat orders to a physician; have your partner check the drug and dose; use tape to distinguish between look-alike drugs; use a pocket or electronic reference guide.
c. Choosing the proper airway device: Use reflection in action; monitor the effects of the intervention; question assumptions (the most advanced airway is not always the best airway for each situation).
(Objective 12)

STUDENT SELF-ASSESSMENT

29. d. This act, passed in 1966, required states to develop effective EMS programs or lose federal construction funds. It enabled large amounts of money to be spent for development of EMS and advanced life support (ALS) pilot programs. *Accidental Death and Disability: the Neglected Disease of Modern Society* (the "white" paper) was not an act but a report published by the National Academy of Sciences–National Research Council through its Committee on Trauma and Shock. The committee's recommendations paved the way for the Highway Safety Act of 1966. The EMSS act of 1973 developed regional EMS organizations. It identified 15 required components of the EMS system. The Consolidated Omnibus Reconciliation Act (COBRA) eliminated federal funds for EMS and redistributed them under state block grants.
(Objective 1)

30. b. Consumers are at the heart of the EMS system.
(Objective 2)

31. a. National EMS Certification is designed to ensure that candidates demonstrate a minimum level of skill and knowledge to earn certification. Certification is a requirement for licensure in most states.
(Objective 3)

32. c. Certification authorizes a person who has met specific qualifications to participate in an activity. Licensure grants a license to practice a profession. Registration is the act of enrolling a person's name in a book of record.
(Objective 6)

33. d
(Objective 5)

34. b. Other personnel should assume patient care and administrative and maintenance duties. The primary role of the EMS physician medical director is to ensure quality patient care.
(Objective 10)

35. a. Online medical direction should be contacted to attempt to arbitrate the situation. If this is impossible, police intervention may be recommended. Written policies addressing this issue should be prepared by the medical director so that actions to be taken in this situation are clearly defined.
(Objective 10)

36. a. The continuing education program can be offered to introduce new material, concepts, or skills so that appropriate patient care is delivered when that knowledge or skill is needed. This is done to ensure quality before a problem occurs. Direct observation of care is a concurrent method of CQI, and review of records and tapes is done after the actual care is delivered (retrospectively).
(Objective 11)

37. b. Reflection in action means you are thinking during the event so you can modify your actions if they are not producing the desired results or to stop yourself from performing an incorrect action.
(Objective 12)

38. a. Each of the other answers reflects good practices to reduce medication errors; however, taping the medication is the only environmental measure listed.
(Objective 12)

39. d. Ambulance vehicle collisions remain the highest risk activity for both the patient and the crew.
(Objective 11)

WRAP IT UP

1. Citizens recognized the emergency, called 9-1-1 and provided information to responding EMS units.
(Objective 2)

2. Dispatch identified the nature of the emergency, dispatched the proper apparatus to the correct location, dispatched the helicopter and an additional ambulance when directed, and updated the scene crew on the status of the helicopter.
(Objective 2)

3. Although no online medical direction was identified on this call, undoubtedly the crews notified online medical direction of their status. In addition, online medical direction should have had a role in determining the treatment protocols used, the protocol for using air medical services, and the protocol determining use of the trauma center. Medical direction also should be involved in a review of the call at a later time to monitor quality of care.
(Objective 10)

4. c. Most systems provide for dispatch of air medical crews when prolonged extrication is likely and the patient's condition warrants it. In other situations, even when the patient's condition is critical, the time to the appropriate hospital and other factors would be considered and should be established by protocol in collaboration with medical direction.
(Objective 2)

Chapter **1** **EMS Systems: Roles, Responsibilities, and Professionalism**

5. a. Protocols should define when patients are taken to a trauma center. Typically, these are based on the mechanism of injury, the anatomical injuries involved, and the patient's physiological status. Definitive care (surgery) for the trauma can be most effectively delivered at a trauma center, where appropriate resources (personnel and equipment) are readily available.
   (Objective 2)

6. c. In many states, advanced invasive skills such as intubation and vascular access are not within the scope of practice of an EMT.
   (Objective 5)

7. Responses will vary by individual opinion; however, careful delivery of service, time management, self-confidence, and communication likely would rank very high on this type of call.
   (Objective 7)

8. All attributes are critical for the paramedic; however, responses will vary by individual opinion. The following attributes are more likely to be ranked higher.
   a. Yes. Communication, respect, empathy, and patient advocacy
   b. Yes. Empathy, respect, and careful delivery of service
   c. Yes. Careful delivery of service, communication, teamwork and diplomacy, and appearance and personal hygiene
   (Objective 7)

9. All of these roles and responsibilities are used on this call.
   (Objective 8)

2 Well-Being of the Paramedic

READING ASSIGNMENT

Chapter 2, pages 24-49, in *Mosby's Paramedic Textbook*, ed. 4.

OBJECTIVES

Upon completion of this chapter, the paramedic student will be able to do the following:

1. Describe the components of wellness and associated benefits.
2. Discuss the paramedic's role in promoting wellness.
3. Outline the benefits of specific lifestyle choices that promote wellness, including proper nutrition, weight control, exercise, sleep, and smoking cessation.
4. Identify risk factors and warning signs of cancer and cardiovascular disease.
5. List measures to take to reduce the risk of infectious disease exposure.
6. Outline actions to be taken after a significant exposure to a patient's blood or other body fluids.
7. Identify preventive measures to minimize the risk of work-related illness or injury associated with exposure, lifting and moving patients, hostile environments, vehicle operations, and rescue situations.
8. List signs and symptoms of addiction and addictive behavior.
9. Describe guidelines for working effectively in a diverse workplace.
10. Distinguish between normal and abnormal anxiety and stress reactions.
11. Give examples of stress-reduction techniques.
12. Outline the 10 components of critical incident stress management.
13. Given a scenario involving death or dying, identify therapeutic actions you may take based on your knowledge of the dynamics of this process.

SUMMARY

- Wellness has two main aspects: physical well-being and mental and emotional health.
- As health care professionals, paramedics have a responsibility to serve as role models in disease prevention.
- Persons who are overweight tend to be at risk for developing certain illnesses. A healthful diet includes a variety of foods that are low in fat, saturated fat, and cholesterol. The calories in the diet should be regulated to prevent unwanted weight gain.
- *Physical fitness* can be described as a condition that helps individuals look, feel, and do their best.
- Sleep helps to rejuvenate a tired body.
- Steps to reduce cardiovascular disease include the following: improving cardiovascular endurance, eliminating cigarette smoking, controlling high blood pressure, maintaining a normal body fat composition, maintaining a good ratio of total cholesterol to high-density lipoprotein cholesterol, monitoring triglyceride levels, controlling diabetes, avoiding excessive alcohol, eating healthy foods, reducing stress, and making a periodic risk assessment.
- Most common cancers are linked to one of three environmental risk factors: smoking, sunlight, and diet.
- The paramedic's duty is to be familiar with laws, regulations, and national standards that address issues of infectious disease. The paramedic also must take personal protective measures to guard against exposure.
- Actions to take after significant exposure include disinfection, documentation, incident investigation, screening, immunization, and medical follow-up.
- Injuries on the job can be minimized. Knowledge of body mechanics during lifting and moving is helpful. Also, being alert for hostile settings is key. Prioritization of personal safety during rescue situations is wise. In addition, paramedics must practice safe vehicle operation. They must use safety equipment and supplies as well.

- The misuse and abuse of drugs and other substances may lead to chemical dependency (addiction). This may have a wide range of effects on physical and mental health.
- The concept of diversity encompasses acceptance and respect of other people. It is important to realize that each person is unique and to recognize individual differences.
- "Good" stress is eustress. Eustress is a positive response to stimuli and is considered protective. "Bad" stress is distress. Distress is a negative response to environmental stimuli and is the source of anxiety and stress-related disorders.
- Adaptation is a process in which persons learn effective ways to deal with stressful situations. This dynamic process usually begins with using defense mechanisms. Next, one develops coping skills followed by problem solving and culminating in mastery.
- Critical incident stress management is designed to help emergency personnel understand their reactions to a call or event that had a major emotional impact. The process reassures them that what they are experiencing is normal and may be common to others involved in the incident.
- Often news of a sudden death must be given to a family. The paramedic's initial contact can influence the grief process greatly.
- The five stages of dying identified by Dr. Elizabeth Kübler-Ross are denial, anger, bargaining, depression, and acceptance.

REVIEW QUESTIONS

Complete the following table to describe your wellness behaviors, analyze risks or benefits associated with those behaviors, and identify opportunities to improve them.

Behavior	Current Practice	Risk or Benefit of This Behavior	Improvement Plan
Diet (fats, vitamins, carbohydrates)			
Weight			
Cardiovascular endurance			
Strength and flexibility			
Sleep (hours/day)			
Cardiovascular disease risk factors			
Cancer risk factors			
Injury prevention			
Substance abuse			
Smoking			

Match the defense mechanism in column II with the appropriate example in column I. Use each defense mechanism only once.

Column I

1. _________ A rape victim cannot recall anything from the time she was abducted until the police find her

2. _________ A paramedic was passed over for a promotion states that the boss always plays favorites

3. _________ A paramedic is upset by a violent death and washes all the vehicles in the garage

4. _________ A victim of an automobile accident refuses to acknowledge that he cannot move his legs

5. _________ An EMT who gave poor care complains about the patient's hospital treatment

6. _________ A 10-year-old begins to suck his thumb en route to the hospital after sustaining a fracture from a fall

Column II

a. Compensation
b. Denial
c. Isolation
d. Projection
e. Rationalization
f. Reaction formation
g. Regression
h. Repression
i. Substitution

Questions 7 to 11 pertain to the following case study:

You respond to a call for an assault. Police on the scene tell you that an 18-year-old man has been stabbed. You find the patient, who is your nephew, at a party on the fourth floor of an apartment complex that has no working elevators. The patient is alert and crying and has a briskly bleeding puncture wound in the midaxillary line. He complains of having severe difficulty breathing and abdominal pain, and he has a rapid radial pulse. Oxygen is administered, and as you prepare for rapid transport and treatment, some party goers become belligerent.

7. Describe three measures you should take to reduce the risk of work-related illness and injury on this type of call in each of the following areas:

   a. Infectious disease

   ____

   b. Lifting and moving

   ____

   c. Hostile environments

   ____

   d. Vehicle operation

   ____

Chapter **2** **Well-Being of the Paramedic**

8. Briefly explain how each area of the body labeled in Fig. 2-1 responds to stress during the alarm reaction in this type of situation.

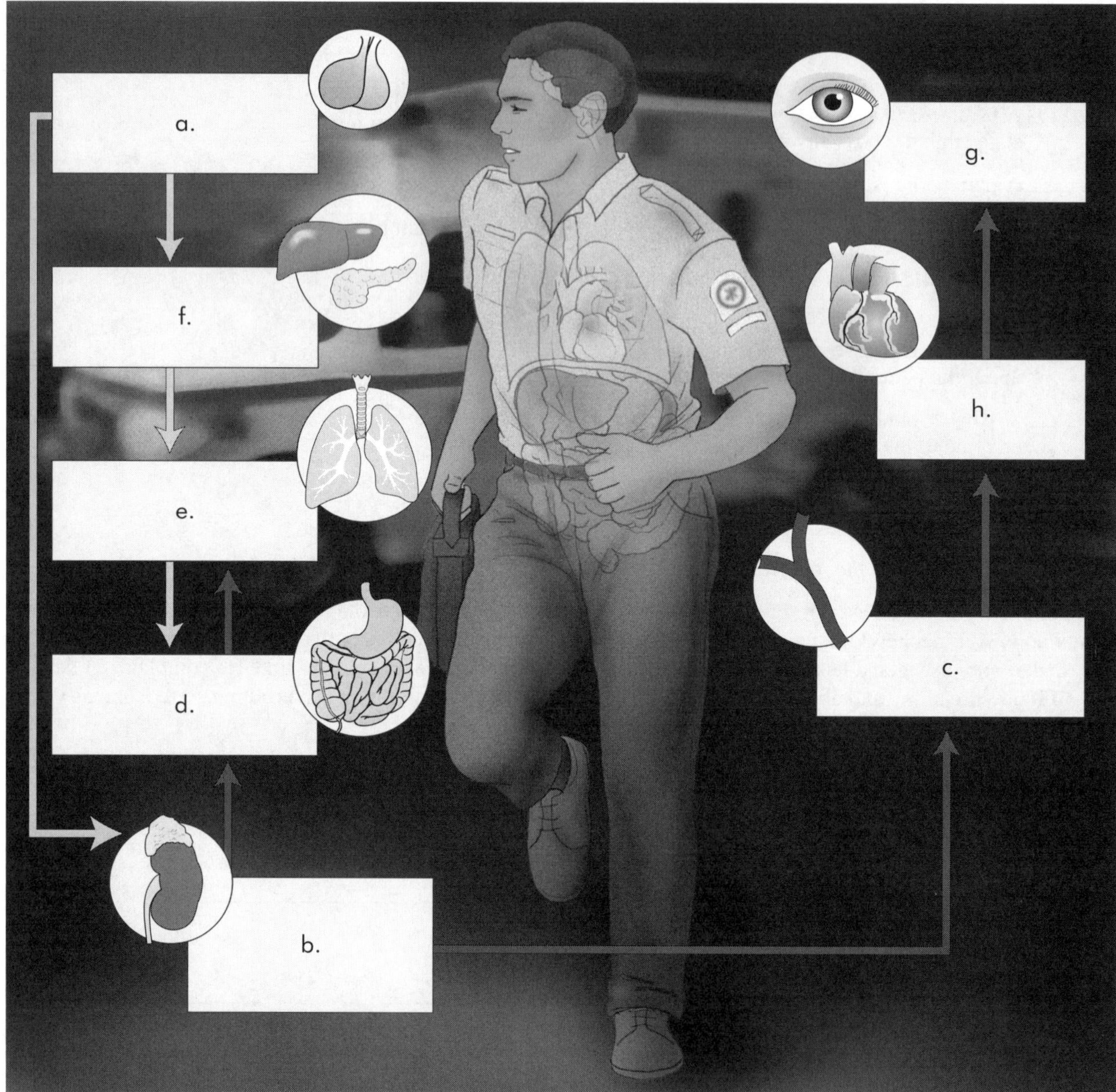

Figure 2-1

a. ____

b. ____

c. ____

d. ____

e. ____

f. ____

g. ____

h. ____

Chapter **2** **Well-Being of the Paramedic**

9. Describe two daily wellness practices that may benefit you as a paramedic when you respond to this type of situation.

   a. ____

   b. ____

10. List two reasons you, your crew, or both might use the services of the critical incident stress debriefing team after this call.

   ____

   ____

11. Which of the services that can be provided by a critical incident stress debriefing team may be of benefit after this call?

   ____

12. List five causes of stress that are job related and five that are not job related.

   a. Job-related stressors:

   ____

   b. Non–job-related stressors:

   ____

13. List three potential symptoms of decompensation from the effects of long-term stress.

   a. ____

   b. ____

   c. ____

14. Name five effective stress-management techniques that can minimize the effects of EMS job-related stress. (After you complete this, survey paramedics you know to see what strategies they use.)

   a. ____

   b. ____

   c. ____

   d. ____

   e. ____

Questions 15 to 17 pertain to the following case study:

You arrive at a family gathering where you find a 46-year-old man in full cardiopulmonary arrest. His mother is crying and begging, "Please, Lord, don't take him; take me." His wife is distraught, pacing, and saying, "It's going to be OK; it's not as bad as it seems." The brother yells at you as you enter, "What took you so long? Hurry up! What are you waiting for?"

15. Identify which of the stages of grief described by Dr. Kübler-Ross each family member is exhibiting in this situation.

   a. Mother: ____

b. Wife: ____

c. Brother: ____

16. How should you care for these family members to promote normal grieving?

____

____

____

17. How can you deal with the pent-up emotions you must suppress while caring for dying patients and their families on calls like this?

____

____

18. Identify which of the following situations represents an exposure to blood or body fluids. If exposure is involved, describe a measure that could have prevented it.

a. After using a lancet to obtain a blood sample from your patient for dextrose measurement, you puncture your hand with the lancet. Exposure? Yes/No

Preventive measure:

____

b. Blood sprays from a patient's endotracheal tube, hitting you in the face. You think it got in your eyes. Exposure? Yes/No

Preventive measure:

____

c. Your bare forearm brushes against a bloody sheet. You have no open wounds on your arm. Exposure? Yes/No

Preventive measure:

____

d. You put the IV bag in your mouth to hold it up as you move the patient, and your partner points out that blood is splattered over the bag. Exposure? Yes/No

Preventive measure:

____

19. At the scene of a motor vehicle collision, glass punctures your glove and cuts your finger. The patient's blood penetrates the glove and comes in contact with your cut. List at least four actions you should take after this exposure.

a. ____

b. ____

c. ____

d. ____

20. Which of the following is true regarding a healthy diet?
- **a.** Amino acids are produced by the body in the liver.
- **b.** Fats should be completely eliminated from the diet.
- **c.** Vitamin supplements are necessary for normal health.
- **d.** Water is one of the most important nutrients.

21. Which of the following is true regarding a routine physical fitness program?
- **a.** A decrease in muscle mass and metabolism will occur.
- **b.** A decrease in resting blood pressure may occur.
- **c.** A decrease in resistance to injury will occur.
- **d.** It should not be done if you have any preexisting illness.

22. Which of the following is a lifestyle modification associated with a decreased risk of heart disease?
- **a.** Reducing cigarette smoking
- **b.** Maintaining blood pressure at 120/80 mm Hg
- **c.** Reducing the very-low-density lipoprotein (VLDL) triglyceride level to 400 mg/dL
- **d.** Maintaining the low-density lipoprotein (LDL) cholesterol level at 190 mg/dL

23. Which of the following signs or symptoms is commonly listed as a warning sign of cancer?
- **a.** Indigestion or change in bowel habits
- **b.** Irregular heart beats or palpitations
- **c.** Lifelong presence of warts or moles
- **d.** Persistent nasal congestion

24. Actions that may prevent you from becoming infected with a communicable disease while practicing as a paramedic include which of the following?
- **a.** Annual skin testing for tuberculosis
- **b.** Frequent hand washing during all patient care activities
- **c.** Recapping of needles after patient use
- **d.** Use of body substance isolation for high-risk patients

25. How can you minimize your risk of injury while lifting or moving patients?
- **a.** Bend at the hips and knees.
- **b.** Hold the load 18 inches from your body.
- **c.** Lift with your back, not your legs.
- **d.** Move backward rather than forward.

26. Which of the following may indicate the potential for addiction or addictive behavior?
- **a.** Your partner asks you to drive him home from a bar because he believes he has had too much to drink.
- **b.** Your partner tells her husband she only had six beers instead of the 12 she actually drank.
- **c.** Your partner mentions that he is going out to have a few beers with some friends after work.
- **d.** Your partner says she can't handle booze the way she used to and now prefers beer to hard liquor.

27. You are called to a scene to assume care from a rescue unit. You immediately recognize the paramedic caring for the patient as an individual with whom you consistently disagree over patient care issues. What type of stress is this call likely to produce?
- **a.** Environmental
- **b.** Managerial
- **c.** Personality
- **d.** Psychosocial

28. What are generalized feelings of apprehension called?
- **a.** Anxiety
- **b.** Phobias
- **c.** Reaction formation
- **d.** Stress

29. A paramedic student has just failed his practical examination station because of improper airway management technique. He states, "Well, I would have done it, but we never practiced it in class this way." This is an example of which defense mechanism?
- **a.** Projection
- **b.** Rationalization
- **c.** Regression
- **d.** Sublimation

30. Critical incident stress debriefing is most helpful for which of the following?
   a. New employees after every critical patient situation
   b. Selected high-risk employees with psychological problems
   c. Mass casualty incidents involving more than 10 patients
   d. Situations in which a high degree of stress is perceived

31. When dealing with the family of a patient who is dying, you can best interact with them by doing which of the following?
   a. Reassuring them that no one you ever care for dies
   b. Changing the subject every time someone brings up death
   c. Allowing the family to remain with the patient if possible
   d. Avoiding direct communication with the immediate family

32. Which response to the death of a close family member would *not* be expected in a preschool child?
   a. The child acts as though nothing has happened.
   b. The child asks when the family member will come back.
   c. The child fears that other family members will also die.
   d. The child thinks that he or she was responsible for the death.

33. School-age children (7 to 12 years old) believe that death
   a. Is temporary and reversible
   b. Happens to others, not themselves
   c. Is a punishment for their bad thoughts
   d. Is the same as severe illness

34. Which of the following is an appropriate action to take after a needle-stick injury of the finger?
   a. Complete the exposure report and turn it in at the end of your shift.
   b. Determine whether the patient is high risk to decide whether you need to report the incident.
   c. Report the exposure to your supervisor and the receiving facility immediately.
   d. Squeeze out as much blood as possible and suck on your finger.

35. Which strategy promotes success when caring for patients in a culturally diverse environment?
   a. Assume that everyone believes as you do and would want to be cared for as you do.
   b. Ignore the differences because they really will not influence your care anyway.
   c. Have your partner deal with the patient and family if you are uncomfortable.
   d. Evaluate how cultural influences might affect patient choices about their care.

WRAP IT UP

Today is your worst nightmare. At about 1430, you are dispatched to a government building for a report of an explosion. It's your third day of a 72-hour shift, and you were just joking about taking the world record for most hours without sleep. En route, you see a plume of thick black smoke in the direction you are headed, and dispatch updates that there have been multiple calls and it appears there is major damage. You begin to review triage principles in your head, and you notice that your mouth is dry and you can feel your own heart pounding—sensations you haven't felt since your first rides as a paramedic student. Arriving on the scene, you see a multistory commercial structure with half of the side blown off. Command directs you and your partner to begin triage. There is mass confusion; people are moving all over the place. You attempt to set up a triage area, but bystanders are everywhere, rushing out with patients. Seven long hours later, 125 patients, some critically injured, have been triaged, treated, and transported. Among the casualties were your overweight captain, who was taken to the hospital with chest pain, and an out of shape coworker, who strained his shoulder trying to free a trapped patient.

After the incident, things just got worse. One of your best friends just seems to be falling apart; she's drinking too much and in jeopardy of losing her job because of tardiness, frequent "sick" call-ins, and poor work performance. She keeps blaming everything on others and won't admit that she has a problem. The first few days after the incident, everyone pulled together, but now the stress level at work is high. Some people just keep to themselves, others are blaming coworkers for things that go wrong, and many of your colleagues don't even want to talk about the call.

   1. What caused the dry mouth and palpitations that the paramedic experienced en route to this call?
   a. Cardiac irregularity
   b. Panic attack
   c. Parasympathetic release
   d. Stress reaction

2. After the incident, which defense mechanisms were observed in the paramedic's coworkers? (Check all that apply.)

________ Compensation   ________ Denial

________ Isolation   ________ Projection

________ Rationalization   ________ Reaction formation

________ Regression   ________ Repression

________ Substitution

3. What wellness activities may have reduced the chance of workplace illness or injury on this call?
   a. Balanced diet
   b. Cardiovascular endurance exercises
   c. Stretching and weight training
   d. All of the above

4. What stress reduction techniques might be helpful
   a. Before a call such as this:

____

   b. After a call such as this:

____

5. What strategies can paramedics use to increase their chance of sleep between calls on long shifts?

____

____

CHAPTER 2 ANSWERS

REVIEW QUESTIONS

   1. h
   2. e
   3. i
   4. b
   5. d
   6. g
   (Questions 1–6: Objective 10)

7. a. To reduce the risk of acquiring an infectious disease, the paramedic should obtain appropriate immunizations; maintain good personal health and hygiene; use universal precautions during patient care (in this case gloves, goggles or mask, and gown if there is a risk of splash or spray); avoid recapping needles; dispose of contaminated sharps in an appropriate container; wash hands thoroughly after completing patient care; and appropriately dispose of soiled linens, equipment, and trash.
   b. To reduce the risk of injury from moving and lifting this patient, the paramedic should maintain good physical conditioning, obtain assistance in moving the patient if the person's size is too great for the paramedic and a partner, pay attention when walking, move forward when possible, take short steps, bend at the knees and hips, lift with the legs, keep the load close to the body, keep the patient's body in line when moving, and use the appropriate device for the situation (e.g., stair chair versus long backboard).
   c. To reduce the risk of injury when providing care in a hostile environment, the paramedic should coordinate activities with law enforcement, scan the area for the fastest escape route, stay alert and move the patient out of the hostile area as quickly as possible, and leave the area if the situation becomes too dangerous. The best policy is to avoid entering the scene until the police have it under control.

d. To ensure maximum safety when leaving this scene and transporting the patient to the hospital, the paramedic should use lights and sirens as dictated by local policy, proceed carefully through intersections, and maintain due regard for the safety of others.
(Objectives 5, 7)

8. (a) The pituitary gland releases adrenocorticotropic hormone, stimulating the sympathetic nervous system. (b) Adrenal glands release epinephrine and norepinephrine, which (c) cause a rise in blood pressure by increasing systemic vascular resistance; (d) slow the digestive tract; (e) dilate the bronchioles, allowing deeper breathing; (f) stimulate glucose production in the liver; (g) dilate the pupils; and (h) increase the rate and strength of the heart's contractions.
(Objective 10)

9. Good physical conditioning permits rapid movement of the patient out of this hostile situation with reduced risk of injury to the paramedic. Good emotional health practices facilitate the use of healthy coping mechanisms in dealing with the personal stressors involved in this call.
(Objective 2, 3)

10. Situations that pose a threat to rescuers' lives may be perceived as stressful, depending on the situation and the individuals involved. Having a critically injured patient who is a close relative or acquaintance often creates a very stressful situation.
(Objective 12)

11. Individual consultation may be necessary if only one person was overwhelmed by the call. If the event was perceived as very stressful by the whole group, defusing immediately after the incident, critical incident stress debriefing within 24 to 72 hours, and follow-up services after debriefing may be needed.
(Objective 12)

12. a. Working in hazardous situations; dealing with injured or dying children; working in an uncontrolled, unpredictable environment; dealing with emotionally upset, unpredictable patients; needing to make life and death decisions quickly. b. Physical illness of oneself or a close family member, loss of a job or starting a new job, personal financial troubles, the death of a loved one, and marital troubles, among others.
(Objective 10)

13. Irritability, apathy, chronic fatigue, feelings of not being appreciated, difficulty sleeping, drinking or drug abuse, decline in social activities, appetite changes, desire to quit work, and physical complaints
(Objective 10)

14. Early recognition of signs and symptoms of stress, awareness of personal limitations, peer counseling, group discussions, proper diet, sleep, exercise, and pursuit of positive activities outside EMS
(Objective 11)

15. a. Bargaining: The mother is bargaining her life for her son's life. b. Denial: The wife is denying the severity of the problem. c. Anger: The brother's anger is directed at the EMS personnel.
(Objective 13).

16. You should tell the family that the patient is critically ill and that you are going to do everything possible to help him. Remain calm and try to let the family remain close if patient care is not compromised. Assign tasks to the angry brother (e.g., stay with his mother and care for her).
(Objective 13)

17. Paramedics should be encouraged to talk about particularly distressing situations with other crew members and to avail themselves of resources available through medical direction and employee assistance programs.
(Objective 11)

18. a. Yes. Use accessible sharps containers and safety lancets.
b. Yes. Wear a mask, eye protection, gloves, and gown when there is a risk of splash or spray.
c. No exposure was involved. You should wash your arm thoroughly.
d. Yes. Do not place objects in your mouth when biohazards are present.
(Objectives 5, 7)

19. a. Wash the area thoroughly.
   b. Document the exposure.
   c. Immediately report to the appropriate personnel.
   d. Complete the medical follow-up.
   (Objective 6)

STUDENT SELF-ASSESSMENT

20. d. Cellular function depends on a fluid environment. Amino acids are essential for body growth and cellular life and are not produced by the body. Polyunsaturated fats can help reduce high blood cholesterol levels if included as part of a low-fat diet.
(Objective 1)

21. b. An increase in muscle mass, metabolism, and resistance to injury should be anticipated with a carefully planned fitness program. Fitness programs can be tailored to accommodate the needs of individuals with preexisting medical conditions (e.g., arthritis, heart disease) and are encouraged.
(Objective 1)

22. b. Cigarette smoking should be eliminated to reduce the risk of heart disease. The triglyceride level should not exceed 200 to 300 mg/dL, and the LDL cholesterol level should be below 160 mg/dL.
(Objective 2, 3)

23. a. The other signs listed by the American Cancer Society are a sore throat, unusual bleeding or discharge, thickening or a lump in the breast or elsewhere, obvious change in a wart or mole, and a nagging cough or hoarseness.
(Objective 4)

24. b. Annual skin testing is an excellent measure for detecting exposure to tuberculosis so that it can be appropriately treated; however, it does not prevent infection. Needle recapping is never advised because this greatly increases the risk of injury and exposure. Body substance isolation measures should be used for all patients, not just those who might be high risk.
(Objective 5)

25. a. To minimize the risk of injury, you should also hold the load close to your body, lift with your legs (not your back), and move forward rather than backward when possible.
(Objective 7)

26. b. Lying about using a substance indicates guilt about using the substance; this is a warning sign.
(Objective 8)

27. d. Environmental stress results from factors such as siren noise and weather. Personality stress relates to the way individuals feel about themselves. Managerial stress is not a distinct entity.
(Objective 10)

28. a. Phobias are unrealistic fears. Reaction formation is a defense mechanism in which unacceptable desires are suppressed by accentuating opposite behaviors. Stress is a generalized response to certain situations.
(Objective 10)

29. b. Projection occurs when one's own undesirable feelings are attributed to someone else. Regression is a return to an earlier stage of emotional adjustment. Sublimation occurs when unacceptable urges are modified to become socially acceptable.
(Objective 10)

30. d. New paramedics may be at greater risk for high stress after a critical call; however, veterans continue to be vulnerable to unusually stressful calls. Multiple-patient situations may not always trigger stress responses in rescuers; it depends on the individual situation. A high-risk employee with psychological problems probably will require care in addition to the critical incident stress debriefing program.
(Objective 10)

31. c. If the family raises the issue of death, a realistic description of the seriousness of the patient's condition should be briefly given. Direct eye contact and touch, if appropriate, may be used to convey concern and caring.
(Objective 13)

32. a. The family should watch for behavioral changes at home and at school, as well as difficulty eating or sleeping, and should encourage the child to express his or her feelings.
(Objective 10)

33. b. School-age children have begun to understand the concept of the finality of death; however, they still believe that it happens only to others.
(Objective 13)

34. c. All needle-stick injuries should be reported immediately so that appropriate source testing and follow-up can be completed in a timely manner.
(Objective 6)

35. d. Cultural influences may impact the patient's decisions and views regarding health care. Your patient may choose different health care than you would. Listen carefully so you can determine the best approach.
(Objective 9)

WRAP IT UP

1. d. These are normal sympathetic responses to stress.
(Objective 10)

2. Denial, rationalization, and substitution (the paramedic who shows poor performance), isolation (co-workers who keep to themselves), and repression (responders who don't want to talk about the call)
(Objective 10)

3. d. Diet and exercise can reduce weight and improve cardiovascular fitness. Musculoskeletal injuries can be reduced by improving strength and flexibility.
(Objective 7)

4. a. Exercise, meditation, and positive social connections can help in the management of stress on a daily basis.
b. Critical incident stress debriefing, one-on-one counseling, exercise, reframing, controlled breathing, progressive relaxation, guided imagery, proper diet, and sleep are all techniques that may assist in the management of stress.
(Objective 11)

5. Take some quiet time to relax before trying to sleep (reading, meditation, exercise); avoid stimulants; eat simple carbohydrates to release serotonin; select a dark sleeping area; try to pick a "normal" nap time (often difficult at work).
(Objective 2)

3 Injury Prevention and Public Health

READING ASSIGNMENT

Chapter 3, pages 50-62, in *Mosby's Paramedic Textbook,* ed. 4.

OBJECTIVES

Upon completion of this chapter, the paramedic student will be able to do the following:

1. Identify roles of the emergency medical services (EMS) community in injury prevention.
2. Describe the epidemiology of trauma in the United States.
3. Define *injury.*
4. Describe Haddon's matrix and the injury triangle.
5. Describe public health goals and activities.
6. Outline the aspects of the EMS system that make it a desirable resource for involvement in community health activities.
7. Describe essential activities for the active participation of EMS in community wellness activities.
8. List situations in which paramedics may participate in injury prevention.
9. Differentiate among primary, secondary, and tertiary health prevention activities.
10. Evaluate a situation to determine opportunities for injury prevention.
11. Identify resources necessary to conduct a community health assessment.
12. Relate how alterations in the epidemiological triangle can influence injury and disease patterns.
13. Describe strategies to implement a successful injury prevention program.

SUMMARY

- Emergency medical services (EMS) providers are members of the community health care system. They can be an important resource in injury prevention.
- Unintentional injuries are the fifth leading cause of death. This cause is exceeded only by heart disease, cancer, stroke, and chronic obstructive pulmonary disease.
- The United States has more than 600,000 EMS personnel. This valuable human resource plays a major role in public education. This component of health promotion seems only fitting.
- For paramedics to play an active role in the health of a community is crucial. Thus, the community must protect EMS workers from injury. The community also needs to provide education to paramedics. The community should supply support and promote the collection and use of injury data as well. In addition, the community must obtain resources for primary injury prevention activities. Last, the community needs to empower paramedics to conduct primary injury prevention.
- Paramedics must have a basic knowledge of personal injury prevention. They also should know about maladies and injuries common to various age groups, recreation activities, workplaces, and other facilities in the community.
- Paramedics need to spot the signs and symptoms of abuse and abusive situations. In addition, paramedics should notice exposure to danger.
- Paramedics should identify and use outside community resources. They should document primary injury data properly. Moreover, they should identify and properly use teachable moments.
- Paramedics must maximize time and resources. Thus, paramedics should identify targets for community health education. Paramedics can do this by performing a community health assessment.
- To identify community education goals, paramedics must understand several factors: (1) illness or injury is related to the extent or exposure to an agent; (2) illness or injury also is related to the strength of the agent; (3) illness or injury is linked to the susceptibility of the individual (host); and (4) illness or injury is related to the biological, social, and physical environment.
- Primary injury prevention involves preventing an injury from occurring. Secondary and tertiary prevention help to prevent further problems from an event that has already occurred.

- A good injury prevention program must serve the whole target population in a community. An effective program also takes into account reading level and age. These aspects are the mark of a successful program. Paramedics can provide community health education in diverse ways, such as verbal, written or static, and dynamic visual materials.

REVIEW QUESTIONS

Questions 1 to 9 pertain to the following case study:

At 1400, the tones sound, and you are dispatched to the home of an elderly resident who has slipped and fallen. On arrival at the emergency department, the physician confirms your suspicion—the patient's hip is broken. As you ride back to the base, you remark to your partner that this is the fourth patient you've transported this month with a broken hip. These calls really bother you because your own grandmother was institutionalized and then died of pneumonia shortly after a similar injury just 6 months ago. By the time you arrive back at your station, you have resolved to do something about the problem. You approach the chief, who listens to your idea to develop a fall prevention program. He tells you to return when you have some solid information about the target population, the magnitude of the problem, your goals, and the cost involved.

1. Why should the paramedic be concerned about the magnitude of injury in this country?

   ____

2. The initial visit to the emergency department for this type of injury has a high price. List two other "costs" associated with this type of injury.

   ____

   ____

3. Give at least three reasons why EMS is ideally suited to perform community prevention activities with elderly adults.

   a. ____

   b. ____

   c. ____

4. What additional information would you need to be able to provide prevention for this type of injury in this group?

   ____

5. What will you need from your boss before moving ahead with this project?

   ____

6. List three community resources you may need to contact to identify the number of elderly individuals living in your district, the incidence of hip fractures, the morbidity and mortality rates associated with this injury, and the costs associated with such fractures.

   a. ____

   b. ____

   c. ____

7. You decide that fall injuries in elderly adults are most likely the result of the host and environmental factors of the epidemiological triangle. List two host and two environmental factors that may contribute to falls in elderly adults.

   Host:

   a. ____

   b. ____

   Environmental:

   a. ____

   b. ____

   After careful evaluation of the problem, you decide that the best plan would be to have EMS crews visit elderly residents' homes with a checklist that would identify risk factors for falls in the home. A brief educational pamphlet with specific recommendations would then be given to the resident.

8. Is your plan an example of a primary, secondary, or tertiary intervention?

   ____

9. List at least four factors you should consider in preparing the written educational materials to be distributed to the community.

   ____

   ____

   Each of the examples in questions 10 to 18 represents a factor that could cause or increase susceptibility to illness and injury. Indicate whether the example is an agent factor (causative), a host factor (influences exposure, susceptibility, or response to agents), or an environmental factor (influences existence of the agent, exposure, or susceptibility).

Example	Agent, Host, or Environmental Factor
10. Fatigue	
11. Firefighter	
12. Carbon monoxide	
13. Gender	
14. Hepatitis	
15. Malnutrition	
16. Poor personal hygiene	
17. Flood	
18. Cholesterol	

19. List at least four injury prevention strategies a paramedic might use to help reduce neurologic injury.

   a. ____

   b. ____

   c. ____

   d. ____

20. Ten people in your EMS district have been killed in motor vehicle collisions thus far this year. Where do deaths from unintentional causes such as this rank in the United States?
- **a.** First
- **b.** Third
- **c.** Fifth
- **d.** Seventh

21. The number of drownings in your community rose last year. The health department asks your EMS agency to assist with an educational plan to help reduce the incidence of drowning. Why are EMS providers ideal for this type of program?
- **a.** They have more time than other health care providers to teach these programs.
- **b.** Paramedics and EMTs are welcomed into homes and public places to present educational programs.
- **c.** EMS agencies have abundant financial resources to fund these programs.
- **d.** EMS providers are the best authorities on preventing such tragedies.

22. How can EMS safety be enhanced during emergency care and transportation?
- **a.** Educate the crews to wear their seatbelt responding to every call.
- **b.** Ticket people who fail to yield to emergency traffic.
- **c.** Establish a policy of parking upwind from all HAZMAT spills.
- **d.** Ensure that police assume all responsibility for scene safety.

23. How can EMS agencies promote the involvement of staff members in community wellness programs?
- **a.** Penalize those who decline to participate.
- **b.** Ask everyone on duty to participate.
- **c.** Offer it as an alternative to a less desirable chore.
- **d.** Provide a salary for off-duty injury prevention work.

24. You respond to a call for domestic violence. You find a woman with bruising around her face, and she and her husband are yelling at each other. She screams at you to leave her alone when you try to examine her, and he is staggering and cursing at you. What is your primary goal in this situation?
- **a.** Restrain the patient and ask medical direction for permission for involuntary transport.
- **b.** Ak the police to arrest both of them so that they can be contained in a controlled space.
- **c.** Maintain the safety of your crew and to diffuse the situation calmly without violence.
- **d.** Forcibly remove the man from the situation so the woman will not be afraid of treatment.

25. Which of the following patient situations would likely present a teachable moment?
- **a.** A hysterical mother being transported with her child, who just fell down a flight of stairs
- **b.** An elderly patient who refuses care after falling in a dimly lit stairway and injuring her wrist
- **c.** A child with minor injuries who was struck by a car that crossed the median onto the sidewalk
- **d.** A cyclist without a helmet who fell off his bike during a race and is confused during transport

26. You believe that you are running many more calls related to heart problems in elderly individuals. What community resources can you use as sources of information to determine whether the makeup of your community is changing?
- **a.** Census data
- **b.** Chamber of commerce
- **c.** Fire service
- **d.** Local newspaper

27. It is a cold, wintry day, and the trees are glistening after the ice storm last night. Your crew alone has run four calls to the local sledding hill to care for patients with injuries ranging from broken extremities to lumbar fractures. Which element in the epidemiological triangle is most likely having the greatest influence on the injuries you are seeing in this situation?
- **a.** Physical environment
- **b.** Social setting
- **c.** Strength of the agent
- **d.** Susceptibility of the host

28. Which of the following is an example of a primary health prevention activity with which a paramedic may be involved?
- **a.** You check the blood pressure of residents diagnosed with hypertension each week.
- **b.** You coordinate a stop smoking program for a group of your fellow employees.
- **c.** You coordinate a drunk-u-drama at the high school before prom week.
- **d.** You arrange a support group for EMS personnel recovering from alcohol abuse.

29. You are preparing a presentation on drug use for the young people in your area. How can you make sure your audience will understand your message?
    a. You test it on a teen patient during an EMS call.
    b. You ask your crew if it appeals to them.
    c. You include slides to increase the likelihood of retention.
    d. You make sure the language and reading level suit the audience.

30. Which of the following injury prevention strategies is associated with the greatest reduction in injury and death after a vehicle crash?
    a. Automatic airbag deployment on crash impact
    b. Driver education programs for senior citizens
    c. Fines for driving without wearing seatbelts
    d. Television advertising promoting safe driving techniques

31. What is the primary goal of public health activities?
    a. Intervention to treat disease
    b. Preventing illness and injury
    c. Sexually transmitted disease care
    d. Enforcing laws and regulations

WRAP IT UP

As you arrive on the scene of a "pedestrian struck" call, you observe a child whose life has changed forever. The 8-year-old boy, who had been riding his bike without a helmet, careened down a hill into an intersection and was struck by a small truck. The distraught driver tells you the boy flew up and hit the windshield with his head. You note that the windshield is starred and the front quarter panel of the truck is dented. It's immediately evident that the child is seriously injured. He has a forehead laceration and is combative. You quickly immobilize him and load him into the ambulance while maintaining the airway. En route to the local trauma center, you continue your assessments, assist ventilation, insert an intravenous (IV) line, and notify the trauma team of your assessment and your estimated time of arrival (ETA). The boy's condition worsens as you roll him into the trauma room. Later, during the postincident review, you are told that although he survived, he will have severe cognitive impairment. He is in rehabilitation, and it is unclear whether he will ever function normally again. You are angry and frustrated. You have many long discussions about the call with your captain. After much thought and with the captain's approval, you decide to start a helmet program in your community. You plan to hold clinics at which you will properly fit helmets for those who have one and sell helmets for $5 (your cost to buy them) to those who don't. You also plan to develop brochures and deliver presentations in the local elementary schools.

1. a. What is the goal of a program such as this?

   ____

   ____

   b. Is this goal consistent with the mission of an EMS organization?

   ____

   ____

2. Why would EMS providers be suitable professionals to initiate such a program?

   ____

   ____

3. Where can you find information to justify the cost of this program to your chief?

   ____

   ____

Chapter 3 Injury Prevention and Public Health

4. How could you tie in on-scene education to a program like this?

____

____

5. Place a ✓ beside the components of a community health assessment that could be helpful in your research for this program.

___________ Population demographics   ___________ Morbidity statistics

___________ Mortality statistics   ___________ Crime and fire information

___________ Community resource allocation   ___________ Hospital data

___________ Senior citizen needs   ___________ Education standards

___________ Recreational facilities   ___________ Environmental conditions

___________ Other factors

6. Would this program be a primary, secondary, or tertiary community health intervention?

____

____

7. Where can you seek funding to support your program?

____

____

8. What must you consider in developing your brochure and your presentation?

____

____

CHAPTER 3 ANSWERS

REVIEW QUESTIONS

1. Injury affects young adults, results in a lot of death and disability, costs the society a huge amount, and uses valuable resources.
(Objective 2)

2. In addition to the initial ED visit, other costs related to injury include lost quality of life, loss of income, and long-term hospitalizations and care.
(Objective 2)

3. EMS providers are ideally suited for educating elderly people in their community because EMS providers are welcomed into the home. Also, they are viewed as experts who are medically educated, they are considered to have people's best interests at heart, and they may be the first to identify situations that pose a risk.
(Objectives 1, 6)

4. Injury prevention material specific to falls in elderly adults would need to be obtained.
(Objective 11)

5. You will need financial support, endorsement of your agency, and possibly assistance from your boss to identify other community resources.
(Objective 13)

6. Census data should reflect the number of elderly adults, the area health department should have statistics on mortality and injury frequency and type, your own EMS system could provide information about the number of elderly patients transported as a result of fall-related injuries, and national agencies such as the Centers for Disease Control and Prevention (CDC) and the National Safety Council can provide cost data and are accessible either through the Internet or the library.
(Objective 11)

7. Host: Poor eyesight, impaired balance secondary to medication use, decreased sensation. Environmental: poor lighting, loose area rugs, absence of or poorly maintained railings, icy walkways.
(Objective 4)

8. This is a primary intervention if it involves people who have not had injuries from a fall.
(Objective 9)

9. You will need to consider the following factors: the cost of the materials (who will pay for them), whether someone in the community already has materials you could use (e.g., hospital, health department), the reading levels of the audience, whether you need to prepare bilingual materials if you have a large group that does not read English, and the type size of the material (to accommodate clients with poor vision).
(Objective 11)

10. Host. Fatigue may result in a shortened attention span, which may lead to an injury.

11. Environment. Firefighters are placed in hostile environments by their work, which increases their susceptibility to injury or illness.

12. Agent. Carbon monoxide is a poisonous gas that can cause illness or death.

13. Host. Certain diseases are more prevalent in one gender than the other (e.g., rheumatoid arthritis is more prevalent in women).

14. Agent. Hepatitis is a virus that causes disease.

15. Host. Malnutrition deprives the body of essential nutrients necessary to maintain health.

16. Host. Poor personal hygiene predisposes an individual to infection.

17. Environmental. Floods may cause water contamination and increase the risk of the epidemic spread of disease.

18. Agent. Excess cholesterol is associated with an increased risk of heart disease.
(Questions 10–18: Objective 4)

19. Helmet, seatbelt, senior fall prevention, safe bicycle riding programs
(Objective 8)

20. c. Unintentional injuries are the top cause of death for persons between 1 and 38 years of age and the fifth leading cause of death overall.
(Objective 2)

21. b. Residents of a community usually have a high level of trust in EMS providers and will let them in to speak about these issues. The amount of time paramedics have in any given EMS system depends on the call volume and other commitments, such as training or other departmental duties. EMS agencies do not always have financial resources but may have a community partner to fund the support materials for the program. EMS providers often have baseline knowledge about injury prevention but can be educated on specific injury prevention materials.
(Objective 6)

22. a. Ticketing people who fail to yield may be helpful, but it affects only those who may have caused injury to EMS providers or their patients. Education is more desirable.
(Objective 13)

23. d. Penalizing personnel or forcing them to participate in an activity may be necessary, but it does not promote maximum participation in activities. Rewards and incentives are helpful.
(Objective 13)

24. c. Situations involving domestic violence are volatile and complicated. Measures to diffuse, rather than escalate, the situation should be used unless the circumstances pose an immediate danger to your crew, your patient, or the police.
(Objective 8)

25. b. This patient is calm and cooperative, but she probably realizes that her injury could have been more serious. A few words about appropriate lighting and specific recommendations for accomplishing it would likely be taken quite seriously at that moment. For the child hit by a car, calming may be a greater priority, and there is no evidence of a need to teach him anything specific to related to this incident. In a and d, the parent or patient is not in an appropriate mental state to be taught.
(Objective 10)

26. a. Census data, which may be obtained through the Internet or the library, provide information about population demographics, including age and income levels. The area health department can give you specific information about deaths in your community and their causes. The local paper may refer you to information sources but won't likely have specifics. Fire departments have very specific call data related to fires and whether they also provide EMS and illness or injury information. The chamber of commerce has economic data and information about industry, religious organizations, and cultural opportunities in a community.
(Objective 11)

27. a. The icy conditions undoubtedly are having the greatest influence on the situation. The ice prevented the host from controlling the speed or direction of the sled, and it caused the crash.
(Objective 12)

28. c. The drunk-u-drama will attempt to teach students how to prevent injuries from occurring. You are performing secondary interventions on the hypertensive group and the smokers; both these groups already have a condition you are attempting to control or stop. Tertiary activities, designed to rehabilitate, would include the support group activities.
(Objective 9)

29. d. Although brief opportunities for teaching occur during an EMS call, a formal educational plan wouldn't be appropriate. Your crew members may think the program is great, but the target audience may not relate to it at all. Slides are appropriate, but depending on your audience and your message, they may not be desirable or possible. For example, if your program is to be delivered to youth groups on a street corner, you would have to choose a different method.
(Objective 13)

Chapter **3** **Injury Prevention and Public Health**

30. a. Engineering safety controls, which do not offer the user a choice whether to use them, are more effective.
   (Objective 13)

31. b. Public health activities and policies do involve treatment and enforcement, but their primary goals are to intervene to prevent illness and injury.
   (Objective 5)

WRAP IT UP

1. a. The goal would be to reduce injury and death for those riding bicycles and other wheeled recreational toys.
   b. For most EMS agencies, this goal should be consistent with their mission, which is to reduce death and disability.
   (Objective 1)

2. EMS providers are medically educated, are high-profile role models, are welcome in schools and homes, and are considered "experts" on injury and prevention. Therefore, they are ideal providers of injury prevention programs.
   (Objective 6)

3. Information on the costs of unintentional injuries can be obtained from National Safety Council statistics, some state data, trauma centers, and trauma organizations.
   (Objective 11)

4. On-scene education could be included in such a program by (1) giving helmets to children who have been in collisions while on bikes, scooters, or roller blades; (2) offering to properly fit them for a helmet; or (3) encouraging them to wear their helmet (or wear them properly).
   (Objective 10)

5. Population demographics, mortality statistics, morbidity statistics, hospital data, recreational facilities (e.g., a skateboard park in your district), and other factors (e.g., funding sources, a local police bicycle rodeo at which you could implement your program) could be helpful in creating your presentation.
   (Objective 11)

6. This is mainly a primary injury prevention program; it prevents the injury from happening.
   (Objective 9)

7. Funding could be sought through federal grants, local service clubs (Kiwanis, Lions, Optimists, Rotary), SafeKids coalitions, and hospitals. If you can establish the program with seed money and then sell your helmets for cost, the program may perpetuate itself, with little additional funding needed.
   (Objectives 11, 13)

8. In developing the materials for your program, you must consider (1) the money available; (2) the reading level of the target audience; (3) the likes and dislikes of the target audience; (4) the attention span of the target audience; and (5) ethnic, cultural, and religious considerations for the target audience. After the program has been put together, someone from your target audience should "preview" the material and give you their opinion.
   (Objective 11, 13)

4 Documentation

READING ASSIGNMENT

Chapter 4, pages 63-72, in *Mosby's Paramedic Textbook,* ed. 4.

OBJECTIVES

Upon completion of this chapter, the paramedic student will be able to do the following:

1. Identify the purpose of the patient care report (PCR).
2. Describe the uses of the PCR.
3. Outline the components of an accurate, thorough PCR.
4. Describe the elements of a properly written emergency medical services document.
5. Describe an effective system for documenting the narrative section of a prehospital patient report.
6. Identify differences necessary when documenting special situations.
7. Describe the appropriate method to make revisions or corrections to the PCR.
8. Recognize consequences that may result from inappropriate documentation.

SUMMARY

- The patient care report (PCR) is used to document the key elements of patient assessment, care, and transport.
- The three primary reasons for written documentation are that the medical community involved in the patient's care uses it, it is a legal record, it is important for reimbursement, and it is essential to data collection.
- The PCR should include dates and response times, difficulties encountered, observations at the scene, previous medical care provided, a chronological description of the call, and significant times.
- A properly written emergency medical services (EMS) document is accurate, legible, timely, unaltered, and free of nonprofessional or extraneous information.
- Many approaches for writing the narrative can be used. The paramedic should adopt only one approach. The paramedic should use this approach consistently to avoid omissions in report writing.
- Special documentation is necessary when a patient refuses care or transport. Such documentation also is needed in cases when care or transportation is not needed. Special documentation also is needed for mass casualty incidents.
- Most EMS agencies have separate forms for revisions or corrections to the PCR.
- Documentation that is inappropriate may have medical and legal implications.

REVIEW QUESTIONS

Questions 1 and 2 pertain to the following case study:

You are a paramedic working on Unit 4017 and are dispatched to a private residence on a call for a "person down." When you arrive at the scene at 1400, you find a 20-year-old woman lying on the lawn in front of the house. She is awake but is saying inappropriate words. The patient's husband tells you that his wife is diabetic and takes insulin, but she missed lunch. He says he found her confused in the yard. Her skin is pale, cool, and diaphoretic; her respiratory rate is 20 breaths per minute and unlabored with clear breath sounds in all fields; her radial pulse is 120 per minute; and her blood pressure is 110/70 mm Hg. While your partner initiates an intravenous (IV) line in the right antecubital space at 1406, you measure the patient's blood glucose level, which is 50 mg/dL. Following your standing orders, you begin an IV of normal saline and then at 1408 administer 25 g (50 mL) of D50W through the IV. Within 2 minutes the patient looks at you and asks, "Why are you here?" She is now alert and answering appropriately, and by the time her husband reminds her what has happened, she is oriented completely to person, place, and time. She agrees to be transported to General Hospital, and the ambulance departs the scene at 1413. While en route, you call a report to Dr. Smith, and at 1416, another set of vital signs reveals the following: BP 118/74, P 96/min, and R 20/min with warm, dry, pink skin. She denies allergies to medicine and states she took 10 units of regular and 20 units of Lente insulin at 0700. On arrival to the hospital at 1420, there is no change in the patient's condition, and you note that 100 mL of the IV fluid has been infused. Your partner restocks your bag with the supplies used, which include a 250-mL bag of normal saline, macrodrip IV tubing, an 18-gauge IV catheter, and D50W.

1. Write a narrative documenting your findings on this patient as you would on your state patient care report (assuming there is no check-box format on your report).

2. List at least four uses for your patient care report from this call.

3. Describe the appropriate method to complete documentation for each of the following situations:

   a. Your patient lacerated his hand. The wound is deep and gaping, and he cannot move two of his fingers. He is refusing care and says he will go to his doctor tomorrow.

b. You are responding to a call for a "full arrest." Before you arrive on the scene, the dispatcher notifies you to disregard the call. You go back in service and return to your station.

____

____

____

c. More than 100 patients are complaining of burning eyes and throats and difficulty breathing after an industrial gas release. You are providing care in the treatment sector.

____

____

____

d. You have just returned to your engine house from the hospital when you realize that you did not document some essential information about the patient's history on the patient care report.

____

____

____

4. What is a possible consequence of failure to document the following information in a patient care report?

a. The trauma patient reports an allergy to tetanus vaccine. He is unconscious when you arrive in the emergency department.

____

____

____

b. You administered the maximum dosage of lidocaine to a patient who was in ventricular tachycardia but neglected to document it on your patient care report.

____

____

____

c. The patient fell earlier in the day and is unconscious on arrival to the emergency department. You do not document that the patient takes warfarin (Coumadin) daily.

____

____

____

d. You fail to document that a patient had numbness in his arm before spinal immobilization.

____

____

____

5. What does the patient care report document?
   a. Patient assessment
   b. Patient care
   c. Patient transport
   d. All of the above

6. Which of the following is an appropriate use of the prehospital patient care report?
   a. Administrative and billing information
   b. Looking up information for your family member
   c. Research document for the local press
   d. Documenting equipment maintenance issues

7. Which of the following should be documented on the patient care report?
   a. Chronological description of events that occurred during the call
   b. Circumstances documenting that the paramedic fell during care of this patient
   c. Statements such as: "The patient was rude and difficult to work with"
   d. A note that the hospital staff was rude on arrival to the ED

8. If the respiratory rate section is not completed on the ambulance reporting form, what should the physician assume about patient respirations?
   a. They were not an important vital sign assessment.
   b. They were not pertinent in this patient section.
   c. They were not assessed specifically by the paramedic.
   d. They were within normal limits for the patient age group.

9. When a patient refuses care, what must the paramedic document?
   a. Advice given to the patient regarding the condition
   b. Nothing as long as the patient was alert and oriented
   c. The detailed physical examination
   d. The patient's insurance information

10. What should you document when your response is canceled en route to the scene?
   a. Canceling authority and time of cancellation
   b. No documentation is needed in this situation.
   c. Scene size-up information
   d. You must still respond and obtain a refusal.

11. You are leaving work and suddenly realize you forgot to document a crucial piece of information about patient care on a patient record. What should you do?
   a. Ask your supervisor to fill in the essential information.
   b. Note the date and time the correction was made on the appropriate form.
   c. Wait until you return to work after your 4-day break to finish it.
   d. You may not add anything after the report is complete.

It seems odd that you would be nervous today. Normally, you are the one who is calm, cool, and collected even on the most serious trauma calls. As you sit waiting to testify at the deposition, you go over the events of the call in your mind. At the time you thought you'd never forget them, but after 5 years, the details tend to fade. Thankfully, your attorney says that you will have the benefit of your patient care report to refer to during your testimony. The plaintiff was thrown off of a motorcycle while apparently intoxicated and is alleging that your care led to the long-term disability he is experiencing from nerve damage to his badly fractured leg. You sit around the table with your attorney; the prosecuting attorney; and a court reporter, who swears you in. The attorney begins by asking you why your response to the scene of the collision was so slow based on the location from which you responded. You explain, as you documented, that traffic was diverted that evening because of highway construction, resulting in an unavoidable delay in response. He queries you about your statements that the patient was "drunk." You respond that you did not document that the patient was drunk. Rather, you noted that there was a strong odor resembling alcohol on the patient's breath, that he had slurred speech, and that he repeatedly moved his clearly fractured extremity despite repeated requests for him to hold still so he would not injure it further until appropriate immobilization could be completed. The attorney asks if that behavior was consistent with a head injury also, and you state that yes it would be; however, as you detailed in your report, the mechanism of injury was not consistent with head injury as evidenced by bystander reports that his leg had been pinned between the bike and a car, and his head never struck the ground. You also note that his helmet was undamaged. The attorney then makes the allegation that you did not follow proper care to his client's injured leg and wonders why you scratched out the word "traction" before splint. You state that, as you noted in your report, there was gross deformity to his lower leg and ankle; however, before, during, and after splinting, there was a good dorsalis pedis and posterior tibial pulse with the last check you noted after you moved the patient to the cot in the resuscitation room at the trauma center. Furthermore, you review with him the policy of your department when an error is made on the report as was done here. Evidently, the word "traction" was written mistakenly, so you crossed through it with a single line and placed your initials beside the strikeout. You also had documented the numbness that the patient reported in his toes and his ability to move them during those pulse checks. In response to his questions regarding your apparently long scene time, you point to your note regarding the patient's repeated attempts to get off the cot and run away. With each series of questions, you were able to answer accurately and thoroughly based on your documentation. After the deposition, your attorney notifies you that although his client's suit is still proceeding against the hospital, the prosecuting attorney will be dropping your name and your service from the client's claims.

1. List five uses of this patient care report aside from the one already mentioned.

____

____

____

____

2. Place a check mark beside the components of an accurate, complete patient care report that were mentioned in this case.
   a. _________ Dates
   b. _________ Response times
   c. _________ Difficulties en route
   d. _________ Communication difficulties
   e. _________ Scene observations
   f. _________ Reasons for extended on scene time
   g. _________ Previous care provided
   h. _________ Time of extrication
   i. _________ Time of patient transport
   j. _________ Reason for hospital selection

3. Which is true regarding the correction of a patient care report that was done in this case?
   a. It would have been better to black out the error completely.
   b. It should have been explained thoroughly in the narrative.
   c. It was completed properly.
   d. Individual strikeouts should not be done; the entire sentence should be rewritten.

  Chapter **4** **Documentation**

CHAPTER 4 ANSWERS

1. At 1400, 4017 arrived to the scene of a residence. Found a 20-year-old woman supine on the lawn, saying inappropriate words. Her husband states she is a diabetic. He found her in the yard confused. Patient's skin is pale, cool, and diaphoretic. Vital signs are BP 110/70, P 120/min, R 20/min with clear breath sounds. Blood glucose determined to be 50 mg/dL. 1406 IV 250 mL NS initiated in the right antecubital space by paramedic Ward. 1408 25 g (50 mL) D50W given IVP by paramedic McKenna. 1410 Patient states, "Why are you here?" 1412 Patient is alert and oriented to person, place, and time. Patient states she took 10 units of regular and 20 units of Lente insulin at 0700 today. 1413 Ambulance en route to General Hospital. Report called to Dr. Smith. No further orders requested. 1416 BP 118/74, P 96/min, R 20/min. Skin is pink, warm, and dry. 1420 Arrival to General Hospital. 100 mL NS infused.

On some patient report forms, check boxes or tables will permit documentation of many of the items included in this narrative report. In that instance, it is often unnecessary to repeat the information in the narrative. (Objectives 3, 4, 5)

2. Medical continuity of care, quality improvement, legal record, supply tracking, performance evaluation, state reporting, education, and skill tracking (Objective 2)

3. a. Document the patient's level of consciousness, your advice to the patient (including possible consequences of refusal), medical direction advice to the patient, signatures of the patient and witnesses as required in your system, a narrative description of your exam that you told patient to call 9-1-1 again if he changes his mind, and the events that occurred.
   b. Note the name of the person or agency that canceled your response and the time the response was terminated. Ensure that this falls within the scope of your departmental policies.
   c. Document care on the appropriate mass casualty incident (MCI) forms (often on triage tags). Record the patient's condition and disposition on the appropriate tracking form (may be done by the sector leader).
   d. Note the purpose of the revision or correction and why the information did not appear on the original document as soon as possible using the appropriate departmental form. Ensure that the correction is made by the original author. Send a copy of the revision to the appropriate parties.
   (Objective 6)

4. a. If tetanus vaccine is administered to the patient in the hospital, he will likely have an allergic reaction and be harmed. You could face legal repercussions.
   b. If additional lidocaine is administered at the hospital, the patient may have a toxic reaction. When the chart is audited for quality purposes, it will appear that you did not perform a procedure that was indicated. If drug inventory is tracked from the patient report, it will not be replaced, and you may run short. If the patient's bill is itemized, he or she will not be charged for this intervention, and your department may lose revenue needed for operations.
   c. The patient's condition could deteriorate quickly, and the medical staff would not recognize the increased risk of bleeding. You could face legal repercussions.
   d. If the patient alleges that the numbness developed as a result of your care, you would have no documentation to substantiate your claim that the patient was symptomatic before your care; you could be successfully sued.
   (Objective 8)

5. d. All of these elements should be recorded in an accurate, legible, understandable manner. (Objective 1)

6. a. The records should be maintained confidentially and only released to parties other than the hospital after patient consent is given. (Objective 2)

7. a. This is documented on the appropriate department incident report. (Objective 3)

8. c. In a court of law, the assumption is that if it is not documented, it was not done. (Objective 4)

9. a. Advice to the patient, including risks of refusal and benefits of treatment, should be noted. Additionally, you should document that the patient was instructed to call back if the condition worsened or if he or she reconsidered. A detailed examination generally is not performed on a patient who refuses (document it if it is done).
(Objective 6)

10. a. A special form may be required to document these situations. You should always keep a record in case subsequent liability results.
(Objective 6)

11. b. Some agencies and states require separate reports. Patient care information should be completed only by the paramedic on the call. Corrections and revisions should be made as soon as possible.
(Objective 7)

WRAP IT UP

1. Medical audit, quality improvement, billing and administration, data collection, written record for other health care professionals to reference
(Objective 2)

2. Dates, response times, difficulties en route, scene observations, reasons for extended on scene time, time of patient transport
(Objective 3)

3. c. Local and state policy for report correction should be followed.
(Objective 7)

5 EMS Communications

READING ASSIGNMENT

Chapter 5, pages 73-87, in *Mosby's Paramedic Textbook*, ed. 4.

OBJECTIVES

Upon completion of this chapter, the paramedic student will be able to do the following:

1. Outline the phases of communications that occur during a typical emergency medical services (EMS) event.
2. Describe the role of communications in EMS.
3. Outline the basic model of communication.
4. Define common EMS communications terms.
5. Describe how to communicate effectively using the primary modes of EMS communication.
6. Outline the elements of an EMS communications system.
7. Describe the characteristics of EMS communications operation modes.
8. Describe the role of dispatching as it applies to prehospital emergency medical care.
9. Outline techniques for relaying EMS communications clearly and effectively.
10. Describe how EMS communications are regulated.
11. Distinguish between EMS frequency ranges.
12. Outline procedures for EMS communications.

SUMMARY

- Communications regarding emergency medical services (EMS)refers to the delivery of information. The patient and scene information is delivered to other key members of the emergency response team.
- There are five phases of typical EMS events, which are occurrence of the event; detection of the need for emergency services; notification and emergency response; EMS arrival, treatment, and preparation for transport; and EMS preparation for the next response.
- Communication is the process by which one person or group transmits meaning to others. The sender encodes a message that the receiver decodes. Four barriers to communication include attributes of the receiver, selective perception, semantic problems, and time pressures.
- Proper verbal and written communications allow the delivery of information among the members of the emergency team, the patient, and the community. Communications should be brief, clear, and confidential.
- EMS communications include simple and complex systems. The simple system includes a desktop transceiver and two-way radio. Complex systems include high-power communication capabilities.
- Operation modes used in EMS communication include simplex mode, which permits only one person to talk at a time; duplex mode, which allows two people to converse at the same time; multiplex mode, which can transmit telemetry and voice simultaneously; and trunked systems, which use five or more repeaters to provide communication channels in busy systems.
- The functions of an effective dispatch communications system include receiving and processing calls for EMS assistance, dispatching and coordinating EMS resources, relaying medical information, and coordinating with public safety agencies. Some emergency dispatchers provide pre-arrival instructions for patient care.
- In the United States, the Federal Communications Commission (FCC) regulates communications over the radio. The paramedic must be familiar with the regulatory agencies. Paramedics must follow their guidelines as well.
- EMS frequency ranges include VHF, UHF, and 800 MHz.
- A standard format of transmission of patient information is a wise idea. The standard allows for the best use of communications systems, allows physicians to receive details quickly about the patient, and decreases the chance of omitting any critical details.

Match the communication term in Column II with the appropriate definition in Column I. Use each answer only once.

Column I

1. _________ A unit of frequency equal to one cycle per second

2. _________ The ability to transmit or receive in one direction at a time

3. _________ A grouping of radio equipment that includes a transmitter and receiver

4. _________ Radio frequencies between 300 and 3000 MHz

5. _________ The ability to transmit and receive simultaneously through two different frequencies

6. _________ A unit of frequency equal to 1 million cycles per second

7. _________ Radio frequencies between 30 and 300 MHz

8. _________ A unit that receives transmissions from a mobile radio and retransmits them at higher power on another frequency

Column II

a. Base station
b. Duplex
c. Hertz
d. Kilohertz
e. Megahertz
f. Mobile station
g. Remote console
h. Repeater
i. Simplex
j. UHF
k. VHF

9. A person is stabbed with a knife. List the five phases of communications that occur on most EMS calls such as this.

a. ____

b. ____

c. ____

d. ____

e. ____

10. A man is injured seriously at a rural site. Describe the communication process from the time of his injury until the EMS crew returns to service.

____

____

____

____

11. List three common causes of environmental interference with radio transmissions.

a. ____

b. ____

c. ____

12. Briefly describe four responsibilities of an EMS dispatcher.

a. ____

b. ____

c. ____

d. ____

13. List three essential pieces of information that the dispatcher must obtain from a bystander who calls in to report a motor vehicle crash.

a. ____

b. ____

c. ____

14. Identify three ways in which the Federal Communications Commission directly influences EMS.

a. ____

b. ____

c. ____

15. Describe six actions paramedics may take to ensure clear and understandable radio transmissions.

a. ____

b. ____

c. ____

d. ____

e. ____

f. ____

Johnny Smith, a paramedic who works on City Unit 7, is called to an industrial site. He finds a 30-year-old patient lying on his back on the grass, where he landed after falling 20 feet from a painting platform. When the paramedic arrives at 1 PM, the patient's vital signs are as follows: blood pressure, 120/80 mm Hg; pulse, 116 per minute; and respirations, 20 per minute. The patient states he became dizzy and fell. When Smith palpates, the patient complains of pain in the lumbar region of the back and on both heels, which are swollen. Distal pulses, sensation, and movement are present in all extremities. Lung sounds are clear and equal bilaterally. The patient gives Smith his name and knows the date and time and where he is. His skin is warm and dry. The patient weighs about 100 kg and takes ibuprofen prescribed by Dr. Jones for back pain. Smith places him on 100% oxygen via a non-rebreather mask; positions him on a backboard with a cervical collar; and notifies Dr. Kane, the online medical physician, of the patient's condition and the 15-minute estimated arrival time to City Hospital. Vital signs at 1:25 PM are unchanged. The patient's condition remains the same en route.

16. Write a concise, complete radio report to communicate the appropriate information regarding this patient to the base hospital.

____

____

____

____

____

____

____

____

____

____

____

____

____

17. What is manipulation of the intended idea for communication known as?
   a. Decoding
   b. Encoding
   c. Feedback
   d. Receiving

18. After being called to an airplane crash with two seriously injured patients, the first arriving EMS crew tells online medical direction, "There are people [meaning bystanders] everywhere." The physician interprets this to indicate a mass casualty situation and activates the mass casualty incident plan. What type of communication error occurred here?
   a. Attributes of the receiver
   b. Selective perception
   c. Semantic problems
   d. Time pressures

19. Which of the following is a component of a simple communication system?
   a. Remote console
   b. Microwave links
   c. Mobile unit
   d. Satellite receivers

20. What is a radio receiver circuit used for suppressing the audio portion of unwanted radio noises or signals called?
   a. Decibel
   b. Frequency modulation
   c. Squelch
   d. Tone

21. What is the term for the number of repetitive cycles per second completed by a radio wave?
   a. Amplitude modulation
   b. Frequency
   c. Range
   d. Wattage

22. What is transmission and reception of electrocardiograms over the radio or telephone called?
   a. Coverage   **c.** Patch
   b. Hotline   **d.** Telemetry

23. What are the HEAR and EACOM radios used to tie hospitals together and receive and transmit tone pulses known as?
   a. Cellular telephones   **c.** Microwave transmitters
   b. Decoders and encoders   **d.** Satellite dishes

24. Which component of a communication system receives transmissions from a low-power portable radio on one frequency and simultaneously retransmits it at a higher power on another frequency?
   a. Mobile transceivers   **c.** Remote console
   b. Portable radios   **d.** Repeaters

25. How is the strongest signal selected when numerous satellite receivers are used?
   a. Base stations   **c.** Decoders
   b. Cellular lines   **d.** Voting systems

26. What are dispatch services located away from base stations that facilitate communications with field personnel known as?
   a. Complex systems   **c.** Portable transceivers
   b. Mobile transceivers   **d.** Remote consoles

27. What is an advantage of communication with cellular telephones?
   a. They allow unlimited channel access.
   b. They permit uninterrupted communication.
   c. They provide a secure link between EMS and the hospital.
   d. They transmit simultaneous calls in disaster situations.

28. Which of the following is a responsibility of the dispatcher?
   a. Follow-up on patient condition
   b. Coordinating with public safety services
   c. Investigating patient care complaints
   d. Providing offline medical control

29. What is a function of pre-arrival instructions?
   a. To allow EMS personnel to be disregarded
   b. To determine whether the call is unfounded
   c. To provide life-saving instructions
   d. To allow the EMS crew more time to respond

30. What is the role of the Federal Communications Commission?
   a. To consult with EMS agencies regarding radio equipment
   b. To develop new radio technologies
   c. To monitor frequencies for appropriate usage
   d. To train dispatchers in pre-arrival instructions

31. Which of the following is a technique for effective radio communication?
   a. Speak at a range of 6 to 8 inches from the microphone.
   b. Speak slowly and clearly and enunciate words distinctly.
   c. Show emotion to demonstrate the urgency of critical situations.
   d. Take your time and include all patient information available.

32. Which of the following is a component of the SOAP format for patient reports?
   a. Assessment data   **c.** Patient information
   b. Overall impression   **d.** Signs and symptoms

At 0130, the pre-alert tone sounds in your engine house, and the lights go on as you hear the dispatcher say, "4017 respond to number 12 Avid Court, chest pain." As you roll out of your bunk, the call is repeated, and then you hear the dispatcher recite the call numbers. Your partner pulls the run direction card as a backup because the computer was down earlier. You are attending this call, so you read the directions and tap the responding key of your on-board computer screen as you pull out of the engine room. The instructions on the screen note the patient's previous heart history. You pull up the global positioning system map to ensure you are proceeding in the correct direction. The dispatcher sends you a note indicating that there is a large dog that the caller has been instructed to secure in a bedroom. You tap the arrival button on your computer screen and proceed in to care for the patient. Based on your patient assessment, you suspect the patient is having an acute myocardial infarction, and you perform 12-lead electrocardiography (ECG). Your partner connects your monitor to the telephone line, and you transmit a copy of the ECG to medical direction. Then, when you contact medical direction using the cellular telephone for orders, they agree with your interpretation of inferior myocardial infarction. You notify dispatch that you are departing the scene to transport to Central Medical Center. They notify you that the local hospital diversion program indicates that they are on diversion and cannot accept the patient, so you elect to go the other direction to a medical center an equal distance and contact them on your UHF radio with a patient report. You indicate your arrival at the hospital on your dispatch screen. After giving a verbal report to the receiving RN, you call times to your computer from dispatch. Then you complete your report following the prompts on the screen and type in the narrative. The patient is now in the cardiac catheterization lab and unable to sign the consent and notice of receipt of the HIPAA forms, so you document that and give the privacy notice to the family member. You obtain the nurse's signature, print your report, and then touch your computer screen to notify dispatch that you are returning to service. As you pull into your station, you press the upload key on your computer, and the report is sent to a secure server, where it will be accessible to only the privacy officer, the hospital, the billing department, and a few designated officers.

1. List all the persons and agencies with which the EMS crew communicated on this call.

2. What key information did the dispatcher provide on this call?

3. What modes of communication were used on this EMS call?

4. Identify problems that could have been encountered on this call if any of the following communication errors had occurred.

Communication Error	**Potential Problems**

   a. Dispatcher fails to identify or transmit correct address.

   b. Dispatcher fails to give instructions regarding dog.

c. Computer fails and no backup system is available.

____

____

d. Incorrect or incomplete information is reported to medical direction.

____

____

e. Fail to report all medications given to receiving RN.

____

____

f. Forget to notify dispatch when returning in service.

____

____

5. List five roles communication played on this call.

a. ____

b. ____

c. ____

d. ____

e. ____

CHAPTER 5 ANSWERS

REVIEW QUESTIONS

1. c
(Objective 4)

2. i
(Objective 4)

3. a
(Objective 4)

4. j
(Objective 11)

5. b
(Objective 4)

6. e
(Objective 4)

7. k
(Objective 11)

8. h
(Objective 4)

9. a. Occurrence of the event
   b. Detection of the need for emergency services
   c. Notification and emergency response
   d. EMS arrival, treatment (including consultation with medical direction), and preparation for transport
   e. Preparation of EMS for the next emergency response
   (Objective 1)

10. EMS response is initiated by bystanders by telephone to a communications center or public safety answering point. The communications specialist obtains the necessary information (often accompanied by digital information) about the origin of the call. The call taker then passes the information by digital technology (if available) to the telecommunicator, who dispatches appropriate emergency personnel and equipment. The EMS crew notifies the communications center while en route and obtains additional information. The EMS crew notifies the communications center on arrival to scene. The EMS crew contacts medical direction for orders and reports. Care is rendered, and the patient is prepared for transport; the EMS crew notifies the communication center when they depart from the scene and arrive at the receiving facility. The ambulance is made ready for the next emergency call, and communications is notified when it is available for another call.
(Objective 3)

11. Mountains, dense foliage, and tall buildings
(Objective 7)

12. a. To receive calls for EMS assistance
   b. Dispatch and coordinate EMS resources
   c. Relay medical information
   d. Coordinate with public safety agencies
   (Objective 8)

13. a. Name and callback number of individual who placed the call
   b. Address of emergency and directions, including specific landmarks because of the possible rural location
   c. The nature of the emergency (Is the victim trapped, how seriously is he or she injured, and is he or she accessible to the EMS crew?)
   (Objective 8)

14. Licensing and frequency allocation, establishing technical standards for radio equipment, and establishing and enforcing rules and regulations
(Objective 10)

15. Speak 2 to 3 inches away from and across the microphone, speak slowly and clearly, speak without emotion, be brief, avoid codes (unless approved by system), and advise the receiving party when the transmission has been completed.
(Objective 9)

16. City Unit 7, paramedic Smith calling City Hospital. We are on the scene at an industrial site with a patient who fell approximately 20 feet onto a grassy area. The patient is a 30-year-old male weighing approximately 100 kg. Patient's chief complaint is back pain. Also complaining of bilateral heel pain. Patient states he became dizzy and fell. Medical history of back pain for which he takes ibuprofen. Patient is awake, alert, and oriented times 3. Lungs are clear bilaterally; skin is warm and dry. Tenderness to palpation in lumbar region of back and bilaterally on heels. Soft tissue swelling present bilaterally at calcaneus. Distal pulse, sensation, and movement present in all extremities. V/S are BP 120/80, P 116, R 20. Patient placed on 100% oxygen by complete non-rebreather mask

and immobilized on a backboard with cervical collar. Private physician is Dr. Jones. ETA will be 15 minutes. Standing by for any additional orders, over.
(Objective 9)

17. b. Decoding is interpretation of a message. Feedback is the response to the initial idea. Receiving indicates the receiver got the message.
(Objective 3)

18. c. The word *people* was mistakenly interpreted as *patients*.
(Objective 5)

19. c. All other equipment listed is part of a complex system.
(Objective 4)

20. c. A decibel is a unit of measurement for signal power levels. Frequency modulation is a deviation in carrier frequency resulting in less noise. A tone is a unique carrier wave used to signal a receiver selectively.
(Objective 4)

21. b. Amplitude modulation is a radio frequency that fluctuates according to the applied audio. Range refers to the general perimeter of signal coverage. A watt measures power output.
(Objective 4)

22. d. Coverage refers to the area where radio communication exists. A hotline is a dedicated line activated by merely lifting the receiver. Patching permits communication between different communication modes.
(Objective 4)

23. b. These tones can be set to all-call for efficient disaster communication. Cellular telephones are used for ambulance-to-hospital contact in some areas. Satellite dishes and microwave transmitters extend transmission distance.
(Objective 6)

24. d. Mobile transceivers usually are mounted on the vehicle and operate at lower outputs than base stations. Portable radios are handheld devices used when working away from the emergency vehicle. Remote center consoles are located away from base stations and are connected by dedicated telephone line, microwave, or other radio means.
(Objective 6)

25. d. Voting systems automatically select the strongest or best audio signal among numerous satellite receivers.
(Objective 6)

26. d. Remote consoles control all base station functions and are connected by dedicated telephone lines.
(Objective 6)

27. c. No dedicated cell channels exist for EMS, so lines may be busy when an emergency call is being made. In some areas, the cell coverage is not good, and communication may be terminated abruptly. This does not allow simultaneous communication.
(Objective 7).

28. b.
(Objective 8)

29. c. Pre-arrival instructions complement EMS care but do not include call screening.
(Objective 8)

30. c. They also are responsible for licensure and allocation of frequencies. They establish technical standards for radio equipment and establish and enforce rules and regulations for equipment operation.
(Objective 10)

31. b. You should speak 2 to 3 inches from the microphone, converse without emotion, and be brief.
(Objective 9)

32. a. Assessment data is a component.
(Objective 9)

WRAP IT UP

1. Partner, dispatch, patient and family, medical direction, receiving facility, receiving RN
(Objective 1)

2. Location of call, nature of call, previous information known about patient, presence of dog, diversion status of hospital, times
(Objective 8)

3. Radio voice, tones, light, computer (dispatch of call); fax (ECG); cellular telephone (medical direction); radio (dispatch, receiving facility); face to face (patient, partner, family, receiving RN)
(Objective 6)

4. a. Determining the correct location of a call is a critical element in your response time. Failure to do so could delay your response significantly.
(Objective 8)

b. Scene safety could have been compromised.
(Objective 8)

c. Response delays if no backup directions are available.
(Objective 6)

d. Inappropriate and even dangerous orders may be given if the report to medical direction is not accurate.
(Objective 9)

e. Duplicate administration of medications is possible if an incomplete report is given. This could cause serious side effects.
(Objective 9)

f. A call might be given to a more distant unit, delaying response time and leaving their zone without coverage.
(Objective 6)

5. a. Dispatch served as primary intake for notification of emergency event.
b. Dispatch notifies EMS of the nature and location of calls.
c. Communication between dispatcher and ambulance tracked call status
d. Transmission of voice and data from the scene to the hospital
e. Verbal and written report of the events of the call
(Objective 2)

Medical and Legal Issues

READING ASSIGNMENT

Chapter 6, pages 88-108, in *Mosby's Paramedic Textbook*, ed. 4.

OBJECTIVES

Upon completion of this chapter, the paramedic student will be able to do the following:

1. Describe the basic structure of the legal system in the United States.
2. Relate how laws affect the paramedic's practice.
3. List situations that the paramedic is legally required to report in most states.
4. Describe the four elements involved in a claim of negligence.
5. Describe measures paramedics may take to protect themselves from claims of negligence.
6. Describe the paramedic's responsibilities regarding patient confidentiality.
7. Outline the process for obtaining expressed, informed, and implied consent.
8. Describe legal complications relating to consent.
9. Describe actions to be taken in a refusal-of-care situation.
10. Describe legal considerations in situations that require the use of force.
11. Describe legal considerations related to patient transportation.
12. Outline legal implications related to resuscitation and patient death.
13. List the paramedics' responsibilities on a crime scene.

SUMMARY

- The structure of the legal system in the United States is composed of five types of law: legislative, administrative, common, criminal, and civil law. The law requires that paramedics perform within their scope of practice and follow all legal guidelines applicable to their practice.
- To safeguard against litigation, paramedics must be knowledgeable of legal issues. Paramedics also must know about the effects of these issues.
- Paramedics and health care workers may be required by law to report some cases. These include cases of abuse or neglect of children and older adults and spouse abuse. They also include cases that involve rape, sexual assault, gunshot wounds, stab wounds, animal bites, and some communicable diseases.
- Some state and federal regulations require notification of emergency medical services (EMS) exposure to infectious disease, include immunity statutes, and have laws that describe special crimes against EMS personnel.
- Lawsuits related to patient care usually result from civil claims of negligence. This refers to the failure to act as a reasonable, prudent paramedic would act in such circumstances.
- Most legal authorities stress that protection against claims of negligence has three elements. The first is training, the second is competent patient care skills, and the third is full documentation of all patient care activities.
- For the most part, confidential information includes any details about a patient that are related to the patient's history. Any assessment findings also are included. Any treatment given is included as well. As a rule, the release of these details requires written permission from the patient or legal guardian. (There are some exceptions.)
- A mentally competent adult with decisional capacity has the right to refuse medical care. This is the case even if the decision could result in death or permanent disability.
- Four other legal complications related to consent are abandonment, false imprisonment, assault, and battery.
- An adult patient with decisional capacity has certain rights. The patient has the right to decide what medical care (and transportation) to receive. This is a basic concept of law and medical practice.
- Legal responsibilities for the patient continue until patient care is transferred to another member of the health care system (or it is clear that the patient no longer requires care). Legal issues related to patient transport include level of care during transportation, use of the emergency vehicle operating privileges, choice of patient destination, and payer protocols.
- Resuscitation issues that relate directly to EMS include withholding or stopping resuscitation, advance directives, potential organ donation, and death in the field.

55

- EMS play two important roles when responding to crime scenes: (1) focusing on patient care and (2) preserving evidence at the scene when possible.
- In the legal field, the general belief is that "if it was not written down, it was not done." Thus, thoroughness and attention to detail are vital in documentation.

REVIEW QUESTIONS

Match the legal term in column II with its definition in column I. Use each answer only once.

Column I

1. ______ Forcefully restraining the arm of an alert, competent patient while an intravenous line is placed

2. ______ As a joke, advising the emergency department staff that the patient is a prostitute

3. ______ Telling a friend that you treated a nurse you both know for a drug overdose

4. ______ Restraining an alert, conscious adult with an obvious fracture and transporting him by ambulance against his will

5. ______ Documenting that the patient is homosexual and remarking, "Now let's see them get insurance."

6. ______ Leaving a patient in the emergency department to go on another call before you have an opportunity to give a report to the nurse or physician on duty

Column II

a. Abandonment
b. Assault
c. Battery
d. False imprisonment
e. Libel
f. Invasion of privacy (libel)
g. Malpractice
h. Slander

7. Violations of state motor vehicle codes by a paramedic can result only in civil lawsuits. True/False. If you answered false, explain why.

____

____

8. Good Samaritan legislation may protect off-duty EMS providers from litigation if no negligence or reckless disregard is involved. True/False. If you answered false, explain why.

____

____

9. Group insurance policies protect EMS providers from lawsuits arising from negligent acts. True/False. If you answered false, explain why.

____

____

56

10. List four situations that most states require a paramedic to report to the authorities.

a. ____

b. ____

c. ____

d. ____

11. List the four elements necessary to prove negligence.

a. ____

b. ____

c. ____

d. ____

12. A 40-year-old patient involved in a motor vehicle collision complains of mild neck pain and tingling in her fingers. She is quickly assessed and signs a refusal of care form at the urging of the paramedic crew. Later that day she loses sensation and movement in all extremities, stops breathing, and dies. Which, if any, of the four elements in question 11 could be used to prove negligence in this situation and why?

____

____

____

13. Name three effective means by which the paramedic can avoid claims of liability when providing patient care.

a. ____

b. ____

c. ____

14. You are called to treat an alert, 72-year-old patient who is experiencing chest pain. The patient exhibits classic signs and symptoms of myocardial infarction. You explain to him that he needs to go to the hospital because you believe his symptoms could be those of a heart attack, and proper medicine could be given to help his condition. He states that he wants his wife to drive him instead of going by ambulance. You advise him that if his condition worsens in the car, his wife would be unable to help him, and he might die. You again urge him to come with you. Fill in the blanks below with the type of consent that best applies to the situation.
The patient can now make a(n)

a. _____________________ consent. He tells you that he has decided to go in the ambulance. This constitutes a(n)

b. _____________________ consent. If he had lost consciousness before agreeing to ambulance transport, his consent is said to be a(n)

c. _____________________ consent, and treatment could be rendered.

15. You respond to the scene of an automobile collision, where you find an awake, alert, 24-year-old man complaining of neck pain and tingling in his right arm. His vital signs are stable. The patient's vehicle was struck from behind and sustained considerable damage. The patient refuses transport to the hospital. What five things should be done or explained to this patient and documented on the patient care report regarding his refusal of care?

    a. ____

    b. ____

    c. ____

    d. ____

    e. ____

Questions 16 to 21 refer to the following case study:

You are dispatched to an expensive rural home for an "accidental injury." When you arrive, you find a man and a woman. The man, who appears to be approximately 30 years old, apparently had been shot in the head at close range. He had been found pulseless and breathless by a family member, who found both patients 20 minutes before your arrival. The male patient has a large exit wound with brain matter extruding. After your initial assessment, you decide not to resuscitate him. The female patient is a woman who you recognize as a local celebrity. She has a gunshot wound to the abdomen, is unconscious, and has no radial pulse. You note a plastic bag of white powder and a hypodermic needle next to her. A handgun is lying on the floor next to the man. The family wants you to take the woman to the closest local hospital so they can "keep things quiet." The nearest trauma center is an equal distance away.

16. What type of consent applies in this situation?

____

17. List four facts you must document about the male patient to ensure legal compliance.

    a. ____

    b. ____

    c. ____

    d. ____

18. Describe actions you should take to preserve evidence at this scene with regard to the following:

    a. Clothing

____

    b. Weapon

____

    c. Blood on the floor

____

58

d. Documentation of the scene

e. Positioning of the ambulance

19. Should you transport the patient to the hospital the family wants or to the trauma center? Explain your answer.

20. Why shouldn't you document, "Drugs found lying next to patient"?

21. To which of the following personnel is it appropriate to tell the facts of this case?
- **a.** Police officers assigned to the case — Yes/No
- **b.** A paramedic from another service — Yes/No
- **c.** The press — Yes/No
- **d.** Medical personnel caring for the patient — Yes/No
- **e.** Hospital staff in the smokers' area — Yes/No

STUDENT SELF-ASSESSMENT

22. Which branch of law is also referred to as tort law?
- **a.** Administrative law
- **b.** Civil law
- **c.** Criminal law
- **d.** Legislative law

23. In which of the following situations may abandonment be alleged when a paramedic relinquishes care to an EMT?
- **a.** A patient being transferred with an infusion of blood
- **b.** A patient going from a nursing home to a hospital for a wrist injury
- **c.** A hysterical, uninjured patient from a mass casualty situation
- **d.** A dialysis patient being transported for routine care

24. Which of the following is necessary for successful prosecution of a criminal law case?
- **a.** Criminal intent must be proved.
- **b.** Injury must be demonstrated.
- **c.** A patient must sue for financial gain.
- **d.** A statute must be violated.

25. You are called to a private residence, where you find an elderly man experiencing heat-related illness. The family evidently left this chronically confused individual at home with no air conditioning and all of the windows closed. What legal issue must you remember on this call?
- **a.** To preserve the chain of evidence, do not remove the patient's clothes.
- **b.** This patient can't consent, so you must contact the family before transport.
- **c.** Writing the neighbors' statements in the patient care report may constitute libel.
- **d.** You are required to report this situation to the appropriate legal or social agency.

26. The Ryan White Act provides protection for the paramedic with regard to which of the following?
- **a.** Good Samaritan acts
- **b.** Governmental immunity
- **c.** Infectious disease
- **d.** Violent acts

    Chapter **6**   **Medical and Legal Issues**

27. A paramedic finds an unconscious patient who has a strong odor resembling alcohol on the breath. No care is initiated, and during transport, the patient aspirates. At the hospital, the patient is found to have a dangerously low blood sugar level, and a lengthy hospitalization ensues. Why could this patient claim negligence?
   a. The paramedic violated a law while providing care.
   b. The paramedic committed malfeasance while providing care.
   c. The patient experienced damage from the negligent act.
   d. Evidence existed of conflicting views of causation.

28. Patient confidentiality would be breached in most states if a paramedic discussed the patient's comments and care with which of the following?
   a. Lawyers in court
   b. Emergency department personnel
   c. Personal friends
   d. A quality assurance committee

29. What type of consent occurs when a patient agrees to treatment verbally or in writing?
   a. Expressed
   b. Implied
   c. Informed
   d. Referred

30. You are caring for an elderly patient who experienced a syncopal episode. He now refuses care. What actions must you take to ensure legal compliance during this refusal process?
   a. Force the patient to sign the refusal form before release.
   b. Tell the patient that if he changes his mind, he can call you again.
   c. Do not give the patient any additional advice or you may be liable.
   d. Transport the patient against his will because he lost consciousness.

31. What do EMS traffic right-of-way privileges usually include?
   a. The right to travel as fast as necessary to get to the hospital quickly
   b. The ability to proceed without slowing through intersections
   c. The right to override the directions of a traffic officer
   d. Definitions of appropriate use of lights and sirens

32. According to the American Heart Association, what criteria must be met to stop resuscitation in the prehospital setting after you have initiated advanced life support procedures?
   a. Persistent asystole or agonal rhythm is present, and no reversible causes are identified.
   b. The family assures you that there is a "do not resuscitate" order, but it can't be found.
   c. Endotracheal intubation and IV access can't be established; therefore, you are unable to give drugs.
   d. Trauma is a factor, and your transport time will be 20 minutes or longer.

33. You respond to a stabbing. What actions should you take to preserve evidence?
   a. Cut the clothing through the knife hole to minimize other damage.
   b. Give the clothes to a bystander so evidence will remain at the scene.
   c. Move the knife, if present, so EMS personnel will not step on it.
   d. Follow the same path to and from the ambulance and patient.

WRAP IT UP

Your ambulance is dispatched at 0500 to a party at a local bar. The patient is a 35-year-old woman who was involved in a fight. She has a large laceration, made by a broken bottle, that extends into her eye. You control the bleeding with 5 × 9 dressings and a Kerlix wrap. The patient is awake and alert and oriented to person, place, and time. She refuses transport. You recognize the seriousness of her wound because of its depth and involvement with her eye, and you attempt at length to persuade her to be transported. She is rude and belligerent and persistently refuses care. You decide to take her forcibly because of the seriousness of her wound. You and your partner pick her up and carry her to the ambulance, secure her with straps and soft wrist restraints, and take her to the hospital. Patients are lined up three deep in the halls in the emergency department (ED). You wait 30 minutes to give a report to a nurse, but they are all busy. Finally, because it is a busy night and you must get back into service, you give the patient care report and your verbal report to the registration clerk along with your phone number so the nurse can contact you with any questions. You call an acquaintance who you know is a coworker of this patient because you know that the woman will need a ride home from the hospital because of her impaired vision. After you leave the ED, the patient, who you left restrained supine, vomits and aspirates. This results in pneumonia, which requires a 2-week hospitalization.

1. Explain whether the actions of the paramedic related to patient consent were proper in this case.

____

____

____

2. Is the paramedic protected under the Good Samaritan rules in this case? If not, why not?

____

____

____

3. Is the paramedic protected by immunity statutes in this case? If not, why not?

____

____

____

4. Is her assault a mandatory reportable situation under most state laws?

____

____

____

5. Place a ✓ beside any term that may describe a legal rule the paramedic may have violated in this situation. Explain each violation.

__________ Abandonment	__________ Negligence
__________ Assault	__________ Battery
__________ False imprisonment	__________ Libel
__________ Slander	__________ Civil rights violation

REVIEW QUESTIONS

1. c. Physical force against individuals against their will and without legal justification is battery.

2. h. Making statements about a person with malicious intent is slander.

3. f. You released information about the nurse that could cause ridicule, embarrassment, or notoriety.

4. d. Forcible restraint and confinement against one's will is false imprisonment.

5. e. Making false written statements about a person with malicious intent is libel.

6. a. Failure to appropriately turn over care of the patient to a qualified individual may be considered abandonment.
   (Questions 1–6: Objectives 2, 6, 8)

7. False. If a criminal law is violated, a paramedic could be charged under that statute as well. For example, in the past, EMS personnel have been charged with manslaughter when someone died as a result of a vehicular collision involving the ambulance.
   (Objective 2)

8. True.
   (Objective 5)

9. False. The lawsuit may be filed regardless of the presence of insurance. However, the insurance may protect the paramedic's personal assets. This is controversial; some sources advise against carrying insurance.
   (Objective 5)

10. Child abuse or neglect, elder abuse or neglect, rape, animal bites, gunshot or stab wounds
    (Objective 3)

11. Duty to act, breach of duty, damage to the patient, and proximate cause are the four elements that must be proven to win a negligence suit.
    (Objective 4)

12. Duty to act: The unit was on duty and was called to care for this patient.
    Breach of duty: The standard of care would have indicated immobilizing and transporting this patient; the crew failed to act as the standard of care dictated.
    Damage to the patient: The patient lost movement, stopped breathing, and died after being abandoned by the paramedic crew.
    Proximate cause: The patient apparently died from spinal cord damage; the paramedic crew did not immobilize and protect the cervical spine, which might have prevented death.
    (Objective 4)

13. The paramedic may reduce the risk of liability claims by obtaining appropriate training, delivering competent patient care, and ensuring thorough documentation.
    (Objective 5)

14. a. Informed
    b. Expressed
    c. Implied
    (Objective 7)

15. You must document the following: the patient's level of consciousness (awake and alert); that you explained to the patient the risks of refusing care, including paralysis or death; that you had the patient sign a refusal form, noting any witnesses; any follow-up instructions you gave the patient; and that you told the patient to call EMS again if his condition worsened or he changed his mind.
(Objective 9)

16. Implied consent is assumed because the patient is unconscious.
(Objective 7)

17. The absence of a heart rate (ECG) strip in several leads; the absence of respirations, pulse, and spontaneous movement; fixed and dilated pupils; and the condition of the body (specifically the wounds) should be documented. In addition, the known time that the patient was breathless and pulseless with no care before your arrival should be documented.
(Objective 12)

18. a. You should take care not to cut the clothing through the bullet hole. If the clothes are removed, you should not shake them. If removed on the scene, the clothes should be given only to the police. If removed in the ambulance, the clothes should be placed in a paper bag and given to a police officer at the hospital, if possible.
b. You should not touch the weapon unless it poses a danger to your crew.
c. Try not to step in the blood on the floor, if possible.
d. Carefully and objectively document your findings on the scene. Note the specific location and position of both patients and the location of the weapon. Any other unusual scene findings should also be listed.
e. Your ambulance should be parked away from any obvious evidence if it does not interfere with scene safety.
(Objective 13)

19. Typically, you may override a family's wishes for specific cases when state protocols indicate that patients may be taken to specialty centers such as trauma centers, which are known to improve survival for specific injuries.
(Objective 12)

20. Unless you have proof that the bag contains drugs, you should note only what you specifically observed, that is, that a bag containing a white powdery substance and a syringe with a needle were found to the right of the patient.
(Objective 13)

21. a. Yes
b. No, not unless the paramedic has a legitimate medical or legal reason to know the information.
c. No. Specific department regulations about information to be released to the press should be followed.
d. Yes. Medical direction needs to know the facts of the case for quality improvement reasons.
e. No. Only hospital staff directly involved in the patient's care should be informed of the details of the case.
(Objective 6)

STUDENT SELF-ASSESSMENT

22. b. Administrative law refers to regulations that are developed by a government agency to provide details about the process of the law. Criminal laws are enacted by federal, state, or local government to protect society. Legislative laws are made by legislative branches of government and are determined by statutes and constitutions.
(Objective 1)

23. a. A patient who needs continuing advanced care should not be released by a paramedic to someone with lesser training.
(Objective 11)

24. d. Criminal law violations need not involve injury or criminal intent. The patient sues for damages in civil suits. A criminal law violation is based on proof that a statute has been violated.
(Objective 1)

25. d. If you have any suspicion of elder abuse or neglect, you are obligated to report it. You should remove clothing if necessary for care. Implied consent is indicated on this call.
(Objective 3)

26. c. The Ryan White Comprehensive AIDS Resources Emergency Act of 1990 (PL 101-381), the Ryan White Treatment Modernization Act of 2006 (PL 109-415) (revised in 2008) describes reporting requirements for hospitals to EMS providers who have been exposed to certain communicable diseases and lists other organizational responsibilities for infectious disease reporting.
(Objective 2)

27. c. The patient experienced damage, as evidenced by the long hospitalization. This could result in loss of income if the person was employed. This was more likely a breach of duty or nonfeasance (failure to perform a required act or duty) rather than malfeasance (performing a wrongful or unlawful act). Although the potential exists that the paramedic's actions violated EMS law, the failure to provide standard of care is usually not legislated.
(Objective 4)

28. c. Privileged patient information should never be given to personnel with no legal right to know it.
(Objective 6)

29. a. Implied consent permits a paramedic to render lifesaving care if the patient is unable to agree because of a lack of mental competence. Informed consent means that the patient has been told the implications of the injury and illness, the treatment needed, and potential complications. There is no such thing as referred consent.
(Objective 7)

30. b. You should ask the patient to sign a refusal of care form; however, if he refuses to do so, document his refusal and witness it. Be sure to advise the patient about further care for his condition. If he is awake and alert now, he may legally refuse transport.
(Objective 8)

31. d. EMS agencies are typically permitted to travel moderately faster (often 10 mph) than regular traffic; however, excessive speed is hazardous. Crews should slow down or stop until they are certain that traffic has stopped and then proceed cautiously though intersections. Traffic officers' instructions should be followed. If a dispute occurs, supervising officers should be contacted immediately.
(Objective 11)

32. a. In most cases, a written rather than verbal "do not resuscitate" order is required to stop resuscitation. If airway or IV access can't be established, resuscitation efforts should not be terminated in the field. In some cases, specific time limits may be placed on the provision of resuscitation; these should be determined in cooperation with medical direction, and they usually are used only with very long transports.
(Objective 12)

33. d. Do not cut through the stab hole. Do not give clothing to bystanders other than authorized law enforcement personnel. Do not move the knife unless it is essential for crew safety.
(Objective 13)

WRAP IT UP

1. The actions related to the patient's consent were not proper. This patient was an adult and apparently had decisional capacity and therefore had the right to refuse care. Forcing her transport against her will with restraint may subject you to claims of assault, battery, and false imprisonment.
(Objective 7, 8)

2. No. Good Samaritan protections do not typically extend to those on duty.
(Objective 2)

3. No. Immunity statutes typically apply only to government agencies and do not always protect individual employees of those agencies.
(Objective 2, 5)

4. No. Most states would not consider this type of assault "reportable"; however, for the safety of the EMS crew, it is prudent to have law enforcement present on all scenes that involve a violent crime. Assaults involving firearms are almost always required to be reported.
(Objective 3)

5. Abandonment: The paramedic crew left the patient in the care of a clerical employee, not a person of equal or higher license.
Negligence: The paramedics had a duty to act (monitor a restrained patient until relieved by a qualified person), they breached that duty (turned the patient over to the registration clerk), there was injury (pneumonia secondary to aspiration), and there was proximate cause (the plaintiff likely could prove that the injury was caused by the paramedics' restraint and abandonment of the patient).
    Assault: The paramedics told the patient they would transport her against her will.
    Battery: The paramedics forcibly restrained the patient against her will.
    False imprisonment: The paramedics restrained the patient to the stretcher against her will.
    Slander: The paramedic called the patient's coworker to tell her of the situation.
(Objectives 2, 4, 6, 8)

READING ASSIGNMENT

Chapter 7, pages 109-117, in *Mosby's Paramedic Textbook,* ed. 4.

OBJECTIVES

Upon completion of this chapter, the paramedic student will be able to do the following:

1. Define *ethics* and *bioethics*.
2. Distinguish between professional, legal, and moral accountability.
3. Outline strategies to use to resolve ethical conflicts.
4. Describe the role of ethical tests in resolving ethical dilemmas in health care.
5. Discuss specific prehospital ethical issues, including allocation of resources, decisions surrounding resuscitation, confidentiality, and consent.
6. Identify ethical dilemmas that may occur related to care in futile situations, obligation to provide care, patient advocacy, and the paramedic's role as physician extender.

SUMMARY

- *Ethics* is the discipline relating to right and wrong, moral duty and obligation, moral principles and values, and moral character. *Bioethics* is the science of medical ethics. *Morals* refers to social standard or customs.
- Paramedics must meet a standard established by their level of training and regional practice. Paramedics must abide by the law when ethical conflicts occur.
- A paramedic must act in a way that is seen as morally acceptable.
- The rapid approach to ethical issues is a process. The process involves reviewing past experiences; deliberation (if possible); and performing the impartiality test, universalizability test, and interpersonal justifiability test to reach an acceptable decision.
- Two concepts of ethical health care are to provide patient benefit and to do no harm.
- All resources must be allocated fairly. This is an accepted bioethical value.
- Advance directives, living wills, and other self-determination documents can help the paramedic to make decisions about the appropriateness of resuscitation in the prehospital setting.
- A health care professional is not allowed to reveal details supplied by the patient to others without the patient's consent. This is the principle of confidentiality.
- In some cases, patients refuse lifesaving care. These cases can produce legal and ethical conflicts.
- Other areas that are likely to raise ethical questions in the prehospital setting include providing care in futile situations, the paramedic's obligation to provide care, patient advocacy, and the paramedic's role as physician extender.

REVIEW QUESTIONS

Match the term in column II with its description in column I. Use each term only once.

Column I

1. _________ Working to benefit others

2. _________ The study of right, wrong, and morality

3. _________ To do no harm

4. _________ A person's ability to make rational decisions independently

5. _________ Moral duty or obligation related to medicine

6. _________ Maintaining the privacy of personal patient information

Column II

a. Autonomy
b. Beneficence
c. Bioethics
d. Confidentiality
e. Ethics
f. Nonmaleficence
g. Rationality

Questions 7 to 9 pertain to the following case study.

A fellow paramedic who is a close friend calls you and is very upset. Her daughter was involved in a vehicle collision. She is fine, but a person in the other car was injured and has been taken to the hospital. You transported the injured patient, and your friend wants to know the extent of injuries, what the patient said, and details related to the crash.

7. a. What should you tell your friend about the patient's injuries?

____

   b. Is your decision ethically correct with regard to the patient and your friend?

____

Your friend's daughter has been charged with reckless driving. You believe that the patient you transported was intoxicated; in fact, he admitted to using alcohol and cocaine before the incident. Despite his serious injuries, he was laughing and making inappropriate comments.

8. Will this affect your decision about disclosing patient information? Why or why not?

____

____

9. Did you make your decision about this problem based on professional, legal, or moral accountability?

____

____

10. Think about how you would respond to each of the following situations and state whether professional, legal, or moral accountability issues would prompt your actions.

   a. You are leaving the hospital after transporting a patient. You notice that your partner has picked up some towels, although you didn't use any on the patient. He says, "Oh, these are for me. I want to wash my car this afternoon."

____

____

   b. As you depart from a scene, you hear your partner make an inappropriate racial comment about the patient.

____

____

   c. You notice that an on-duty coworker has an alcoholic drink while attending your annual department awards banquet.

____

____

d. Your partner administers a slightly different dose of pain medicine than that ordered by medical direction because he believes that the doctor was being "too conservative."

____

____

e. Your teenage niece is experiencing severe vomiting in her first trimester of pregnancy. It is clear that she needs IV fluids to relieve her dehydration, but she has no insurance, and you know it will cost your brother hundreds of dollars if she is seen in the emergency department. He asks whether you can get some supplies from work and come to the house to give her the fluids.

____

____

Question 11 pertains to the following case study:

You and your partner are caring for a 55-year-old patient who is in respiratory arrest. You have called for assistance and are told it will be 10 minutes. After intubation, the patient is stable as long as you ventilate regularly. You are preparing for transport when suddenly your partner collapses and is pulseless.

11. a. The circumstances allow you to care for only one patient or the other. Who will you choose to resuscitate? Why?

____

____

b. How did you reach the above decision? Try using the ethical tests in the rapid approach to emergency medical problems to see whether they would assist you in this situation.
   (1) Have you experienced a similar problem in the past?
   (2) Can you buy time for deliberation or to consult with others?
   (3) Would you accept the action if you were in the patient's place?
   (4) Would you feel comfortable having the action performed in all similar circumstances?
   (5) Can you provide good reasons to justify and defend your actions to others?

12. State which of the following factors is the cause of the ethical dilemma in each of the following situations. Then give an action you could take.

Allocation of resources	Care in futile situations
Decisions regarding resuscitation	Obligation to provide care
Confidentiality	Physician extender role
Consent	

a. You request pain medicine to care for your patient's very painful single extremity injury. Online medical direction refuses.

Cause of ethical dilemma: ____

Possible action: ____

____

b. Your patient has a severe headache, is vomiting, and has a numb right hand. The patient's blood pressure is 220/140 mm Hg. Despite your detailed explanations, the patient is refusing treatment or transport.

Cause of ethical dilemma: ____

Possible action: ____

____

c. You are triaging at a mass casualty situation. You evaluate a child, the same age as yours, whose skin is warm. Bystanders say she just stopped breathing a few moments ago.

Cause of ethical dilemma: ____

Possible action: ____

____

d. You respond to a private residence. The patient has a legally executed living will. Hysterical family members are begging you to resuscitate the patient.

Cause of ethical dilemma: ____

Possible action: ____

____

STUDENT SELF-ASSESSMENT

13. What are the standards of honorable behavior to which paramedics are expected to conform in the EMS profession?

   a. Certifications   **c.** Laws
   b. Ethics   **d.** Morals

14. Which of the following determines moral accountability in the practice of EMS?

   a. Laws and regulations
   b. Personal beliefs and values
   c. Professional licensure
   d. Standards related to education and skills

15. During a call, you find yourself in a situation that involves an ethical dilemma. What strategy can you use to resolve the problem?

   a. Let the patient's family tell you what to do even if the patient disagrees.
   b. Ask yourself which action you would prefer if you were in the patient's place.
   c. Abide by your partner's opinion in the situation.
   d. Rely on your policies and procedures for guidance.

16. Which of the ethical tests can help correct for your personal bias about a situation?

   a. Would you accept the action if you were in the patient's place?
   b. Would you feel comfortable having this action performed under similar circumstances?
   c. Can you justify and defend your actions to others?
   d. Have you experienced a similar problem in the past?

17. On a call, you are faced with an unusual situation that falls just on the fringe of your legal and professional boundaries. You decide to take action because you are able to provide clear reasons explaining and defending your actions to others. What type of ethical test have you used?

   a. Autonomy   **c.** Interpersonal justifiability
   b. Impartiality   **d.** Universalizability

70

18. Which of the following situations involves an ethical decision? The patient has a living will and is pulseless.
   a. The family asks you to abide by the living will.
   b. The patient is cold and has rigor mortis.
   c. A signature is in the wrong place on the living will document.
   d. The nursing home staff think that a living will exists but cannot locate it.

19. You are transporting a patient and her doctor from an outpatient surgery center to the hospital because a complication has occurred. The patient's respirations are very slow, and her chest is barely moving. You note the need to ventilate, but the physician strongly disagrees. If you elect to proceed, you are acting on which ethical principle?
   a. Allocation of resources   **c.** Care in futile situations
   b. Autonomy   **d.** Patient advocacy

WRAP IT UP

You are dispatched at 1500 to a home in a quiet residential neighborhood to "check the welfare with possible forcible entry." Out-of-town adult family members report that they have been unable to contact their father for a day and a half, and they are concerned for his health. On arrival, you note that the man's car is in the garage. Two newspapers are in the driveway, and neighbors tell you that they haven't seen him in 2 days. You circle the home, knocking loudly and looking in windows. Through the kitchen window, you are able to see feet protruding from behind the counter. The captain elects to force a door to gain entry. Once in, you find a 79-year-old man who tells you he slipped and fell 2 days ago and is unable to get up. You examine him and are unable to find any injuries, although he appears somewhat dehydrated, his heart rate is elevated, and his clothing is soaked with urine. He is very thin, and when you check the refrigerator and cabinets, you find little food.

The patient is alert and oriented; however, he seems slow to respond, his speech is slightly slurred, and he has weakness on the left side. He tends to repeat information. He adamantly refuses to be transported. According to your protocol, you can't forcibly transport him based on the information you have provided. Repeated attempts to reach medical control are not successful.

1. Why does this call present an ethical conflict?

   ____

   ____

2. Answer all the tests of ethical decision making to see how they would apply to this situation. Explain your answers.
   a. Impartiality test: Would you accept this action if you were in the patient's place?

   ____

   ____

   b. Universalizability test: Would you feel comfortable having this action performed in all relevantly similar circumstances?

   ____

   ____

   c. Interpersonal justifiability test: Are you able to provide good reasons to justify and defend your actions to others?

   ____

   ____

3. Answer the following ethical questions regarding this call.

    a. What is the patient's best interest?

    b. What are the patient's rights?

    c. Does the patient understand the issues at hand?

    d. What is the paramedic's professional, legal, and moral accountability?

    a. ____

    b. ____

    c. ____

    d. ____

4. a. Put a ✓ beside the bioethical values you would be following if you leave the patient unattended at the scene.

    b. Put an X beside the bioethical values you would be following if you arrange either for someone to come and provide temporary care for the patient or for the Division of Aging to come and evaluate him within 12 hours.

________ Autonomy	________ Beneficence
________ Confidentiality	________ Allocation of resources
________ Nonmaleficence	________ Personal integrity

CHAPTER 7 ANSWERS

REVIEW QUESTIONS

1. b
(Objective 4)

2. e
(Objective 1)

3. f
(Objective 4)

4. a
(Objective 4)

5. c
(Objective 4)

6. d
(Objective 1)

7. a. You can disclose nothing about the patient's injuries except what is permitted by departmental policy.
b. Your feelings about whether this is ethical will be personal.

72

8. Your legal obligation would not change regardless of your decision.

9. Your legal obligation prevents you from disclosing information.
(Questions 7–9: Objective 2)

10. a. Legal (theft), professional, and moral conflicts may come into play here.
    b. Professional and moral conflicts may be involved as you make a decision about how to respond to this situation.
    c. Legal (working and driving while under the influence), professional, and moral standards are involved in the paramedic's actions and in your response to them.
    d. Professional and moral issues are involved in this situation.
    e. Legal (theft of equipment), professional (actions without medical direction), and moral (allocation of resources) issues are involved in this situation.
(Objective 2)

11. The answers to each of these questions are personal. Discuss your answers with a fellow student. How do your views compare?
(Objective 3)

12. a. Physician extender role. Possible actions: Clarify and repeat request for orders. Ask for a call review or critique to discuss the issue.
    b. Consent. Possible actions: Have online medical direction speak to the patient. Talk to the family to see if they can convince the patient. If not, provide detailed follow-up instructions and try to leave the patient in the supervised care of family or friends.
    c. Allocation of resources. Possible actions: Reevaluate your resources to determine whether resuscitation should proceed. Ask for a change of assignment if possible.
    d. Decisions regarding resuscitation. Possible actions: Contact medical direction. Remove the family from the area and calmly explain the wishes of their loved one.
(Objectives 3-5)

STUDENT SELF-ASSESSMENT

13. b. Certification is a professional standard. Laws are legal standards. Morals are social standards.
(Objective 1)

14. b. Laws and regulations relate to legal accountability. Professional licensure and standards relate to education. Skills relate to professional accountability.
(Objective 2)

15. b. This is known as the impartiality test.
(Objective 3)

16. b. This is known as the universalizability test.
(Objective 3)

17. a. The impartiality test can correct partiality or personal bias. The universalizability test helps eliminate moral decision difficulty. The interpersonal justifiability test requires reasons for your actions and approval from others of those reasons.
(Objective 4)

18. c. If the family concurs and the living will is legal, no ethical question exists. If the patient has obvious signs of death, no ethical dilemma exists. If the living will document cannot be produced, legally it cannot be recognized.
(Objective 5)

19. d. Allocation of resources is an issue when the patient's health care needs can't be met because of inadequate resources. Autonomy is a person's ability to make decisions. Care in futile situations arises when the care you are about to give serves no purpose.
(Objective 6)

1. An ethical conflict exists because a disparity clearly exists between what you can legally do and what you know needs to be done for this man.
   (Objective 2)

2. a. Assuming the patient is lucid, he may not accept it.
   b. This is a question each student should answer individually.
   c. Could you justify your actions? What rationale would you use? Are other options available?
   (Objective 4)

3. a. Do you have enough information to determine whether this is in the patient's best interest?
   b. An alert, oriented patient has the right to refuse care. Are other social service agencies available that you could involve that might help make the determination whether the patient is presently competent to make this decision? Can local police assist you?
   c. Did you explain and have the patient verbalize his understanding of the risks of leaving him alone?
   d. Professionally, you have a responsibility to care for patients and to ensure their safety; however, you also have a responsibility to follow protocols. Legally, your state law and your local protocols may state that the patient has the right to refuse. Moral questions will be answered individually. Involve medical direction to help resolve the situation online.
   (Objective 2)

4. a. Autonomy, possibly personal integrity
   (Objective 5)
   b. Beneficence, nonmaleficence
   (Objective 5)

8 | Research Principles and Evidence-Based Practice

READING ASSIGNMENT

Chapter 8, pages 118-127, in *Mosby's Paramedic Textbook,* ed. 4.

OBJECTIVES

Upon completion of this chapter, the paramedic student will be able to do the following:

1. Explain the importance of EMS research.
2. Distinguish the differences between types of EMS research.
3. Outline the 10 steps to perform research identified in this chapter.
4. Define *evidence-based practice*.
5. Describe criteria to evaluate when reading a research paper.

SUMMARY

- The paramedic must be familiar with research principles. This knowledge is needed to conduct research, collect research data, and interpret published studies.
- Research is essential to improve patient care.
- Two main types of research methods are descriptive and experimental. Data are collected by various methods. These methods may be prospective, retrospective, or cross-sectional.
- Ten steps of EMS research include prepare a question, write a hypothesis, decide what to measure and how to measure it, define the population, identify study limitations, seek IRB approval, obtain informed consent, gather data after conducting pilot trials, analyze the data, and present the data.
- Descriptive statistics does not try to infer anything about a subject that goes beyond the data.
- Qualitative analysis provides a non-numerical description of the population. Quantitative data analysis evaluates the data using numbers.
- Inferential statistics infers whether the relationships seen in a sample are likely to occur in the larger population. In this type of study, researchers develop a null hypothesis.
- Emergency medical services (EMS) care should be evidence based. This means that there should be proof that interventions and procedures have benefit for the patient.
- Paramedics should read research articles critically to determine if they are relevant to their practice.

REVIEW QUESTIONS

Questions 1 to 9 pertain to the following research abstract, which was published in *Prehospital Emergency Care*, 2(3), 1998. Read the abstract carefully and then answer each question.

Efficacy of Midazolam for Facilitated Intubation by Paramedics
Authors: Edward T. Dickinson, MD, NREMT-P
Jason E. Cohen, BA, EMT-P
C. Crawford Mechem, MD

Affiliation: Department of Emergency Medicine, University of Pennsylvania School of Medicine, Philadelphia, Pennsylvania

Objective: The use of pharmacological agents by paramedics to facilitate endotracheal intubation (ETI) is becoming increasingly common. This study was done to determine the efficacy of intravenous midazolam, a short-acting benzodiazepine, as a drug to facilitate ETI in patients resistant to conventional ETI.

Methods: The study was conducted in a suburban municipal EMS system over a 22-month period. All paramedics were trained in the use of midazolam for facilitated intubation prior to allowing the use of midazolam in the system. All calls in which midazolam was used were reviewed on a monthly basis by investigators via retrospective review of the prehospital care reports.

Results: During the study period, 13,212 emergency responses occurred, resulting in 154 ETIs by paramedics. Midazolam was used to facilitate 20 (13%) of these ETIs. "Clenched teeth" and failed intubation attempt were the most commonly cited indications for facilitated intubation. Eleven patients had medical complaints, and nine were trauma patients. Successful ETI with midazolam was achieved in 17 of 20 (85%) cases. In 88% (15 of 17) of these cases, a single dose of midazolam was sufficient for ETI; mean dose 3.6 mg (standard deviation [SD] 1.1 mg). The three patients with failed ETI received multiple doses of midazolam; mean dose 5 mg (SD 2 mg).

Conclusion: The prehospital use of single-dose IV midazolam is generally effective in accomplishing facilitated ETI in patients resistant to conventional (nonpharmacological) endotracheal intubation.

1. What was the purpose of this study (i.e., what problem or question are the authors trying to solve)?

   ____

   ____

2. Is the hypothesis stated in this abstract? _____________________ If you answered yes, what is it? If you answered no, what do you think it is?

   ____

3. What is the study population?

   ____

4. What are the sample and sample size for this research?

   ____

5. Was a random sampling procedure used? Yes/No Explain your answer.

   ____

6. Did this study use a qualitative or quantitative approach?

   ____

7. The study indicates a standard deviation for the mean dose of 1.1 mg. What does this mean?

   ____

8. What are some weaknesses or unanswered questions related to this research?

   ____

9. Are the findings of this study important to the EMS community?

   ____

Match the terms in Column II that describe types of research with the appropriate description in Column I.

Column I

10. _________ You review patient care reports from last year to find causes of falls.

11. _________ You interview an EMS group to find trends in feelings about violence.

12. _________ You use a new piece of equipment for 1 month to determine its effectiveness.

13. _________ You will evaluate burn assessment using a new tool for the next year.

14. _________ You evaluate the average turn-out time for each EMS station.

15. _________ You compare patient pain when standard treatment is alternated randomly with a new drug.

Column II

a. Cross-sectional
b. Descriptive
c. Experimental
d. Prospective
e. Qualitative
f. Retrospective

STUDENT SELF-ASSESSMENT

16. You want your medical director to adopt a new medicine to treat nausea and vomiting. Which of the following demonstrates an evidence-based approach to this project?
    a. Ask your EMS colleagues to email the medical director to say why they want the change.
    b. Do an analysis to see which of the medicines will be most cost effective.
    c. Search peer-reviewed journals for scientific research related to this topic.
    d. Call other agencies to see which medication they are using for this problem.

17. In an unblinded study when the paramedic is assessing the patient's response to a new drug that relieves pain, who would know when the study treatment is being given as opposed to the control treatment?
    a. The patient, paramedic, and researcher
    b. None of them
    c. The patient and the researcher but not the paramedic
    d. The researcher and paramedic but not the patient

18. You are conducting research for a drug to treat cardiac arrest. Only you and your partner have been trained to gather the data, so the drug will be used only on days that you work. This type of subject selection is called which of the following:
    a. Alternative time sampling
    b. Convenience sampling
    c. Statistical table sampling
    d. Systemic sampling

19. You are doing a study on the variability of scene response times according to time of day. Here are the data you collected (in minutes) for one group: 1, 2, 3, 4, 4, 4, 4, 4, 5, 5, 5, 5, 6, 6, 6, 7, 7, 8, 9. What is the mode for this set of data?
    a. 4
    b. 5
    c. 6
    d. 7

20. Before your research is approved by an institutional review board, what must you prove?
    a. Consent will be obtained.
    b. The hypothesis is true.
    c. No risks will be incurred.
    d. Your sample is large enough.

Chapter **8** **Research Principles and Evidence-Based Practice**

21. Which section of a research article describes step-by-step processes to conduct the research?
   a. Discussion
   b. Introduction
   c. Methods
   d. Results

22. Which type of statistical analysis has findings that suggest the results in the sample could be generalized to the entire population?
   a. Cross-sectional
   b. Descriptive
   c. Inferential
   d. Prospective

23. What is the primary goal of the institutional review board?
   a. Assessing value
   b. Cost analysis
   c. Determining merit
   d. Patient safety

24. Which type of consent would be most common when performing cardiac arrest studies?
   a. Consent at a distance
   b. Cohort consent
   c. Deferred consent
   d. Stepped consent

WRAP IT UP

You work for an urban EMS agency that runs 20,000 ambulance calls per year. Your department wants to participate in a research study to compare the effectiveness of dextrose 25% as opposed to dextrose 50% when treating adult patients who have symptomatic hypoglycemia. Patients who take oral diabetic agents or those who are not known to be diabetic will be excluded.

1. Write a hypothesis that describes your research question for this study.
2. What should you measure to conduct this research?
3. What are some limitations to this study?
4. Why might you have difficulty getting IRB approval for this study?
5. What additional step should you take after IRB approval before you formally begin your study?
6. When you analyze the data, what would you look for?
7. Where might you publish your research if your findings are significant?
8. Why do you think this study would or would not be important to the broader EMS community?

CHAPTER 8 ANSWERS

REVIEW QUESTIONS

1. To determine the efficacy of IV midazolam to aid in prehospital intubations that failed conventional methods (Objective 3)

2. No. No hypothesis is stated. The hypothesis could have been that the use of midazolam will facilitate intubation in patients who could not be intubated by conventional means. (Objective 3)

3. The study population is the 154 ETIs that occurred within the study period. (Objective 3)

4. The sample is the patients who could not be intubated by conventional means (sample size is 20 patients). (Objective 3)

5. No. Random sampling was not done. All patients who met the criterion (failed intubation) were included. (Objective 2)

6. Descriptive statistics were used to report the findings in this quantitative paper. (Objective 2)

7. This means that about 65% of the patients received 3.6 mg ± 1.1 mg of midazolam in the successful ETI group. (Objective 3)

8. Many other things could be considered. For example, did the age of the patients affect the success? Were the missed patients trauma or medical patients, and did that influence success rates? Is 20 a large enough sample size to make a broad generalization to all EMS patients? What was the experience level of the paramedics in the "success" group versus the "fail" group? (Objective 3)

9. The use of any drug is associated with potential risks and complications. Objective data on the effectiveness of drugs, especially in the unique prehospital environment, support the standards and practice of paramedic care. (Objective 1)

10. f

11. e

12. a

13. d

14. b

15. c
(Questions 10–15, Objective 2)

STUDENT SELF-ASSESSMENT

16. c. Review of current scientific research in peer-reviewed publications is important in evidence-based practice. (Objective 4)

17. a. In a blinded study, one or more of the persons who are involved will not know when a treatment is being given. (Objective 2)

18. b. Alternative time sampling selects participants based on a predetermined time interval (e.g., day of the week, month). Sampling using a statistical table involves selection of patients based on a table that predetermines which patient will be following a selected protocol. Systemic sampling enrolls patients in the order in which they are encountered. For example, it may be established that every other patient encountered gets the test intervention. (Objective 10)

19. a. The number 4 occurs most frequently. The mean, or average of the sum of the times, is 5, as is the median, or middle of the group. (Objective 10)

20. a. Although traditional informed consent is not always possible, an acceptable alternative must be demonstrated to the IRB before your project is approved. The purpose of the research is to prove or disprove the hypothesis; this can be determined only after the study is completed. If risks are associated with the research, you must demonstrate that the potential benefit of the study warrants the risk. The primary responsibility of the IRB is to consider ethical, not procedural, issues with the research. (Objective 11)

21. c. The introduction sets the stage for the need for research and provides a review of existing related literature. The results section outlines data analysis to support or refute the research findings. The discussion provides the author's interpretation of the findings.
(Objective 5).

22. c. Cross-sectional research is research conducted within a short, specified amount of time. Descriptive statistics present the "what is" of a given situation without inferring implications for a larger population. Prospective research indicates a plan to conduct the research at a future date.
(Objective 2)

23. d. Patient safety and ethical treatment is the number one concern of an IRB.
(Objective 3)

24. c. Consent at a distance occurs when a physician explains the protocol and obtains consent over the phone or radio. Cohort consent involves asking a group of patients to consent to a future study. Stepped consent occurs when paramedics provide a brief description of the protocol in the ambulance with verbal consent and then a full description is provided later.
(Objective 3)

WRAP IT UP

1. There are many possible hypotheses for this study. Some examples are:
Dextrose 25% increases blood glucose to normal levels as effectively as dextrose 50%.
Or Dextrose 25% is as effective as dextrose 50% to treat hypoglycemia in adults with type 1 diabetes.
(Objective 3)

2. Measurements for this research could include blood glucose levels before treatment, blood glucose levels at selected time intervals after treatment, Glasgow Coma Scale score before treatment, Glasgow Coma Scale score at selected intervals after treatment, patient transports after each treatment, repeat EMS calls after treatment, or complications after each treatment.
(Objective 3)

3. Limitations of the study include the fact that only adults are included and people with type 2 diabetes are not included. Other limitations may include characteristics of the overall patient population such as poverty or other factors that may mean you cannot generalize your findings to all cases of hypoglycemia.
(Objective 2, 3)

4. IRB approval may be difficult because patients who are hypoglycemic usually do not have decision-making capacity because of altered mental status. This will make obtaining informed consent for research more difficult. You will need to seek an alternative type of consent or prove to the IRB that the treatment has little risk of harm to the patient.
(Objective 3)

5. Before you begin the study, conduct a pilot study with a small sample of patients. This will identify problems with your research protocol or questionnaire that you can fix before you begin collecting data on your larger group of patients.
(Objective 3)

6. When you analyze the data, you will be looking for the range of increase of blood glucose in each patient group, mean increase in blood glucose in each patient group, time to return to normal in each patient group, transports in each patient group, number of return calls in each patient group, and any complications in each patient group.
(Objective 3)

7. This would be published in a peer-reviewed EMS journal with a readership that has interest in clinical topics related to prehospital care such as *Prehospital Emergency Care* or *Annals of Emergency Medicine*.
(Objective 3)

8. Significant findings related to the topic would be of broad interest in the EMS community because (1) it relates to both AEMT and paramedic practice, (2) EMS treat many patients with this condition, (3) patients with this diagnosis are found in all geographic areas.
(Objective 2)

9 Medical Terminology

READING ASSIGNMENT

Chapter 9, pages 128-138, in *Mosby's Paramedic Textbook*, ed. 4.

OBJECTIVES

Upon completion of this chapter, the paramedic student will be able to do the following:

1. Describe what medical terms are used to describe.
2. Explain the role of a prefix, root word, combining vowels, and suffixes in a medical term.
3. Interpret selected examples of medical prefixes, root words, combining vowels, and suffixes.
4. Distinguish between singular and plural forms of medical terms.
5. Use accepted medical abbreviations appropriately.
6. Discriminate between similar medical terms and abbreviations.

SUMMARY

- Medical terminology is the language of medicine. It is important to know the language to communicate and interpret patient information with other health care personnel.
- Medical terms are used to describe body structures, systems and functions; anatomical regions and locations; diseases and other health problems: medical and surgical procedures: diagnostic tests; and medical instruments
- Medical terms are broken down into several parts. These parts include prefixes, suffixes, root words, and some combining vowels.
- A prefix is a root syllable at the beginning of a word that describes location or intensity.
- A suffix occurs at the end of a word and describes a patient's condition or diagnosis.
- Root words describe a structure or condition. Root words may be combined with other root words, a prefix, or a suffix (or any combination of these).
- Combining vowels join syllables in medical terms to make them easier to pronounce.
- Interpret medical terms by analyzing each word part and then combining them to determine the meaning.
- There are specific rules to convert medical terms from singular to plural. For example, vertebra becomes vertebrae, diagnoses becomes diagnoses, phalanx becomes phalanges, and alveolus become alveoli.
- Medical abbreviations, acronyms, and symbols are a form of medical shorthand. It is important to use abbreviations approved within your EMS system.
- It is important to pronounce medical terms correctly so your intended meaning will be communicated clearly.

REVIEW QUESTIONS

Match the general descriptive terms in Column II with the medical term in Column I. You may use each descriptive term more than once.

Column I

1. _________ Proximal

2. _________ Cholecystectomy

3. _________ Lymph/o

4. _________ Myopathy

5. _________ Laryngoscope

6. _________ Oximetry

Column II

a. Body structure or system
b. Anatomical region or location
c. Disease or health problem
d. Medical or surgical procedure
e. Diagnostic test
f. Medical instrument

7. _________ Ophthalm/o

8. _________ Anemia

9. _________ Thoracostomy

10. _________ Medial

11. For each of the following medical terms, note the meaning of the prefix, suffix, and root word, if present.

Medical Term	Prefix (with Meaning)	Root Word (with Meaning)	Suffix (with Meaning)
a. splenomegaly			
b. polymyalgia			
c. pericardiocentesis			
d. periorbital			
e. nephrectomy			
f. pneumothorax			
g. hepatitis			

12. State whether each of the following medical terms represents the singular or multiple form.

a. pleura ____

b. coxae ____

c. ovum ____

d. testes ____

e. bronchi ____

f. alveolus ____

13. Rewrite the following sentences substituting the proper medical abbreviations.
a. The patient has congestive heart failure related the rheumatic heart disease he had as a child.

____

b. The patient had severe peripheral vascular disease and diabetes, which indicated the potential for hypertension, coronary artery disease (including acute myocardial infarction), and cerebrovascular accident.

____

86

c. The basic life support unit obtained vital signs and a history and physical exam.

____

d. The patient took an overdose of pills. Her blood pressure was 100/60 mm Hg, her heart rate was 100 beats/min, and her oxygen saturation was 95%.

____

e. The patient had paroxysmal atrial tachycardia after taking an over-the-counter medicine.

____

f. The patient was in ventricular fibrillation. After defibrillation, the patient had return of spontaneous circulation, but his heart rate was 48 beats/min, so we began transcutaneous pacing.

____

14. Circle the correct term on the right to match the description provided to the left.

a. An internal organ	Viscus or viscous?
b. Related to the ear	Aural or oral?
c. The volume of drug to give	Milligrams or milliliters?
d. Part of the tibial bone	Malleolus or malleable?
e. Membrane lining the abdominal cavity	Perineum or peritoneum?

STUDENT SELF-ASSESSMENT

15. What is the most important reason a paramedic should use proper medical terminology when giving a hand-off report to other medical professionals?
a. So the exact meaning is clear
b. To appear more professional
c. So the patient will not understand
d. To improve reimbursement claims

16. What the suffix in the medical term _pancreatitis_ tell you about the organ it relates to?
a. Size
b. Inflammation
c. Growth
d. Pain

17. What does the root word in _ophthalmoscope_ describe about the instrument?
a. Its size
b. Its function
c. How it is used
d. Where it is used

18. What is the purpose of a combining vowel in medical terms?
a. To note direction
b. They make pronunciation easier
c. To explain the nature of illness
d. They describe the disease process

19. How does a medical term that ends in "is" change to its plural form?
a. Drop the "s" and add "des."
b. Add an "e."
c. Change the "i" to "e."
d. Convert "is" to "ex."

20. What does the abbreviation CO mean?
a. Capnography
b. Carbon dioxide
c. Carbon monoxide
d. Chronic obstruction

21. If you saw the abbreviation grav II on a woman's chart, what would it denote?
a. Two deliveries
b. Two pregnancies
c. Two antinausea medications
d. Two levels on the pain scale

Chapter **9** **Medical Terminology**

It is early in the shift when the call comes out for a "person unresponsive" at the local skilled nursing facility. When you arrive, you find a 72-year-old man who withdraws slightly to painful stimulus. His vital signs are BP 110/72 P 128 BPM and **temperature** 102°F (38.9°C). The nurse tells you he was awake earlier and complained of a slight **headache**. Other than slight **dyspnea on exertion** he seemed fine. His medical history includes <u>DJD, CHF,</u> **hepatitis C virus, and myocardial infarction**. He was hospitalized recently and had an *angiogram* and *bronchoscopy*. He was found to have *cardiomegaly*. You apply **oxygen** and start an <u>IV</u> of <u>NS TKO</u>. When you apply the <u>ECG</u> leads, you note an <u>AICD</u>. His 12-lead ECG shows a <u>LBBB</u>. His face seems to be drooping, so you wonder if this could be a <u>CVA</u>, possibly caused by a <u>SAH</u>. En route to the **emergency department,** the patient has a seizure, and you administer diazepam **intravenous push**.

1. Convert all of the bolded terms to their appropriate abbreviations.

____

____

2. Convert all of the underlined abbreviations to their full terms

____

____

____

3. Break down each italicized word and describe the meaning of each root word and suffix.

____

____

____

CHAPTER 9 ANSWERS

REVIEW QUESTIONS

1. b. Closer to the heart

2. d. Removal of the gall bladder

3. a. Pertaining to the lymphatic system or organs

4. c. Disease of the muscle

5. f. Lighted blade to visualize the vocal cords in the larynx

6. e. Measuring oxygen saturation

7. a. Pertaining to the eyes

8. c. Decreased red blood cells

9. d. Creating an opening into the chest

10. b. Toward the middle
    (Questions 1-10; Objective 1)

11.

Medical Term	Prefix (with Meaning)	Root Word (with Meaning)	Suffix (with Meaning)
a. splenomegaly	None	Splen- Pertaining to the spleen	-megaly Enlarged
b. polymyalgia	Poly- Many	My- Pertaining to the muscles	-algia Pain
c. pericardiocentesis	Peri- Around	Cardio- Pertaining to the heart	-centesis Drain or puncture
d. periorbital	Peri- Around	Orbital Bony cavity surrounding the eye	-al Pertaining to
e. nephrectomy	None	Nephr- Pertaining to the kidney	-ectomy Surgical removal of
f. pneumothorax	Pneumo- Containing air	Thorax Pertaining to the chest cavity	None
g. hepatitis	None	Hepat- Pertaining to the liver	-itis Inflammation

(Objective 3)

12. a. pleura: singular
 b. coxae: plural
 c. ovum: singular
 d. testes: pleural
 e. bronchi: singular
 f. alveolus: singular
(Objective 4)

13. a. The patient has CHF related to the RHD he had as a child.
 b. The patient had severe PVD and diabetes, which indicated the potential for HTN, CAD, including AMI and CVA.
 c. The BLS unit obtained VS and an H&P.
 d. The patient took an OD of pills. Her BP was 100/60 mm Hg, her heart rate was 100 BPM, and her O_2 saturation was 95%.
 e. The patient had PAT after taking an OTC medicine.
 f. The patient was in VF. After defibrillation, the patient had ROSC, but his heart rate was 48 BPM, so we began TCP.
(Objective 5)

14. a. Viscus. *Viscous* means thick.
 b. Aural. *Oral* refers to the mouth.
 c. Milliliters. *Milligrams* refers to weight, not volume.
 d. Malleolus. *Malleable* means flexible or bendable.
 e. Peritoneum. The perineum is the area on the body surface between the anus and the scrotum or vulva.
(Objective 6)

STUDENT SELF-ASSESSMENT

15. a. Proper use of medical terminology also makes the paramedic appear more professional. (Objective 1).

16. b. "Itis" refers to inflammation. (Objective 3)

17. d. "Ophthalm" refers to the structures of the eye. (Objective 3).

18. b. Combining vowels make it easier to say the terms. (Objective 2).

19. c. For example, one diagnosis versus many diagnoses. (Objective 4)

20. c. The abbreviation for carbon dioxide is CO_2 (Objective 5, 6)

21. b. Two deliveries would be para II (Objective 5)

WRAP IT UP

1. Convert all of the bolded terms to their appropriate abbreviations.
Temperature: T
Headache: HA
dyspnea on exertion: DOE
hepatitis C virus: HCV
myocardial infarction: MI
oxygen: O_2
emergency department: ED
intravenous push: IVP
(Objective 5)

2. Convert all of the underlined abbreviations to their full terms.
BP: blood pressure
P: pulse
BPM: beats per minute
°F: degrees Fahrenheit
°C: degrees centigrade
DJD: degenerative joint disease
CHF: congestive heart failure
IV: intravenous
NS: normal saline
TKO: to keep open
ECG: electrocardiogram
AICD: automated implanted cardioverter defibrillator
LBBB: left bundle branch block
CVA: cerebrovascular accident
SAH: subarachnoid hemorrhage
(Objective 5)

3. Angiogram: angio (pertains to the blood vessels) + gram (imaging)
Bronchoscopy: broncho (pertains to the bronchi in the lungs) + scopy (using a camera to visualize
Cardiomegaly: cardio (pertains to the heart) + megaly (enlargement)
(Objective 3)

10 Review of Human Systems

READING ASSIGNMENT

Chapter 10, pages 139-210, in *Mosby's Paramedic Textbook,* ed. 4.

OBJECTIVES

Upon completion of this chapter, the paramedic student will be able to do the following:

1. Discuss the importance of human anatomy as it relates to the paramedic profession.
2. Describe the anatomical position.
3. Properly interpret anatomical directional terms and body planes.
4. List the structures that comprise the axial and appendicular regions of the body.
5. Define the divisions of the abdominal region.
6. List the three major body cavities.
7. Describe the contents of the three major body cavities.
8. Discuss the functions of the following cellular structures: the cytoplasmic membrane, the cytoplasm (and organelles), and the nucleus.
9. Describe the process by which human cells reproduce.
10. Differentiate and describe the following tissue types: epithelial tissue, connective tissue, muscle tissue, and nervous tissue.
11. For each of the 11 major organ systems in the human body, label a diagram of anatomical structures, list the functions of the major anatomical structures, and explain how the organs of the system interrelate to perform the specified functions of the system.
12. For the special senses, label a diagram of the anatomical structures of the special senses, list the functions of the anatomical structures of each sense, and explain how the structures of the senses interrelate to perform their specialized functions.

SUMMARY

- Paramedics must understand human anatomy fully. This understanding will help them to organize a patient assessment by body region. Knowledge of anatomy also will help paramedics to communicate well with medical direction and other members of the health care team.
- The anatomical position refers to a patient standing erect with the palms facing the examiner.
- Directional terms are expressed in anatomical terminology. Examples of these are *up* or *down, front* or *back*, and *right* or *left*. These terms always refer to the patient, not the examiner. Internal body structure is classified into anatomical planes of the human body. These planes can be thought of as imaginary straight-line divisions.
- The appendicular region of the body includes the limbs, or extremities. The axial region consists of the head, neck, thorax, and abdomen.
- The abdomen usually is divided into four quadrants: upper right, lower right, upper left, and lower left.
- The three major cavities of the human body are the thoracic cavity, the abdominal cavity, and the pelvic cavity.
- The thoracic cavity contains the trachea, esophagus, thymus, heart, great vessels, lungs, and the cavities and membranes that surround them. The abdominopelvic cavity is surrounded by membranes and contains organs and blood vessels.
- The cytoplasmic membrane encloses the cytoplasm. The membrane forms the outer boundary of the cell.
- Cytoplasm lies between the cytoplasmic membrane and the nucleus. Specialized structures in the cell (organelles) are located in the cytoplasm. These organelles perform functions key to the survival of the cell. The nucleus is a large, membrane-bound organelle. It ultimately controls all other organelles in the cytoplasm.
- All human cells, with the exception of the reproductive (sex) cells, reproduce by a process known as mitosis. In this process, cells divide to multiply.

- Four main types of tissue make up the many organs of the body. These are epithelial, connective, muscle, and nervous. Epithelial tissue covers surfaces and forms structures. Connective tissue is made of cells separated from each other by intercellular material. This material is known as the extracellular matrix. Muscle tissue is contractile tissue and is responsible for movement. The nervous tissue has the ability to conduct electrical signals. These signals are known as action potentials.
- A system is a group of organs arranged to perform a more complex function than any one organ can perform alone. The 11 major organ systems in the body are the integumentary, skeletal, muscular, nervous, endocrine, circulatory, lymphatic, respiratory, digestive, urinary, and reproductive.
- The integumentary system consists of the skin and accessory structures such as hair, nails, and a variety of glands. The functions of the integumentary system include protecting the body against injury and dehydration, defense against infection, and temperature regulation.
- The skeletal system consists of bone and associated connective tissues, including cartilage, tendons, and ligaments. The skeletal system provides a rigid framework for support and protection. It also provides a system of levers on which muscles act to produce body movements.
- The three primary functions of the muscular system are movement, postural maintenance, and heat production.
- The nervous and the endocrine systems are the major regulatory and coordinating systems of the body. The nervous system rapidly sends information. It does this by means of nerve impulses conducted from one area of the body to another. The endocrine system sends information more slowly. It does this by means of chemicals secreted by ductless glands into the bloodstream.
- The heart and cardiovascular system are responsible for circulating blood throughout the body. Blood transports nutrients and oxygen to tissues. Blood carries carbon dioxide and waste products away from tissues. In addition, blood carries hormones produced in endocrine glands to their target tissues. Blood also plays a key role in temperature regulation and fluid balance. Blood also protects the body from bacteria and foreign substances.
- The lymphatic system includes lymph, lymphocytes, lymph nodes, tonsils, the spleen, and the thymus gland. The lymphatic system has three basic functions. The first is to help maintain fluid balance in tissues. The second is to absorb fats and other substances from the digestive tract. The third is to play a role in the immune defense system of the body.
- The organs of the respiratory system and the cardiovascular system move oxygen to cells. They move carbon dioxide from cells to where it is released into the air. The entrance to the respiratory tract begins at the nasal cavity and includes the nasopharynx, oropharynx, laryngopharynx, and larynx. Below the glottis are the structures of the lower airway and lungs. These structures include the trachea, the bronchial tree, the alveoli, and the lungs.
- The digestive system provides the body with water, electrolytes, and other nutrients used by cells. The gastrointestinal tract is an irregularly shaped tube. Associated accessory organs (mainly glands) secrete fluid into the digestive tract.
- The urinary system works with other body systems to maintain homeostasis. It does this by removing waste products from the blood. It also does this by helping to maintain a constant body fluid volume and composition. The contents of the urinary system include two kidneys, two ureters, the urinary bladder, and the urethra.
- The purpose of the male reproductive system is to make and transfer spermatozoa to the female. The purpose of the female reproductive system is to make oocytes and to receive the spermatozoa for fertilization, conception, gestation, and birth. The male reproductive system consists of the testes, epididymis, ductus deferens, urethra, seminal vesicles, prostate gland, bulbourethral glands, scrotum, and penis. The female reproductive organs consist of the ovaries, uterine (or fallopian) tubes, uterus, vagina, external genital organs, and mammary glands.
- Senses provide the brain with information about the outside world. Four senses are recognized as special senses: smell, taste, sight, and hearing and balance.

REVIEW QUESTIONS

Match the cellular structure from column II with its definition in column I. Use each answer only once.

Column I

1. _______ Cytoplasmic "canals" that transport proteins and other substances

2. _______ Phospholipid layer that forms the outer boundary of the cell

3. _______ Organelles that contain enzymes capable of digesting proteins and lipids

4. _______ Mass of a cell that lies between the cytoplasmic membrane and nucleus

Column II

a. Centrioles
b. Cytoplasm
c. Cytoplasmic membrane
d. Endoplasmic reticulum
e. Golgi apparatus
f. Lysosomes
g. Mitochondria
h. Nucleus
i. Ribosomes

5. ________ Sacs that package materials for secretion from the cell

6. ________ Control center of the cell; contains genetic material

7. ________ Structures composed of ribonucleic acid and protein that manufacture enzymes

8. ________ Powerhouse of the cell; produces adenosine triphosphate

9. Label Fig. 10-1 with the appropriate cellular structures listed in column II of question 8.

a. ____

b. ____

c. ____

d. ____

e. ____

f. ____

g. ____

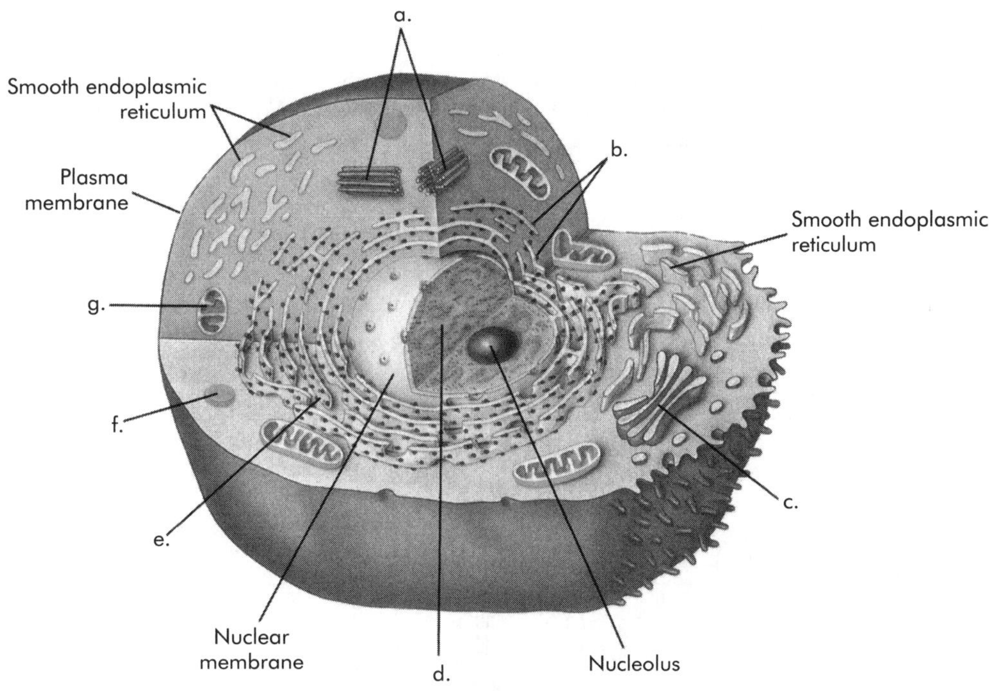

Figure 10-1

10. All human cells divide by the process of mitosis throughout the life of a human organism. True/False. If this is false, explain why.

____

____

11. Describe the anatomical position.

____

93

12. Circle the appropriate directional terms in boldface in the following sentences.

   a. The wrist lies **distal/proximal** to the elbow.

   b. The right nipple is located **medial/lateral** to the sternum.

   c. The cervical spine is **superior/inferior** to the lumbar spine.

   d. The umbilicus is located on the **dorsal/ventral** surface of the body.

13. List the structures that make up the following regions of the body.

   a. Appendicular region:

____

   b. Axial region:

____

14. Name the anatomical landmarks that divide the abdomen into four quadrants.

____

Questions 15 to 19 pertain to the following case study:

You respond to a call for a patient who was burned. You determine that the scene is safe and then approach the patient. She is lying on her right side, moaning, and has burned skin over several areas. You begin your assessment and care and roll her supine. As you carefully remove her clothing, you can better observe the burns, as shown in Fig. 10-2.

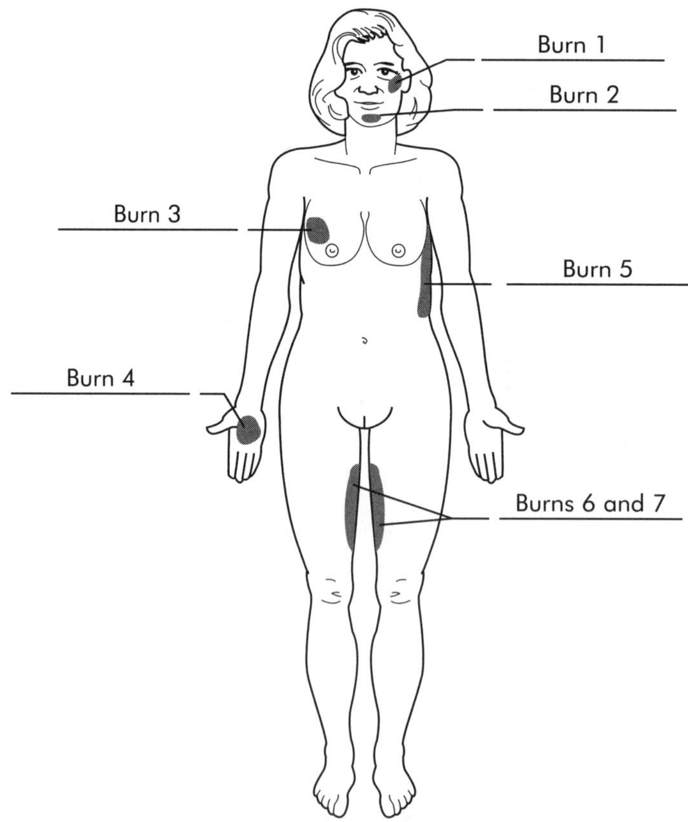

Figure 10-2

15. What directional term describes the patient's position when you arrived?

____

16. Using appropriate directional terms, describe where.

    a. Burn (1) is located relative to the left eye.

____

    b. Burn (2) is located relative to the mouth.

____

    c. Burn (3) is located relative to the nipple.

____

    d. Burn (4) lies relative to the right hand.

____

    e. Burn (5) lies relative to the axilla.

____

    f. Burns (6 and 7) are located.

____

17. Burn (5) encroaches on what abdominal quadrant?

____

18. List the major body cavities under each wound.

    a. Burn (3)

____

    b. Burn (5)

____

19. Have these wounds affected the axial or appendicular regions of the body?

____

20. For each of the following subgroups of tissues, list the tissue type (epithelial, connective, muscle, or nervous), one area of the body where it is found, and at least one specialized function it performs.

Subgroup	Type	Body Area	Function
Striated voluntary tissue			
Bone			
Epithelium			
Adipose tissue			
Hemopoietic tissue			
Striated involuntary tissue			
Neurons			
Cartilage			
Areolar tissue			
Nonstriated involuntary tissue			
Neuroglia			

21. List the 11 major body systems.

a. ____

b. ____

c. ____

d. ____

e. ____

f. ____

g. ____

h. ____

i. ____

j. ____

k. ____

96

22. Label the structures of the skin shown in Fig. 10-3 and list two functions of each.

	Structure	Function
a.		
b.		
c.		

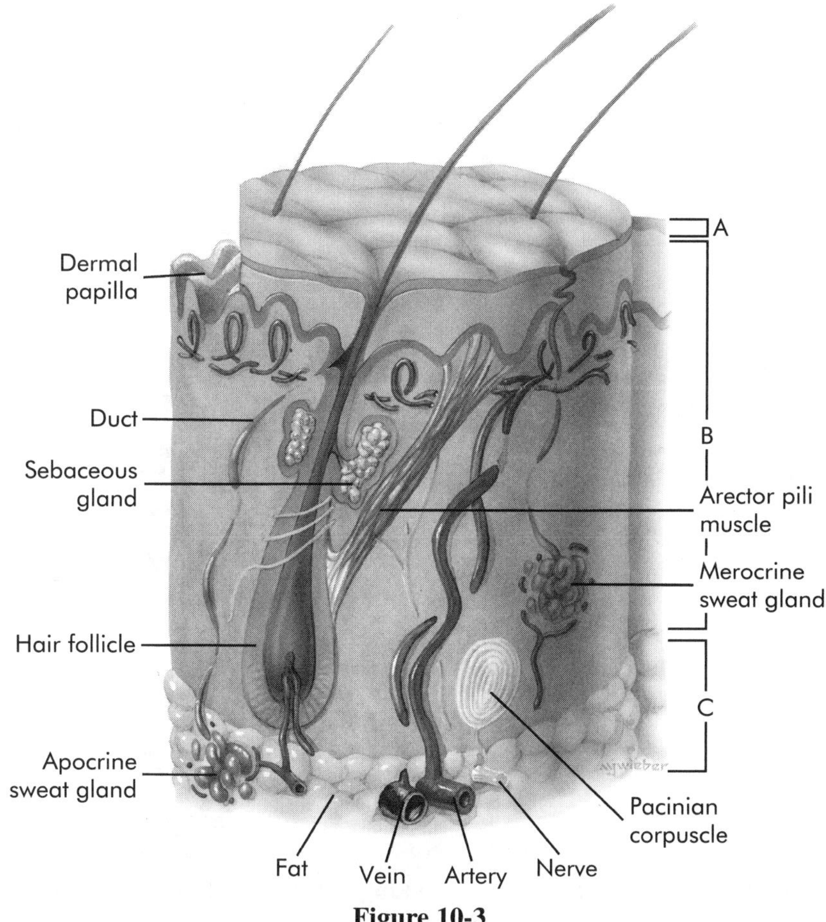

Figure 10-3

23. List three functions of the glands located in the skin.

   a. ____

   b. ____

   c. ____

24. Describe the effect on the skin's function of a large, third-degree (full-thickness) burn that destroys all the layers of the dermis.

____

____

25. Label the bones of the human skull shown in Fig. 10-4.

a. _______________________________   g. _______________________________

b. _______________________________   h. _______________________________

c. _______________________________   i. _______________________________

d. _______________________________   j. _______________________________

e. _______________________________   k. _______________________________

f. _______________________________

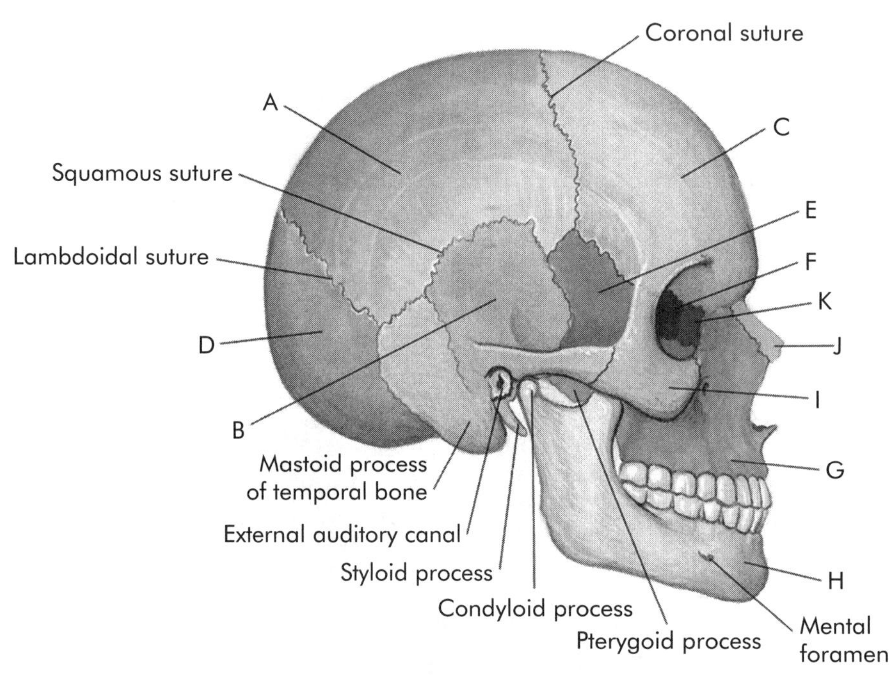

Figure 10-4

26. Label the bony regions of the vertebral column shown in Fig. 10-5 and indicate the number of vertebrae in each region.

Region   **Number of Vertebrae**

a. _______________________________

b. _______________________________

c. _______________________________

d. _______________________________

e. _______________________________

Chapter **10**   **Review of Human Systems**

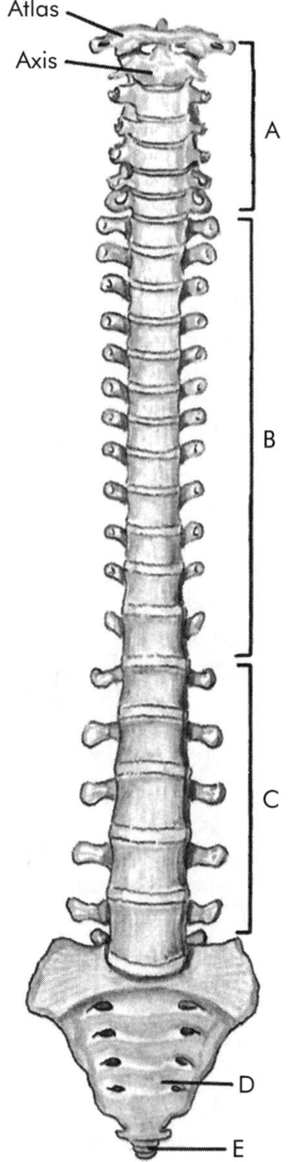

Figure 10-5

27. List two functions of the thoracic cage.

    a. ____

    b. ____

28. Label the structures of the thoracic cage shown in Fig. 10-6.

a. ____

b. ____

c. ____

d. ____

e. ____

f. ____

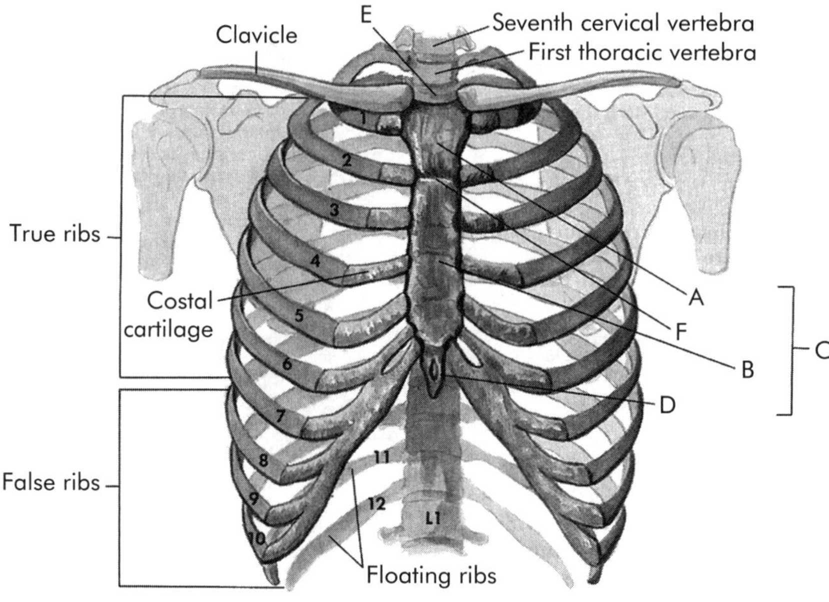

Figure 10-6

29. What problems can occur when a patient sustains a traumatic injury that results in a fractured sternum and multiple fractured ribs?

____

30. Complete the following sentences, which relate to the skeletal system.

The pectoral girdle is composed of the (a) _______________ and (b) _______________. Its function is to

(c) _______________.

The point of attachment of the appendicular and axial skeleton occurs at the (d) _______________ joint.

31. Label the diagram of the upper extremity shown in Fig. 10-7.

a. _______________________________   h. _______________________________

b. _______________________________   i. _______________________________

c. _______________________________   j. _______________________________

d. _______________________________   k. _______________________________

e. _______________________________   l. _______________________________

f. _______________________________   m. _______________________________

g. _______________________________

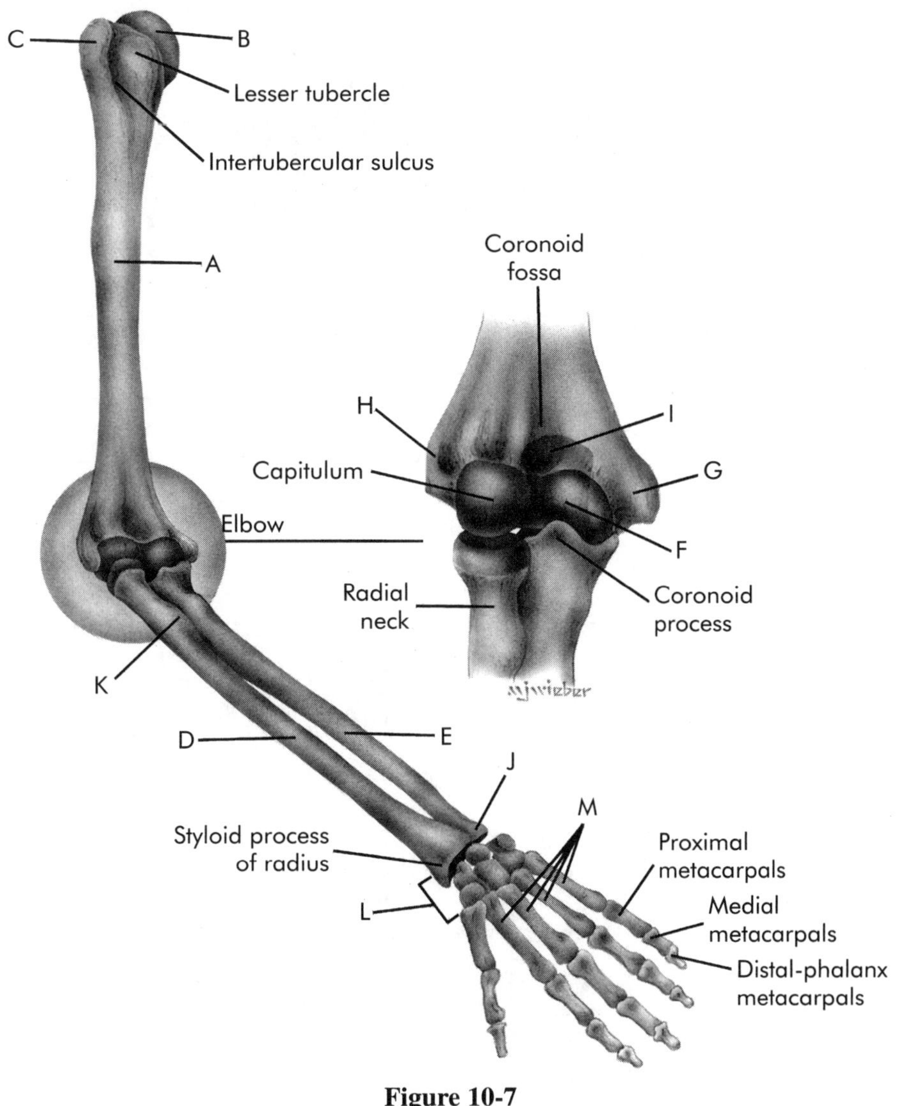

Figure 10-7

32. Label the parts of the pelvic girdle shown in
Fig. 10-8.

a. ___________________________   d. ___________________________

b. ___________________________   e. ___________________________

c. ___________________________

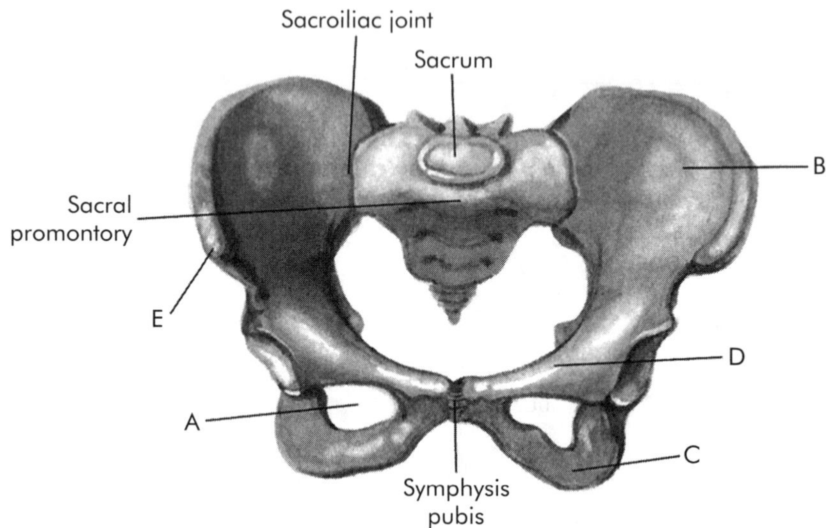

Figure 10-8

33. What are the functions of the pelvic girdle?

____

____

34. Label the bones of the lower extremity shown in
Fig. 10-9.

a. ___________________________   j. ___________________________

b. ___________________________   k. ___________________________

c. ___________________________   l. ___________________________

d. ___________________________   m. ___________________________

e. ___________________________   n. ___________________________

f. ___________________________   o. ___________________________

g. ___________________________   p. ___________________________

h. ___________________________   q. ___________________________

i. ___________________________

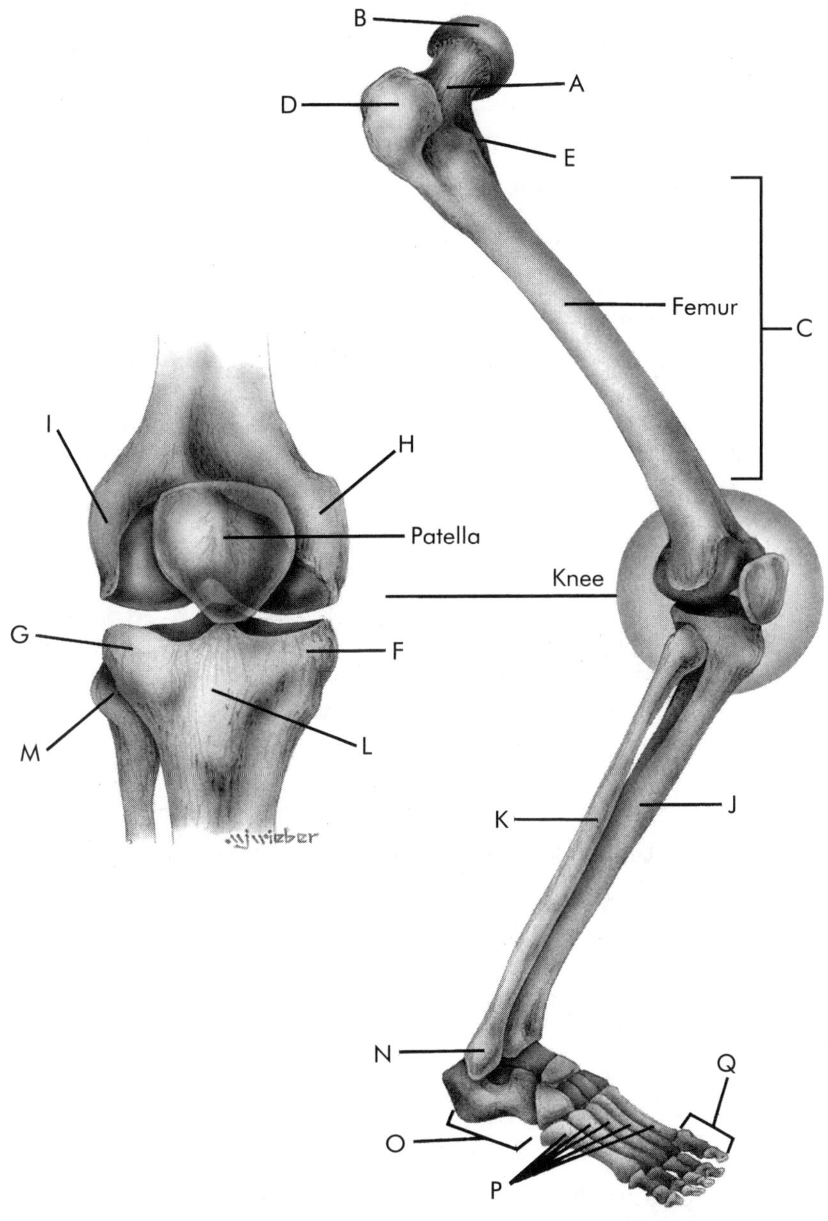

Figure 10-9

35. Complete the blanks in the following statements about joints.

The three major classifications of joints are **(a)** _______________ , _______________ , and _______________.

Fibrous joints have **(b)** _______________ movement. Fibrous joints can be further divided into sutures found

in the **(c)** _______________; syndesmoses found between the **(d)** _______________ and _______________; and

a gomphosis joint, which consists of a peg in a socket, such as the joints between **(e)** _______________ and

_______________. A synchondrosis is a cartilaginous joint that allows only slight movement. One can be found in

the chest between the ribs and the **(f)** _______________. Symphysis joints, another example of cartilaginous joints,

can be found in the chest at the **(g)** _______________ _______________ , in the pelvis at the **(h)** _______________

_______________ , and in the spine at the **(i)** _______________ _______________. Synovial joints are classified

into six divisions, all of which contain **(j)** _______________. Joints consisting of two opposed, flat surfaces, such as the articular processes between vertebrae, are **(k)** ______________ joints. Joints that consist of two saddle-shaped, articulating surfaces that allow movement in two planes (e.g., the carpometacarpal joint in the thumb) are **(l)** ______________ ______________. Joints that consist of a convex cylinder of bone that fits into a corresponding concavity in another bone and permit movement in one plane, such as the elbow and knee, are known as **(m)** ______________ joints. A cylindrical bony process that rotates within a ring composed of bone and ligament, such as the head of the radius where it articulates with the ulna, is a(n) **(n)** ______________ joint. A wide range of motion is permitted by shoulder and hip joints, where the head of one bone fits into the socket of an adjacent bone. These are known as **(o)** ______________ ______________ ______________ joints. The atlantooccipital joint is an example of a modified ball and socket joint known as a(n) **(p)** ______________ joint.

36. Replace the boldface words in the following sentences with the correct terms from the following list. Use each term only once.

Abduction	Excursion	Opposition
Adduction	Extension	Pronation
Depression	Flexion	Rotation
Eversion	Inversion	Supination

   a. The patient has sustained an injury to his elbow and is unable to **rotate his forearm so that the anterior surface is up** or **rotate his forearm so that the anterior surface is down.**

   ____ or

   ____

   b. To determine whether the patient had intact neurologic function, the paramedic had **her move her thumb and little finger toward each other.**

   ____

   c. After he injured his knee, the soccer player had pain when he **bent** and **stretched** out his lower leg.

   ____ and

   ____

   d. An older woman with a hip fracture has a leg that looks shortened and shows **external movement about its axis.**

   ____

   e. A person with a shoulder separation has limited ability to **move the arm from the midline.**

   ____

   f. A patient with a posterior hip dislocation has the following physical findings: the leg is shortened, internally rotated, and slightly **moved toward the midline.**

   ____

   g. Ankle sprains are frequently produced by turning the ankle **inward** or turning it **outward.**

   ____ or

   ____

h. Newer splints for the foot can sometimes make casting unnecessary when the desired effect is to prevent **movement from side to side**.

____

i. The blow to the head with a baseball bat **produced movement of the temporal bone in an inferior direction**.

____

37. List the three primary functions of the muscular system.

a. ____

b. ____

c. ____

38. Complete the following sentences pertaining to the muscular system.

The specialized contractile cells of the muscles are called **(a)** _______________. Each muscle fiber is filled with thick and thin threadlike structures known as **(b)** _______________. These are composed of the proteins **(c)** _______________ and _______________. The contractile unit of skeletal muscle fibers is the **(d)** _______________. During muscle contraction, the two myofilaments slide toward each other and shorten the sarcomere fueled with energy from **(e)** _______________.

39. Define the following terms.

a. Isometric muscle contraction:

____

b. Isotonic muscle contraction:

____

c. Muscle tone:

____

40. Describe the role the muscular system plays in maintaining body temperature.

____

____

41. Briefly describe the function of the nervous system.

____

____

42. List the primary components of the following:

a. Central nervous system:

____

b. Peripheral nervous system:

____

43. List the two subdivisions of the efferent division of the nervous system and briefly describe the function of each.

    a. ____

    b. ____

44. Label the parts of the brain shown in Fig. 10-10.

    a. ________________________________   **e.** ________________________________

    b. ________________________________   **f.** ________________________________

    c. ________________________________   **g.** ________________________________

    d. ________________________________

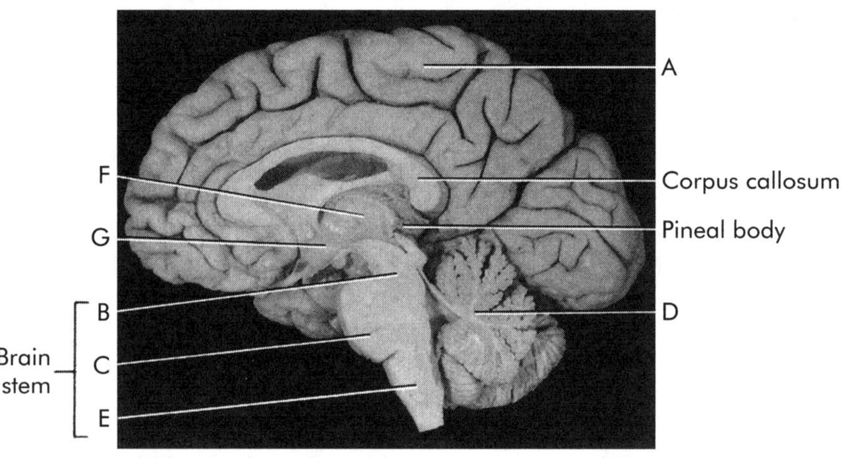

Figure 10-10

45. Briefly describe the functions of each of the following areas of the brain stem.

    a. Medulla:

____

    b. Pons:

____

    c. Midbrain:

____

    d. Reticular formation:

____

106

e. Hypothalamus:

____

f. Thalamus:

____

46. Label the parts of the cerebrum shown in Fig. 10-11 and list one important function of each area.

Area	Function
a.	
b.	
c.	
d.	

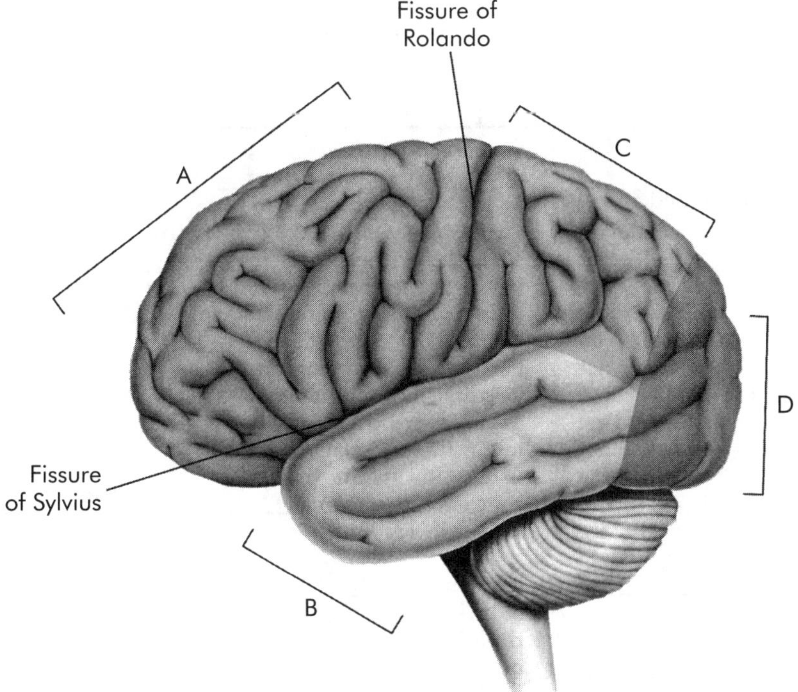

Figure 10-11

47. Briefly describe the major functions of the cerebellum.

____

____

48. List two functions of the spinal cord.

a. ____

b. ____

49. Complete the following sentences about the meninges.

Cerebrospinal fluid bathes and cushions the **(a)** _______________ and _______________. It is formed in a network

of brain capillaries known as the **(b)** _______________.

50. List the three functional categories of the 12 cranial nerves.

a. ____

b. ____

c. ____

51. For each of the following organs or body systems, describe the effects of stimulation by each division of the autonomic nervous system.

Affected Organ	Sympathetic	Parasympathetic
Heart		
Lungs		
Pupils		
Intestine		
Blood vessels		

52. Describe the function of the endocrine system.

____

____

53. For each of the following hormones, list the primary target tissue(s) and one action the hormone may have on the tissue(s).

Hormone	Target	Action
Epinephrine		
Aldosterone		
Antidiuretic hormone		
Parathyroid hormone		
Calcitonin		
Insulin		
Glucagon		
Testosterone		
Thymosin		
Oxytocin		
Thyroid hormone		

54. Describe how hormones reach their target tissues.

____

____

55. List five functions of the circulatory system.

a. ____

b. ____

c. ____

d. ____

e. ____

56. Complete the following sentences regarding the components of blood.

About 95% of the formed elements in blood are red blood cells, also known as **(a)** _______________. The primary component of red blood cells is **(b)** _______________. This gives blood its red color and allows it to transport **(c)** _______________ from the lungs to the tissues and to transport **(d)** _______________ from the tissues to the lungs. The remaining 5% of the formed elements in blood consists of white blood cells, called **(e)** _______________ and platelets, known as **(f)** _______________. The primary function of white blood cells is **(g)** _______________ Platelets help prevent blood loss by activating the formation of **(h)** _______________ to seal off wounds in the blood vessels. The pale yellow fluid that surrounds these formed elements is **(i)** _______________.

57. Label the structures of the heart indicated on Fig. 10-12 and draw arrows to show the path taken by the blood from the point where it enters the heart from the body until it returns to the body from the heart.

a. ____

b. ____

c. ____

d. ____

e. ____

f. ____

g. ____

h. ____

i. ____

j. ____

k. ____

l. ____

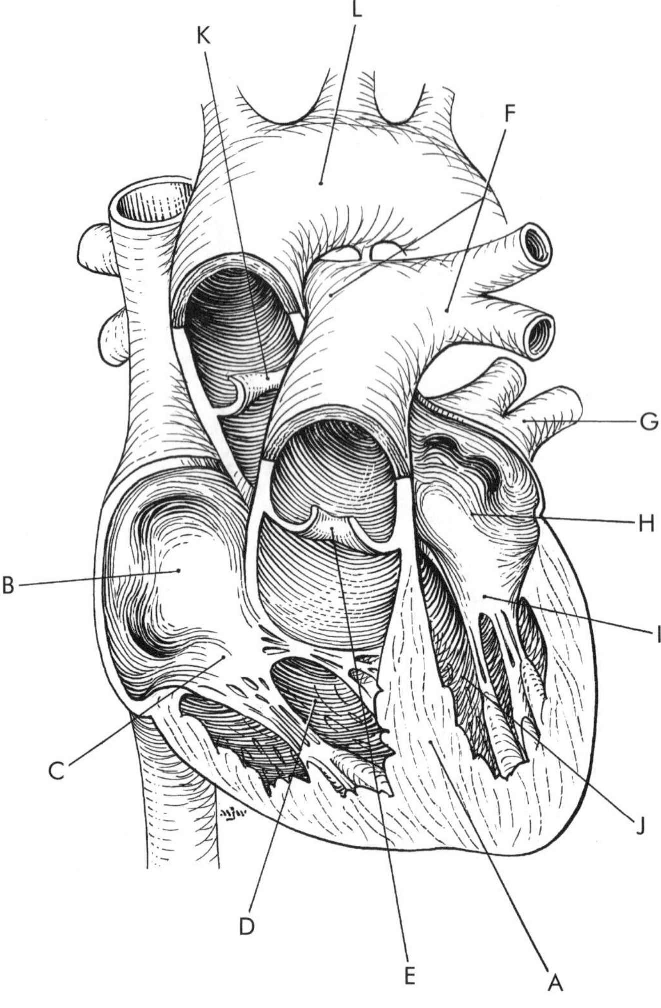

Figure 10-12

58. Name the branches of the circulatory system from the aorta to the cellular level and back to the vena cava.

____

____

59. Briefly describe the characteristics of blood vessels that permit vasodilation and vasoconstriction.

____

____

60. What structural feature of some veins inhibits the back flow of blood?

____

61. What is the purpose of an arteriovenous anastomosis (arteriovenous shunt)?

____

____

110

62. List the three basic functions of the lymphatic system.

a. ____

b. ____

c. ____

63. Describe the flow of lymph from its beginning in the tissues until it empties into the circulatory system.

____

____

64. Label the parts of the upper airway shown in Fig. 10-13 and list one function of each structure.

Structure	Function
a.	
b.	
c.	
d.	
e.	
f.	

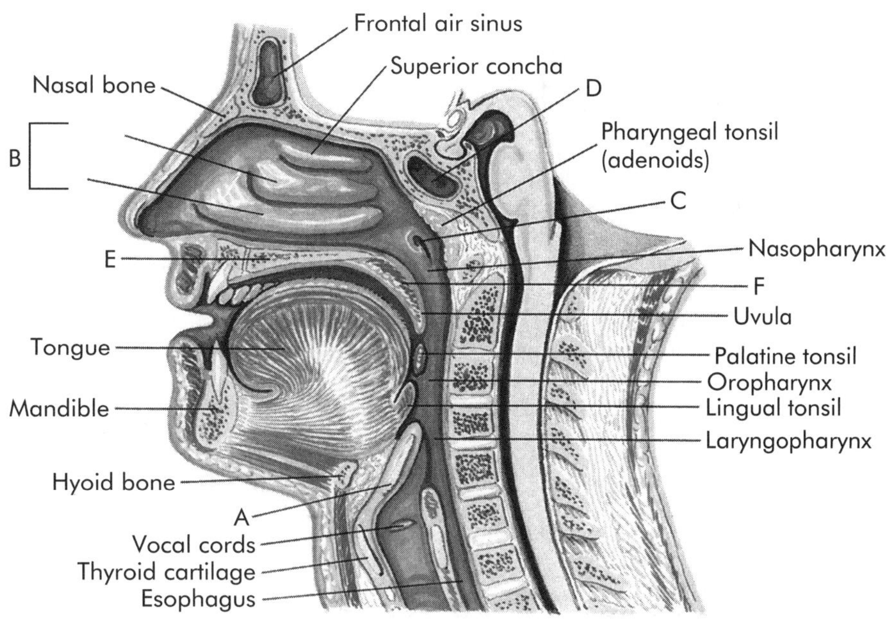

Figure 10-13

65. Label the parts of the larynx shown in Fig. 10-14.

a. _______________________________ d. _______________________________

b. _______________________________ e. _______________________________

c. _______________________________

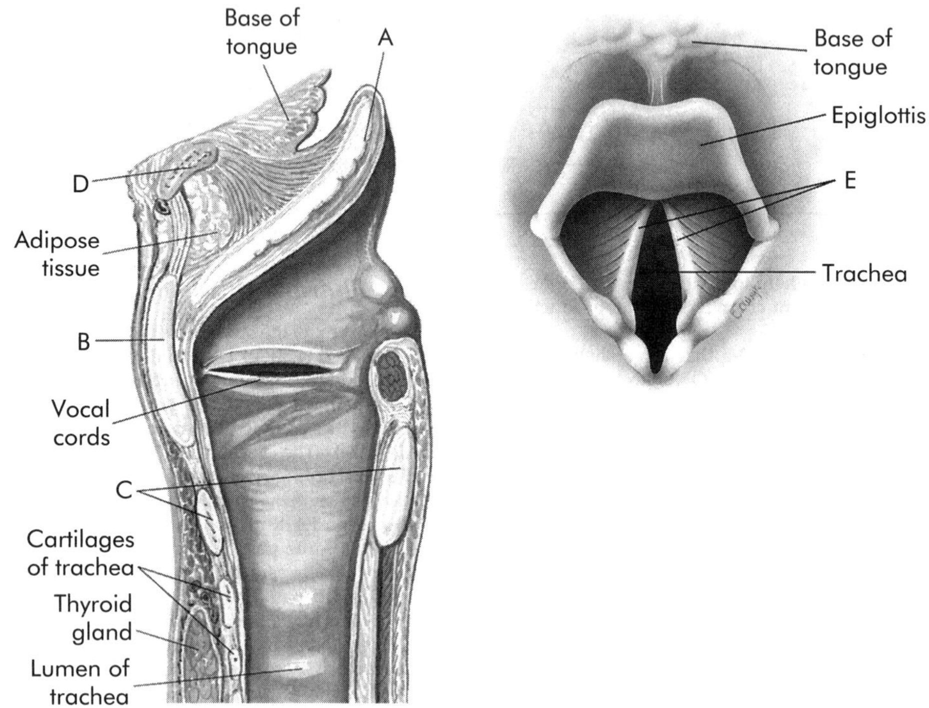

Figure 10-14

66. Label the parts of the lower airway shown in Fig. 10-15.

a. ____

b. ____

c. ____

d. ____

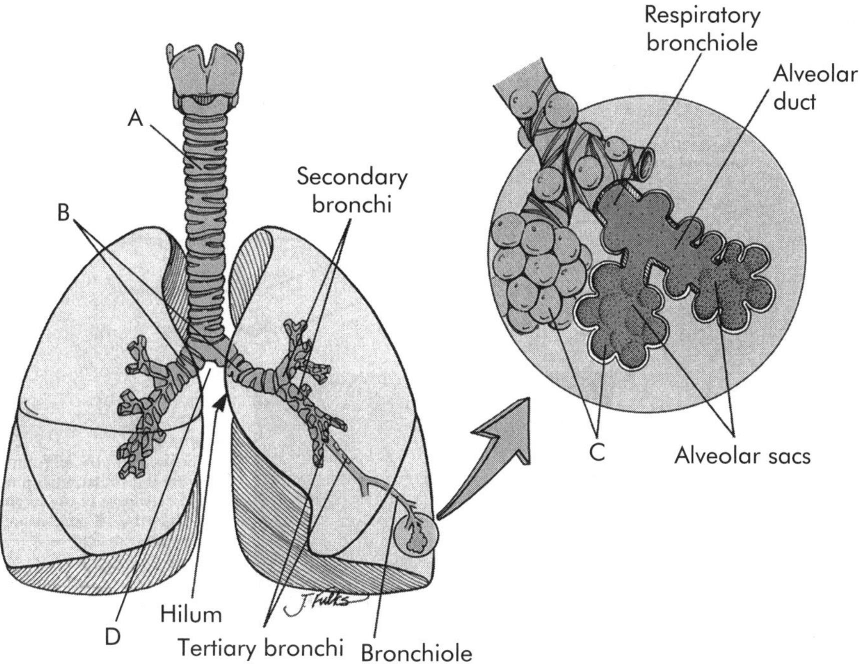

Figure 10-15

67. Describe how the structure of the trachea protects the airway.

____

____

68. Describe what happens to the bronchioles that causes wheezing during an asthma attack.

____

____

69. Describe the anatomical feature of the alveoli that performs the following functions.

    a. Permits the movement of oxygen to the blood and carbon dioxide (CO_2) from the blood:

____

    b. Prevents collapse of the alveoli:

____

70. Describe the location of the lungs in the chest cavity.

____

____

71. List the divisions of the following:

    a. Right lung:

____

    b. Left lung:

____

72. Describe the functions of the following:

    a. Pleural space:

____

    b. Pleural fluid:

____

73. List the functions of the digestive system.

____

74. As a cheeseburger passes through the digestive tract, many digestive juices act on it to convert the food into a usable form for the body. For each area of the digestive tract listed, name a digestive juice excreted and briefly describe its function.

Area	Digestive Juice	Function
Mouth		
Stomach		
Pancreas		
Liver		
Large intestine		

75. List the functions of the urinary system.

____

____

76. List two specific functions of the kidneys in addition to urine production.

    a. ____

    b. ____

77. The basic functional unit of the kidney is the **(a)** _______________. It produces urine by a three-step process:

    (b) _______________, **(c)** _______________ and **(d)** _______________

78. State whether each of the following increases or decreases urine production.

    a. Aldosterone: ____

    b. Atrial natriuretic factor: _______________________________________

    c. Large increase in blood pressure: _______________________________

    d. Shock: ____

79. Label the parts of the male reproductive system shown in Fig. 10-16.

    a. ____________________________   **f.** ____________________________

    b. ____________________________   **g.** ____________________________

    c. ____________________________   **h.** ____________________________

    d. ____________________________   **i.** ____________________________

    e. ____________________________

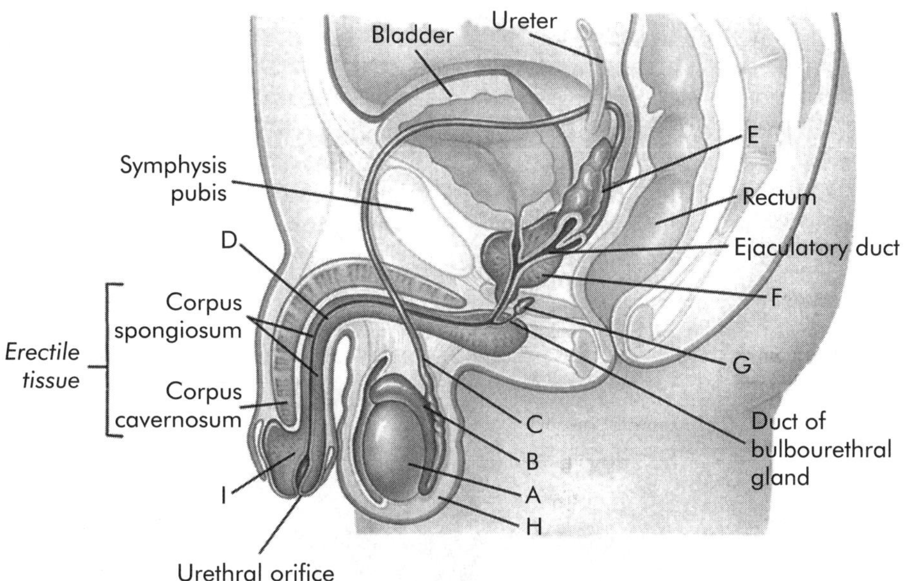

Figure 10-16

80. Label the parts of the female reproductive system shown in Fig. 10-17.

    a. ____________________________   **d.** ____________________________

    b. ____________________________   **e.** ____________________________

    c. ____________________________   **f.** ____________________________

    Chapter **10** **Review of Human Systems**

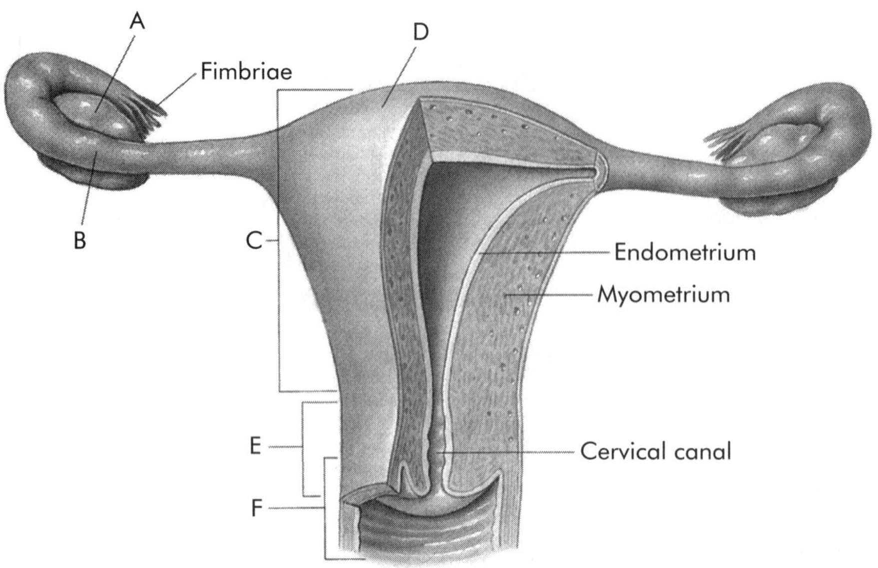

Figure 10-17

81. Label the parts of the female perineum shown in Fig. 10-18.

a. _______________________   e. _______________________

b. _______________________   f. _______________________

c. _______________________   g. _______________________

d. _______________________

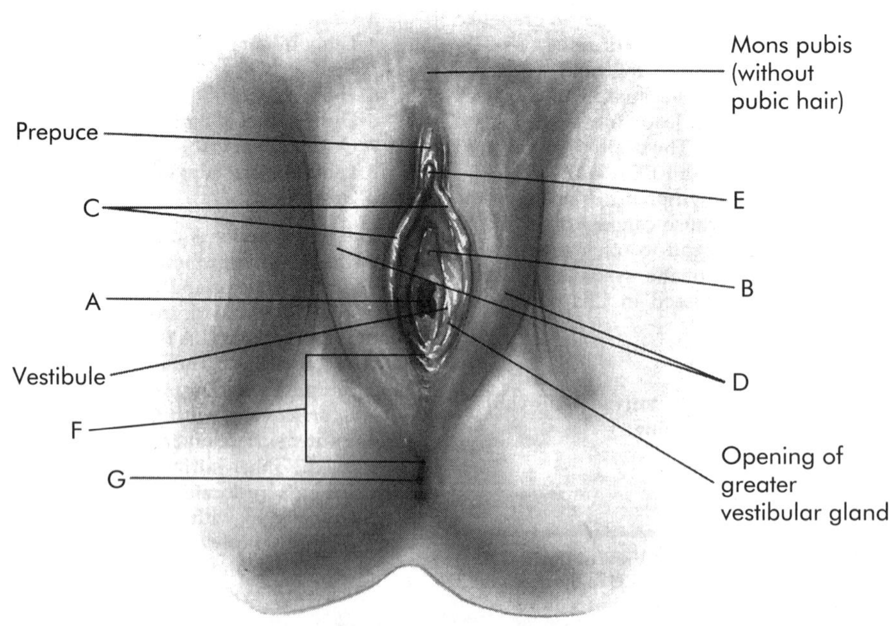

Figure 10-18

Chapter **10**   **Review of Human Systems**

82. Complete the following sentences pertaining to the olfactory sense.

Receptors for the olfactory nerves lie in the upper part of the **(a)** _____________ cavity. When olfactory cells are stimulated by airborne molecules, the nerve impulses travel in the olfactory bulb and **(b)** _____________. The brain interprets the impulses as specific odors in the **(c)** _____________ and **(d)** _____________ centers.

83. Complete the following sentences pertaining to the sense of taste.

Sensory structures that detect taste stimuli in the mouth are **(a)** _____________ _____________. Taste buds are most commonly found in the mouth on the **(b)** _____________. However, they are also found on the **(c)** _____________ , _____________ , and _____________. The four basic tastes that are detected are **(d)** _____________ , _____________ , _____________ , and _____________.

84. Complete the following sentences pertaining to the sense of vision.

The sensation of vision is transmitted from the eye to the brain by way of the **(a)** _____________ nerve.

Impulses that travel from the brain to control the movements of the eye are relayed by the **(b)** _____________ nerve. The avascular, transparent structure that bends and refracts light as it enters the eye is the **(c)** _____________. The size of the pupil and therefore the amount of light that enters the eye through it is controlled by the **(d)** _____________. The inner sensory layer of the retina contains two types of photoreceptor cells. The receptors responsible for night vision are the **(e)** _____________, and the receptors that permit daytime and color vision are the **(f)** _____________. The eye has two compartments. The anterior chamber is filled with **(g)** _____________ humor, and the posterior chamber contains **(h)** _____________ humor. The humor in both chambers helps maintain **(i)** _____________ _____________.

85. List the function of each of the following accessory structures of the eye.

   a. Eyebrows:

   ____

   b. Eyelids:

   ____

   c. Lacrimal glands:

   ____

86. Complete the following sentences pertaining to the tissues associated with hearing and balance.

The external and middle ear are involved in **(a)** _____________, and the inner ear plays a role in **(b)** _____________ and _____________. The senses of hearing and balance are transmitted by the **(c)** _____________ nerve. Sound is picked up by the external ear prominence, known as the **(d)** _____________, and transmitted through the external auditory meatus into the **(e)** _____________ canal. At the end of the canal, vibration of the **(f)** _____________ _____________ is produced. These vibrations are picked up and transmitted to the oval window by the auditory ossicles of the middle ear. These three bones are the **(g)** _____________ , _____________ , and _____________. Finally, in the inner ear inside the cochlea lies the hearing sense organ, called the **(h)** _____________. The two other structures in the inner ear involved in balance are the **(i)** _____________ and **(j)** _____________ _____________.

87. You find your patient lying face up on his back. Which position is this?
   a. Anatomical
   b. Lateral recumbent
   c. Prone
   d. Supine

88. A teenage football player collapsed after a sharp blow to the left upper quadrant of the abdomen. You suspect injury to which of the following?
   a. Appendix
   b. Gallbladder
   c. Liver
   d. Spleen

89. Which of the following structures is located in the mediastinum?
   a. Diaphragm
   b. Lungs
   c. Thyroid
   d. Trachea

90. Cardiac muscle cells are which of the following?
   a. Striated voluntary
   b. Striated involuntary
   c. Nonstriated voluntary
   d. Nonstriated involuntary

91. Which of the following are the actual conducting cells of the nervous system?
   a. Dendrites
   b. Neuroglia
   c. Neurons
   d. Synapses

92. Which of the following is a function of the integumentary system?
   a. Collection of lymph
   b. Movement
   c. Production of vitamin C
   d. Temperature regulation

93. Which structure is comprised of the scapula and clavicle?
   a. Pectoral girdle
   b. Pelvic girdle
   c. Thorax
   d. Vertebral disks

94. An indoor soccer player has sustained an injury resulting in marked swelling and pain at the inner aspect of the ankle. You would describe this to an online physician as pain and swelling in which area?
   a. Lateral malleolus
   b. Medial malleolus
   c. Olecranon
   d. Patella

95. Muscle fiber contractions are initiated when stimulated by which of the following?
   a. Actin and myosin
   b. Motor neurons
   c. Myofilaments
   d. Sarcomeres

96. What is the primary action of the frontal lobe of the cerebral cortex?
   a. Receive and integrate visual input
   b. Evaluate olfactory and auditory input
   c. Receive and interpret sensory information
   d. Initiate voluntary motor function

97. The spinal cord ends at which vertebra?
   a. Twelfth thoracic
   b. Second lumbar
   c. Sacral
   d. Coccygeal

98. What is the innermost meningeal layer (mater), which adheres to the brain and spinal cord?
   a. Arachnoid
   b. Choroid
   c. Dura
   d. Pia

99. Which component of the endocrine system transmits information from the gland to its target body part?
   a. Enzyme
   b. Hormone
   c. Neurotransmitter
   d. Synapse

100. Which formed element in blood contains hemoglobin and carries oxygen?
  a. Erythrocyte
  b. Immunoglobulin
  c. Leukocyte
  d. Platelet

101. Which blood vessel (or vessels) carries blood from the heart to the systemic circulation?
  a. Aorta
  b. Pulmonary arteries
  c. Pulmonary veins
  d. Vena cava

102. Cardiac electrical impulse conduction is normally initiated in which of the following structures?
  a. Atrioventricular node
  b. Bundle of His
  c. Purkinje fibers
  d. Sinoatrial node

103. Lymph nodes filter foreign substances and are located in all the body regions listed below *except* which?
  a. Axillary
  b. Cervical
  c. Inguinal
  d. Temporal

104. Which of the following is the airway division that is involved in the production of speech and that serves as a protective sphincter to prevent liquids and solids from entering the lungs?
  a. Larynx
  b. Retropharynx
  c. Pharynx
  d. Trachea

105. Which of the following is the functional unit of the respiratory system where gas exchange occurs between the lungs and the blood?
  a. Alveolus
  b. Bronchus
  c. Capillary
  d. Trachea

106. What is the major site of nutrient absorption in the intestines?
  a. Colon
  b. Duodenum
  c. Ileum
  d. Jejunum

107. Which of the following is a liver function?
  a. Glucagon production
  b. Drug detoxification
  c. Hormone secretion
  d. Platelet synthesis

108. Which of the following statements is true with regard to renal function?
  a. All fluid filtered from the glomerulus becomes urine.
  b. Healthy people produce 180 L of urine per day.
  c. Water and other nutrients are reabsorbed in the tubules.
  d. Potassium and ammonia are secreted into the blood.

109. Which of the following hormones influences urine production?
  a. Aldosterone
  b. Glucagon
  c. Oxytocin
  d. Testosterone

110. Where does sperm production occur?
  a. Epididymis
  b. Prostate
  c. Seminal vesicle
  d. Testes

111. When the nasal receptors of the olfactory neurons are stimulated, messages are sent for interpretation to the olfactory and ______ centers of the brain.
  a. Frontal
  b. Medullary
  c. Pontine
  d. Thalamic

112. The hearing sense organ is which of the following?
  a. Cochlea
  b. Organ of Corti
  c. Semicircular canal
  d. Vestibule

You are dispatched to a rural emergency department to transfer a patient to the regional trauma center. The nurse gives you the following patient report: The 27-year-old female patient was thrown off her all-terrain vehicle (ATV) and struck a tree. She is lying on her back in full spinal immobilization. She has a laceration on her forehead above her right eyebrow, a fracture of her right forearm, a fracture in her right upper thigh, a pelvic fracture, several rib fractures on the left anterior side of her chest, and possible internal abdominal injuries. The nurse also tells you that the patent's erythrocyte count is low; her urine output is 10 mL/hour, which is draining through the urinary catheter; she has a nasogastric tube because she vomited earlier; and she is receiving high-concentration oxygen because her oxygen saturation level dropped and she was dyspneic. The woman is conscious but slightly confused and can't feel anything below her umbilicus. She is unable to move below her waist but can bend and straighten her arms.

1. Fill in the appropriate anatomical terms to describe this patient.

   She is lying **(a)** ________________ on the long spine board. Her laceration is **(b)** ________________ to her

   eyebrow. Her forearm fracture is **(c)** ________________ to her elbow and could be in one of two long bones, the

   (d) ________________ or ________________. The fracture in her upper thigh is in the **(e)** ________________ , and the

   bones of the pelvis that could be fractured are the **(f)** ________________ , ________________ , ________________ , or

   ________________.

2. What structures lie under the fractured ribs and could also be injured?

   ____

3. List the abdominal organs that could be involved if the patient's injuries are in the following places.

   a. Upper right quadrant: ____

   b. Upper left quadrant: ____

   c. Lower right quadrant: ____

   d. Lower left quadrant: ____

4. What region of the brain lies under her facial injury? ________________________________

5. **a.** What are erythrocytes?

   ____

   b. What is the significance of a low erythrocyte count?

   ____

6. The loss of sensation below her umbilicus signals likely injury to what level of the spinal cord?

   ____

7. **a.** Is she producing too much, too little, or a normal amount of urine?

   ____

   b. What could cause a change in urine output?

   ____

8. The urinary catheter passes through what anatomical structures?

____

9. What medical terms could you substitute for "can bend and straighten her arms"?

____

10. Put a ✓ beside the body systems that are affected in some way by this patient's condition (either directly or by the body's compensatory mechanisms).

_______ Integumentary system	_______ Skeletal system
_______ Muscular system	_______ Nervous system
_______ Endocrine system	_______ Circulatory system
_______ Lymphatic system	_______ Digestive system
_______ Urinary system	_______ Reproductive system
_______ Respiratory system	

CHAPTER 10 ANSWERS

REVIEW QUESTIONS

1. d

2. c

3. f

4. b

5. e

6. h

7. i

8. g
(Questions 1–8: Objective 8)

9. a. centrioles; b. ribosomes; c. Golgi apparatus; d. nucleus; e. endoplasmic reticulum; f. lysosome;
g. mitochondrion
(Objective 8)

10. False. Some cells, such as those of the nervous system, divide only until birth.
(Objective 9)

11. The person is standing erect with palms and feet facing the examiner.
(Objective 2)

12. a. Distal; b. lateral; c. superior; d. ventral
(Objective 3)

13. a. Extremities and their girdles; b. head, neck, thorax, and abdomen
(Objective 4)

14. Horizontally through the umbilicus and vertically from the xiphoid process through the symphysis pubis
(Objective 5)

15. You initially found the patient in the right lateral recumbent position.
(Objective 3)

16. a. Burn (1) is inferior and lateral to the left eye.
b. Burn (2) is inferior to the mouth.
c. Burn (3) is superior and lateral to the right nipple.
d. Burn (4) is on the ventral aspect (or palmar surface) of the hand.
e. Burn (5) is inferior to the axilla.
f. Burns (6) and (7) are on the medial aspect of both thighs.

17. Burn (5) encroaches on the left upper quadrant of the abdomen.
(Objective 5)

18. a. Burn (3) overlies the thoracic cavity.

b. Burn (5) overlies the thoracic and abdominal cavities.

19. The wounds affect both the axial and appendicular regions of the body.
(Objective 4)

20. Conduction of action potentials

Subgroup	Type	Body Area	Function
Striated voluntary tissue	Muscle	Skeletal muscle	Movement of bones
Bone	Connective	Bones of body	Support and protection
Epithelium	Epithelial	Skin, glands	Protection, lining of body cavities
Adipose tissue	Connective	Subcutaneous tissue	Insulation, protection, storage of energy
Hemopoietic tissue	Connective	Marrow cavities, spleen, tonsils	Formation of blood and lymph cells
Striated involuntary tissue	Muscle	Cardiac muscle	Contraction of the heart
Neurons	Nervous	Nervous system	Conduction of action potentials
Cartilage	Connective	Articulating surface	Smooth movement of bones; ear, nose
Areolar tissue	Connective	Around organs, under skin	Cushioning and affixing
Nonstriated involuntary tissue	Muscle	Smooth muscle of viscera	Vegetative muscle functions
Neuroglia	Nervous	Nervous system	Support cells, nourishment, protection, insulation

(Objective 10)

21. Integumentary, skeletal, muscular, nervous, endocrine, circulatory, lymphatic, respiratory, digestive, urinary, and reproductive
(Objective 11)

22. a. Epidermis: barrier against infection, protection, prevention of fluid loss
b. Dermis: sense organ, contains sweat glands
c. Subcutaneous layer: insulation, storage of energy, shock layer, absorption
(Objective 11)

23. Lubrication to prevent drying, excretion of water and wastes, and temperature regulation
(Objective 11)

24. Decreased ability to perceive pain, decreased ability to regulate temperature, and decreased ability to preserve body fluids
(Objective 11)

25. a. Parietal; b. temporal; c. frontal; d. occipital; e. sphenoid; f. ethmoid; g. maxilla; h. mandible; i. zygomatic; j. nasal; k. lacrimal
(Objective 11)

26. a. Cervical spine (7); b. thoracic spine (12); c. lumbar spine (5); d. sacrum (1 fused); e. coccyx (1 fused)
(Objective 11)

27. Protection for the organs of the thorax (and some abdominal organs) and maintenance of lung inflation
(Objective 11)

28. a. Manubrium; b. body; c. sternum; d. xiphoid process; e. jugular notch; f. sternal angle
(Objective 11)

29. Injury to underlying organs, impaired ventilation, and blood loss
(Objective 11)

30. a. Scapula; b. clavicle; c. attach the upper extremity to the axial skeleton; d. sternoclavicular joint
(Objective 11)

31. a. Humerus; b. head; c. greater tubercle; d. radius; e. ulna; f. trochlea; g. medial epicondyle; h. lateral epicondyle; i. olecranon; j. styloid process; k. radial tuberosity; l. carpals; m. metacarpals
(Objective 11)

32. a. Obturator foramen; b. ilium; c. ischium; d. pubis; e. anterior superior iliac spine
(Objective 11)

33. Protection of the pelvic organs and point of attachment for the lower extremity to the axial skeleton
(Objective 11)

34. a. Neck; b. head; c. shaft; d. greater trochanter; e. lesser trochanter; f. medial condyle; g. lateral condyle; h. medial epicondyle; i. lateral epicondyle; j. tibia; k. fibula; l. tibial tuberosity; m. head of fibula; n. lateral malleolus; o. tarsal bones; p. metatarsals; q. phalanges
(Objective 11)

35. a. Fibrous, cartilaginous, synovial; b. little or no; c. skull; d. radius, ulna; e. teeth, mandible (or maxilla); f. sternum; g. sternal angle; h. symphysis pubis; i. intervertebral disks; j. synovial fluid; k. plane (or gliding); l. saddle joints; m. hinge; n. pivot; o. ball and socket; p. ellipsoid
(Objective 11)

36. a. Supinate (supination) or pronate (pronation); b. opposition; c. flexion and extension; d. rotation; e. abduction; f. adduction; g. inversion or eversion; h. excursion; i. depression
(Objective 11)

37. Movement, muscle tone, and heat production
(Objective 11)

38. a. Muscle fibers; b. myofilaments; c. actin, myosin; d. sarcomere; e. adenosine triphosphate (ATP)
(Objective 11)

39. a. Isometric muscle contraction maintains constant length of the muscles in the body. b. During an isotonic
contraction, the amount of muscle tension is constant, but the length of the muscle changes, causing movement of
a body part. c. Muscle tone is the constant tension of muscles responsible for posture and balance.
(Objective 11)

40. Excess energy from adenosine triphosphate in a muscle contraction is released as heat. If the body temperature
falls below a certain level, muscles begin shivering, which can increase heat production up to 18 times the normal
resting level.
(Objective 11)

41. Regulation and coordination of the body to maintain homeostasis
(Objective 11)

42. a. Brain and spinal cord; b. nerves and ganglia
(Objective 11)

43. The somatic division transmits impulses from the central nervous system to skeletal muscle. The autonomic
division transmits impulses from the central nervous system to smooth muscle, cardiac muscle, and certain glands.
(Objective 11)

44. a. Cerebral cortex; b. midbrain; c. pons; d. cerebellum; e. medulla; f. thalamus; g. hypothalamus
(Objective 11)

45. a. Serves as conduction pathway for ascending and descending nerve tracts and regulates heart rate, blood vessel
diameter, breathing, swallowing, vomiting, coughing, and sneezing. b. Ascending and descending nerve tracts
pass through and relay information from cerebrum to cerebellum and sleep and respiratory center. c. Involved
in hearing and visual reflexes and regulates some automatic functions, such as muscle tone. d. Important for
arousal and consciousness and the sleep/wake cycle. e. Temperature regulation, water balance, sleep cycle control,
appetite, sexual arousal. f. Relays information from sense organs to the cerebral cortex and influences mood.
(Objective 11)

46. a. Frontal lobe: voluntary motor function, motivation, aggression, and mood. b. Temporal lobe: olfactory and
auditory input; memory. c. Parietal lobe: reception and evaluation of sensory information (except smell, hearing,
and vision). d. Occipital lobe: reception and integration of visual input.
(Objective 11)

47. Coordination; balance; and smooth, flowing movement
(Objective 11)

48. Reflex center; also transmits impulses to and from the brain and the rest of the body
(Objective 11)

49. a. Brain, spinal cord; b. choroid plexus
(Objective 11)

50. Sensory, somatomotor and proprioception, and parasympathetic
(Objective 11)

51. Affected

Affected Organ	Sympathetic	Parasympathetic
Heart	Increased rate, contractility	Decreased rate and electrical activity contractility conduction speed
Lungs	Bronchodilation	Bronchoconstriction
Pupils	Dilation	Constriction
Intestine	Decreased peristalsis	Increased peristalsis
Blood vessels	Constriction	No effect

(Objective 11)

52. Coordinates with the nervous system to regulate and control multiple body functions, including metabolic activities and body chemistry
(Objective 11)

53.

Hormone	Target Tissue	Action
Epinephrine	Heart, blood vessels, liver, lungs	Increases heart rate, contractility, blood flow to heart and release of glucose and fatty acids into blood
Aldosterone	Kidneys	Regulates water and electrolyte balance
Antidiuretic hormone	Kidneys	Stimulates water retention by kidneys
Parathyroid hormone	Bone, kidney	Increases bone breakdown, helps maintain blood calcium levels
Calcitonin	Bone	Decreases breakdown of bone; maintains blood calcium levels
Insulin	Liver	Promotes glucose entry into cells
Glucagon	Liver	Increases blood glucose by glycogenolysis
Testosterone	Most cells	Produces male sex characteristics, behavior, spermatogenesis
Thymosin	Immune tissues	Promotes development of immune system
Oxytocin	Uterus, mammary gland	Causes uterine contractions, milk expulsion from breasts
Thyroid hormone	Most cells	Increases metabolic rate

(Objective 11)

54. Hormones are secreted into blood and travel to all tissues of the body but act only on the target tissues.
(Objective 11)

55. Transports nutrients, carries hormones, transports wastes, regulates temperature and fluid balance, and provides protection from bacteria
(Objective 11)

56. a. erythrocytes; b. hemoglobin; c. oxygen; d. carbon dioxide; e. leukocytes; f. thrombocytes; g. defense; h. clots; i. plasma
(Objective 11)

57. a. septum; b. right atrium; c. tricuspid valve; d. right ventricle; e. pulmonic valve; f. pulmonary arteries; g. pulmonary veins; h. left atrium; i. mitral or bicuspid valve; j. left ventricle; k. aortic valve; l. aorta
(Objective 11)

Chapter **10** **Review of Human Systems**

58. Aorta, smaller arteries, arterioles, capillaries, venules, veins, venae cavae, and right atrium
(Objective 11)

59. Blood vessels have smooth muscle walls; this allows them to dilate (increasing their diameter) or constrict
(decreasing their diameter). This allows blood flow to be directed away from less vital organs to the heart and
brain during emergencies.
(Objective 11)

60. Many veins, especially in the lower extremities, have valves that prevent the back flow of blood in this low-
pressure system.
(Objective 11)

61. The arteriovenous shunt can selectively allow blood to bypass the capillaries. This is useful to help maintain body
temperature.
(Objective 11)

62. Maintains tissue fluid balance, absorbs fats and other substances from the digestive tract, and enhances the body's
defense system
(Objective 11)

63. Lymph is gathered from the tissues by lymph capillaries that have one-way valves to prevent the back flow of
lymph into tissues. It flows to larger lymph capillaries that resemble veins. Then it passes through the lymph
nodes (in the groin, axilla, and neck), where microorganisms and foreign substances are removed. The lymph
vessels meet to enter the right or left subclavian vein, where the lymph reenters the blood.
(Objective 11)

64. a. Epiglottis: protection of lower airway; b. conchae and turbinates: warming and filtering of air; c. eustachian and
auditory tube: joining of nasopharynx to ear; d. sinuses: production of sound and mucus; e. hard palate: separation
of oropharynx from sinuses; f. soft palate: prevents food from entering nasal cavities.
(Objective 11)

65. a. Epiglottis; b. thyroid cartilage (or Adam's apple); c. cricoid cartilage; d. hyoid bone; e. vocal folds
(Objective 11)

66. a. Trachea; b. bronchi; c. alveoli; d. carina
(Objective 11)

67. Cartilage rings maintain patency of the airway. Goblet cells in the ciliated epithelium of the trachea sweep mucus,
bacteria, and other small particles toward the larynx.
(Objective 11)

68. The small bronchioles are surrounded by smooth muscle. Irritants cause constriction of that muscle, the airway
size decreases, and a wheeze is produced as air is forced through a very tight airway.
(Objective 11)

69. a. Alveoli are only one cell thick, allowing gases to diffuse easily from within them into the pulmonary capillaries.
b. Pulmonary surfactant reduces surface tension in the alveoli, which inhibits collapse of the alveoli.
(Objective 11)

70. The bases of the lungs rest on the diaphragm; the apex extends to a point 2.5 cm superior to the clavicles.
(Objective 11)

71. a. Three lobes, which are further divided into 10 lobules; b. Two lobes, which are further divided into nine lobules
(Objective 11)

72. a. A potential space that forms a vacuum and causes the lung to adhere to the chest wall and remain expanded; b. a lubricant that allows the pleural membranes to slide across one another and that helps the visceral and parietal pleurae to adhere to one another.
(Objective 11)

73. Provides the body with water, nutrients, and electrolytes
(Objective 11)

74.

Area	Digestive Juice	Function
Mouth	Salivary amylase	Begins digestion of carbohydrates
Stomach	Hydrochloric acid, mucus	Produces chyme (intrinsic factor, gastrin, semisolid mixture), pepsinogen
Pancreas	Amylase, sodium bicarbonate	Neutralizes stomach acid, continues digestion
Liver	Bile	Dilutes stomach acid, emulsifies fat
Large intestine	Mucus	Aids movement of feces

(Objective 11)

75. Removes wastes from the body and helps maintain normal body fluid volume and composition
(Objective 11)

76. Control of red blood cell production and vitamin D metabolism
(Objective 11)

77. a. Nephron; b. filtration; c. reabsorption; d. secretion
(Objective 11)

78. a. Decreases; b. increases; c. increases; d. decreases
(Objective 11)

79. a. Testis; b. epididymis; c. ductus deferens and vas deferens; d. urethra; e. seminal vesicles; f. prostate gland; g. bulbourethral glands; h. scrotum; i. penis
(Objective 11)

80. a. Ovary; b. fallopian tube; c. uterine body; d. fundus; e. cervix; f. vagina
(Objective 11)

81. a. Vagina; b. urethra; c. labia minora; d. labia majora; e. clitoris; f. clinical perineum; g. anus
(Objective 11)

82. a. Nasal; b. olfactory tract; c. thalamic; d. olfactory
(Objective 12)

83. a. Taste buds; b. tongue; c. palate, lips, throat; d. sweet, sour, bitter, salt
(Objective 12)

84. a. Optic; b. oculomotor; c. cornea; d. iris; e. rods; f. cones; g. aqueous; h. vitreous; i. intraocular pressure
(Objective 12)

85. a. Shade eyes from direct sun and prevent perspiration from entering eyes; b. protect against foreign objects; c. moisten the eye, lubricate the eyelids, and wash away foreign objects
(Objective 12)

86. a. Hearing; b. hearing, balance; c. vestibulocochlear; d. pinna; e. auditory; f. tympanic membrane; g. incus, stapes, malleus; h. organ of Corti; i. vestibule; j. semicircular canals
(Objective 12)

87. d. The anatomical position is standing erect with the palms forward. A person lying in the lateral recumbent position is reclining on the right or left side. The prone position refers to lying on the stomach. (Objective 2)

88. d. The liver and gallbladder are located in the right upper quadrant, and the appendix is in the right lower quadrant. (Objective 5)

89. d. The lungs are found in the thoracic cavity, and the diaphragm separates the thoracic cavity from the abdominal cavity. The thyroid gland is found in the neck. (Objective 7)

90. b. Striated voluntary muscle is skeletal muscle, and nonstriated involuntary muscles are found in the viscera. Nonstriated muscles are always involuntary. (Objective 10)

91. c. A dendrite is a component of the neuron. Neuroglia are types of nerve cells that support the cells in the nervous system. Synapses are the gaps or spaces between nerve cells or effector tissues. (Objective 10)

92. d. Lymph is collected by the lymphatic system and drains into the circulatory system. Movement is a function of the musculoskeletal system. Vitamin C is ingested by food sources. A form of vitamin D is produced in the skin when exposed to light. (Objective 11)

93. a. (Objective 4)

94. b. The lateral malleolus is on the outside of the ankle, the olecranon is at the elbow, and the patella is over the knee. (Objective 3)

95. b. Actin and myosin are the actual myofilaments (thin, threadlike structures) that pull together to cause movement. A sarcomere is the contractile unit that contains actin and myosin. (Objective 10)

96. d. The other actions described are attributed to the occipital lobe (a), temporal lobe (b), and parietal lobe (c). (Objective 11)

97. b (Objective 11)

98. d. The layers, from innermost to outermost, are the pia, arachnoid, and dura. The choroid plexus is where the cerebrospinal fluid is manufactured. (Objective 11)

99. b (Objective 11)

100. a. Immunoglobulins are antibodies, leukocytes are white blood cells, and platelets are cell fragments that aid in hemostasis. (Objective 11)

101. a. Pulmonary arteries carry deoxygenated blood from the heart to the lungs. Pulmonary veins carry oxygenated blood from the lungs to the heart, and the vena cava carries blood from the systemic circulation to the heart. (Objective 11)

102. d. Sinoatrial node impulses travel to the atrioventricular node, to the bundle of His, and then to the Purkinje fibers.
(Objective 11)

103. d.
(Objective 11)

104. a.
(Objective 11)

105. a. The trachea and bronchus convey air to the alveoli. The capillary is not part of the respiratory system.
(Objective 11)

106. d. Absorption occurs in the other areas of the small intestine (duodenum and ileum) and to a much lesser extent in the colon; however, the primary site of absorption is the jejunum.
(Objective 11)

107. b
(Objective 11)

108. c. Roughly 180 L per day is filtered from the glomerulus; however, all but approximately 2 L of this is reabsorbed into the blood. Potassium and ammonia are secreted from the blood into the urine.
(Objective 11)

109. a. Glucagon promotes conversion of glycogen stored in the liver back to glucose. Oxytocin is a female sex hormone that stimulates uterine contractions and plays a role in lactation. Testosterone is the male sex hormone responsible for male sexual characteristics.
(Objective 11)

110. d. Final maturation (but not production) of sperm occurs in the epididymis. The prostate and seminal vesicle produce seminal fluid.
(Objective 11)

111. d. Thalamic
(Objective 12)

112. b. The organ of Corti lies within the cochlea. The semicircular canals and vestibule are involved in balance.
(Objective 12)

WRAP IT UP

1. a. supine; b. superior; c. distal; d. radius, ulna; e. femur; f. sacrum, pubis, ilium, ischium
(Objectives 2, 3, 11)

2. aorta, lungs, heart, spleen
(Objective 7)

3. a. liver, intestines; b. spleen, stomach, liver, pancreas, intestines; c. intestines; d. intestines
(Objectives 5 through 7)

4. Frontal
(Objective 11)

5. a. red blood cells; b. A drop in the number of red blood cells reduces the blood's ability to carry oxygen to the cells. It is an indication of blood loss.
(Objective 11)

6. Injuries to the lower thoracic or upper lumbar vertebrae can cause these symptoms.
   (Objective 11)

7. a. There is too little urine output. Normal urine output should be approximately 40 to 80 mL/hour (1–L/day).
   b. Urine production could be reduced by increased secretion of aldosterone or antidiuretic hormone (ADH); by a
   drop in arterial blood pressure; or by sympathetic nervous stimulation.
   (Objective 11)

8. The urinary catheter passes through the urethra and into the urinary bladder.
   (Objective 11)

9. Flex and extend
   (Objective 3)

10. Integumentary system (wound above her eye), skeletal system (fractures), muscular system (damage surrounding
    fractures), nervous system (motor and sensory deficit in her lower extremities), endocrine system (hormone
    secretion to limit urine output), lymphatic system (if splenic injury is present), respiratory system (increased
    respiratory rate to compensate for decrease in red blood cells and circulatory shock), digestive system (decreased
    peristalsis), urinary system (decreased urinary output)
    (Objective 11)

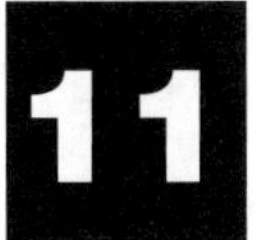 **General Principles of Pathophysiology**

READING ASSIGNMENT

Chapter 11, pages 211-256, in *Mosby's Paramedic Textbook*, ed. 4.

OBJECTIVES

Upon completion of this chapter, the paramedic student will be able to do the following:

1. Describe the normal characteristics of the cellular environment and the key homeostatic mechanisms that strive to maintain an optimal fluid and electrolyte balance.
2. Outline pathophysiological alterations in water and electrolyte balance and list their effects on body functions.
3. Describe the treatment of patients with particular fluid or electrolyte imbalances.
4. Describe the mechanisms in the body that maintain normal acid–base balance.
5. Outline pathophysiological alterations in acid–base balance.
6. Describe the management of a patient with an acid–base imbalance.
7. Describe the changes in cells and tissues that occur with cellular adaptation, injury, neoplasia, aging, or death.
8. Outline the effects of cellular injury on local and systemic body functions.
9. Describe changes in body functions that can occur as a result of genetic and familial disease factors.
10. Outline the causes, adverse systemic effects, and compensatory mechanisms associated with hypoperfusion.
11. Describe the ways in which the inflammatory and immune mechanisms respond to cellular injury or antigenic stimulation.
12. Explain how changes in immune status and the presence of inflammation can adversely affect body functions.
13. Describe the impact of stress on the body's response to illness or injury.
14. Describe factors that influence disease.

SUMMARY

- Two facts illustrate the importance of body water. First, body water is the medium in which all metabolic reactions occur. Second, the precise regulation of the volume and composition of body fluids is essential to health. Water follows osmotic gradients established by changes in sodium concentrations. Thus, sodium and water balance are closely related.
- Two abnormal states of body fluid balance can occur. If the water gained exceeds the water lost, a state of water excess, or overhydration, exists. If the water lost exceeds the water gained, a state of water deficit, or dehydration, exists.
- In addition to fluid imbalances, disturbances in the balance of electrolytes (other than sodium) may occur. These electrolytes include potassium, calcium, and magnesium. Imbalances of these electrolytes can interfere with neuromuscular function. They may even cause cardiac rhythm disturbances.
- The treatment of isotonic dehydration may include volume replacement with isotonic or occasionally hypotonic solutions. The treatment of hypotonic dehydration may involve intravenous (IV) replacement with normal saline or lactated Ringer solution. Occasionally, hypertonic saline (e.g., in seizures caused by hyponatremia) is used. Interventions for overhydration depend on the cause. These interventions may include water restriction; administration of a diuretic; or if hyponatremia is present, administration of saline.
- In-hospital treatment of hypokalemia involves IV or oral potassium replacement. Management of hyperkalemia may involve potassium restriction; enteral administration of a cation exchange resin; or IV administration of glucose and insulin, sodium bicarbonate, or calcium.
- Treatment of hypocalcemia involves IV administration of calcium ions. The management of hypercalcemia may include controlling the underlying disease; hydration; and, occasionally, drug therapy such as with furosemide and other calcium-lowering drugs.
- Hypomagnesemia typically is corrected by the administration of IV magnesium sulfate. The most effective treatment for hypermagnesemia is hemodialysis. Calcium salts that antagonize magnesium may also be given.
- he healthy body is sensitive to changes in the concentration of hydrogen ions (pH). It tries to maintain the pH of extracellular fluid at 7.4. This is accomplished through three interrelated compensatory mechanisms: carbonic acid–bicarbonate buffering, protein buffering, and renal buffering.
- Metabolic acidosis occurs when the amount of acid generated exceeds the body's buffering capacity. The four most common forms of metabolic acidosis encountered in the prehospital setting are lactic acidosis, diabetic ketoacidosis, acidosis resulting from renal failure, and acidosis caused by ingestion of toxins. Treatment for metabolic acidosis is aimed at correcting the underlying cause.

131

- Loss of hydrogen is the initial cause of metabolic alkalosis. This may be caused by vomiting (hydrochloric acid loss), gastric suction, or increased renal excretion of hydrogen ion in the urine. Treatment is directed at correcting the underlying condition. Volume depletion, if present, should be corrected with isotonic solutions.
- Respiratory acidosis is caused by the retention of carbon dioxide. This leads to an increase in the Pco_2. This condition usually is caused by an imbalance in the production of carbon dioxide and its elimination through alveolar ventilation. Treatment for respiratory acidosis involves improving ventilation quickly to eliminate carbon dioxide.
- Hyperventilation may produce respiratory alkalosis by decreasing the Pco_2. Treatment of respiratory alkalosis is directed at correcting the underlying cause of the hyperventilation. An initial approach is to place the patient on low-concentration oxygen. Another is to provide calming measures to assist the patient with slow, controlled breathing.
- An understanding of the processes of disease is crucial. This requires knowledge of the structural and functional reactions of cells and tissues to injurious agents. Changes in cells and tissues can be caused by adaptation, injury, neoplasia, aging, or death.
- An injured cell may have an abnormal physical shape or size. Cell injury has both cellular and systemic indications.
- Certain factors cause disease. For the most part, these factors may be classified as genetic or environmental. However, a strong interaction occurs between the two.
- The term *hypoperfusion* is used to describe inadequate tissue circulation. Hypoperfusion may result from decreased cardiac output. Decreased cardiac output can lead to shock, multiple organ dysfunction syndrome, and other disease states associated with impaired cellular metabolism. Negative feedback mechanisms important in maintaining cardiac output and tissue perfusion are baroreceptor reflexes, chemoreceptor reflexes, the central nervous system ischemia response, hormonal mechanisms, reabsorption of tissue fluids, and splenic discharge of stored blood.
- The external barriers are the body's first line of defense against illness and injury. These barriers include the skin and the mucous membranes of the digestive, respiratory, and gastrointestinal tracts. When these barriers are breached, chemicals, foreign bodies, or microorganisms are allowed to penetrate cells and tissues. Then the second and third lines of defense are activated. These are the inflammatory response and the immune response. Both the external barriers and the inflammatory response respond to all organisms using the identical nonspecific mechanism. The immune response is specific to individual pathogens.
- Immune responses usually are protective. They help to protect the body from harmful microorganisms and other injurious agents. At times these responses may be inappropriate. They may even have undesirable effects. Examples of inappropriate responses include hypersensitivity and immunity or inflammation deficiencies.
- Many immune-related conditions and diseases are associated with stress. However, the exact mechanisms causing these illnesses have not yet been clearly defined. It is believed that the immune, nervous, and endocrine systems communicate through complex pathways and that they may be affected by factions involved in the stress reaction.
- Factors that cause disease are complex. They may involve genetic or environmental factors or a combination of both. Age and gender also influence illness.

REVIEW QUESTIONS

Match the mechanism of cellular injury in column I with the appropriate cause in column II.

Column I

1. _______ Inadequate perfusion of oxygenated blood to an organ

2. _______ Group of proteins that kill or help kill bacteria

3. _______ Presence of air or oxygen

4. _______ Amount of blood returning to the ventricle

5. _______ Total resistance against which blood is pumped

6. _______ Substance that causes an antibody to form

7. _______ Osmotic concentration of a solution

8. _______ Ion with a negative charge

9. _______ Volume of blood ejected from a ventricle with each heart beat

Column II

a. Aerobic
b. Afterload
c. Anaerobic
d. Anion
e. Antigen
f. Complement system
g. Ischemia
h. Osmolality
i. Preload
j. Stroke volume

Match the mechanism of cellular injury in column I with the appropriate cause in column II.

Column I

10. _______ Skin burns resulting from prolonged contact with gasoline

11. _______ Bruising caused by a blow from a tire iron

12. _______ Unconsciousness resulting from a drop in blood sugar

13. _______ Death secondary to septic shock

14. _______ Tissue death in a leg after occlusion of a blood vessel

15. _______ Severe wheezing that develops after a bee sting

Column II

a. Chemical injury
b. Genetic factors
c. Hypoxic injury
d. Immunological injury
e. Infectious injury
f. Nutritional imbalances
g. Physical agents

16. Complete the following sentences, which refer to the fluid compartments of the body.

The water found outside the cells that includes the water in plasma, bone, tendon, and fascia is the

(a) _________________ fluid. The water outside the vascular bed that lies between the tissue cells is known as

(b) _________________ fluid. The fluid found inside the cells of the skeletal muscle, intestine, viscera, bone

marrow, glands, and red blood cells is the **(c)** _________________ fluid.

17. For each of the following ions, state its name, indicate whether it is a cation or an anion and state where it is most plentiful in the body (extracellular fluid [ECF] or intracellular fluid [ICF]).

Ion	Name	Cation or Anion	ECF or ICF
PO_4^-			
K^+			
Na^+			
HCO_3^-			
Mg^{++}			
Cl^-			

18. Briefly define the following terms:

a. Cell membrane permeability:

____

____

b. Diffusion:

____

____

Chapter **11** **General Principles of Pathophysiology**

c. Concentration gradient:

____

____

d. Osmosis:

____

____

e. Active transport:

____

____

f. Facilitated diffusion:

____

____

19. For each of the following patient situations, choose the suspected fluid or electrolyte imbalance from the list provided and describe appropriate assessments, interventions, or both.

a. You are transporting an older patient for chest pain. After an intravenous (IV) line has been inserted, 500 mL is accidentally infused rapidly. The patient becomes very short of breath, and evaluation reveals moist crackles in the lungs.

Imbalance: Hyponatremia, hypermagnesemia, or overhydration?

____

Management:

____

____

b. Your patient is a 65-year-old adult who complains of vomiting and diarrhea. Home medications include a diuretic. The physical examination reveals a blood pressure of 100/70 mm Hg, a weak pulse, decreased reflexes, and shallow respirations.

Imbalance: Hyperkalemia, hypocalcemia, or hypokalemia?

____

Management:

____

____

c. You are called to the airport to evaluate an obviously malnourished child flown to the United States from India for adoption. The chaperone reports that the child has shown abnormal behavior and complains of muscle cramps, abdominal cramps, and tingling of the extremities. As you begin to assess the vital signs, the patient has a grand mal seizure.

Imbalance: Hypernatremia, hypocalcemia, or hypomagnesemia?

____

Management:

____

____

d. A father calls you to evaluate an infant who has been vomiting for 36 hours. The father states that the child has not had a wet diaper in 8 hours. The anterior fontanelle is depressed, and the skin and mucous membranes are dry.

Imbalance: Hypercalcemia, hypermagnesemia, or isotonic dehydration?

____

Management:

____

____

e. Your patient is a 13-year-old bulimic girl who admits to frequent use of water enemas for weight control. You were called for a chief complaint of abdominal pain; however, on arrival, you find the patient diaphoretic with a rapid, thready pulse and cyanosis. There is no indication of bleeding.

Imbalance: Hyperkalemia, hyponatremic dehydration, or overhydration?

____

Management:

____

f. The family of an older patient with chronic renal failure says that she is confused and very weak. The physical examination reveals shallow, slow respirations that become progressively worse.

Imbalance: Hypermagnesemia, hypocalcemia, or hypokalemia?

____

Management:

____

____

20. Describe the mode of action of the three acid–base buffer systems in the body. Begin with the fastest mechanism and end with the slowest one.

a. ____

b. ____

c. ____

d. ____

21. For each case presented, indicate which one of the four acid–base disturbances listed below is the cause. State at least one prehospital intervention for management of the imbalance.

Respiratory acidosis   Respiratory alkalosis

Metabolic acidosis   Metabolic alkalosis

a. A 17-year-old student complains of dizziness and tingling in the hands and around the mouth during a college entrance examination. The medical history and physical examination are unremarkable. The respiratory rate is 28 breaths/min and deep.

Imbalance: ____

Intervention: ____

b. A 72-year-old resident of an extended care facility has been treated with gastric suction.

Imbalance: ____

Intervention: ____

c. A 30-year-old diabetic woman has had influenza. She has taken no insulin in 2 days and appears dehydrated. Respirations are deep and rapid.

Imbalance: ____

Intervention: ____

d. A 46-year-old patient who took an overdose of a barbiturate has shallow respirations at a rate of 8 breaths/min.

Imbalance: ____

Intervention: ____

22. The following arterial blood gas values were obtained in a patient who had had a stroke. State whether each is normal or abnormal. Discuss any action that may be taken in the field to correct any abnormalities identified.

a. pH: 7.25   Normal/Abnormal

Actions: _________________________

b. Po_2: 60 mm Hg   Normal/Abnormal

Actions: _________________________

c. Pco_2: 53 mm Hg   Normal/Abnormal

Actions: _________________________

23. For each of the following cellular adaptations, give the cause, the effect on the cell, and an example.

Adaptation	Cause	Effect on Cell	Example
Atrophy			
Dysplasia			
Hyperplasia			
Hypertrophy			
Metaplasia			

24. For each of the following situations, explain why cardiac output will increase or decrease in an otherwise healthy individual.

a. The patient has had a myocardial infarction with necrosis of 50% of the heart muscle.

____

____

b. A dehydrated patient is given 500 mL of normal saline intravenously.

____

____

c. The patient's normal heart rate is 80 and suddenly drops to 40.

____

____

d. A paramedic student enters a testing station.

____

____

25. Describe the physiological effects of the baroreceptor response to compensate in each of the following situations.

a. A 47-year-old adult has a sudden increase in blood pressure to 170/110 mm Hg.

____

____

b. A 22-year-old adult is thrown from a horse and sustains a pelvic fracture. The paramedic's findings are significant internal bleeding and a sudden drop in blood pressure to 60 mm Hg systolic by palpation.

____

____

26. Describe the physiological effects of chemoreceptor stimulation in the following situations.

   a. A 36-year-old adult has a massive hemothorax from a gunshot wound. Blood pressure is 76/60 mm Hg.

   ____

   ____

   b. A 17-year-old patient who took a drug overdose has a shallow respiratory rate of 8 breaths/min. Arterial blood gas tests reveal a Pco_2 of 60 mm Hg

   ____

   ____

27. A 47-year-old man who had a large inferior myocardial infarction has progressively deteriorated. He is now unconscious and has a weak carotid pulse and no obtainable blood pressure. Describe the physiological effects that ensue when the central nervous system ischemia response is initiated.

____

____

28. A 65-year-old alcoholic man states that he had a sudden onset of vomiting. The emesis contains bright red blood, and he continues to vomit. Vital signs are blood pressure, 94/78 mm Hg; pulse, 132 beats/min (bpm); and respirations, 28 breaths/min. Describe the effects of the following three hormonal mechanisms, which will be activated.

   a. Adrenal medullary mechanism

   ____

   ____

   b. Renin-angiotensin-aldosterone mechanism

   ____

   ____

   c. Vasopressin mechanism

   ____

   ____

29. Multiple organ dysfunction syndrome (MODS) begins with **(a)** ______________ _____________ damage caused by **(b)** _____________ and _____________, which are released into the circulation. This causes the vascular **(c)** _____________ to become **(d)** _____________, which allows fluid and cells to leak into the **(e)** _____________ spaces, increasing **(f)** _____________ and _____________. Three plasma enzyme cascades are then activated. They are **(g)** _____________, _____________, and _____________/_____________. Phagocytes cause further damage to the endothelium, causing uncontrolled **(h)** _____________ and the formation of microvascular **(i)** _____________ and tissue ischemia. Bradykinin contributes to low **(j)** _____________ _____________ _____________. The overall effect of the three complement systems is **(k)** _____________ formation, **(l)** _______________, and **(m)** _______________ _______________. Initially, the body compensates for these changes, but ultimately tissue hypoxia causes **(n)** _______________ _______________, _______________ _______________. Finally, multiple **(o)** _______________ failure occurs.

30. Your partner is off sick with a diagnosis of strep throat. Describe whether the following signs and symptoms experienced during this illness are local or systemic and give at least one inflammatory mechanism that causes the sign or symptom.

Sign or Symptom	Local or Systemic Response	Cause
Edematous throat		
Purulent drainage		
Fever		
Red throat		
Difficulty swallowing		

31. For the following patient blood types, list all safe donor types.

Blood Type	Donors
a. A positive	
b. O negative	
c. AB positive	
d. B negative	

32. For each statement below, note which one of three types of altered immunological reaction has occurred: allergy, autoimmunity, or isoimmunity.

a. Your patient is agitated and complains of severe low back pain a few moments after you begin to transfuse a unit of blood. _______________

b. You are dispatched to a private residence to care for a 46-year-old woman who began to experience dyspnea, a swollen face, and hives after taking a penicillin tablet prescribed by her dentist. _______________

c. You are transferring a patient to a dialysis center for care after his body rejected his kidney transplant. _______________

d. You notice that your eyes water and get puffy and your hands become very red and itchy when you wear Latex gloves at work. _______________

e. Your patient, a 30-year-old woman, is having chest pain. The family tells you she has systemic lupus erythematosus with cardiac and pulmonary involvement. _______________

Chapter **11** **General Principles of Pathophysiology**

Match the probable cause of immune suppression in column II with the statement in column I.

Column I

33. _______ An elderly woman develops pneumonia several months after the death of her husband.

34. _______ A cancer patient becomes septic after a course of chemotherapy.

35. _______ A young girl with anorexia nervosa repeatedly becomes ill with viral illness.

36. _______ A patient infected with the human immunodeficiency virus (HIV) develops Kaposi sarcoma.

Column II

a. Acquired immune deficiency
b. Deficiencies caused by stress
c. Deficiencies caused by trauma
d. Iatrogenic deficiencies
e. Nutritional deficiencies

37. Fill in the missing information relating to the stress response.

Hormone or Receptor	Location	Action
a.	Found in plasma	Stimulates gluconeogenesis; suppresses inflammation
Alpha$_1$-receptors	Postsynaptic located on effector organs	b.
Beta$_1$-receptors	c.	Increased pulse rate
d.	Lungs and arteries	Bronchodilation

38. For each of the following diseases, list a factor that may contribute to its development. Identify whether the factor is environmental or genetic.

Disease	Factor	Environmental or Genetic
Stroke		
Cervical cancer		
Oral cancer		
Melanoma (skin cancer)		
Depression		

39. Which mechanism of cellular transport moves substances against a concentration gradient and requires the use of energy?
  a. Active transport
  b. Diffusion
  c. Facilitated diffusion
  d. Osmosis

40. Which of the following electrolytes is found predominantly in the intracellular fluid?
  a. Bicarbonate
  b. Chloride
  c. Potassium
  d. Sodium

41. Which type of solution has a concentration of solute particles equal to that inside the cells?
  a. Atonic
  b. Hypertonic
  c. Hypotonic
  d. Isotonic

42. Which of the following causes the normal flow of fluid through the interstitial space?

  a. Capillary hydrostatic pressure filters fluid from the interstitial space through the capillary wall.
  b. Oncotic pressure exerted by blood proteins attracts fluid from the vascular space back into the interstitial space.
  c. Capillary permeability determines the ease with which fluid can pass through the capillary wall.
  d. The lymphatic channels close to prevent entry of capillary fluid pushed out by hydrostatic pressure.

43. Your patient is being transferred from a nursing home to a hospital for admission for an intestinal obstruction. His skin is dry, and his tongue has furrows. What fluid and electrolyte imbalance do you suspect?
  a. Hypernatremic dehydration
  b. Hyponatremic dehydration
  c. Isotonic dehydration
  d. Osmotic dehydration

44. You are called to transport a 56-year-old patient with a history of renal failure who missed his last dialysis session. He complains of nausea, abdominal distension, weakness, and irritability. Which of the following do you suspect?
  a. Hypercalcemia
  b. Hyperkalemia
  c. Hypernatremia
  d. Hyperuria

45. Which of the following is true regarding hypomagnesemia?
  a. It is often accompanied by hypercalcemia.
  b. It results from antacid abuse.
  c. It causes hypoactive reflexes.
  d. It causes cardiac dysrhythmias.

46. Your patient has metabolic acidosis. Which of the following compensatory mechanisms uses proteins in an attempt to rapidly restore normal acid–base balance?
  a. Carbonic acid–bicarbonate buffering
  b. Excretion of hydrogen ions to acidify the urine
  c. Exhalation of excess carbon dioxide
  d. Recovery of bicarbonate in the renal tubules

47. Which acid–base disturbance would you anticipate in a patient with severe flail chest?
  a. Metabolic acidosis
  b. Metabolic alkalosis
  c. Respiratory acidosis
  d. Respiratory alkalosis

48. Lactic acidosis is harmful to the body because it
  a. Increases the basal metabolic rate
  b. Decreases the force of cardiac contraction
  c. Increases the response to catecholamines
  d. Can cause severe hypertension

49. Increasing the rate of ventilations for a patient with metabolic acidosis and inadequate stroke volume typically causes which of the following?
  a. Decreased pH and decreased Pco_2
  b. Decreased pH and increased Pco_2
  c. Increased pH and decreased Pco_2
  d. Increased pH and increased Pco_2

     Chapter **11** **General Principles of Pathophysiology**

50. Which cellular change, which may occur with aging, results in shrinkage of the brain and may cause a delay in the signs and symptoms associated with subdural hematoma (blood clot on the brain)?
    a. Atrophy
    b. Dysplasia
    c. Metaplasia
    d. Hypertrophy

51. What is the process of cellular self-destruction known as?
    a. Autolysis
    c. MODS
    b. Necrosis
    d. Osmosis

52. Which of the following changes would be expected early after cellular injury?
    a. Accelerated cellular reproduction
    b. Decreased intracellular hydrostatic pressure
    c. Increased intracellular oxygen accumulation
    d. Swelling of cells from increased osmosis

53. Sympathetic vasoconstriction during shock results in which of the following?
    a. Tachycardia
    b. Pupil dilation
    c. Increased container size
    d. Pale, cool skin

54. What triggers activation of the central nervous system ischemic response?
    a. Blood pressure falls below 90 mm Hg systolic.
    b. Aortic and carotid chemoreceptors are stimulated.
    c. Bradycardia and vasodilation are present.
    d. Blood flow decreases in the vasomotor center.

55. Which of the following hormonal mechanisms increases urine production?
    a. Adrenal medullary mechanism
    b. Atrial natriuretic mechanism
    c. Renin–angiotension–aldosterone mechanism
    d. Vasopressin mechanism

56. An elderly patient calls 9-1-1 complaining of chest discomfort and difficulty breathing. Electrocardiographic changes on arrival at the hospital are consistent with acute myocardial infarction. The patient is showing signs of hypoperfusion. What type of shock does this likely represent?
    a. Anaphylactic
    b. Cardiogenic
    c. Hypovolemic
    d. Septic

57. Which of the following situations represents natural immunity in a fellow paramedic?
    a. Immunity to feline leukemia virus
    b. Immunity to measles after immunization
    c. Immunity to chicken pox after having them
    d. Immunity to hepatitis after immunoglobulin administration

58. Which of the following is true regarding hypersensitivity?
    a. It occurs only when the body encounters foreign antigens.
    b. The response always occurs immediately after exposure to the antigen.
    c. It may produce either minor or life-threatening consequences.
    d. It is a normal immune response resulting from exposure to an antigen.

59. Which hormone increases the level of blood glucose and acts as an immunosuppressant by reducing the number of selected leukocytes?
    a. Cortisol
    b. Dopamine
    c. Epinephrine
    d. Norepinephrine

You are dispatched to an industrial accident where people are trapped. When you arrive, the incident commander tells you a floor collapsed during erection of a high-rise building. A worker is trapped under the rubble, and the rescue squad is attempting to free him. The commander allows one person to approach the scene. You ask your partner to set up the ambulance and then meet you with a stretcher as close as he can approach the scene. You take the long spine board, immobilization supplies, an airway kit, and your primary resuscitation bag and move carefully toward the patient. He is conscious but very pale and complains of a burning pain in his lower extremities. The extrication is dangerous; with every piece of debris removed, the entire pile becomes more unstable. It is 4 hours before the patient is released. You immobilize him and quickly move him to the ambulance. His skin is pale and cool, he is breathing rapidly, and he has a puncture wound of unknown depth over his right upper abdomen. His lower extremities are gray and pale, but no crepitus or deformity is noted. His vital signs are BP, 80/56 mm Hg; P, 136/min; R, 32/min; and an oxygen saturation (Sao_2) that won't register a reading. The monitor shows a sinus tachycardia with tall-tented T waves. You administer oxygen by non-rebreather mask at 15 L/min, initiate two large-bore IVs and infuse them at a rapid rate, and quickly begin transport to the trauma center.

1. What fluid should be started on this patient? Explain your answer.
   a. D_5W
   b. D_5NS
   c. LRS
   d. NS

   Explanation:

   ____

   ____

2. a. If the electrocardiographic (ECG) change indicates excessive amounts of potassium in the blood, what additional signs or symptoms might this patient experience?

   ____

   b. What could explain this patient's hyperkalemia?
      (1) Abdominal puncture releases potassium into the blood.
      (2) Crushed cells release potassium into the blood.
      (3) Lack of oxygen related to shock causes the release of potassium.
      (4) Potassium production is stimulated during hypoperfusion.

3. What acid–base imbalance will this patient most likely experience? Explain your answer.
   a. Metabolic acidosis
   b. Metabolic alkalosis
   c. Respiratory acidosis
   d. Respiratory alkalosis

   Explanation:

   ____

   ____

4. How will the body attempt to compensate for this acid–base imbalance?

   ____

   ____

  Chapter **11** **General Principles of Pathophysiology**

5. For each of the following compensatory mechanisms used by the body during shock, put a on the line if the mechanism directly increases heart rate or contractility, put an X if it acts directly on the blood vessels to cause constriction, and put an M if it conserves body water.

_________ Parasympathetic stimulation   _________ Sympathetic stimulation

_________ Adrenal medullary mechanism   _________ Renin–angiotensin–aldosterone mechanism

_________ Vasopressin mechanism   _________ Tissue fluid reabsorption

_________ Splenic discharge of blood

6. What stage of shock does this patient's signs and symptoms appear to indicate?
   a. Compensated
   b. Multiple organ dysfunction syndrome
   c. Terminal
   d. Uncompensated

CHAPTER 11 ANSWERS

REVIEW QUESTIONS

1. g
   (Objective 10)

2. f
   (Objective 11)

3. a
   (Objective 5)

4. i
   (Objective 10)

5. b
   (Objective 10)

6. c
   (Objective 11)

7. h
   (Objective 1)

8. d
   (Objective 5)

9. j
   (Objective 10)

10. a

11. g

12. f

13. e

14. c

144

15. d

(Questions 10–15: Objective 7)

16. (a) Extracellular; (b) interstitial; (c) intracellular

(Objective 1)

17. PO_4^-: phosphate, anion, intracellular; K^+: potassium, cation, intracellular; Na^+: sodium, cation, extracellular; HCO_3^-: bicarbonate, anion, extracellular; Mg^{++} magnesium, cation, intracellular; Cl^-: chloride, anion, extracellular

(Objective 1)

18. a. The property of a cell membrane that freely permits the passage of water but selectively allows the passage of solute particles. This permits the cell to maintain a relatively constant internal environment. b. A passive process that allows molecules or ions to move from an area of higher concentration to an area of lower concentration in an attempt to achieve a state of equilibrium. c. A situation in which the solute concentration is greater at one point than another in a solvent. Solutes diffuse from the area of higher concentration to the area of lower concentration until equilibrium is achieved. d. The diffusion of water across a selectively permeable membrane from an area of higher water concentration to an area of lower water concentration. e. A rapid, carrier-mediated process that can move a substance across a selectively permeable membrane from an area of low concentration to an area of high concentration. This process requires energy. f. A carrier-mediated process (faster than diffusion) that can move a substance from an area of higher concentration to an area of lower concentration. This process does not require energy.

(Objective 1)

19. a. Overhydration; fluid restriction, normal saline given intravenously to keep the vein open

  b. Hypokalemia; lactated Ringer solution given intravenously to keep the vein open, preparation to assist ventilations, and high-flow oxygen. In-hospital treatment may include oral or IV potassium

  c. Hypocalcemia; possibly calcium ions (calcium chloride) given intravenously, airway management, seizure precautions, IV anticonvulsant therapy

  d. Isotonic dehydration; evaluation of airway, breathing, and circulation; assessment for shock; IV therapy with an isotonic solution

  e. Hyponatremic dehydration; evaluation of the effectiveness of ventilations, high-flow oxygen, IV therapy with lactated Ringer solution or normal saline, and evaluation of vital signs. Occasionally, hypertonic saline may be administered

  f. Hypermagnesemia; open airway, assistance with ventilations as necessary, high-flow oxygen, evaluation of vital signs, IV line with normal saline, furosemide 1 mg/kg if dialysis is not available, and possibly IV calcium salts. The most effective treatment is hemodialysis.

(Objective 2)

20. a. Buffers produce an immediate response to changes in the hydrogen ion concentration (pH). They represent the body's ability to adjust the concentration of bicarbonate and carbon dioxide in the blood to maintain a relationship of 1 mEq of carbonic acid to 20 mEq of base bicarbonate. If this relationship is maintained, the pH stays within normal limits.

  b. The respiratory system can increase alveolar ventilation within minutes in response to an increase in the hydrogen ion concentration. Hydrogen ions combine with bicarbonate to form carbonic acid, which in turn breaks down into carbon dioxide and water. Therefore, by increasing the amount of carbon dioxide the body eliminates, the process can be accelerated and the hydrogen ion concentration reduced.

  c. The renal system takes hours to days to act. It restores normal pH by reabsorbing or excreting bicarbonate or hydrogen ions.

(Objective 4)

21. a. Respiratory alkalosis; treat the cause of underlying hyperventilation.

  b. Metabolic alkalosis; initiate IV administration of lactated Ringer solution or normal saline.

  c. Metabolic acidosis; initiate IV administration of normal saline.

  d. Respiratory acidosis; assist ventilations.

(Objectives 5, 6)

22. a. Abnormal; for acidosis caused by an increase in the Pco_2, increase ventilations.
    b. Abnormal; increase oxygen delivery to the patient.
    c. Abnormal; increase rate of ventilations.
(Objective 6)

23.

Adaptation	Cause	Effect on Cell	Example
Atrophy	Diminished function, inadequate hormonal or nervous stimulation, reduced blood supply	Decrease or shrinkage in cellular size	Shrinkage of muscle size in a casted limb or from neuromuscular disease; brain atrophy in old age
Dysplasia	Chronic irritation or inflammation	Abnormal changes in mature cells	Precancerous changes of the cervix or lungs
Hyperplasia	Response to an increase in demand	Increase in the number of cells in a tissue or organ	Cellular or endometrial hyperplasia
Hypertrophy	Increased demand for work by a cell	Increase in the size (but not number) of cells	Large muscles of a body builder or enlarged hear or kidneys
Metaplasia	Cellular adaptation to adverse conditions	Conversion or replacement of normal cells by other cells	Bronchial metaplasia secondary to cigarette smoke

(Objective 7)

24. a. Muscle is lost, so contractility and stroke volume decrease, lowering cardiac output.
    b. The additional fluid volume improves preload, thereby increasing stroke volume and cardiac output.
    c. A sudden drop in the heart rate results in a decrease in cardiac output.
    d. Fear and anxiety cause a rise in heart rate and stroke volume, which in turn increases cardiac output.
(Objective 10)

25. a. The vasoconstrictor center of the medulla is inhibited, and the vagal center is excited, resulting in peripheral vasodilation and a decrease in heart rate and the strength of contraction. This results in a decrease in blood pressure.
    b. Vagal stimulation is reduced, resulting in a sympathetic response that causes an increase in peripheral vasoconstriction and in the heart rate and strength of contraction. This results in an increase in blood pressure.
(Objective 10)

26. a. The low pressure results in a decrease in oxygen to the chemoreceptor cells; this in turn stimulates the vasomotor center of the medulla, resulting in peripheral vasoconstriction.
    b. Chemoreceptors are also stimulated by an increase in the Pco_2, which causes vasoconstriction and an increase in blood flow to the lungs, enhancing their ability to eliminate carbon dioxide.
(Objective 10)

27. The central nervous system ischemic response is initiated when blood pressure drops below 50 mm Hg; it triggers intense vasoconstriction in an attempt to improve perfusion to the brain. If the ischemia lasts longer than 10 minutes, the vagal center may be activated, resulting in peripheral vasodilation and bradycardia.
(Objective 10)

28. a. Increased sympathetic stimulation causes the adrenal medulla to release epinephrine and norepinephrine, which results in an increase in heart rate, stroke volume, and vasoconstriction.
    b. Low flow to the kidneys results in a release of renin, which by a series of chemical reactions causes plasma proteins to synthesize angiotensin II. Angiotensin II causes vasoconstriction and initiates the release of aldosterone. Aldosterone causes increased retention of sodium and water by the kidneys.
    c. The hypothalamic neurons are stimulated by a drop in blood pressure or an increase in plasma solutes, and the secretion of antidiuretic hormone (vasopressin) is increased. This results in vasoconstriction and a decreased rate of urine production.
(Objective 10)

146

29. (a) vascular endothelial
   (b) endotoxins, inflammatory mediators
   (c) endothelium
   (d) permeable
   (e) interstitial
   (f) hypotension, hypoperfusion
   (g) complement, coagulation, kallikrein/kinin
   (h) coagulation
   (i) thrombus
   (j) systemic vascular resistance
   (k) edema
   (l) cardiovascular instability
   (m) clotting abnormalities
   (n) cellular acidosis, impaired cellular function
   (o) organ
   (Objective 10)

30.

Sign or Symptom	Local or Systemic Response	Cause
Edematous throat	Local	Cellular accumulation of sodium causes edema. Also, hyperemia increases filtration pressure and capillary permeability, causing fluid to leak into interstitial spaces
Purulent drainage	Local	Bacteria are destroyed by phagocytosis. Then macrophages clear and destroy tissues of dead cells. Destruction of leukocytes is initiated by phagocytosis. Dead tissues plus dead leukocytes plus fluid that leaks into the area form pus.
Fever	Systemic	Mast cell degranulation and an increase in the metabolic rate caused by the inflammatory process
Red throat	Local	Dilation of arterioles, venules, and capillaries in the area of cellular injury
Difficulty swallowing	Local	A consequence of the edema described above

(Objective 11)

31. a. O positive, O negative, A positive, A negative; b. O negative; c. O positive, O negative, A positive, A negative, B positive, B negative, AB positive; AB negative; d. O negative, B negative
   (Objective 11)

32. a. Isoimmunity. The body is reacting to beneficial foreign cells.
   b. Allergy. The body is responding to the introduction of a foreign protein (antigen) that it recognizes as harmful.
   c. Isoimmunity. The body rejects helpful foreign tissue that it sees as harmful.
   d. Allergy. The body may be reacting to the protein (antigen) in the Latex.
   e. Autoimmunity. It is thought that systemic lupus erythematosus and other diseases such as dermatomyositis, periarteritis nodosa, scleroderma, and rheumatoid arthritis may be caused by an autoimmune response.
   (Objective 12)

33. b. Prolonged emotional or psychological stress can result in physical illness.

34. d. Patients undergoing chemotherapy or radiation therapy for cancer may experience significant suppression of the immune system.

     Chapter **11** **General Principles of Pathophysiology**

35. e. Severe deficits in calorie or protein intake can seriously impair the immune system.

36. a. The human immunodeficiency virus (HIV) attacks the immune system, making the body easy prey for opportunistic infections and malignancies.
(Questions 33–36: Objective 10)

37. a. Cortisol
b. Vasoconstriction
c. Heart
d. Beta-2 receptors

38.

Disease	Factor	Environmental or Genetic
Stroke	Hypertension, high cholesterol, smoking	Environmental
Cervical cancer	Infection with gonorrhea	Environmental
Oral cancer	Chewing smokeless tobacco	Environmental
Melanoma (skin cancer)	Excessive exposure to sun Familial tendency	Environmental Genetic
Depression	Metabolic disturbance, drug reaction, nutritional disorder, situational crisis	Environmental

(Objective 14)

STUDENT SELF-ASSESSMENT

39. a. Diffusion is a passive process involving the movement of molecules from an area of high concentration to an area of lower concentration. Facilitated diffusion uses a carrier molecule to move molecules rapidly down a concentration gradient. Osmosis is a process that causes the movement of fluid from an area of low solute concentration to an area of high solute concentration.
(Objective 1)

40. c. All others are found chiefly in the extracellular fluid.
(Objective 1)

41. d. Atonic means without tone. A hypertonic solution has a greater solute concentration than that inside the cells; a hypotonic solution is less concentrated than that inside the cells.
(Objective 1)

42. c. Capillary hydrostatic pressure filters fluid from the blood through the capillary wall. Oncotic pressure exerted by blood plasma proteins attracts fluid from the interstitial space into the blood. The lymph channels open and collect some of the fluid forced out of the capillaries by hydrostatic pressure and return it to the circulation.
(Objective 2)

43. c. Hypernatremic dehydration is associated with an intake of sodium that exceeds sodium losses. Hyponatremic dehydration typically manifests with cramps, seizures, a rapid, thready pulse, diaphoresis, or cyanosis. There is no such classification as osmotic dehydration.
(Objective 3)

44. b. A patient in renal failure is frequently hypocalcemic, not hypercalcemic.
(Objective 2)

45. d

(Objective 2)

46. c. Both hydrogen and carbon dioxide bind to hemoglobin, which carries them to the lungs for exhalation.

(Objective 4)

47. c. Ventilation (caused by a reduced tidal volume) is frequently severely decreased in these patients. This inhibits the excretion of carbon dioxide from the lungs, causing an increase in carbonic acid and a decrease in the pH.

(Objective 5)

48. b. Lactic acid reduces the peripheral response to catecholamines and can cause severe hypotension.

(Objective 5)

49. c. A decreased pH and increased Pco_2 are signs of respiratory acidosis. An increased pH and decreased Pco_2 are signs of respiratory alkalosis. An increased pH and increased Pco_2 are signs of metabolic alkalosis.

(Objective 6)

50. a. The decrease in cell size that occurs secondary to atrophy of brain cells causes the brain to shrink in size. Dysplasia is an abnormal change in a mature cell. Metaplasia is the substitution of one cell type for another. Hypertrophy is an increase in cell size that results in an increase in organ size.

(Objective 7)

51. a. MODS is the progressive failure of two or more organ systems secondary to severe illness or injury. Necrosis refers to the cellular changes that occur after local cell death. Osmosis is the movement of water across a semipermeable membrane.

(Objective 7)

52. d. Sodium rushes into the injured cells, increasing the osmotic pressure, which draws more water into the cell.

(Objective 8)

53. d. Tachycardia and pupil dilation are sympathetic responses but do not occur secondary to vasoconstriction. The container size should decrease because of vasoconstriction.

(Objective 10)

54. d. When blood flow to the vasomotor center of the medulla is reduced to the point of ischemia, this response initiates profound vasoconstriction.

(Objective 10)

55. b. All other mechanisms decrease urinary output to conserve blood volume.

(Objective 10)

56. b. If sufficient cardiac muscle is destroyed in myocardial infarction, the stroke volume and therefore cardiac output can be markedly decreased. Anaphylactic shock occurs secondary to exposure of a sensitized individual to an allergen, resulting in dyspnea, wheezing, shock, urticaria, erythema, angioedema, and other dramatic signs and symptoms. Septic shock occurs secondary to a bacterial infection that releases harmful endotoxins.

(Objective 10)

57. a. Feline leukemia virus is a disease to which humans have a natural immunity. Acquired immunity occurs after immunization for measles and after having chicken pox (for most patients). Temporary acquired immunity is conferred if hepatitis B immunoglobulin is administered, but vaccination is needed to ensure acquired long-term immunity.

(Objective 11)

58. c. Hypersensitivity can occur secondary to foreign antigens (allergy, isoimmune reactions) or, in the case of autoimmunity, when the body attacks its own tissues. The response may be immediate or delayed up to several days. Hypersensitivity represents an abnormal immune response.

(Objective 12)

59. a. Dopamine exerts effects on the blood vessels. It causes renal and mesenteric dilation at low levels, beta effects at midrange levels, and strong alpha stimulation at high levels. Epinephrine stimulates alpha and beta cells, causing an increase in the heart rate and contractility and in bronchiolar dilation; it also increases blood glucose by glycogenolysis. It does not suppress white blood cells, as cortisol does. Norepinephrine exerts effects similar to those of epinephrine; however, its alpha effects predominate.
(Objective 13)

WRAP IT UP

1. d. Normal saline (NS) is an isotonic fluid that remains in the intravascular space, available for the heart to pump longer than either of the fluids containing dextrose (D_5W, D_5NS). Lactated Ringer solution (LRS) contains potassium, which would not be indicated in this patient.
(Objective 3)

2. a. Cardiac conduction disturbances, irritability, abdominal distension, nausea, diarrhea, oliguria, weakness, or paralysis
(Objective 3)

b. (2). Intracellular potassium levels are very high. When cells break open, such as during an extensive crush injury or electrical injury, large amounts of potassium are released into the blood.
(Objective 3)

3. a. The prolonged crush forces causes anaerobic metabolism in the affected areas. This creates an accumulation of lactic acid in the tissues that is released into the general circulation when the patient is freed. In addition, the presence of systemic hypoperfusion creates anaerobic metabolism in some tissues, resulting in the production of lactic acid.
(Objective 5)

4. The respiratory rate will increase, the kidneys will excrete hydrogen ions, and the carbonic acid–bicarbonate buffering system will try to compensate for the metabolic acidosis.
(Objective 4)

5. Parasympathetic stimulation: None
Sympathetic stimulation: Increases heart rate and contractility, constricts blood vessels
Adrenal medullary mechanism: Increases heart rate and contractility, constricts blood vessels
Renin–angiotensin–aldosterone mechanism: Constricts blood vessels, conserves body water
Vasopressin mechanism: Constricts blood vessels, conserves body water
Tissue fluid reabsorption: Moves fluid from interstitial to intravascular space (doesn't conserve it)
Splenic discharge of blood: Releases blood from spleen (doesn't conserve it) (Objective 10)

6. d. The blood pressure is low; therefore, the compensatory mechanisms are no longer sufficient to resolve the patient's hypoperfusion.
(Objective 10)

12 Life Span Development

READING ASSIGNMENT

Chapter 12, pages 257-274, in *Mosby's Paramedic Textbook,* ed. 4.

OBJECTIVES

Upon completion of this chapter, the paramedic student will be able to do the following:

1. Describe the normal vital signs and body system characteristics of the newborn, neonate, infant, toddler, preschooler, school-aged child, adolescent, young adult, middle-aged adult, and older adult.
2. Identify the psychosocial features of the infant, toddler, preschooler, school-aged child, adolescent, young adult, middle-aged adult, and older adult.
3. Explain the effect of parenting styles, sibling rivalry, peer relationships, and other factors on a child's psychosocial development.
4. Discuss the physical and emotional challenges faced by the older adult.

SUMMARY

- A newborn is a baby in the first hours of life. A neonate is a baby younger than 28 days. An infant is a child 28 days to 1 year of age.
- A newborn normally weighs 3 to 3.5 kg (7–8 pounds). This weight typically triples in 9 to 12 months. The infant's head accounts for about 25% of the total body weight.
- At birth, structures unique to fetal circulation constrict and normally close within the first year of life. Fluid is expelled from the lungs during the first few breaths. Respiratory muscles and alveoli are not fully developed.
- Infants are born with protective reflexes related to breathing, eating, and stress or discomfort.
- At birth, the anterior and posterior fontanels are open. Bone growth occurs at the epiphysis of the bones.
- Some passive immunity is conferred at birth and through the mother's breast milk.
- The caregiver is the major factor in the infant's psychosocial development.
- Temperament is a person's behavioral style. It is the way the person interacts with the environment.
- Toddlers are children 1 to 3 years of age. Preschoolers are 3 to 5 years of age.
- The hemoglobin level in toddlers and preschoolers approaches that of adults. The brain in this age group is about 90% of the adult brain weight. Muscle mass and bone density increase. Walking occurs by age 2 years, and fine motor skills develop. Control of bowel and bladder are achieved.
- Parenting styles can be described as authoritarian, authoritative, or permissive.
- Sibling rivalry, peer relationships, divorce, and exposure to aggression and violence affect a child's development.
- School-aged children range from 6 to 12 years of age. Physical growth slows, but brain function and the ability to learn quickly develop in this age group. Many children reach puberty during this time. Self-esteem and moral development are critical at this age.
- Adolescents are 13 to 19 years of age. The growth of bone and muscle mass is nearly complete in this age group. Reproductive maturity has been reached. Adolescence often involves some emotional turmoil, and antisocial behavior may be seen.
- Early adulthood spans the period from 20 to 40 years of age. Lifelong habits and routines develop. Body systems are at their optimal performance.
- Middle adulthood extends from 41 to 60 years of age. The physiological aspects of aging become more apparent in this age group. Menopause in women occurs during this stage.
- People reach late adulthood at 61 years of age. Body system changes vary widely from person to person, but the systemic changes of aging become apparent. Some adults in this age group face financial, physical, and emotional challenges.

Match the age range in Column I with the appropriate age in Column II.

Column I

1. _________ Infant

2. _________ Neonate

3. _________ Newborn

4. _________ Preschool

5. _________ School age

6. _________ Toddler

Column II

a. First few hours of life
b. Younger than 28 days
c. 28 days to 1 year
d. 1 to 3 years
e. 3 to 5 years
f. 6 to 12 years

Match the reflex in Column II with the appropriate description in Column I.

Column I

7. _________ Head turns toward facial stimulation.

8. _________ Lips pucker when mouth contacts nipple.

9. _________ Toes spread up and out when sole stroked.

10. _________ Mouth opens if palm is pressed when supine.

11. _________ Infant stretches and then hugs self after loud noise.

Column II

a. Babinski
b. Babkin
c. Moro
d. Palmar grasp
e. Rooting
f. Stepping
g. Sucking

Circle toddler (1 to 3 years) or preschooler (3 to 5 years) to indicate the most common age that children achieve the following social milestones.

12. Can state name of friend   Toddler or Preschooler

13. Speech is understandable to strangers   Toddler or Preschooler

14. Follows directions   Toddler or Preschooler

15. Shows sympathy when appropriate   Toddler or Preschooler

16. Points to a named part of the body   Toddler or Preschooler

17. Fill in the blanks related to the physiological changes associated with late adulthood.

Blood pressure rises as blood vessels **(a)** _________________, **(b)** _______________ resistance increases, and **(c)** _________________ sensitivity decreases. Blood flow to organs **(d)** _________________.

Increased workload on the heart causes **(e)** _________________, changes in the mitral and aortic **(f)** _________________, and decreased **(g)** _________________ elasticity. The number of pacemaker cells in the heart **(h)** _____________, resulting in **(i)** _________________. Blood volume, red blood cells, and platelet count **(j)** _________________. Lung function and lung capacity **(k)** _______________.

Pain **(l)** _______________ and reaction **(m)** _________________ decrease. Secretion of **(n)** _________________ and gastric juices decreases. Intestinal sphincters lose **(o)** _________________. About 50% of the nephrons in the **(p)** _________________ are lost.

18. List two causes of each of the following stressors that affect the older adult's lifestyle.

   a. Financial burdens:

____

____

b. Physical and emotional challenges:

____

____

19. A heart rate of 140 beats/min at rest would be considered normal for what age range?
   a. Newborn
   b. Preschool
   c. School age
   d. Toddler

20. Which of the following physiological changes occurs at birth?
   a. The ductus venosus dilates.
   b. Pulmonary vascular resistance decreases.
   c. Right ventricular pressure increases.
   d. Systemic vascular resistance decreases.

21. Which is true regarding the infant's respiratory system?
   a. Bones are the primary chest support.
   b. Body heat and fluids can be lost through respirations.
   c. The number of alveoli is close to that of adults.
   d. Tracheal bifurcation occurs lower than that of adults.

22. Which is a protective survival reflex in the infant?
   a. Babinski's
   b. Moro
   c. Palmar grasp
   d. Rooting

23. For which type of temperament might low intensity of reactions and a negative mood be observed?
   a. Difficult
   b. Easy
   c. Slow to warm up
   d. Temperamental

24. Which statement is true regarding toddlers?
   a. Hemoglobin approaches adult levels.
   b. Ear, nose, and throat structures are similar to those in adolescents.
   c. Passive immunity protects children of this age.
   d. Visual acuity averages 20/20.

25. Which parenting style tends to produce children who are responsible, assertive, and self-reliant?
   a. Authoritarian
   b. Authoritative
   c. Permissive
   d. Traditional

26. Which is true regarding the development of peer relationships in the toddler or preschool age group? They are formed with others _______________________.
   a. At the same age level
   b. Of same school age
   c. Who are adult caregivers
   d. Younger than they are

27. Which is true regarding school-age children?
  a. Growth rates are faster than in toddlers.
  b. Lymphatic tissue is small relative to adults.
  c. Primary tooth growth is beginning.
  d. Skull growth is 95% complete.

28. Conventional reasoning is a stage in which phase of the psychosocial development of a child?
  a. Moral
  b. Peer relationships
  c. Self-concept
  d. Self-esteem

29. What stimulates the release of hormones that initiate the physical changes of puberty in girls?
  a. Gonadotropin
  b. Follicle-stimulating hormone
  c. Luteinizing hormone
  d. Progesterone

30. Which is true regarding psychosocial issues in teenagers?
  a. Anorexia nervosa is a depressive disorder seen in this age group.
  b. Appearance is not a major concern for teens.
  c. Suicide is the leading cause of death in gay and lesbian teens.
  d. Depression rarely is seen in this age group.

31. On which developmental issue do early adults often focus?
  a. Losing weight
  b. Health concerns
  c. Retirement planning
  d. Selecting a mate

32. Which health-related concern is common in middle-aged adults?
  a. Dementia
  b. Diverticulitis
  c. Hypercholesterolemia
  d. Stroke

WRAP IT UP

You find yourself in a difficult situation. You are the only paramedic on the rescue squad at the scene of a fire at a home day care and have been assigned to care for a group of children until the next ambulances arrives; estimated time of arrival (ETA) is 20 to 30 minutes. The caregiver, a 60-year-old woman, and one child sustained significant smoke inhalation and are being rushed to the hospital. You are left with four children: a 5-week-old infant, a 13-month-old boy, a 3-year-old girl, and a 5-year-old girl. The baby is sleeping quietly, and the other children are upset and crying. You obtain the following vital signs with the help of another firefighter:

5-week-old infant: BP 78/60 mm Hg, P 124/min, R 28/min, SaO_2 99%
13 month-old boy: BP 80/64 mm Hg, P 120/min, R 28/min, SaO_2 100%
3-year-old girl: BP 94/66 mm Hg, P 112/min, R 24/min, SaO_2 98%
5-year-old girl: BP 96/68 mm Hg, P 104/min, R 20/min, SaO_2 98%

The 5-week-old infant is pink with a 1-second capillary refill and is using the abdominal muscles to breathe. You can feel a soft diamond-shaped depression at the top of his skull that appears to pulsate with each heartbeat. When he awakens, he turns his face toward you, and he tries to suck when you stroke his cheek, but he does not cry or seem upset.

The 13-month-old boy wants nothing to do with you. He screams when you approach him and tries to run but falls, striking his head on the corner of the bench on which you are seated. His abdomen is protruding, and you note that he has a wet diaper.

The 3-year-old girl is calm by the time you try to examine her. She asks what happened to her caregiver, "Mo-Mo," and you explain that there was a fire and the smoke made her sick.

154

The 5-year-old girl is trying to be helpful, watching the younger children. She denies feeling sick or hurt and wants her parents to come. You explain that you will call them to come and get her as quickly as they can, but it may take a few minutes.

You continue to monitor the children until the ambulance arrives.

1. Place a check mark beside the age groups for which you were responsible on this call.

   a. _________ Newborn   **d.** _________ Toddler

   b. _________ Neonate   **e.** _________ Preschooler

   c. _________ Infant   **f.** _________ School age

2. Identify the abnormal findings that you encountered in each of the following children:

   a. 5-week-old infant

   ____

   ____

   b. 13-month-old boy

   ____

   ____

   c. 3-year-old girl

   ____

   ____

   d. 5-year-old girl

   ____

   ____

3. Which of the following is true regarding the 5-week-old infant's behavior?
   a. He should have cried when he awoke and did not recognize you.
   b. He should be able to track your finger with his eyes.
   c. He should grasp your finger if you place it in his hand.
   d. He should be saying some single-syllable words.

CHAPTER 12 ANSWERS

REVIEW QUESTIONS

1. c

2. b

3. a

4. e

5. f

6. d
(Objective 1)

7. e
(Objective 1)

8. g
(Objective 1)

9. a
(Objective 1)

10. b
(Objective 1)

11. c
(Objective 1)

12. Preschooler
(Objective 2)

13. Preschooler
(Objective 2)

14. Toddler
(Objective 2)

15. Preschooler
(Objective 2)

16. Toddler
(Objective 2)

17. a. Thicken
b. Peripheral
c. Baroreceptor
d. Decreases
e. Cardiomyopathy
f. Valves
g. Myocardial
h. Decreases
i. Dysrhythmias
j. Decrease
k. Decreases
l. Perception
m. Time
n. Saliva
o. Tone
p. Kidney
(Objective 1)

18. a. Reduced income at retirement; increased health care costs (insurance, drugs); costs of assisted living needs
(Objective 4)

b. Decreased mobility; disease processes; cognitive loss; death of a companion
(Objective 4)

19. a. The heart rate for each of the other ages can increase to 140 beats/min during serious illness or injury. (Objective 1)

20. b. The ductus venosus constricts, right ventricular pressure decreases, and systemic vascular resistance increases at birth. (Objective 1)

21. c. The bones are not fully formed, so muscles provide much support to the chest. Infants have significantly fewer alveoli than adults. The tracheal bifurcation is higher in infants. (Objective 1)

22. d. The rooting reflex allows the baby to move toward food. (Objective 1)

23. c. Easy children are characterized by regularity of body functions and acceptance of new situations. Difficult children display intense reaction and withdrawal from new stimuli. (Objective 2)

24. a. The ear, nose, and throat structures are shorter and more susceptible to infection than in adolescents. Passive immunity wanes early in infancy. Visual acuity is typically 20/30 in this age group. (Objective 1)

25. b. Authoritarian parenting style tends to produce children who have low motivation and self-esteem. Children reared by permissive parents may be discontented, distrustful, and self-centered. (Objective 3)

26. a. Peer relationships are formed with children near the same age and level of maturity. (Objective 2)

27. d. Growth rates are slower than infants and toddlers. Lymphatic tissue is larger relative to adults until about age 10 years. Primary teeth are lost, and replacement with permanent teeth begins. (Objective 1)

28. a. One theory of moral development lists three stages: preconventional reasoning, conventional reasoning, and postconventional reasoning. Self-concept, self-esteem, and peer relationships are also critical in the development of children. (Objective 2)

29. b. Gonadotropin is released from the hypothalamus and subsequently stimulates the release of luteinizing and follicle-stimulating hormones from the pituitary. These in turn stimulate the release of progesterone (breast development and menstrual cycle) and estrogen (female secondary sex characteristics). (Objective 1)

30. c. Suicide is the third leading cause of death for teens 15 to 19 years, but gay and lesbian teens are two to three times more likely to attempt suicide. Anorexia nervosa is an eating disorder. Depression is common. Appearance is important to teens. (Objective 1)

31. d. Other key issues in this age group include rearing children, managing a home, finding a social group, leisure activities, and selecting a stable occupation. (Objective 2)

32. c. Dementia, diverticulitis, and stroke can occur in this age group but are much more common in older adults. (Objective 2)

1. c, d, e, f
(Objective 1)

2. No abnormal findings were identified in any of the children.
(Objectives 1 and 2)

3. c. This is known as the palmar grasp reflex.
(Objective 1)

158

13 Principles of Pharmacology and Emergency Medications

READING ASSIGNMENT

Chapter 13, pages 275-337, in *Mosby's Paramedic Textbook,* ed. 4.

OBJECTIVES

Upon completion of this chapter, the paramedic student will be able to do the following:

1. Explain what a drug is.
2. Identify the four types of drug names.
3. Outline drug standards and legislation and the enforcement agencies pertinent to the paramedic profession.
4. Distinguish between characteristics of routes of drug administration.
5. Discuss factors that influence drug absorption, distribution, and elimination.
6. Describe how drugs react with receptors to produce their desired effects.
7. List variables that can influence drug interactions.
8. Distinguish among drug forms.
9. Describe the paramedic's responsibilities to understand drug profiles.
10. Identify special considerations for administering pharmacological agents to pregnant patients, pediatric patients, and older patients.
11. Outline drug actions and care considerations for a patient who is given drugs that affect the nervous, cardiovascular, respiratory, endocrine, and gastrointestinal systems.
12. Explain the meaning of drug terms that are necessary to interpret information in drug references safely.

SUMMARY

- A drug is any substance taken by mouth; injected into a muscle, blood vessel, or cavity of the body; or applied topically to treat or prevent a disease or condition.
- Drugs can be identified by four types of names. These include the chemical name; generic or nonproprietary name; trade, brand, or proprietary name; and official name.
- The Drug Enforcement Agency is the sole legal drug enforcement body in the United States. Other regulatory bodies or services include the Food and Drug Administration; the Public Health Service; the Federal Trade Commission; in Canada, the Health Protection Branch of the Department of National Health and Welfare; and for international drug control, the International Narcotics Control Board.
- Drugs do not confer any new functions on a tissue or organ; they only modify existing functions. A drug that interacts with a receptor to stimulate a response is known as an agonist. A drug that attaches to a receptor but does not stimulate a response is called an antagonist.
- Pharmacokinetics is the study of how the body handles a drug over a period of time.
- The degree to which drugs attain pharmacological activity depends partly on the rate and extent to which they are absorbed. Absorption in turn depends on the ability of the drug to cross the cell membrane. The rate and extent of absorption depend on the nature of the cell membrane the drug must cross, blood flow to the site of administration, solubility of the drug, pH of the drug environment, drug concentration, and drug dosage form.
- The route of drug administration influences drug absorption. These routes can be classified as enteral, parenteral, pulmonary, and topical.
- Distribution is the transport of a drug through the bloodstream to various tissues of the body and ultimately to its site of action. After absorption and distribution, the body eliminates most drugs. The body first biotransforms the drug and then excretes the drug. The kidney is the primary organ for excretion; however, the intestine; lungs; and mammary, sweat, and salivary glands also may be involved.
- The blood–brain barrier and the placenta are barriers to distribution of some drugs.
- Many factors can alter the response to drug therapy, including age, body mass, gender, pathological state, time of administration, genetic factors, and psychological factors.

- Most drug actions are thought to result from a chemical interaction. This interaction is between the drug and various receptors throughout the body. The most common form of drug action is the drug–receptor interaction.
- Many variables can influence drug interactions, including intestinal absorption, competition for plasma-protein binding, biotransformation, action at the receptor site, renal excretion, and alteration of electrolyte balance.
- Paramedics are held responsible for the safe and effective administration of drugs. In fact, they are responsible for each drug they provide to patients. They are legally, morally, and ethically responsible.
- Elements of the drug profile paramedics should know include the drug names, classification, mechanism of action, indications, pharmacokinetics, side or adverse effects, dose, route of administration, contraindication, special considerations, and storage requirements.
- Alterations in drug administration may be needed when caring for children, pregnant patients, and older adults.
- Autonomic drugs mimic or block the effects of the sympathetic and parasympathetic divisions of the autonomic nervous system. These drugs are classified into four groups: cholinergic (parasympathomimetic) drugs, cholinergic blocking (parasympatholytic) drugs, adrenergic (sympathomimetic) drugs, and adrenergic blocking (sympatholytic) drugs.
- Narcotic analgesics relieve pain. Narcotic antagonists reverse the narcotic effects of some analgesics. Nonnarcotic analgesics interfere with local mediators released when tissue is damaged in the periphery of the body. These mediators stimulate nerve endings and cause pain.
- Anesthetic drugs are central nervous system (CNS) depressants that have a reversible effect on nervous tissue. Antianxiety agents are used to reduce feelings of apprehension, nervousness, worry, or fearfulness. Sedatives and hypnotics are drugs that depress the CNS. They produce a calming effect. They also help induce sleep. Alcohol is a general CNS depressant that can produce sedation, sleep, and anesthesia.
- Antianxiety agents are used to reduce feelings of apprehension, nervousness, worry, or fearfulness. Sedatives and hypnotics are drugs that depress the CNS, produce a calming effect, and help induce sleep. Alcohol has characteristics of both of these drug groups.
- Anticonvulsant drugs are used to treat seizure disorders. Most notably, they treat epilepsy.
- All CNS stimulants work to increase excitability. They do this by blocking activity of inhibitory neurons or their respective neurotransmitters or by enhancing the production of the excitatory neurotransmitters.
- Psychotherapeutic drugs include antipsychotic agents, antidepressants, and lithium. These drugs are used to treat psychoses and affective disorders, especially schizophrenia, depression, and mania.
- Movement disorders such as Parkinson's disease can result from an imbalance of dopamine and acetylcholine. Drugs that inhibit or block acetylcholine are referred to as anticholinergic. Three classes of drugs affect brain dopamine: those that release dopamine, those that increase brain levels of dopamine, and dopaminergic agonists.
- Skeletal muscle relaxants can be classified as central acting, direct acting, and neuromuscular blockers.
- Cardiac drugs are classified by their effects on specialized cardiac tissues. Cardiac glycosides are used to treat congestive heart failure and certain tachycardias. Antidysrhythmic drugs are used to treat and prevent disorders of cardiac rhythm. The pharmacological agents that suppress dysrhythmias may do so by direct action on the cardiac cell membrane (lidocaine), by indirect action that affects the cell (propranolol), or both. The four classes of antidysrhythmic drugs are sodium channel blockers, beta blockers, potassium channel blockers, and calcium channel blockers.
- Antihypertensive drugs used to reduce blood pressure are classified into four major categories: diuretics, sympathetic blocking agents (sympatholytic drugs), vasodilators, calcium channel blockers, angiotensin-converting enzyme (ACE) inhibitors, and angiotensin II receptor antagonists.
- Antihemorrheologic agents are used to treat peripheral vascular disorders. These disorders are caused by pathological or physiological obstruction (e.g., arteriosclerosis). These agents improve blood flow to ischemic tissues.
- Drugs that affect blood coagulation may be classified as antiplatelet, anticoagulant, or fibrinolytic agents. Drugs that interfere with platelet aggregation are known as antiplatelet or antithrombic drugs. Anticoagulant drug therapy is designed to prevent intravascular thrombosis. The therapy decreases blood coagulability. Fibrinolytic drugs dissolve clots after their formation. These drugs work by promoting the digestion of fibrin.
- Hemophilia is a group of hereditary bleeding disorders. These disorders involve a deficiency of one of the factors needed for the coagulation of blood. Replacing the missing clotting factor can help manage hemophilia.
- Hemostatic agents speed up clot formation, thus reducing bleeding. Systemic hemostatic agents are used to control blood loss after surgery. They work by inhibiting the breakdown of fibrin. Topical hemostatic agents are used to control capillary bleeding. They are used during surgical and dental procedures.
- The treatment of choice in managing a loss of blood or blood components is to replace the blood component that is deficient. Replacement therapy may include transfusing whole blood (rare), packed red blood cells, fresh-frozen plasma, plasma expanders, platelets, cryoprecipitate, fibrinogen, albumin, or gamma globulins.

- Antihyperlipidemic drugs sometimes are used along with diet and exercise to control serum lipid levels, which may include high cholesterol and triglycerides.
- Bronchodilator drugs are the primary form of treatment for obstructive pulmonary disease such as asthma, chronic bronchitis, and emphysema. These drugs may be classified as sympathomimetic drugs and xanthine derivatives.
- Mucokinetic drugs are used to move respiratory secretions, excessive mucus, and sputum along the tracheobronchial tree.
- Oxygen is used chiefly to treat hypoxia and hypoxemia.
- Direct respiratory stimulant drugs act directly on the medullary center of the brain. These drugs are analeptics. They increase the rate and depth of respiration.
- A cough may be prolonged or result from an underlying disorder. In such a case, treatment with antitussive drugs may be indicated.
- The main clinical use of antihistamines is for allergic reactions. They also are used to control motion sickness or as a sedative or antiemetic.
- Drug therapy for the gastrointestinal (GI) system can be divided into drugs that affect the stomach and drugs that affect the lower GI tract. Antacids buffer or neutralize hydrochloric acid in the stomach. Antiflatulents prevent the formation of gas in the GI tract. Digestant drugs promote digestion in the GI tract. They do this by releasing small amounts of hydrochloric acid in the stomach. Drugs used to treat nausea and vomiting include antagonists of histamine, acetylcholine, and dopamine and other drugs the actions of which are not understood clearly.
- Cytoprotective agents and other drugs are used to treat peptic ulcer disease by protecting the gastric mucosa. H_2 receptor antagonists block the H_2 receptors. They also reduce the volume of gastric acid secretion and its acid content. Proton pump inhibitors decrease hydrochloric acid secretion by inhibiting the actions of the parietal cells
- Two common conditions of the lower GI tract may require drug therapy: constipation and diarrhea. Drugs used to manage these conditions include laxatives and antidiarrheals.
- Drugs used to treat eye disorders include antiglaucoma agents, mydriatics, cycloplegics, antiinfective and antiinflammatory agents, and topical anesthetics.
- Drugs used to treat disorders of the ear include antibiotics, steroid and antibiotic combinations, and miscellaneous preparations.
- The endocrine system works to control and integrate body functions. A number of drugs are used to treat disorders of the anterior and posterior pituitary, the thyroid and parathyroid glands, and the adrenal cortex.
- The pancreatic hormones play a key role in regulating the amount of certain nutrients in the circulatory system. The two main hormones secreted by the pancreas are insulin and glucagon. Imbalances in either of these may call for drug therapy. This therapy is meant to correct metabolic derangements. Oral hypoglycemic agents help lower blood glucose by a variety of mechanisms.
- Drugs that affect the female reproductive system include synthetic and natural substances such as hormones (estrogen and progesterone), oral contraceptives, ovulation stimulants, and drugs used to treat infertility.
- The male sex hormone is testosterone. Adequate amounts of this hormone are needed for normal development and maintenance of male sex characteristics.
- Erectile dysfunction drugs are used to enhance sexual function.
- Antineoplastic agents are used in cancer chemotherapy to prevent the increase of malignant cells.
- Antibiotics are used to treat local or systemic infection. This group includes penicillin, cephalosporins, and related products; macrolide antibiotics; tetracyclines; fluoroquinolones; and miscellaneous antibiotic agents.
- Persons can be infected by bacterial organisms, fungi, and viruses. Examples of antifungal drugs include tolnaftate (Tinactin), fluconazole (Diflucan), and nystatin (Mycostatin).
- Few drugs exist for use in any viral infections. One antiviral drug is acyclovir (Zovirax). This drug is effective against herpes infection. Another one is zidovudine (Retrovir, AZT), which currently is used to treat human immunodeficiency virus infection.
- Drugs used to treat inflammation or its symptoms may be classified as analgesic–antipyretic drugs and nonsteroidal antiinflammatory drugs. A number of medications have both properties.
- Immunosuppressant drugs reduce the activity of the immune system. They do this by suppressing the production and activity of lymphocytes. These drugs are prescribed after transplant surgery. They can help to prevent the rejection of foreign tissues. They also are sometimes given to halt the progress of autoimmune disorders.
- Immunomodulating agents are drugs that help the immune system to be more efficient. They do this by activating the immune defenses and by modifying a biological response to an unwanted stimulus.
- Serum contains agents of immunity. These are antibodies. The antibodies can protect against an organism if the serum is injected into someone else. This forms the basis for passive immunization. Vaccines are composed of killed or altered microorganisms. These are administered to a person to produce specific immunity to a disease-causing bacterial toxin, virus, or bacterium (active immunization).

163

Match the appropriate drug form in Column II with its description in Column I. Use each drug form only once.

Column I

1. _______ Semisolid medicine in a greasy base externally applied to the skin

2. _______ A sweetened alcohol and water solution

3. _______ Drug ground into loose granules

4. _______ Drug compressed into small disks

5. _______ Drug dissolved in sugar and water suspension (magma)

6. _______ Flat or round medicine held in the mouth until dissolved

7. _______ Gelatin-covered, dry drug preparation

8. _______ Suspension of fat or oil in water with an agent that decreases surface tension

9. _______ Suspension of insoluble particles in water

Column II

a. Capsule
b. Elixir
c. Emulsion
d. Extract
e. Liniment
f. Lotion
g. Aqueous
h. Ointment
i. Tablets
j. Powder
k. Aqueous solution
l. Troche

10. Complete the following sentences by listing the appropriate drug name:

    The precise composition and molecular structure of a drug are described in its **(a)** ___________________________

    name. The name that is not protected by law and denotes pharmacologically similar drugs is known as the

    (b) _______________________ name. The trademarked name of the drug designated by the company

    that manufactures it is the **(c)** _______________________ name. The initials USP or NF follow the

    (d) _______________________ name.

11. In one sentence, describe how the following drug standards or legislation influence medication administration and distribution in the United States:

    a. Pure Food and Drug Act (1906):

    ____

    b. Federal Drug and Cosmetic Act (1938):

    ____

    c. Harrison Narcotic Act (1914):

    ____

12. List the agency responsible for each of the following aspects of drug control:

    a. It has the power to suppress false or misleading advertising regarding drugs to the general public.

    ____

    b. It is responsible for enforcing the federal Food, Drug, and Cosmetic Act.

    ____

c. It monitors the distribution of controlled substances.

____

d. It regulates biological products like antitoxins.

____

13. Refer to a drug reference source to find the answers to the following questions.

a. What is the indication for the drug beclomethasone?

____

b. List the contraindications and side effects of this drug.

____

Questions 14 to 17 pertain to the following case study:
Dispatch alerts you to respond to a call for an "accidental injury." A 35-year-old man stumbled and fell, injuring his wrist. There is deformity, swelling, crepitus, and tenderness proximal to his right hand. After application of the appropriate splint and ice, you decide that medication for pain is indicated.

14. What eight points are critical to ensure that you meet your legal, moral, and ethical obligations for safe, effective medication administration to this patient?

a. ____

b. ____

c. ____

d. ____

e. ____

f. ____

g. ____

h. ____

After eliciting a careful history and consultation with medical direction, you initiate an intravenous (IV) line in the uninjured extremity and administer ketorolac tromethamine (Toradol) IV push. Several moments after administration, the patient becomes anxious and states that he feels like his "throat is going to close in." His skin appears flushed, and a large, flat, raised rash is erupting. The patient states he has never taken this drug before.

15. What type of reaction is this patient having?

____

16. List two emergency drugs that may be used to treat this patient's signs and symptoms.

____

165

After you arrive at the emergency department, the patient admits to the physician that he had a reaction to aspirin in the past (although during your history, he denied any allergic reactions). The physician tells you that there is a reported cross-reactivity between aspirin and ketorolac tromethamine.

17. How would you have known that this type of reaction was possible?

____

18. Select the appropriate drug term from the following list to complete the sentences:

Antagonism	Potentiation
Contraindications	Side effect
Cumulative action	Stimulant
Depressant	Summation
Drug allergy	Synergism
Drug dependence	Therapeutic action
Drug interaction	Tolerance
Idiosyncrasy	Untoward effect

    a. An abnormal or peculiar response to a drug that possibly is caused by a genetic deficiency is

    _______________________________.

    b. Caffeine and methylphenidate (Ritalin) are examples of drugs that exhibit a(n) _______________________

    _______________________ effect.

    c. A drug action caused by an immunological response to a previous exposure is a(n) _______________________

    _______________________ reaction.

    d. The desired effect of naloxone on narcotics is attributed to _______________________________________.

    e. The enhancement of the effects of one drug caused by the concurrent administration of a second drug is

    _______________________________________.

    f. An undesirable effect of a drug that is harmful to the patient is a(n) _______________________________.

    g. The combined action of two drugs that is greater than the sum of each individual agent acting

    independently is _______________________________________.

    h. The intense physical or emotional disturbance possibly resulting when a narcotic is withheld from a person

    who frequently uses it is a result of _______________________________.

    i. A drug that diminishes a person's central nervous system function is a _______________________________.

    j. The ability of atropine to increase the heart rate is known as the desired effect, or _______________________.

    k. The list of factors used to describe situations when medication administration would be harmful is the ________

    _______________________________.

l. Concurrent administration of drugs such that one agent modifies the actions of the other is ___________________

___________________________________.

m. A decreased response to a drug after repetitive doses, which necessitates higher doses to achieve the desired effect, is _______________________________________.

n. When repeat administration of drugs results in absorption that exceeds metabolism and excretion, the increased effect that results is known as ____.

19. List six factors that influence the rate and extent to which a drug is absorbed in the body.

a. ____

b. ____

c. ____

d. ____

e. ____

f. ____

20. List four groups of drugs that are associated with a high incidence of drug–drug interactions.

a. ____

b. ____

c. ____

d. ____

21. You need to administer acetaminophen to a child who has been vomiting repeatedly. What enteral route will you choose?

____

22. When giving epinephrine to an asthmatic patient, a slow and sustained effect is desirable to minimize side effects and prolong the effects of the drug. You will administer the drug by the _______________________________ route.

23. Your 76-year-old patient has a heart rate of 34 and a blood pressure of 70 mm Hg by palpation. You wish to give atropine to increase the heart rate. What route will you choose? _______________________________

24. A 3-month-old infant is in hemorrhagic shock after sustaining a gunshot wound to the abdomen. After intravenous attempts are unsuccessful, what route will you consider for fluid volume resuscitation?

____

   Chapter **13** **Principles of Pharmacology and Emergency Medications**

25. Is the rate of drug absorption by the pulmonary route faster or slower than the subcutaneous route?

____

26. List the two physiological barriers to drug distribution within the body.

a. ____

b. ____

27. Circle the appropriate response regarding drug effects in children.

a. The blood–brain barrier in infants is **less/more** effective than in adults; therefore, the central nervous system effects of drugs will be **less/more**.

b. The newborn has a(n) **decreased/increased** ability to metabolize drugs; therefore, drug toxicity is **less/more** likely to occur.

28. List three physiological factors that may result in altered drug absorption, distribution, biotransformation, or elimination in older adults.

a. ____

b. ____

c. ____

29. You are called to a sparsely furnished, one-room apartment to care for a 79-year-old woman complaining of difficulty breathing. She states that she has a history of heart disease and "swelling," and she hands you a sack of empty medication bottles that contained furosemide, digoxin, and potassium. She thinks she last took them 5 or 6 days ago. Discuss three possible reasons for the patient's medication noncompliance.

a. ____

b. ____

c. ____

DRUG CLASSIFICATIONS

30. When given the following description and drug name, identify the drug group to which it belongs and give one additional example of another drug from the same group.

a. Your patient says he takes lorazepam (Ativan) to help him relax.

Drug group: ________________________________ Example: ___________________________

b. You arrive in the rural emergency department with a 65-year-old woman experiencing an acute myocardial infarction. Immediately, the emergency department staff administers reteplase (Retavase) in an attempt to dissolve the clot.

Drug group: ________________________________ Example: ___________________________

c. Before your Mediterranean cruise, you take dimenhydrinate (Dramamine) to prevent seasickness.

Drug group: ________________________________ Example: ___________________________

d. During a cardiopulmonary arrest or in selected cases of shock, drugs such as epinephrine (Adrenalin) may be used to stimulate the heart.

Drug group: _______________________ Example: _______________________

e. Your 45-year-old patient is complaining of chest pain. His only home medication is hydrochlorothiazide (HCTZ) for hypertension.

Drug group: _______________________ Example: _______________________

f. An older patient is taking captopril (Capoten) for her congestive heart failure.

Drug group: _______________________ Example: _______________________

g. A 30-year-old patient with a seizure disorder is taking phenobarbital (Luminal).

Drug group: _______________________ Example: _______________________

h. A 52-year-old hospice patient is taking hydromorphone (Dilaudid) to control his pain.

Drug group: _______________________ Example: _______________________

i. Diltiazem (Cardizem) is used by a patient who states that she takes it to control a fast heart rhythm.

Drug group: _______________________ Example: _______________________

j. A person at risk for developing clots that may cause heart attack or stroke may be prescribed clopidogrel (Plavix).

Drug group: _______________________ Example: _______________________

k. People with asthma may have a large number of home medicines that may include albuterol (Proventil).

Drug group: _______________________ Example: _______________________

l. You observe a patient in the emergency department who is drowsy and having difficulty speaking moments after she has been given etomidate (Amidate).

Drug group: _______________________ Example: _______________________

m. You will have increased vigilance for evidence of bleeding if a patient tells you he is taking warfarin sodium (Coumadin).

Drug group: _______________________ Example: _______________________

n. A 35-year-old patient is experiencing complications after an outpatient surgical procedure. Her only home medication is pentazocine (Talwin).

Drug group: _______________________ Example: _______________________

o. People with asthma may be taking a variety of drugs besides bronchodilators in an attempt to control their disease. Examples of these include cromolyn sodium (Intal), beclomethasone dipropionate (Vanceril Qvar Inhaler), and ipratropium (Atrovent).

Drug group: _______________________ Example: _______________________

   Chapter **13** **Principles of Pharmacology and Emergency Medications**

p. You are dispatched to a call for an unconscious person. The patient is awake but confused and combative when you arrive and has a medication list that includes ethosuximide (Zarontin).

Drug group: _________________________ Example: _________________________

q. You are treating a young woman with a history of depression. She has taken all 20 of her fluoxetine (Prozac) in a suicide attempt.

Drug group: _________________________ Example: _________________________

r. When you arrive at the emergency department with a combative, psychotic patient in restraints, the nurse gives the patient an intramuscular injection of haloperidol (Haldol).

Drug group: _________________________ Example: _________________________

s. A patient with a chronic pain disorder is taking amitriptyline (Elavil).

Drug group: _________________________ Example: _________________________

t. Medications for management of gastroesophageal reflux disease may include esomeprazole (Nexium).

Drug group: _________________________ Example: _________________________

u. During your annual physical, a blood test reveals that you have high cholesterol. The doctor prescribes atorvastatin (Lipitor).

Drug group: _________________________ Example: _________________________

v. A patient with Parkinson's disease is taking levodopa (Larodopa).

Drug group: _________________________ Example: _________________________

w. Your patient is vomiting blood. His home medicines include ranitidine (Zantac).

Drug group: _________________________ Example: _________________________

31. List the generic name of one drug and its general mechanism of actions for each of the following groups of antidysrhythmic drugs.

Group	Generic Name	Actions
IA		
IB		
IC		
II		
III		
IV		

32. Fill in the missing information about hypertensive medications in the following table:

Classification	Generic Name	Actions
	Furosemide, hydrochlorothiazide, spironolactone with hydrochlorothiazide (Aldactazide)	
Beta-blocking agents		
		Block sympathetic stimulation, have multiple sites of action
	Diazoxide, hydralazine, minoxidil (arteriolar dilator), sodium nitroprusside, amyl nitrite, isosorbide dinitrate, nitroglycerin (arteriolar and venous dilator drugs)	
Angiotensin II receptor antagonists	Irbesartan (Avapro), losartan (Cozaar), valsartan (Diovan), candasartan (Atacand)	
Calcium channel blockers		Decrease peripheral resistance by inhibiting blockers, decreasing the contractility of vascular smooth muscle

33. Match the drug listed in Column II with the endocrine gland that it affects in Column I. Use each drug only once.

Column I

________ Adrenal cortex

________ Ovary

________ Pancreas

________ Parathyroid

________ Pituitary

________ Testes

________ Thyroid

Column II

a. Clomiphene citrate (Clomid)
b. Dexamethasone (Decadron)
c. Iodine products
d. Methyltestosterone (Metandren)
e. Glimepiride (Amaryl)
f. Vasopressin
g. Vitamin D

STUDENT SELF-ASSESSMENT

34. What is the term that describes any substance taken by mouth; injected into a muscle, blood vessel, or cavity of the body; or applied topically to treat or prevent a disease or condition?
a. Antidote
b. Drug
c. Parenteral
d. Vaccine

35. What Schedule is morphine as regulated under the Controlled Substance Act of 1970?
a. I
b. II
c. III
d. IV

36. Which of the following substances can pass through the blood–brain barrier and placental barrier?
a. Antibiotics
b. Lipid-soluble drugs
c. Undissociated drugs
d. Water-soluble drugs

37. Agonists are drugs that do which of the following?
a. Bind to a receptor and cause a specific response
b. Bind to a receptor and cause no response
c. Cause duplication of specific receptors
d. Prevent chemicals from reaching the receptor sites

38. The measurement of the relative safety of a drug is which of the following?
   a. Biological half-life
   b. Median effective dose
   c. Median lethal dose
   d. Therapeutic index

39. Which of the following drugs can be administered by endotracheal tube?
   a. Amiodarone
   b. Hydroxyzine
   c. Diazepam
   d. Naloxone

40. Which of the following drug administration routes delivers the most rapid effects?
   a. Oral
   b. Intramuscular
   c. Subcutaneous
   d. Transtracheal

41. Which of the following is the route of choice for drug administration in a patient who is in profound shock after myocardial infarction?
   a. Intramuscular
   b. Intravenous
   c. Oral
   d. Subcutaneous

42. Which of the following is an opioid antagonist?
   a. Butorphanol tartrate
   b. Naloxone hydrochloride
   c. Oxycodone hydrochloride
   d. Pentazocine hydrochloride

43. Which of the following drugs has anticonvulsant properties?
   a. Lidocaine
   b. Magnesium sulfate
   c. Cocaine
   d. Morphine

44. You are transporting a patient with a history of narcolepsy. What drugs might you find that he is taking to reduce his symptoms of this disorder?
   a. Methamphetamine (Desoxyn)
   b. Methylphenidate (Ritalin)
   c. Pemoline (Cylert)
   d. Phenmetrazine (Preludin)

45. What condition are drugs such as levodopa (Larodopa) and carbidopa–levodopa (Sinemet) that enhance brain dopamine levels used to treat?
   a. Depression
   b. Hypotension
   c. Myasthenia gravis
   d. Parkinson's disease

46. You are experiencing severe muscle spasms after injuring your back at work. Which antispasmodic medication may be prescribed for you?
   a. Carbamazepine (Tegretol)
   b. Chlordiazepoxide (Librium)
   c. Chlorpromazine (Thorazine)
   d. Cyclobenzaprine (Flexeril)

47. The drugs vecuronium (Norcuron) and succinylcholine (Anectine) may be used for rapid-sequence induction of intubation in a person who has sustained severe head trauma. The primary action of these drugs in this situation is which of the following?
   a. To decrease intracranial pressure
   b. To dry oral secretions
   c. To paralyze the muscles
   d. To provide pain relief

48. Which of the following is an indirect-acting cholinergic drug that may be used in the management of poisoning from atropine?
   a. Glucagon
   b. Lorazepam
   c. Physostigmine
   d. Verapamil

49. What is the chief neurotransmitter for the parasympathetic nervous system?
   a. Acetylcholine
   b. Epinephrine (Adrenalin)
   c. Metaraminol (Aramine)
   d. Norepinephrine

50. Stimulation of the beta$_2$-adrenergic receptors will cause which of the following?
  a. Negative inotropic effect on the heart
  b. Positive inotropic effect on the heart
  c. Bronchiolar dilation
  d. Peripheral vasoconstriction

51. What effects does epinephrine have?
  a. Alpha effects only
  b. Beta effects only
  c. Alpha and beta effects
  d. Neither alpha nor beta effects

52. Drugs that increase the contractility of the heart have a positive __________ effect.
  a. Chronotropic
  b. Cholinergic
  c. Dromotropic
  d. Inotropic

53. An older man is complaining of dizziness, nausea, vomiting, weakness, and yellow vision. When questioned about his home medications, he states that he takes a small tablet to help his "weak heart." His pulse is 45 beats/min. What do you suspect he is experiencing?
  a. Digoxin overdose
  b. Isoproterenol overdose
  c. Tricyclic antidepressant overdose
  d. Verapamil overdose

54. Which of the following is a group IV antidysrhythmic drug?
  a. Amiodarone
  b. Lidocaine
  c. Procainamide
  d. Verapamil

55. The primary mechanism by which antihypertensives reduce blood pressure is by decreasing which of the following?
  a. Cardiac output
  b. Intravascular blood volume
  c. Myocardial contractility
  d. Peripheral vascular resistance

56. Which of the following drugs acts by dissolving a clot that has formed already?
  a. Aspirin
  b. Coumadin
  c. Heparin
  d. Streptokinase

57. Which of the following is a beta$_2$-specific bronchodilator?
  a. Albuterol
  b. Aminophylline
  c. Ephedrine
  d. Ipratropium

58. For which of the following patients are antihistamines indicated?
  a. Petechial rash
  b. Asthma
  c. Heart failure
  d. Nausea and vomiting

59. An elderly patient has a disorder necessitating the use of pilocarpine drops. What is he experiencing?
  a. Conjunctivitis
  b. Glaucoma
  c. Keratitis
  d. Pain

60. Which of the following is true about insulin?
  a. It is secreted by the adrenal glands.
  b. It is secreted only during stress.
  c. It will increase the use of fat for fuel.
  d. It will move glucose into the cells.

61. Your patient states that she is allergic to penicillin. Which of the following drugs can she take safely?
  a. Amoxicillin (Amoxil)
  b. Cefazolin (Ancef)
  c. Dicloxacillin (Dynapen)
  d. Tetracycline (Achromycin)

62. Which of the following is an antiviral drug used in treatment of patients infected with human immunodeficiency virus?

    a. Acyclovir (Zovirax)
    b. Pyrimethamine (Daraprim)
    c. Quinine (Quinamm)
    d. Zidovudine (Retrovir)

63. Isoniazid (INH) and rifampin (Rifadin) are drugs used to treat which of the following?

    a. HIV infection
    b. Leprosy
    c. Malaria
    d. Tuberculosis

WRAP IT UP

You are dispatched to the home of an elderly man who has been "passing out." When you arrive, you find him conscious but confused and unable to give you any history. He is pale and sweaty; has vomited; and has the following vital signs: BP 90/54 mm Hg, P 56/min, and R 16/min. When you listen to his lungs, you hear crackles in the bases on both sides. You find a medication list that indicates he is allergic to penicillin and the following list of current medicines: digoxin (Lanoxin), atenolol, amiodarone, Humulin insulin 70/30, oxycodone, lorazepam, sertraline, cyclobenzaprine, diltiazem, aspirin, furosemide, K-Dur (potassium), ipratropium, albuterol, ranitidine, and azithromycin.

1. What type of medication allergy reaction is penicillin most likely to cause?

    a. Type I, anaphylactic
    b. Type II, cytotoxic
    c. Type III, serum sickness
    d. Type IV, contact dermatitis

2. Which of his home medications have an effect on the autonomic nervous system?

____

3. Which of his home medications are given by the parenteral route?

____

4. One of his medications, Lanoxin, has a very low therapeutic index. Why is that important for you to know?

____

5. What factors may contribute to medication noncompliance in an older adult?

____

6. Which of his home medications could be contributing to his confusion?

____

7. Which of his medications is a(n)

    a. Antihypertensive
    b. Antidysrhythmic (list specific class)
    c. Antiplatelet
    d. Muscle relaxant
    e. Controlled substance
    f. Bronchodilator
    g. Analgesic
    h. H_2 receptor antagonist
    i. Antibiotic

____

8. Because the patient is unable to give you information about his medical history, you must try to determine what medical conditions he could have based on his medication list. What conditions do you suspect he has?

____

____

9. Based on this knowledge and your physical exam of the patient, what are some possible causes for his signs and symptoms today?

____

____

CHAPTER 13 ANSWERS

REVIEW QUESTIONS

1. h

2. b

3. j

4. i

5. k

6. l

7. a

8. c

9. g
(Questions 1–9, Objective 8)

10. a. Chemical
b. Generic or nonproprietary
c. Trade or proprietary
d. Official
(Objective 2)

11. a. Protected the public from mislabeled drugs, prohibited the use of false and misleading claims for medications, and restricted sales of drugs with abuse potential
b. Prevented marketing of drugs until they were tested and required names of all ingredients and directions on labels
c. Controlled the sale of narcotics and established _narcotic_ as a legal term
(Objective 3)

12. a. Federal Trade Commission
b. Food and Drug Administration
c. Drug Enforcement Administration
d. Public Health Service
(Objective 3)

13. a. For chronic control of bronchial asthma
b. Contraindicated in the treatment of acute episodes of asthma or status asthmaticus or if a known hypersensitivity exists (PDR)
(Objective 12)

14. A paramedic's responsibilities relative to drug administration include the following: using correct techniques, observing and documenting effects of drugs, maintaining current knowledge regarding pharmacology, maintaining professional relationships, understanding pharmacology, evaluating drug indications and contraindications, using drug reference materials, taking a patient history, and consulting with medical direction.
(Objective 9)

175

15. The patient is demonstrating signs and symptoms of a type I hypersensitivity allergic reaction.
(Objective 9)

16. The chemicals histamine and slow-reacting substance of anaphylaxis are released during an anaphylactic reaction.
Diphenhydramine and epinephrine are used to treat this.
(Objective 9)

17. Sometimes patients may have an allergic reaction to a drug they have never taken that is chemically similar to
another drug to which they are allergic. This information can be found in the drug profile.
(Objective 9)

18. a. Idiosyncrasy   h. Drug dependence
    b. Stimulant   i. Depressant
    c. Drug allergy   j. Therapeutic action
    d. Antagonism   k. Contraindications
    e. Potentiation   l. Drug interaction
    f. Side effect   m. Tolerance
    g. Synergism   n. Cumulative action.
(Objective 12)

19. The nature of the absorbing surface through which the drug must travel, the blood flow to the site of
administration, the solubility of the drug, the pH of the drug environment, the drug concentration, and the drug
dosage form
(Objective 5)

20. Drug–drug interactions commonly are associated with blood thinners, tricyclic antidepressants, amphetamines,
digitalis glycosides, diuretics, alcohol, antihypertensives, and cigarette smoking.
(Objective 7)

21. Rectal
(Objective 10)

22. Subcutaneous
(Objective 11)

23. Intravenous
(Objective 11)

24. Intraosseous
(Objective 11)

25. Faster
(Objective 5)

26. Placenta and blood–brain barrier
(Objective 5)

27. a. Less, more
    b. Decreased, more
(Objective 10)

28. Decreased renal function, altered nutrition habits, greater consumption of nonprescription drugs, reduced gastric
acid, slowed gastric motility, decreased serum albumin, congestive heart failure, and decreased blood flow
to the liver
(Objective 10)

29. Inability to pay for new drugs, forgetfulness or confusion, lack of symptoms (causing patient to become
noncompliant), and other physical disabilities not mentioned
(Objective 10)

176

30. a. Benzodiazepines: alprazolam (Xanax), chlordiazepoxide (Librium), clorazepate (Tranxene), diazepam (Valium), flurazepam (Dalmane), lorazepam (Ativan), midazolam (Versed), temazepam (Restoril), clonazepam (Klonopin)

    b. Fibrinolytic agents: anisoylated plasminogen streptokinase activator (Eminase), streptokinase (Streptase), tissue plasminogen activator (TPA), tenecteplase (TNKase)

    c. Antiemetics/antihistamines: diphenhydramine hydrochloride (Benadryl), hydroxyzine pamoate (Vistaril), meclizine hydrochloride (Antivert), promethazine hydrochloride (Phenergan)

    d. Adrenergics: dobutamine (Dobutrex), dopamine (Intropin), isoproterenol (Isuprel), norepinephrine (Levophed)

    e. Diuretics: furosemide (Lasix), spironolactone (Aldactone)

    f. Angiotensin-converting enzyme (ACE) inhibitor: enalapril (Vasotec), benazepril (Lotensin), fosinopril (Monopril), lisinopril (Prinivil, Zestril), quinapril (Accupril)

    g. Anticonvulsants, barbiturate: mephobarbital (Gemonil)

    h. Narcotic analgesics: codeine, methylmorphine, meperidine (Demerol), methadone (Dolophine, Methadose), morphine sulfate (Astramorph and others), oxycodone (Percodan, Tylox, Percocet), propoxyphene (Darvon, Dolene), hydrocodone (Lortab)

    i. Class IV antidysrhythmics: verapamil (Isoptin), amlodipine (Norvasc), felodipine (Plendil)

    j. Antiplatelet agents: aspirin, sulfinpyrazone (Anturane), dipyridamole (Persantin), ticlopidine (Ticlid), abciximab (ReoPro)

    k. Beta$_2$-selective bronchodilators: bitolterol (Tornalate), terbutaline sulfate (Brethine, Bricanyl), salmeterol (Serevent), levalbuterol (Xopenex)

    l. Nonbarbiturate anesthetic agents: fentanyl (Sublimaze), sufentanil (Sufenta), alfentanil (Alfenta)

   m. Anticoagulants: heparin sodium (Liquaemin)

    n. Opioid agonist–antagonist agents: nalbuphine hydrochloride (Nubain)

    o. Muscarinic antagonists used to treat respiratory emergencies: glycopyrrolate (Robinul)

    p. Anticonvulsants (succinimides): methsuximide (Celontin), phensuximide (Milontin)

    q. Selective serotonin reuptake inhibitors: sertraline (Zoloft), paroxetine (Paxil), fluvoxamine (Luvox), and citalopram (Celexa)

    r. Antipsychotic agents: chlorpromazine (Thorazine), thioridazine (Mellaril), fluphenazine (Prolixin), molindone (Lidone), loxapine (Loxitane), olanzapine, resperidol

    s. Tricyclic antidepressants: mirtazapine (Remeron), nortriptyline (Pamelor)

    t. Proton pump inhibitors: lansoprazole (Prevacid), omeprazole (Prilosec), pantoprazole (Protonix), rabeprazole (AcipHex)

    u. Antihyperlipidemic drugs: fenofibrate (Tricor), fluvastatin (Lescol), gemfibrozil (Lopid), pravastatin (Pravachol), simvastatin (Zocor)

    v. Drugs that affect brain dopamine (used in treatment of Parkinson's disease): carbidopa–levodopa (Sinemet), amantadine (Symmetrel), bromocriptine (Parlodel), pergolide (Permax)

    w. H2-receptor antagonists: cimetidine (Tagamet), famotidine (Pepcid)

    (Objective 12)

31.

Group	Drug Name	Actions
IA	Quinidine, procainamide	Decrease conduction velocity; prolong electrical potential of cardiac tissue
IB	Lidocaine, phenytoin	Increase or have no effect on conduction velocity
IC	Flecainide, encainide	Profoundly slow conduction
II	Propranolol, metoprolol	Beta-blockers
III	Amiodarone	Antiadrenergic agents; positive inotropic action; terminate reentry dysrhythmias
IV	Verapamil, diltiazem	Block flow of calcium into cardiac and smooth muscle cells; decrease automaticity

(Objective 11)

  Chapter **13 Principles of Pharmacology and Emergency Medications**

32.

Classification	Generic Name	Actions
Diuretics	Furosemide, hydrochlorothiazide, spironolactone with hydrochlorothiazide (Aldactazide)	Increase renal excretion of salt and water; decrease blood volume direct effect on arterioles
Beta-blocking agents	Propranolol, acebutolol, atenolol, metoprolol, labetalol, nadolol	Decrease cardiac output; inhibit renin secretion from kidneys; beta-blockers compete with epinephrine for beta receptor sites and inhibit tissue or organ response to beta stimulation
Adrenergic inhibiting agents	Clonidine (central acting), guanethidine, reserpine (peripheral inhibitors) prazosin hydrochloride, phentolamine, phenoxy benzamine (alpha$_1$- and alpha$_2$- blocking agents, nonselective)	Block sympathetic stimulation; have multiple sites of action
Vasodilator drugs	Diazoxide, hydralazine, minoxidil (arteriolar dilator), sodium nitroprusside, amyl nitrite, isosorbide dinitrate, nitroglycerin (arteriolar and venous dilator drugs)	Act directly on smooth muscle walls of arterioles, veins, or both; lower peripheral resistance and blood pressure
Angiotensin-converting enzyme inhibitors, angiotensin II receptor antagonist	Captopril, enalapril, lisinopril, irbesartan (Avapro), losartan (Cozaar, Hyzaar), valsartan (Diovan)	Inhibit the conversion of angiotensin I to angiotensin II. Angiotensin II is a powerful vasoconstrictor that suppresses the renin–angiotensin–aldosterone system. Selectively inhibit angiotensin receptors that include vasoconstriction, renal tubular sodium reabsorption, aldosterone release, and stimulation of arterial and peripheral sympathetic activity.
Calcium channel blockers	Verapamil, nifedipine, diltiazem	Decrease peripheral resistance by inhibiting blockers and the contractility of vascular smooth muscle

(Objective 11)

33. b, a, e, g, f, d, c
(Objective 11)

34. b. An antidote is a specific drug taken to minimize the adverse effects of an ingested drug or poison. *Parenteral* refers to a drug route. A vaccine is an injection of drug given to prevent disease.
(Objective 1)

35. b
(Objective 3)

36. b. Only selected antibiotics pass through these barriers.
(Objective 5)

37. a. Antagonists block receptor sites and inhibit action.
(Objective 6)

38. d. The median lethal dose is the lethal dose for 50% of animals that took the drug. The median effective dose is the effective dose for 50% of animals that took the drug. The biological half-life is the time required to excrete half of the total amount of drug introduced into the body.
(Objective 5)

39. d. Atropine, lidocaine, and epinephrine also may be given by this route.
(Objective 5)

178

40. d. Then intramuscular, subcutaneous, and oral
(Objective 5)

41. b. All of the other routes listed give unpredictable, slow absorption because of poor perfusion in shock.
(Objective 5)

42. b. Butorphanol tartrate and pentazocine are opioid agonist–antagonists, and oxycodone hydrochloride is an opioid analgesic–agonist.
(Objective 11)

43. b
(Objective 11)

44. a. Methylphenidate (Ritalin) and pemoline (Cylert) are used to manage patients with attention deficit disorder and hyperactivity. Phenmetrazine is an anorexiant.
(Objective 11)

45. d. Depression usually is treated with a tricyclic antidepressant. Hypotension is treated based on the cause. Occasionally, intravenously administered dopamine is used, but it acts in a different manner than the drugs that affect brain dopamine levels. Drugs used to treat myasthenia gravis elevate acetylcholine at the myoneural junctions.
(Objective 11)

46. d. Carbamazepine (Tegretol) is used to treat seizure disorders. Chlordiazepoxide (Librium) and chlorpromazine (Thorazine) are antipsychotic drugs. Baclofen (Lioresal) and diazepam (Valium) are also antispasmodics that may be used to manage muscle spasms.
(Objective 11)

47. c. These drugs paralyze muscles and usually are given concurrently with other drugs that decrease the intracranial pressure during intubation (lidocaine) and sedatives or pain relievers.
(Objective 11)

48. c. Physostigmine is used to manage poisonings. Glucagon is a pancreatic hormone that increases blood glucose, lorazepam is a minor tranquilizer, and verapamil is an antidysrhythmic drug.
(Objective 11)

49. a. Norepinephrine is the primary neurotransmitter for the sympathetic nervous system. Adrenalin is a trade name for epinephrine, and Aramine is the trade name for metaraminol.
(Objective 6)

50. c
(Objective 11)

51. c
(Objective 6)

52. d. Chronotropes increase heart rate; dromotropes increase conduction velocity. Cholinergic drugs increase parasympathetic effects.
(Objective 6)

53. a. Influenza-like symptoms and a variety of dysrhythmias are associated with digoxin toxicity. Tricyclic antidepressant or isoproterenol overdose likely would produce tachyarrhythmias. Verapamil overdose may cause bradycardias and severe hypotension.
(Objective 11)

54. d. Amiodarone is a group III, lidocaine is a group IB, and procainamide is a group IA antidysrhythmic agent.
(Objective 11)

   Chapter **13** **Principles of Pharmacology and Emergency Medications**

55. d. Some also decrease heart rate and contractility; however, the majority achieve their effects by decreasing vascular resistance.
(Objective 11)

56. d. All of the others prevent clot formation.
(Objective 11)

57. a. Ephedrine is a nonspecific beta-agonist, and aminophylline is a xanthine derivative. Ipratropium is an anticholinergic.
(Objective 11)

58. d. Antihistamines may worsen an acute asthma attack by thickening bronchial secretions.
(Objective 11)

59. b. Antiinfective and antiinflammatory agents are used to treat conjunctivitis or keratitis. Topical anesthetic agents are used to treat pain.
(Objective 11)

60. d. Insulin is secreted continually in amounts determined by the needs of the body.
(Objective 11)

61. d. Amoxicillin and dicloxacillin are penicillin drugs. A percentage of persons who are allergic to penicillin have cross-reactivity to cephalosporins such as cefazolin.
(Objective 11)

62. d. Acyclovir (Zovirax) typically is prescribed for herpes infection (some patients infected with human immunodeficiency virus also may take this to treat opportunistic herpes infections). Pyrimethamine (Daraprim) and quinine (Qui-namm) are antimalarial drugs.
(Objective 11)

63. d
(Objective 11)

WRAP IT UP

1. a. The reaction may vary from hives to life-threatening airway compromise. Cytotoxic reactions usually involve hemolysis and result from administration of procainamide or hydralazine. Serum sickness can be caused by penicillins, iodides, sulfonamides, phenytoin, and some antitoxins and can cause a severe inflammatory reaction. Contact dermatitis results from exposure to poison ivy, sunscreens, and other topical ointments.
(Objective 6)

2. Atenolol is a beta-blocker, and albuterol is a $beta_2$-selective stimulant.
(Objective 5)

3. His Humulin insulin is given by subcutaneous injection.
(Objective 5)

4. The margin between the therapeutic dose of digoxin (Lanoxin) and its lethal dose is small. Often patients experience signs and symptoms of digoxin overdose.
(Objective 6)

5. Drug cost may be too much for an older adult; confusion may cause overdosing or underdosing; visual or physical impairment can cause drug errors; or the patient may choose not to follow the prescribed medication plan.
(Objective 11)

6. Oxycodone, lorazepam, sertraline, or cyclobenzaprine could cause some confusion. If his blood sugar is low because of his Humulin insulin administration, it also could cause confusion.
(Objective 12)

180

7. a. Atenolol, diltiazem, furosemide
   b. Digoxin (Lanoxin; cardiac glycoside), atenolol (Class II—beta-blockers); diltiazem (Class IV—calcium channel blockers); amiodarone (Class III—potassium channel blockers)
   c. Aspirin
   d. Lorazepam, cyclobenzaprine
   e. Propoxyphene, lorazepam
   f. Albuterol, ipratropium (indirectly)
   g. Propoxyphene, aspirin
   h. Ranitidine
   i. Azithromycin
   (Objective 12)

8. Based on the medication list that you have found, you can suspect that his medical history may include diabetes (Humulin), hypertension (atenolol, diltiazem, furosemide), cardiac rhythm disturbance (digoxin [Lanoxin], atenolol, amiodarone, diltiazem), risk factors for or history of myocardial infarction or stroke (aspirin), musculoskeletal pain or arthritis (propoxyphene, lorazepam, cyclobenzaprine), chronic obstructive pulmonary disease (ipratropium, albuterol), gastritis or ulcers (ranitidine), and recent infection (azithromycin). (Objective 12)

9. Clues to the cause of his present illness may be found in the physical examination. He could be confused because of his drugs, sepsis, a stroke, chronic dementia, electrolyte imbalance (low sodium or potassium), or hypotension and subsequent decrease in cerebral perfusion. He could be having a stroke, he could have taken too much of his medications, or he may be hypoxic. (Objective 12)

14 Venous Access and Medication Administration

Chapter 14, pages 338-382, in *Mosby's Paramedic Textbook,* ed. 4.

OBJECTIVES

Upon completion of this chapter, the paramedic student will be able to do the following:

1. Convert selected units of measurement into the household, apothecary, and metric systems.
2. Identify the steps in the calculation of drug dosages.
3. Calculate the correct volume of drug to be administered in a given situation.
4. Compute the correct rate for an infusion of drugs or intravenous fluids.
5. List measures for ensuring the safe administration of medications.
6. Describe actions paramedics should take if a medication error occurs.
7. List measures for preserving asepsis during parenteral administration of a drug.
8. Explain drug administration techniques for the enteral and parenteral routes.
9. Describe the steps for safely initiating an intravenous infusion.
10. Identify complications and adverse effects associated with intravenous access.
11. List the steps for safely initiating intravenous access.
12. Describe the steps for safely initiating an intraosseous (IO) infusion.
13. Explain drug administration techniques for percutaneous routes.
14. Identify special considerations in the administration of pharmacological agents to pediatric patients.
15. Explain the technique for obtaining a venous blood sample.
16. Describe the safe disposal of contaminated items and sharps.

SUMMARY

- Three systems for measuring drug dosage are in use today. These are the metric system, the apothecary system (no longer recommended), and the common household system. Each system deals with units of mass and volume. Any of these three systems may be used by a physician when ordering drugs.
- Paramedics should choose a drug calculation method that is precise. It also should be reliable. Paramedics should
  (1) Convert all units of measure to the same size and system.
  (2) Assess the computed dosage to determine whether it is reasonable.
  (3) Use one method of dose calculation consistently.
- Many drug calculations can be performed almost intuitively. Nevertheless, paramedics should never rely on intuitive calculations. Methods of calculation include the basic formula (desire over have), ratios and proportions, and dimensional analysis.
- Intravenous (IV) flow rates can be calculated using the following formula:

$$\text{Drops/min} = \frac{\text{Volume to be infused} \times \text{Drop/mL of infusion set}}{\text{Total time of infusion (min)}}$$

- Safety procedures should be a high priority during the administration of any medication. Paramedics must make sure the *right* patient receives the *right* dose of the *right* drug via the *right* route at the *right* time.
- A medication error may occur. In such a case, paramedics should take responsibility for their actions. They should quickly advise medical direction. They also should assess and monitor the patient for effects of the drug. They must document the error as required by local, state, and medical direction policies. In addition, they must change their personal practice to prevent a similar error in the future.
- Medical asepsis is accomplished by using clean technique, which involves hygienic measures, cleaning agents, antiseptics, disinfectants, and barrier fields.
- Enteral drugs are administered and absorbed through the gastrointestinal tract. They are given by the oral, gastric, and rectal routes. Parenteral drugs are administered outside the intestine. They are usually injected. Parenteral drugs are given by the intradermal, subcutaneous, intramuscular, IV, and IO routes.

- In the prehospital setting, the route of choice for fluid replacement is through a peripheral vein in an extremity. The over-the-needle catheter generally is preferred in this setting.
- Several possible complications are associated with all IV techniques. These include local complications, systemic complications, infiltration, and air embolism.
- Fluids and drugs that are infused by the IO route pass from the marrow cavities into the sinusoids. Next, they pass into large venous channels and emissary veins. Then they pass into the systemic circulation. The site of choice for IO infusions in children is the tibia, one to two fingerbreadths below the tubercle on the anteromedial surface. Other sites for IO infusions include the distal tibia, humerus, and sternum (adults).
- Percutaneous drugs are absorbed through the mucous membranes or skin. These include topical drugs, sublingual drugs, buccal drugs, inhaled drugs, endotracheal drugs, nasal drugs and drugs for the eye and ear.
- Administering drugs to infants and children can be quite difficult. This often is especially true in emergency situations. Paramedics frequently calculate pediatric drug doses by using memory aids. Some of these aids include charts, tapes, and dosage books. Doses also are calculated with the advice of medical direction.
- If possible, venous blood samples should be obtained when IV access is established. They also should be obtained before any fluids are infused. If no IV line is to be used and a blood sample is still needed, it must be obtained with a needle and syringe (or a special vacuum needle and sleeve).
- The Centers for Disease Control and Prevention recommends that needles not be capped, bent, or broken before disposal. Rather, they should be left on the syringe and discarded in an appropriate, clearly marked container that is puncture proof and leak proof.

MATH SKILLS

The following questions present a brief review of basic math skills necessary for drug dose calculation. The review is intended as a refresher. If the student does not understand these concepts, the student should consult references or seek tutoring before proceeding to the next section.

FRACTIONS

A fraction is part of a whole number or one number divided by another number. A fraction consists of two parts, the numerator and the denominator:

$$\frac{a}{b} \quad \frac{a \text{ is the numerator}}{b \text{ is the denominator}}$$

The denominator indicates the number of equal parts into which the whole is separated. The numerator tells how many parts are being considered (Fig. 14-1).

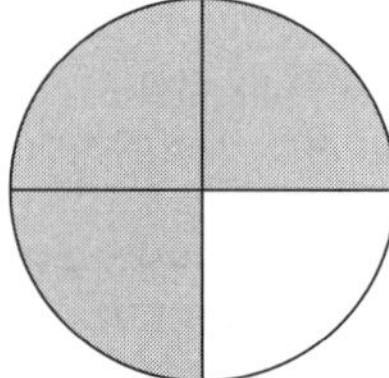

Figure 14-1

Example: $\frac{3}{4}$ $\dfrac{\text{Numerator is 3, so three parts are being used}}{\text{Denominator is 4. There are four equal parts}}$

A fraction that has the same numerator and denominator equals the whole number 1 (Fig. 14-2).

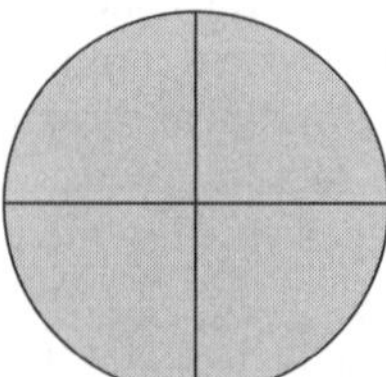

Figure 14-2

Example: $\frac{4}{4} = 1$

184

1. Identify the numerator and denominator of the following fractions.

   a. Example: $\dfrac{7}{8}$ = ——————   b. Example: $\dfrac{6}{13}$ = ——————

   When the numerator and denominator of the fraction are multiplied by the same number, the value of the fraction remains unchanged.

   Example: $\dfrac{1 \times 2}{2 \times 2} = \dfrac{2}{4} = \dfrac{1}{2}$

   A fraction may be reduced to lower terms by dividing the numerator and denominator by the largest whole number that will go evenly into both of them.

   Example: $\dfrac{100}{1000} \times \dfrac{100}{1000} \div \dfrac{100}{1000} = \dfrac{1}{10}$

2. Reduce the following fractions to lowest terms.

a. $\frac{7}{28}$	**d.** $\frac{6}{36}$	**g.** $\frac{24}{120}$	**j.** $\frac{10}{25}$
b. $\frac{9}{12}$	**e.** $\frac{25}{125}$	**h.** $\frac{9}{25}$	**k.** $\frac{17}{23}$
c. $\frac{4}{8}$	**f.** $\frac{18}{72}$	**i.** $\frac{1000}{10,000}$	**l.** $\frac{16}{24}$

   An improper fraction has a larger numerator than denominator.

   Example: $\dfrac{8}{4}$

   To change an improper fraction to a whole number, divide the numerator by the denominator:

   Example: $\frac{8}{4} = 8 \div 4 = 2$ (Whole number)
   $\qquad\quad \frac{7}{4} = 7 \div 4 = 1\frac{3}{4}$ (This is a mixed number because it has a whole number plus a fraction.)

3. Convert the following to whole numbers or mixed fractions.
   a. $\frac{75}{5}$ **b.** $\frac{24}{12}$ **c.** $\frac{12}{4}$ **d.** $\frac{15}{6}$

   To change a mixed number into an improper fraction, multiply the whole number by the denominator of the fraction and add the numerator of the fraction to the result.

   Example: $4\frac{1}{2} = \dfrac{(4 \times 2) + 1}{2} = \dfrac{9}{2}$

4. Change each of the following mixed numbers to improper fractions:
   a. $5\frac{3}{8}$ **b.** $1\frac{3}{4}$ **c.** $3\frac{1}{12}$ **d.** $1\frac{2}{3}$

   To change a fraction to equivalent fractions in which both terms are larger, multiply the numerator and denominator by the same number.

   Example: Enlarge $\frac{2}{5}$ to the equivalent fraction in tenths.

   $$\dfrac{2}{5} \times \dfrac{2}{2} = \dfrac{4}{10}$$

5. Change the following fractions to the equivalent fraction indicated.

   a. $\dfrac{6}{8} = \dfrac{x}{24}$ **b.** $\dfrac{12}{15} = \dfrac{x}{60}$ **c.** $\dfrac{79}{100} = \dfrac{x}{100,00}$

   To compare fractions with different denominators, find the lowest common denominator. The lowest common denominator is the smallest number that is divisible by the denominators.

   Example 1: What is the lowest common denominator of $\frac{1}{2}$, $\frac{3}{5}$, and $\frac{7}{10}$?

   The denominators are 2, 5, and 10. Because 10 is divisible by 2 and 5, it is the lowest common denominator.

     Chapter **14** **Venous Access and Medication Administration**

Example 2: What is the lowest common denominator of ⅓ and ⅖? Because 5 is not divisible by 3, multiply the larger denominator by 2, 3, 4, and so on. Each time, determine whether the product is divisible by 3:

$5 \times 2 = 10$ 10 is not divisible by 3.
$5 \times 3 = 15$ 15 is divisible by 3, so 15 is the lowest common denominator.

6. Find the lowest common denominator.
    a. ⅑ and ⅕   **b.** ⅔ and 1/12   **c.** ⅓, 2/6 and ⅜

7. Circle the correct response:
    a. ⅜ is greater than, less than, or equal to 9/24.
    b. 8/9 is greater than, less than, or equal to ⅝.
    c. ⅖ is greater than, less than, or equal to 7/10.

To add or subtract fractions, do the following:

1. Convert all fractions to equivalent fractions using the lowest common denominator.
2. Add or subtract the numerator and place over the common denominator.
3. Simplify to the lowest terms.

Example: $\dfrac{5}{9} + \dfrac{2}{6} = \dfrac{5(2)}{9(2)} + \dfrac{2(3)}{6(3)} = \dfrac{10}{18} + \dfrac{6}{18} \div \dfrac{2}{2} = \dfrac{8}{9}$

8. Add the following fractions and mixed numbers:
    a. ⅞ + ⅖ + 1/10   **b.** 1¼ + 2 ⅔

9. Subtract the following fractions and mixed numbers:
    a. 1⅗ − 6/10   **b.** 2¾ − ⅚

To multiply fractions, do the following:

1. Change mixed numbers to improper fractions.
2. Multiply numerators.
3. Multiply denominators.
4. Simplify to the lowest terms.

Example: $\dfrac{3}{4} \times \dfrac{4}{5} = \dfrac{12}{20} \div \dfrac{4}{4} = \dfrac{3}{5}$

10. Multiply the following fractions and mixed numbers:
    a. 5/16 × 11/13   **c.** 6⅞ × 2
    b. 8½ × 3   **d.** ⅓ × ⅞

To divide fractions, do the following:

1. Change mixed numbers to improper fractions.
2. Turn the number after the division sign (÷) upside down.
3. Follow the steps for multiplication of fractions.
4. Simplify to the lowest terms.

Example: $\dfrac{4}{5} \div \dfrac{2}{3} = \dfrac{4}{5} \times \dfrac{3}{2} = \dfrac{12}{10} \div \dfrac{2}{2} = \dfrac{6}{5} = 1\tfrac{1}{5}$

11. Divide the following fractions:
    a. ⅜ ÷ 3/10   **b.** 2½ ÷ 7/11

186

All whole numbers are to the left of the decimal; all decimal fractions are to the right of the decimal (Fig. 14-3).

12. Write the decimal notation for the following examples:
    a. 3 and 4 tenths   **b.** 5 and 35 hundredths   **c.** 62 thousandths

To convert a fraction into a decimal, do the following:

  1. Divide the numerator by the denominator.
  2. Place the decimal point in the proper position.

$$\text{Example:} \frac{3}{5} = 3 \div 5 = 5 \overline{) 0.3}^{\,0.6}$$

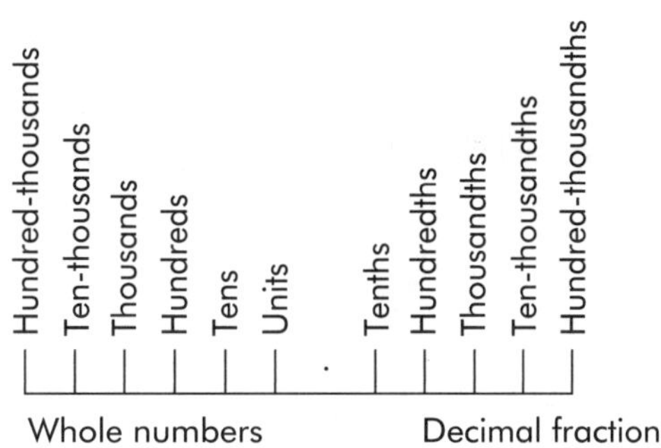

Figure 14-3

13. Change the following fractions to decimals:
    a. $\frac{1}{4}$ **b.** $\frac{7}{25}$ **c.** $\frac{3}{150}$

To convert a decimal to a fraction, do the following:

  1. Write the numerator of the fraction as the numbers expressed in the decimal.
  2. Write the denominator of the fraction as the number 1 followed by the number of zeros as there are places to the right of the decimal point.
  3. Simplify the fraction to the lowest terms.

    Example: 0.234 = x
    Numerator = 234
    Denominator = 1 + three zeros = 1000
    Simplify: $\frac{234}{1000} = \frac{234}{1000} \div \frac{2}{2} = \frac{117}{500}$

14. Change the following decimals to fractions.
    a. 0.5   **b.** 3.24   **c.** 6.007

To add or subtract decimals, do the following:

  1. Line up the decimal points.
  2. Add zeros to make all decimal numbers equal length.
  3. Add or subtract as with whole numbers.
  4. Place the decimal point in the sum.

Example: 0.6 + 4.23 + 1.123 = x

Line up the decimal points:	0.6
	4.23
	<u>1.123</u>
Add zeros:	0.600
	4.230
	<u>1.123</u>
Add as whole numbers:	<u>5.953</u>

Place the decimal point in the sum.

15. Add the following decimals.
    a. 0.03 + 0.12 + 0.32   **b.** 0.26 + 0.01 + 0.75

16. Subtract the following decimals.
    a. 91.5 − 62.5   **b.** 17 − 3.42

To multiply decimals, do the following:

1. Multiply as with whole numbers.
2. Count the total number of decimal places in the decimals multiplied.
3. Place the decimal point in the answer to the left of the total decimal places calculated in step 2.
4. When multiplying a decimal by a power of 10, move the decimal point the same number of places to the right as there are zeros in the multiplier.

Example: $1.25 \times 3.3 = x$
1.25   (two decimal places)
× 3.3   (one decimal place)

4.125   (The decimal point is placed to the left of three decimal places.)

Example: $3.46 \times 10 = 3.4.6 = 34.6$

17. Multiply the following decimals.
    a. 3.62×0.02 **c.** 7.25×0.03 **e.** 2.9×10
    b. 27×0.04 **d.** 4.256×100 **f.** 7.052×1000

To divide decimals, do the following:

1. If the divisor (number you are dividing by) is a whole number, divide as you would with whole numbers. Place the decimal place in the answer in the same place it was in the number to be divided.
2. If the divisor (number you are dividing by) is a decimal, make it a whole number by moving the decimal place to the end of the divisor. Move the decimal in the number being divided by the same number of places.
3. If the divisor is a power of 10, move the decimal point to the left as many places as there are zeros in the divisor.

Example: $25.5 \div 5 = 5\overline{)25.5} = 5.1$

Example: $25.5 \div 0.5 = 0.5\overline{)25.5} = 5\overline{)255} = 51$

Example: $25.5 \div 10 = 2.55\ (2.5.5)$

18. Divide the following.
    a. $0.25 \div 5$ **d.** $0.16 \div 0.04$
    b. $5.16 \div 2$ **e.** $14.237 \div 100$
    c. $4 \div 0.5$ **f.** $0.17 \div 10$

Rounding decimal fractions: Most drug calculations require rounding to the hundredth or greater. This depends on the individual example. To round off, consider the number in the next position to the right. If the number is greater than or equal to 5, increase the number being considered by 1. If it is less than 5, do not increase the number being considered.

Example: Round off 0.74 to the nearest tenths. Because the number in the hundredths column is less than 5, the answer will be 0.7.

Example: Round off 0.24555 to the nearest hundredths. Because the number in the thousandths column is 5, the answer will be 0.25.

19. Round off the following examples to the nearest tenth:
    a. 7.6245   **b.** 0.081   **c.** 0.851

20. Round off the following examples to the nearest hundredth:
    a. 0.10423   **b.** 5.6258   **c.** 892.02975

RATIOS

Ratios indicate the relationship of one quantity to another. They indicate division and may be expressed as the following:

$\frac{a}{b}$, a to b, or a:b

Example: Five gallons of gas for $6 means the ratio of gas to dollars is as follows:

$\frac{5}{6}$, 5 to 6, or 5:6

21. Write the ratio for the following examples.
   a. The heart ejects approximately 5000 mL of blood every 60 seconds.
   b. Approximately 6000 mL of air is moved in and out of the lungs every 60 seconds.
   c. The intravenous line delivers 100 mL every 30 minutes.
   d. There are 100 mg of the drug in 10 mL of solution.

To simplify a ratio that compares two measures, divide the denominator into the numerator to calculate the unit rate.

Example: On a routine transfer, we traveled 120 miles in 2 hours.

The unit rate $= \dfrac{120 \text{ miles}}{2 \text{ hours}} = 60$ miles per hour

The unit rate is 60 miles per hour.

22. Calculate the unit rate for each of the following (based on the examples in Question 21).
   a. How many milliliters of blood are ejected from the heart each second?
   b. How much air is moved in and out of the lungs each second?
   c. How much fluid is being delivered each minute?
   d. How many milligrams are in each milliliter?

A proportion shows the relationship between two different ratios. To determine whether a proportion is true (equivalent), do the following:

1. If the proportion is expressed as a fraction (1/2 = 2/4), multiply the cross products and then determine whether the proportion is equivalent.

   Example: $\dfrac{1}{2} = \dfrac{2}{4} = \dfrac{1}{2} \bullet \dfrac{2}{4} = 1 \times 4 = 4$ and $2 \times 2 = 4$;

   $4 = 4$; therefore the proportion is true.

2. If the proportion is expressed as a ratio (2:5::4:10), multiply the two inside numbers ($5 \times 4 = 20$) and the two outside numbers ($2 \times 10 = 20$); $20 = 20$; therefore the proportion is equivalent.

23. Determine whether each of the following proportions is true:

   a. $\dfrac{5}{10} = \dfrac{1}{2}$ **b.** $\dfrac{4}{6} = \dfrac{8}{10}$ **c.** $\dfrac{25}{75} = \dfrac{1}{3}$

To solve a proportion problem when one of the numbers is unknown (x), do the following:
1. Use either proportion method demonstrated previously.
2. Make x stand alone by dividing both sides of the equation by the number on the side of x.
3. Solve for x.

   Example: $\dfrac{17}{20} = \dfrac{x}{100}$ $2x = 17 \times 100 = \dfrac{20x}{20} = \dfrac{17 \times 100}{20}$

   $$x = \dfrac{17 \times 100}{20}$$

   $$x = 85$$

   Example: $20x = 17 \times 100$

   $$\dfrac{20x}{20} = \dfrac{17 \times 100}{20}$$

      Chapter **14** **Venous Access and Medication Administration**

24. Solve for x in the following problems:

   a. $\frac{2}{4} = \frac{x}{6}$ **c.** $\frac{2}{3} = \frac{7}{x}$ **e.** $3:5::x:45$ **g.** $x:35::80:100$

   b. $\frac{1}{4} = \frac{x}{16}$ **d.** $\frac{5}{4} = \frac{x}{12}$ **f.** $4:9::16:x$ **h.** $1.5:3::x:18$

Simplifying a problem by cancelling common elements will make problem solving easier.

Example: $x = \dfrac{12 \times 10}{20} = 6$ Zeros cancel. Then 2 divides into 12 six times

Example: $x = \dfrac{1\,mg \times 1\,mL}{1\,mg} = 1\,mL.$ The mg in the numerator cancels mg in the

     denominator. 1 mL is left.

25. Simplify the following problems as much as possible and then solve.

   a. $x = \dfrac{10 \times 150}{550}$

   b. $x = \dfrac{25 \times 2}{50}$

   c. $x = \dfrac{2500 \times 500}{20{,}000}$

   d. $x = \dfrac{1g \times 1L}{1\,g}$

   e. $x = \dfrac{2\,mg \times 1\,mL}{10\,mg}$

   f. $x = \dfrac{10\,mg \times 10\,mL}{100\,mg}$

Percentages

Percent (%) is a portion of a whole divided by 100.

1. To change a percent to a decimal, drop the percent sign and move the decimal two places to the left.
   Example: $15.0\% = 0.15$

2. To change a decimal to a percent, move the decimal two places to the right and add the percent sign.
   Example: $0.76 = 76\%$

3. To change a fraction to a percent, convert it to a decimal and follow rule 2.
   Example: $\frac{1}{5} = 0.2 \quad 0.2 = 20\%$

26. Change the following percentages to decimals.

   a. 25%   **b.** 110%   **c.** 0.5%

27. Convert the following decimals to percentages.

   a. 0.34   **b.** 2.29   **c.** 0.07

28. Express the following as percentages:

   a. $\frac{34}{50}$ **b.** $\frac{100}{500}$ **c.** $\frac{3}{7}$

29. Rewrite the following fractions as ratios, decimals, and percentages:

Fraction	Ratio	Decimal	Percentage
a. $\frac{5}{6}$			
b. $\frac{1}{20}$			
c. $\frac{7}{33}$			

30. Solve the following:
    a. 15% of 75   **b.** 0.5% of 250
This concludes the refresher.

MATHEMATICAL EQUIVALENTS AND DRUG DOSE CALCULATIONS

31. In the metric system, the primary unit of volume is the **(a)** ____________, the primary unit of mass (weight) is the

(b) ____________, and the primary unit of length is the **(c)** ____________.

32. List the four metric mass units commonly used in the prehospital environment, beginning with the largest and ending with the smallest.

a. ____

b. ____

c. ____

d. ____

33. Each of the units listed in Question 32 differs in value from the next unit by ____________________.

34. To convert from one unit to the next smallest unit in Question 32, you must move the decimal point three places to

the right or left? ____________________

35. To convert from one unit to the previous unit (example unit 32d to unit 32c), you must move the decimal point

three places to the right or left? ____________________

36. Convert the following units of mass to the units indicated.

    a. 2 kg = ____________ g   **e.** 400 mcg = ____________ mg
    b. 4 mg = ____________ mcg   **f.** 350 mg = ____________ g
    c. 2 g = ____________ mg   **g.** 0.25 mg = ____________ mcg
    d. 600 mg = ____________ kg   **h.** 12.5 g = ____________ mg

37. Convert the following units of volume to the units indicated.

    a. 1 cc = ____________ mL   **c.** 250 mL = ____________ L
    b. 10 mL = ____________ cc   **d.** 0.33 L = ____________ mL

38. The primary unit of mass in the apothecary system is the ____________________.

39. The primary unit of volume in the apothecary system is the ____________________.

Chapter **14** **Venous Access and Medication Administration**

40. If the physician orders acetaminophen gr X, how many milligrams will you give? _____________

41. Your patient has chest pain, and medical direction orders nitroglycerin gr 1/150. How many milligrams will you administer?

(a) _______________________________

When it is time for a second nitroglycerin, the patient's blood pressure is slightly low, so this time the physician orders nitroglycerin gr 1/200. How many milligrams will you give?

(b) _______________________________

42. Convert the following measures in the household system to the units indicated:

a. 1 T = _____________________ tsp   **c.** 1 pt = _____________________ oz   **e.** 1 fl oz = _____________________ T

b. 1 lb = _____________________ oz   **d.** 1 gal = _____________________ qt   **f.** 1 c = _____________________ fl oz

43. Convert the following measures in the household system to the appropriate metric units.

a. 1 tsp = _____________ mL   **c.** 1 fl oz = _____________ mL   **e.** 22 lb = _____________ kg

b. 1 T = _____________ mL   **d.** 1 qt = _____________ mL   **f.** 110 lb = _____________ kg

44. Convert the following measures to the appropriate units indicated.

a. A patient's family tells you that he lost about 1 cup of blood from a head wound. You will relay to medical direction that the estimated blood loss is approximately _____________________ mL.

b. A patient vomits about a quart of coffee-grounds emesis. This is equal to _____________________ mL.

c. The patient took 1 oz or _______ mL of antacid. Then she drank 16 oz of milk. This is equal to

_____________________ mL of milk.

d. A parent reads a drug label and, instead of administering 2 mL of a drug, accidentally gives 2 oz of a drug. How many milliliters in excess of the prescribed dose did the parent give?

_____________________ mL

e. The human body normally contains about 5 L of blood, or _____________________ qt.

f. A pregnant woman states that her membranes have ruptured and about 1 pint of amniotic fluid leaked out. This is equal to _____________________ mL.

g. A premature newborn you have just delivered weighs 2 lb, or _____________ kg (_____________ g).

45. Identify the following information from the drug label or package in Fig. 14-4.

a. Drug name: _____________________   **d.** Total drug: _____________
b. Expiration date: _____________________   **e.** Concentration of drug: _____________
c. Total volume: _____________________

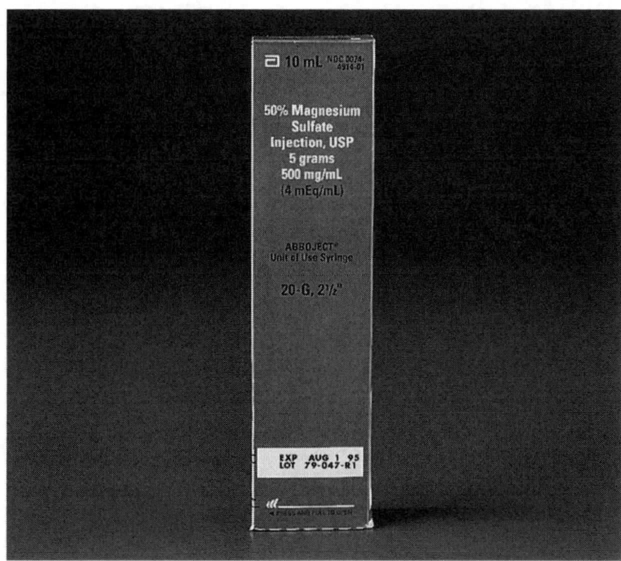

Figure 14-4

46. Convert the following drug concentrations into the total number of grams.

    a. Calcium chloride 10% solution = _________________ g in 100 mL.

    b. Epinephrine 1:1000 solution = _________________ g in 1000 mL.

    c. Magnesium sulfate 10% solution = _________________ g in 100 mL.

    d. Epinephrine 1:10,000 solution = _________________ g in 10,000 mL.

    e. Lidocaine 0.4% solution = _________________ g in 100 mL.

    f. Mannitol 25% solution = _________________ g in 100 mL.

    g. Dextrose 50% solution = _________________ g in 100 mL.

47. Calculate the concentration per milliliter of the following drugs using the following formula: Concentration = Total dose of drug (mg) ÷ Total volume (mL). For example, a 10-mL vial of lidocaine contains 100 mg of the drug. Concentration = 100 mg ÷ 10 mL = 10 mg/ml.

    a. A 40-mg vial of furosemide is in a 4-mL vial. Concentration = _________________ .

    b. A 10-mL vial of epinephrine contains 1 mg of the drug. Concentration = _________________ .

    c. You have 25 g of D50W in 50 mL. Concentration = _________________ .

    d. A 2-mL vial of diphenhydramine contains 50 mg of the drug. Concentration = _________________ .

    e. A 250-mL bag contains 1 g of lidocaine. Concentration = _________________ .

48. Calculate the total dose of a drug to be administered.

    a. Lidocaine 1 mg/kg is ordered for a 100-kg patient who is having many premature ventricular contractions each minute. Dose = _________________ mg.

b. The maximum dose of diltiazem is 0.25 mg/kg and the patient weighs 60 kg. Total dose = _________________ mg.

c. Push sodium bicarbonate 1 mEq/kg during a lengthy cardiac arrest. The patient weighs 80 kg.

Dose = _________________ mEq.

d. Hang a dopamine drip at 5 mcg/kg/min on a hypotensive patient who weighs 50 kg. Dose = _________________ mcg/min.

e. Give epinephrine 0.01 mg/kg to an 11-lb child who is in cardiopulmonary arrest. Dose = _________________ mg.

f. Administer mannitol 1 g/kg to a 176-lb patient with rising intracranial pressure. Dose = _________________ g.

49. Solve the following problems using the following formula:

$$\text{Volume (x)} = \frac{\text{Desired dose (D)} \times \text{Volume on hand (Q)}}{\text{Dose on hand (H)}}$$

a. You wish to give furosemide 20 mg. It is supplied in a 4-mL vial containing 40 mg of the drug.

Volume = _________________ mL.

b. You wish to administer morphine 3 mg. You have a 1-mL pre-filled syringe containing 10 mg of the drug.

Volume = _________________ mL.

c. You wish to give amiodarone 300 mg. You have a 3-mL vial containing 150 mg of the drug.

Volume = _________________ mL.

d. You must give 2.5 mg of diazepam. It is supplied in a 2-mL vial containing 10 mg.

Volume = _________________ mL.

e. You have 50 mg of diphenhydramine in a 1-mL vial. You need to give 12.5 mg of the drug.

Volume = _________________ mL.

f. Your patient needs 0.3 mg of epinephrine (1:1000). You have a 1-mL vial containing 1 mg.

Volume = _________________ mL.

g. Your patient needs 0.5 mg of dopamine. You have a 500-mL bag containing 400 mg of the drug.

Volume = _________________ mL.

50. Solve the following drug dose problems using the following equation:

Desired dose:Desired volume::Dosage on hand:Volume on hand

Example: Give 50 mg of lidocaine. It is supplied in a 10-mL syringe containing 100 mg.

$50 \text{ mg}:x = 100 \text{ mg}:10 \text{ mL}$ Set up the ratio.

$\dfrac{100 \text{ mg} \times x}{100 \text{ mg}} \dfrac{50 \text{ mg} \times 10 \text{ mL}}{100 \text{ mg}}$ Multiply inside (means) and then outside (extremes) numbers.

$x = \dfrac{50 \text{ mg} \times 10 \text{ mL}}{100 \text{ mg}}$ Solve for x.

$x = 5 \text{ mL}$

a. Administer adenosine 6 mg. It is supplied in a 2-mL vial containing 6 mg of the drug.

Desired volume = _________________ mL.

b. Administer diphenhydramine 25 mg. You have a 2-mL vial containing 50 mg of the drug.

Desired volume = ___________________ mL.

c. Give 2.5 mg of verapamil. It is supplied in a 2-mL vial containing 5 mg of the drug.

Desired volume = ___________________ mL.

d. Give 1000 mg of mannitol. You have a 20% solution. Desired volume = ___________________ mL.

51. Calculate the drops per minute needed to deliver the following volumes of fluid over the required time.

a. The physician orders an intravenous fluid to run at 30 mL/hr (drop factor, 60 drops/mL).

Drops/min = ___________________.

b. You want to give a fluid challenge of 200 mL over 20 minutes (drop factor, 10 drops/mL).

Drops/min = ___________________.

c. You need to infuse a drug mixed in 50 mL of fluid over 15 minutes (drop factor, 15 drops/mL).

Drops/min = ___________________.

d. Online medical direction orders 150 mL of lactated Ringer solution to infuse in 2 hours (drop factor, 15 drops/mL). Drops/min = ___________________.

e. You are told to give 275 mL over 2 hours (drop factor, 10 drops/mL). Drops/min = ___________________.

f. The intravenous drug must run in at 0.5 mL/min (drop factor, 60 drops/mL). Drops/min = ___________________.

g. Medical direction advises you to infuse normal saline at 200 mL/hr (drop factor, 10 drops/mL).

Drops/min = ___________________.

h. You have added magnesium sulfate to D5W for a total volume of 100 mL. You must infuse it over 2 minutes to treat your patient's ventricular arrhythmia (drop factor, 10 drops/mL). Drops/min = ___________________.

i. A severely acidotic patient needs bicarbonate. You have added 50 mEq of sodium bicarbonate (50 mL) to 1000 mL of normal saline and are to infuse it over 2 hours (dropfactor, 15 drops/mL). Drops/min =

___________________.

j. You have added 2 mg (2 mL) of epinephrine to a 250-mL bag of normal saline and wish to infuse it at 1 mL/min to your severely bradycardic patient (drop factor, 60 drops/mL). Drops/min = ___________________.

k. Your patient has just converted from ventricular fibrillation. You are hanging a lidocaine drip at 3 mg/min. You have mixed 1 g of lidocaine in 250 mL normal saline. How many drops per minute will you set your IV to deliver the 0.75 mL/min necessary for this dose of drug (drop factor, 60 drops/mL)?

Drops/min = ___________________.

52. Calculate the following problems using any of the methods demonstrated. Ensure that all units are compatible. If the dosage is given in milligrams per kilogram, make the appropriate calculation.

a. You wish to give lidocaine 1 mg/kg to a 75-kg man. The lidocaine is supplied in a 10-mL syringe containing 100 mg of the drug. How many milliliters will you administer?

b. You must give amiodarone 300 mg to a 60-kg woman. You have a 2-mL vial containing 150 mg of the drug. How many mL will you give?

c. You must give 0.5 mg of glucagon to a 90-kg patient. When you mix it up, you have 1 mg in 1 mL of solution. How much will you give?

d. You have 20 mg of etomidate supplied in 10 mL vials. You need to give 0.3 mg/kg. The patient weighs 100 kg. How many mL will you give?

e. You must give 8 mg/kg of calcium chloride. The patient weighs 70 kg. You have a 10% solution. How many milliliters will you give?

f. You need to administer 4 mg of ondansetron. It is supplied in a vial with 2 mg/mL. How many milliliters will you give?

g. Your patient needs a dopamine drip at 5 mcg/kg/min. He weighs 100 kg. You have 400 mg of dopamine in 500 mL of D_5W. How many milliliters per minute will you administer and at how many drops per minute will you set the microdrip intravenous line?

h. You wish to administer a lidocaine drip at 2 mg/min. You have an intravenous bag containing a 0.4% solution of lidocaine. How many milliliters will you give each minute, and how fast will you set your microdrip tubing to deliver this rate?

53. For each of the following situations, calculate the correct volume of solution to be administered using the drug package information illustrated.

a. Give 0.5 mg of atropine (Fig. 14-5). Desired volume = _________________ mL.

b. Give 0.3 mg of epinephrine (Fig. 14-6). Desired volume = _________________ mL.

c. Give lidocaine 0.5 mg/kg to an 80-kg patient (Fig. 14-7). Desired volume = _________________ mL.

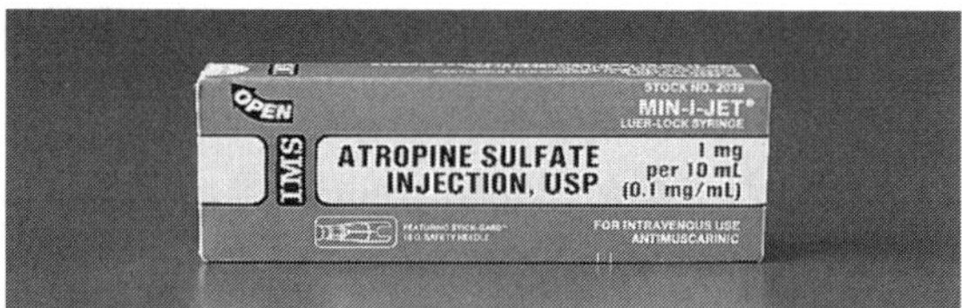

Figure 14-5

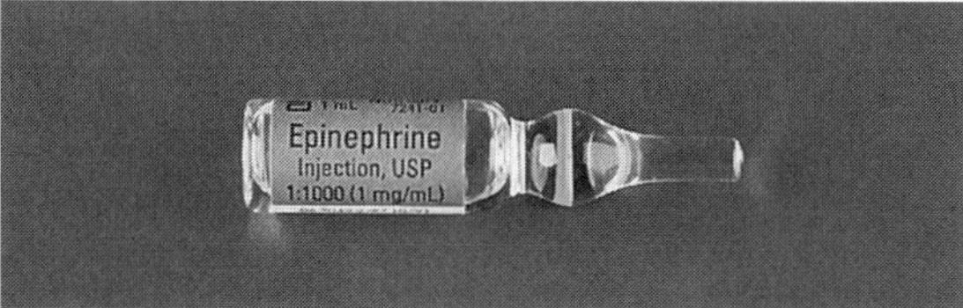

Figure 14-6

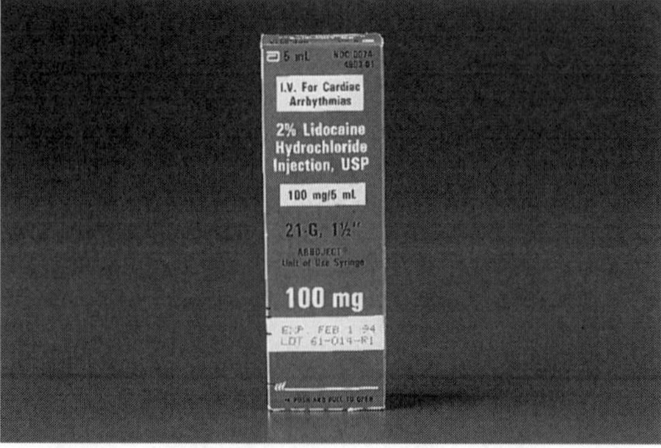

Figure 14-7

54. After determining the correct volume of drug to be administered in the following examples, shade the corresponding syringe in Fig. 14-8 to illustrate the proper amount to be given.

a. Adenosine 6 mg must be given to a patient with paroxysmal supraventricular tachycardia. You have a 2-mL vial containing 3 mg/mL of the drug. How many milliliters will you give?

b. Your patient has had a seizure and needs phenytoin 200 mg. You have a 5-mL vial containing 250 mg of the drug. How much will you give?

c. You have a 10-mL vial of furosemide containing 10 mg/mL of the drug. A total of 70 mg is indicated for your patient, who is in congestive heart failure. What volume will you administer?

d. You wish to administer epinephrine 0.3 mg to a patient experiencing an allergic reaction. The epinephrine is supplied in a 1-mL ampule containing 1 mg of a 1:1000 solution of the drug. How much will you give?

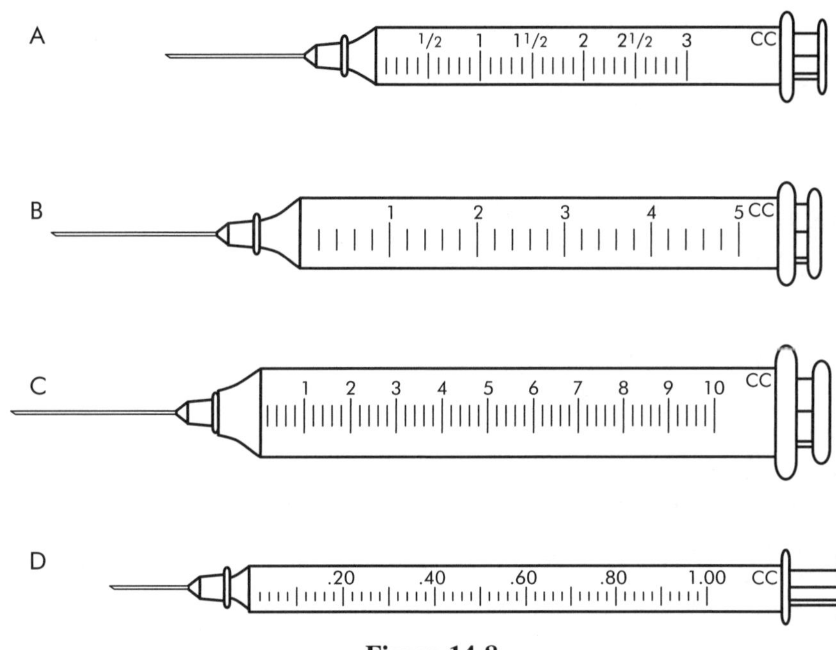

Figure 14-8

DRUG ADMINISTRATION

55. List at least 10 general steps to be taken when administering any drug to avoid errors.

a. ____

b. ____

c. ____

d. ____

e. ____

f. ____

g. ____

h. ____

i. ____

j. ____

56. You intended to deliver the procainamide drip at 1 mL/min during your 15-minute transport, but when you look at the 250-mL bag, the roller clamp has been opened, and almost 150 mL has been infused. List five actions that you should take after this error.

a. ____

b. ____

c. ____

d. ____

e. ____

57. List two methods to ensure medical asepsis when you administer an intramuscular injection.

a. ____

b. ____

58. Complete the following sentences regarding drug administration routes:

Oral medications should be given with the patient in the **(a)** _______________ position. The drug should be swallowed with **(b)** _______________ oz of fluid to ensure that it reaches the **(c)** _______________. Sublingual medications should be placed under the **(d)** _______________ and allowed to **(e)** _______________. They should not be **(f)** _____ because this will delay action of the drug. Parenteral drug administration may cause **(g)** _______________, **(h)** _______________, or **(i)** _______________. The correct needle length and size are important. For subcutaneous injections a **(j)** _______________-inch, **(k)** _______________ -gauge needle should be used. When administering an intramuscular injection, you should select a **(l)** _______________-inch, **(m)** _______________-gauge needle. To minimize the risk of needle-stick injury, you should understand that the use of two-handed needle recapping is **(n)** _______________. Also, all sharp items, including needles, should be placed in **(o)** _______________. When withdrawing medication from a multidose vial, you should cleanse the stopper with alcohol and then inject the same amount of **(p)** _______________ as drug to be withdrawn before aspirating the appropriate amount of medicine into the syringe. To minimize the risk of glass particles entering the injection when aspirating from a glass ampule, use a **(q)** _______________. Subcutaneous injections should be administered at a **(r)** _______________-degree angle. Sites of administration for this route include **(s)** _______________, _______________, and _______________. Intramuscular injections should be administered at a **(t)** _____-degree angle. Administration sites for this route include the **(u)** _______________ and _______________. To prevent drug effects on the rescuer, you should always wear **(v)** _______________ when administering transdermal medicines. Dilution with at least **(w)** _______________ mL of fluid is recommended to ensure maximum absorption of drugs administered by the endotracheal route. Two advantages of drugs administered by inhalation are **(x)** _______________ and fewer _______________.

59. List three complications of intravenous line placement for each of the following approaches:

a. Peripheral site: ____

b. Internal jugular and subclavian sites: ____

c. Femoral site: ____

60. You respond to care for a 3-year-old child who is in cardiac arrest. Attempts to intubate and secure intravenous access are unsuccessful, so you elect to attempt intraosseous infusion. After applying gloves and preparing your equipment, you select the preferred site, located **(a)** _______________. Then you use a syringe filled with **(b)** _______________ to ensure that free flow occurs without resistance. If you detect correct placement, you connect the **(c)** _______________ and infuse the drug at the appropriate rate. To prevent the needle from being dislodged, you should **(d)** _______________ the needle.

STUDENT SELF-ASSESSMENT

61. Your patient's mother states that her child's temperature is 38.5°C. What is her temperature in degrees Fahrenheit?
- **a.** 69.9
- **b.** 99.6
- **c.** 101.3
- **d.** 103.6

62. You must administer a drug that is calculated based on milligrams per kilogram. The patient tells you that he weighs 144 lb. How many kilograms does that convert to (rounded to the nearest kilogram)?
- **a.** 65
- **b.** 72
- **c.** 80
- **d.** 86

63. You wish to administer calcium chloride 10 mg/kg to a 100-kg woman. You have a 10% solution of the drug. How many milliliters will you give?
- **a.** 1
- **b.** 10
- **c.** 100
- **d.** 1000

64. You are going to give epinephrine 0.01 mg/kg to a 6-kg child. The epinephrine is supplied as 1 mg in a 10-mL syringe. How many milliliters will you administer?
- **a.** 0.006
- **b.** 0.06
- **c.** 0.6
- **d.** 6.0

65. Which syringe will you use to withdraw the drug volume that you calculated in Question 64?
- **a.** 1 mL
- **b.** 3 mL
- **c.** 5 mL
- **d.** 10 mL

66. Which measure should be taken to ensure safe administration of drugs?
- **a.** Learn a rapid dose calculation method you can always perform in your head.
- **b.** Set unlabeled syringes in a consistent place so you will know what is in them.
- **c.** Verify the label of the drug selected once before administration.
- **d.** Monitor the patient closely for drug effects for the first 5 minutes after you give them.

67. Your patient suddenly vomits and has chest pain after you administer epinephrine intravenously instead of subcutaneously as ordered for his anaphylaxis. How should this be recorded in the patient care report?
- **a.** Document the correct route only.
- **b.** Document the route ordered and the incorrect route.
- **c.** Document the incorrect route only.
- **d.** Omit the route in the report.

68. What parenteral route would you use to test for allergies?
   a. Intradermal
   b. Intramuscular
   c. Intravenous
   d. Subcutaneous

69. Which muscle is preferred for an intramuscular injection in a 2-year-old child?
   a. Deltoid
   b. Dorsogluteal site
   c. Ventrogluteal site
   d. Vastus lateralis

70. You suspect that your patient has a ruptured ectopic pregnancy. She is in profound shock. Which intravenous catheter will you select?
   a. 14 gauge, 1½ inch
   b. 14 gauge, 3 inch
   c. 18 gauge, 1½ inch
   d. 18 gauge, 3 inch

71. You are transferring a patient with a jugular central line. Suddenly, the patient becomes unconscious, cyanotic, and tachycardic. You note that the intravenous tubing has been disconnected from the central line catheter. How should you position the patient?
   a. Left side with his head down
   b. Left side with his head up
   c. Right side with his head down
   d. Right side with his head up

72. You wish to administer normal saline intravenously at 30 mL/hr. The infusion set delivers 60 drops/mL. How fast will you run it?
   a. 1 drop/min
   b. 30 drops/min
   c. 100 drops/min
   d. 400 drops/min

73. A 200-mL fluid challenge is to be infused over 15 minutes. The drop factor is 10 drops/mL. How fast will you run it?
   a. 35 drops/min
   b. 75 drops/min
   c. 133 drops/min
   d. 150 drops/min

74. Which of the following statements is true regarding intraosseous infusion?
   a. It generally is recommended for children between 1 and 3 years of age.
   b. It is associated with a risk of air embolism if the tubing is disconnected.
   c. Absorption of drugs is irregular and slow through this route.
   d. The procedure should be considered only in critically ill patients.

75. Which of the following is true regarding sublingual drug administration?
   a. The patient may have a sip of water after administration.
   b. This route should not be used if the patient is nauseated.
   c. The drug should be permitted to dissolve under the tongue.
   d. Swallowing the drug will increase its effects.

76. When administering medication into a 2-year old child's ear, you should pull the ear
   a. Down and back
   b. Down and forward
   c. Up and back
   d. Up and forward

77. Which is true regarding administration of medication to young children?
   a. Tell the child to cry and make noise.
   b. Avoid any physical restraint.
   c. Give injections slowly and firmly.
   d. Be honest about painful techniques.

78. Which of the following describes an appropriate procedure for obtaining a blood sample for glucose on an adult patient?
   a. Disconnect the intravenous infusion and withdraw the blood sample.
   b. Insert the intraosseoous needle, flush with normal saline, attach a syringe, and pull back.
   c. Enter the vein with a 24-gauge needle attached to a syringe and withdraw.
   d. Push blood collection tubes into the barrel of the vacutainer and allow it to fill.

You are dispatched to a school for an allergic reaction. On arrival, you find a 66-lb 7-year-old who was stung by a bee and is having an anaphylactic reaction. She has hives, her eyes are swollen, and she is wheezing. You and your partner apply oxygen, and you draw up and administer epinephrine 0.5 mg intramuscularly, give diphenhydramine (1.25 mg/kg) intramuscularly (you carry 50-mg/mL vials), and give albuterol by nebulizer treatment. You initiate an IV and reevaluate her vital signs. Her wheezing has cleared almost completely, and the hives are beginning to dissipate, but she is anxious and tachycardic. Your partner asks how much epinephrine you gave, and you realize that you administered a dose in excess of the 0.01 mL/kg (1:1000) maximum 0.3 mL indicated in your protocol.

1. Convert this child's weight to the metric system. ____________________

2. a. Compute the correct dose of epinephrine that should have been given. ____________________

   b. How much did you overdose or underdose this patient? ____________________

3. a. Compute the correct dose of diphenhydramine. ____________________

   b. How many milliliters should be administered? ____________________

   c. In what location should the intramuscular injection of diphenhydramine be given? ____________________

4. What steps should have been taken before giving the drugs to ensure safe administration? (Five rights of drug administration) ____________________

5. Now that you recognize an error has been made, what should you do? ____________________

6. Fill in the information missing in the table:

Injection Site	Angle of Administration	Max. Volume to be Given
Intradermal		
Subcutaneous		
Intramuscular		

7. Which of the following is true regarding vascular access on this child?
   a. Aseptic technique should be followed.
   b. The external jugular would be the initial site of choice.
   c. Intraosseous infusion should be used.
   d. Vascular access is not needed in this situation.

8. Describe the procedure for administration of nebulized albuterol by aerosol mask.

____

VENOUS ACCESS AND MEDICATION ADMINISTRATION

1. a. 7 is the numerator; 8 is the denominator.
   b. 6 is the numerator; 13 is the denominator.

2. a. $\frac{1}{4}$; b. $\frac{3}{4}$; c. $\frac{1}{2}$; d. $\frac{1}{6}$; e. $\frac{1}{5}$; f. $\frac{1}{4}$; g. $\frac{1}{5}$; h. $\frac{9}{25}$; i. $\frac{1}{10}$; j. $\frac{2}{5}$; k. $\frac{17}{23}$; l. $\frac{2}{3}$

3. a. 15; b. 2; c. 3; d. 2 $\frac{1}{2}$

4. a. 4 $\frac{3}{8}$; b. $\frac{7}{4}$; c. 3 $\frac{7}{12}$; d. 4 $\frac{7}{3}$

5. a. $\frac{18}{24}$; b. $\frac{48}{60}$; c. $\frac{79,000}{100,000}$

6. a. 45; b. 12; c. 24

7. a. Equal to; b. Greater than; c. Less than

8. a. $\frac{13}{8}$; b. 1 $\frac{1}{12}$

9. a. 1; b. 1 $\frac{11}{12}$

10. a. $\frac{55}{208}$; b. 25 $\frac{1}{2}$; c. 13 $\frac{3}{4}$; d. $\frac{7}{24}$

11. a. $\frac{11}{4}$; b. 3 $\frac{13}{14}$

12. a. 3.4; b. 5.35; c. 0.062

13. a. 0.25; b. 0.28; c. 0.02

14. a. $\frac{1}{2}$; b. $\frac{36}{25}$; c. $\frac{67}{1000}$

15. a. 0.47; b. 1.02

16. a. 29; b. 13.58

17. a. 0.0724; b. 1.08; c. 0.2175; d. 425.6; e. 29; f. 7052

18. a. 0.05; b. 2.58; c. 8; d. 4.0; e. 0.14237; f. 0.017

19. a. 7.6; b. 0.1; c. 0.9

20. a. 0.10; b. 5.63; c. 892.03

21. a. 5000:60 (5000 mL:60 seconds); b. 6000:60 (6000 mL:60 seconds); c. 100:30 (100 mL:30 minutes);
    d. 100:10 (100 mg:10 mL)

22. a. 83 mL/sec; b. 100 mL/sec; c. 3 mL/min; d. 10 mg/mL

23. a. True; b. Not true; c. True

24. a. x = 3; b. x = 4; c. x = 10.5; d. x = 15; e. x = 27; f. x = 36; g. x = 28; h. x = 9

25. a. $x = \dfrac{10 \times 150}{50} = \dfrac{\cancel{10} \times \cancel{150}^{30}}{50} = 30$

b. $x = \dfrac{25 \times 2}{50} = \dfrac{{}^{1}\cancel{25} \times \cancel{2}^{1}}{50^{1}} = 1$

c. $x = \dfrac{2500 \times 500}{20{,}000} = \dfrac{\cancel{2500} \times \cancel{500}}{\cancel{20{,}000}} = \dfrac{125}{2}$

d. $x = \dfrac{1\,g \times 1\,L}{1\,g} = \dfrac{\cancel{1\,g} \times 1\,L}{\cancel{1\,g}} = 1\,L$

e. $x = \dfrac{2\,mg \times 1\,mL}{10\,mg} = \dfrac{\cancel{2\,mg} \times 1\,mL}{{}^{5}10\,mg} = \dfrac{1\,mL}{5} = 0.2\,mL$

f. $x = \dfrac{10\,mg \times 10\,mL}{100\,mg} = \dfrac{\cancel{10\,mg} \times \cancel{10\,mL}}{\cancel{100\,mg}} = 1\,mL$

26. a. 0.25; b. 1.1; c. 0.005

27. a. 34%; b. 229%; c. 7%

28. a. 68%; b. 20%; c. 43%

29.

Fraction	Ratio	Decimal	Percentage
a. 5/6	5:6 or 5 to 6	0.83	83%
b. 1/20	1:20 or 1 to 20	0.05	5%
c. 7/33	7:33 or 7 to 33	0.21	21%

30. a. 11.25; b. 1.25

31. a. Liter; b. gram; c. meter
(Objective 1)

32. Kilogram (kg), gram (g), milligram (mg), and microgram (mcg)
(Objective 1)

33. 1000
(Objective 1)

34. Right
(Objective 1)

35. Left
(Objective 1)

36. a. 2000 g; b. 4000 mcg; c. 2000 mg; d. 0.0006 kg; e. 0.4 mg; f. 0.35 g; g. 250 mcg; h. 12,500 mg
(Objective 1)

37. a. 1; b. 10; c. 0.25; d. 330
(Objective 1)

38. Grain (gr)
(Objective 1)

39. Minim
(Objective 1)

40. 600 mg
(Objective 1)

41. a. 0.4 mg; b. 0.3 mg
(Objective 1)

42. a. 3; b. 16; c. 16; d. 4; e. 2; f. 8
(Objective 1)

43. a. 5; b. 15: c. 30; d. 960; e. 10; f. 50
(Objective 1)

44. a. 240; b. 960; c. 30; 480; d. 58; e. 5.2; f. 480; g. 0.9 and 900
(Objective 1)

45. a. Magnesium sulfate; b. Aug. 1, 1995; c. 10 mL; d. 5g; e. 500 mg/mL (4 mEq/mL)
(Objective 2)

46. a. 10; b. 1; c. 10; d. 1; e. 0.4; f. 25; g. 50
(Objective 2)

47. a. 40 mg/4 mL = 10 mg/mL; b. 1 mg/10 mL = 0.1 mg/mL; c. 25 g/50 mL = 25,000 mg/50 mL = 500 mg/mL;
d. 50 mg/2 mL = 25 mg/mL; e. 1 g/250 mL = 1000 mg/250 mL = 4 mg/mL
(Objective 2)

48. a. 100; b. 15; c. 80; d. 250; e. 0.05 (Do not forget to convert to kilograms.); f. 80
(Objective 2)

49. a. $x = \dfrac{20\,mg \times 4\,mL}{40\,mg} = 2\,mL$

b. $x = \dfrac{3\,mg \times 1\,mL}{10\,mg} = 0.3\,mL$

c. $x = \dfrac{300\,mg \times 3\,mL}{150\,mg} = 6\,mL$

d. $x = \dfrac{2.5\,mg \times 2\,mL}{10\,mg} = 0.5\,mL$

e. $x = \dfrac{12.5\,mg \times 1\,mL}{50\,mg} = 0.25\,mL$

f. $x = \dfrac{0.3\,mg \times 1\,mL}{1\,mg} = 0.3\,mL$

g. $x = \dfrac{0.5\,mg \times 500\,mL}{400\,mg} = 0.625\,mL$

(Objective 3)

50. a. 6 mg:x::6 mg:2 mL

$x \times 6\,mg = 6\,mg \times 2\,mL$

$\dfrac{x \times 6\,mg}{6\,mg} = \dfrac{6\,mg \times 2\,mL}{6\,mg}$

$x = 2\,mL$

b. 1 mL

c. 1 mL

d. 1 g:x::20 g:100 mL, x = 5 mL

(Objective 3)

51. a. 30; b. 100; c. 50; d. 19; e. 23; f. 30 g. 33; h. 500; i. 130; j. 60; k. 45
(Objective 4)

52. a. 7.5 mL; b. 4.0 mL; c. 0.5 mL; d. 15 mL; e. 5.6 mL; f. 2 mL; g. 0.625 mL and 38 gtt/min; h. 0.5 mL and 30 gtt/min
(Objectives 3, 4)

53. a. 5; b. 0.3; c. 2.0
(Objective 3)

54.

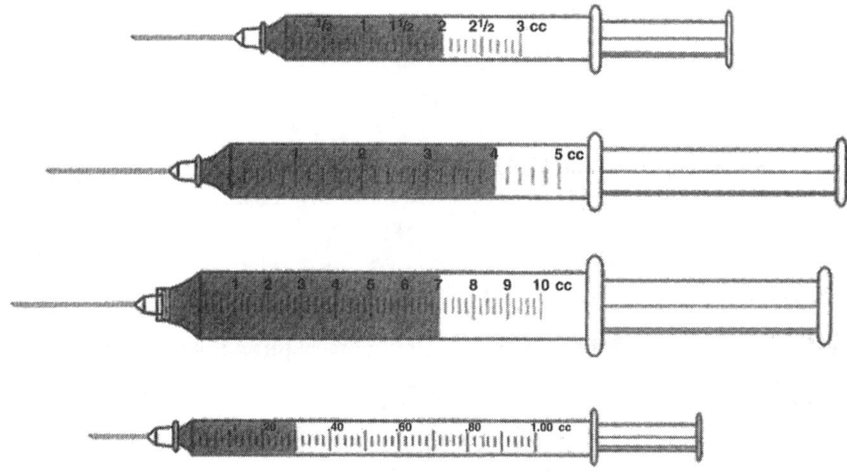

(Objective 3)

55. Avoid distractions; repeat orders to medical direction; verify that you are giving the right patient the right dose of the right drug at the right time by the right route; verify the correct drug on the label at least three times; verify the route of administration; ensure that the labeling information is correct for the drug you want to give; never give drugs from an unlabeled container; verify difficult calculations on paper, with a coworker, or both; label the syringe immediately after withdrawing a drug that will not be completely administered immediately; do not give unlabeled drugs prepared by another person; do not give medications that are outdated or appear discolored, cloudy, or unusual; if the patient or a coworker questions the drug or dose, double check it; monitor the patient for adverse effects after administration; and document carefully.
(Objective 5)

56. a. Stop the infusion.
   b. Evaluate the patient's response to the drug. Perform an assessment that includes level of consciousness, vital signs, and electrocardiogram rhythm.
   c. Advise medical direction and the receiving physician of the amount of drug infused and ask for their treatment advice if you have not yet arrived at the receiving facility.
   d. Document the amount of drug administered on the patient care report objectively. Document all facts surrounding the error on the appropriate confidential departmental quality improvement (incident) form.
   e. Critique the situation with your crew (if appropriate) and identify measures that can be taken to prevent a similar error in the future.
   (Objective 6)

57. a. Wash hands before initiating the procedure.
   b. Cleanse the area with an antiseptic solution before puncturing the skin.
   (Objective 7)

58. a. Upright (sitting)
   b. 4 to 8 oz
   c. Stomach
   d. Tongue

   Chapter **14** **Venous Access and Medication Administration**

e. Dissolve

f. Swallowed

g. h., and i. Infection, lipodystrophy, abscesses, necrosis, skin slough, nerve injuries, prolonged pain, and periostitis

j. 1/2 or 5/8

k. 23 or 25

l. 11/2 to 2

m. 19 or 21

n. Prohibited

o. An appropriate sharps container

p. Air

q. Filter straw

r. 45

s. Upper arm, abdomen, thigh, and back

t. 90

u. Deltoid muscle, dorsogluteal site, vastus lateralis muscle, rectus femoris muscle, and ventrogluteal muscle

v. Gloves

w. 10

x. Rapid onset and side effects

(Objectives 8, 13, and 16)

59. a. Hematoma, cellulitis, thrombosis, phlebitis, sepsis, pulmonary thromboembolism, catheter embolism, fiber embolism, infiltration

b. All complications in (a), plus air embolism, hematoma, damage to arteries or nerves, pneumothorax, hemothorax, and infiltration of fluid into the pleural space or mediastinum

c. All complications in (a), plus hematoma, thrombosis extending to deep veins, and an inability to use the saphenous vein

(Objective 10)

60. a. One to two fingerbreadths below the tubercle on the anteromedial surface of the tibia

b. Saline

c. Intravenous fluid infusion

d. Secure

(Objective 11)

61. c. To convert degrees Celsius to degrees Fahrenheit: $\dfrac{38.5 \times 9}{5} \div 32 = 101.3°F.$

(Objective 1)

62. a. Multiply pounds by 0.45 to convert to kilograms. $144 \times 0.45 = 64.8$. Round to 65 kg.

(Objective 1)

63. b. $\dfrac{1000\,mg \times 100\,mL}{10,000\,mg} = 10\,mL$

(Objective 3)

64. c. $\dfrac{0.06 \times 10}{1} = 0.6$

(Objective 3)

65. a. The 1-mL syringe will permit the most accurate measurements.

(Objective 8)

66. d. Many dose calculations can be done in your head; however, you should always write down any calculation that is difficult or that you question. Do not set down an unlabeled syringe with drug in it. Label the syringe or tape the medicine vial to it. The drug label should be verified at least three times before administration.

(Objective 5)

67. c. On the patient care report, only the actual action taken (the incorrect route) should be documented. The circumstances surrounding the error, including the actual correct route ordered, should be recorded in the appropriate confidential incident (quality improvement) reports.

(Objective 6)

68. a. Slower absorption and fewer systemic effects are achieved in this manner.
(Objective 8)

69. d. The other muscles are not developed adequately in the young child.
(Objective 14)

70. a. The 14-gauge, 1 1/2-inch needle has the widest diameter and is the shortest. Both of these properties allow rapid fluid administration.
(Objective 9)

71. a. The goal is to cause the air to stay in the right side of the heart and away from the cardiac valves.
(Objective 10)

72. b.
(Objective 4)

73. c.
(Objective 4)

74. d. Intraosseous infusion can be used in adults and children. Complications are infrequent but include infiltration of fluid, fat embolism, osteomyelitis, periostitis at the site, infection, or fracture. Absorption of drugs and fluids from a properly placed intraosseous needle is rapid.
(Objective 11)

75. c. Swallowing a sublingual medicine will decrease its effectiveness; therefore, water should not be given.
(Objective 8)

76. a. The angle of the ear canal will promote faster absorption if this technique is used.
(Objectives 13 & 14)

77. d. Recognize the child's fear and allow him or her to express it in appropriate ways such as crying or yelling. Use mild restraint if necessary and firmly stabilize injection sites. Give injections quickly.
(Objective 14)

78. d. Blood should not be drawn from an intravenous catheter if fluids already have been infusing (except under special circumstances and with the authorization of medical direction). Typically, a large 19- or 21-gauge needle should be used; however, in neonates, a smaller needle should be used.
(Objective 15)

WRAP IT UP

1. $66 \div 2.2 = 30\,kg$
(Objective 1)

2. a. $0.01\,mL/kg \times 30\,kg = 0.3\,mL$
b. $0.5\,mL$ given $- 0.3\,mL$ indicated $= 0.2\,mL$ overdose
(Objective 3)

3. a. $1.25\,mg/kg \times 30\,kg = 37.5\,mg$ total dose
b. $37.5\,mg \div 50\,mg \times 1\,mL = 0.75\,mL$
c. Diphenhydramine should be given by deep intramuscular injection into the dorsogluteal or vastus lateralis injection sites.
(Objectives 3, 8 and 14)

4. Ensure that the right patient gets the right dose of the right drug at the right time by the right route.
(Objective 5)

5. After a medication error, advise medical direction and the person receiving the patient; monitor the patient; document the error according to state and local policy; determine how to prevent errors in the future. (Objective 6)

6.

Injection Site	Angle of Administration	Max. Volume to be Given
Intradermal	15 degrees	Less than 0.5 mL
Subcutaneous	45 degrees	Less than 0.5 mL
Intramuscular	90 degrees	Up to 5 mL (less in small children)

(Objective 13)

7. a. Intraosseous infusion could be performed if the child was in critical condition if no venous access site was readily available. A peripheral intravenous site on the arm would be preferred because of its easier access, ability to secure, and complication potential. An intravenous line is indicated to permit drug administration should the child's condition worsen. (Objective 9)

8. Add prescribed drug to nebulizer; attached to oxygen and mask; adjust flow meter to 6 to 8 L/min; place mask on patient; instruct patient to inhale slowly and deeply and hold breath 3 to 5 seconds before exhaling. (Objective 8)

15 Airway Management, Respiration, and Artificial Ventilation

Chapter 15, pages 383-470, in *Mosby's Paramedic Textbook*, ed. 4.

OBJECTIVES

Upon completion of this chapter, the paramedic student will be able to do the following:

1. Describe the anatomy of the airway and respiratory structures.
2. Distinguish between respiration, pulmonary ventilation, and external and internal respiration.
3. Explain the mechanics of ventilation and respiration.
4. Explain the relationship of the partial pressures of gases in the blood and lungs to atmospheric gas pressures.
5. Describe pulmonary circulation.
6. Explain the process of exchange and transport of gases in the body.
7. Describe voluntary, nervous, and chemical regulation of respiration.
8. Discuss the assessment and management of airway obstruction.
9. Describe risk factors and preventive measures for pulmonary aspiration.
10. Outline assessment of airway and breathing.
11. Describe the indications, contraindications, and techniques to deliver supplemental oxygen.
12. Discuss methods of patient ventilation based on the indications, contraindications, potential complications, and use of each method.
13. Describe the use of manual airway maneuvers and mechanical airway adjuncts based on knowledge of their indications, contraindications, potential complications, and techniques for each.
14. Describe effective techniques to verify proper placement of endotracheal and peritracheal airway devices.
15. Explain variations in assessment and management of airway and ventilation problems in pediatric patients.
16. Given a patient scenario, identify possible alterations in oxygenation and ventilation and appropriate interventions to treat those alterations.

SUMMARY

- The upper airway opens at the nose and mouth and extends to the glottic opening.
- Structures of the lower airway include the trachea; right and left bronchus; bronchi; bronchioles; and the functional units of the lungs, the alveoli.
- The base of the lungs rests on the diaphragm. The right lung has three lobes, and the left has two.
- The primary muscles of ventilation are the diaphragm and the intercostal muscles.
- The phrenic nerve enervates the diaphragm.
- Respiration is the exchange of oxygen and carbon dioxide between and organism and the environment. Pulmonary ventilation involves movement of gas into and out of the lungs.
- External respiration is the transfer of gases between the inspired air and pulmonary capillaries. Internal respiration is the transfer of gases between the blood and tissue cells.
- During inspiration, the size of the thoracic cavity increases. This creates negative pressure inside the chest compared with atmospheric pressure, so air rushes into the lungs.
- During exhalation the chest muscles relax passively, and air is forced out of the lungs.
- Work of breathing increases if surfactant is lost, airway resistance increases, or pulmonary compliance decreases.
- The normal adult respiratory rate is 12 to 24 breaths/min.
- No gas exchange occurs in the anatomic dead space. The physiologic dead space includes the anatomic dead space plus and any nonfunctioning alveoli.

- Tidal volume is the amount of gas inhaled or exhaled with each normal breath.
- Respiratory rate multiplied by tidal volume equals minute volume.
- Atmospheric gas contains approximately 79% nitrogen, 21% oxygen, and less than 1% carbon dioxide.
- As the pulmonary capillaries pass the alveoli, carbon dioxide diffuses into the alveoli and oxygen diffuses into the pulmonary capillaries.
- Oxygen is carried in the blood on hemoglobin. A small amount is also dissolved in the plasma. The amount of oxygen dissolved in the blood influences the extent to which oxygen binds with hemoglobin. Normal partial pressure of arterial blood oxygen (ç) is 80 to 100 mm Hg. Venous PO_2 in the lungs is only 40 mm Hg, so oxygen diffuses easily from the alveoli into the pulmonary capillaries.
- The respiratory centers are normally controlled by pH of body fluids, which are related to carbon dioxide levels. Oxygen plays a role in regulation of breathing in abnormal situations.
- Body temperature, medications, pain, emotion, and sleep also influence breathing.
- Modified forms of respiration are protective and include coughing, sneezing, and sighing.
- Older adults experience alterations in ventilation and respiration that lead to a gradual decline in PO_2.
- Respiratory compromise and hypoxia can be caused by interruption of nervous control, structural damage to the thorax, bronchoconstriction, disruption of airway patency, oxygen deprivation, environmental factors, changes in alveolar–capillary gas exchange, ventilation deficiencies, decreases in lung compliance, ventilation–perfusion mismatch, disrupted oxygen transport, disrupted circulation, or cellular disruptions.
- Upper airway obstruction can rapidly cause death if not corrected.
- Aspiration is inhalation of food, fluid, or foreign bodies into the lungs. This can cause airway obstruction and chemical damage with collapse of alveoli.
- Assess rate, regularity, and rhythm of breathing. Also note the patient's position, color, and heart rate. A thorough patient history should be obtained.
- Respiratory distress may be caused by upper or lower airway obstruction, inadequate ventilation, impairment of the respiratory muscles, ventilation–perfusion mismatching, diffusion abnormalities, or impairment of the nervous system.
- Supplemental oxygen is administered to increase oxygen content in pulmonary capillaries and to help the patient compensate.
- Oxygen gas is administered by a variety of devices that regulate the concentration of oxygen delivered to the patient.
- Patient ventilation is provided by several methods. These include rescue breathing (mouth to mouth, mouth to nose, mouth to stoma), mouth-to-mask breathing, bag-mask devices, and automatic transport ventilators.
- Airway management should progress from the least to most invasive methods. Airway management begins with manual maneuvers.
- Oropharyngeal or tracheal suction is used to remove liquids and foreign objects from the airway.
- Gastric distension can impair ventilation and it increases the risk of aspiration. Orogastric or nasogastric tubes are inserted to reduce gastric distension
- After manual airway maneuvers are performed, mechanical adjuncts can be used to maintain the airway. Nasopharyngeal airways are used to maintain the airway in patients with a gag reflex. An oropharyngeal airway is inserted in patients with no gag reflex.
- Advanced airways include those that intubate the trachea and peritracheal airways such as the laryngeal mask airway, King LT-D airway, and esophageal–tracheal Combitube airway.
- Endotracheal intubation permits direct ventilation of the trachea, protection against aspiration, and a route to administer some medications. The endotracheal tube may be inserted orally or nasally (in breathing patients). Adjuncts to assist with intubation include the stylet, tube introducer (bougie), and Magill forceps.
- It is essential to confirm proper placement of the endotracheal tube. Measures include auscultation of breath sounds, absence of gastric sounds, use of an esophageal detector device, and measurement of end-tidal carbon dioxide and oxygen saturation.
- The laryngeal mask airway is inserted blindly into the hypopharynx in unresponsive patients with no gag reflex.
- An esophageal–tracheal Combitube is a twin-lumen airway placed blindly in unconscious patients with no gag reflex. In most cases, the distal lumen is positioned in the esophagus, and inflation of balloons in the hypopharynx permits ventilation through tube number one. In rare cases, when the distal lumen is positioned in the trachea, the patient is ventilated through tube number two.
- Sedation is sometimes used in airway management and ventilation to reduce anxiety, induce amnesia, and decrease the gag reflex.
- In some systems, neuromuscular blocking agents are used with sedation to permit endotracheal intubation.
- When an airway cannot be introduced through the nose or mouth and the patient cannot be ventilated, translaryngeal cannula ventilation or cricothyrotomy may be performed to access the airway by creating an opening in the cricothyroid membrane in the neck.

212

Match the lung volume in Column II with its description in Column I. Use each answer only once.

Column I

1. _______ The air inhaled and exhaled during a normal respiratory cycle (500–600 mL)

2. _______ Quantity of air moved on deepest inspiration and expiration

3. _______ Tidal volume multiplied by respiratory rate

4. _______ Air remaining in respiratory passages after a forceful exhalation

5. _______ Amount of air that can be exhaled forcefully after a normal breath is exhaled

Column II

a. Expiratory reserve volume
b. Inspiratory reserve volume
c. Minute volume
d. Residual volume
e. Tidal volume
f. Vital capacity

6. Pulmonary ventilation is the movement of oxygen and carbon dioxide into and out of the lungs. True/false. If this is false, why is it false?

____

7. pH is a measurement that reflects hydrogen ion concentration. True/false. If this is false, why is it false?

____

8. The pressure regulator attached to an oxygen cylinder permits administration of a specific amount of oxygen. True/false. If this is false, why is it false?

____

9. Describe the *mechanical* process by which air is moved into and out of the lungs.

____

____

____

10. Complete the sentences in the following paragraph: At sea level, atmospheric pressure is

(a) _______________. The pressure in the alveoli is known as the **(b)** _______________ pressure. Changes in this pressure are caused by changes in the **(c)** _______________ size. Whereas during inspiration, the pressure in the alveoli will **(d)** _______________ approximately 1 mm Hg relative to atmospheric pressure, during exhalation, the pressure will **(e)** _______________ by 1 mm Hg. The ability of the lungs to expand during changes in pressure is known as **(f)** _______________. This ability can be impaired by diseases such as **(g)** _______________, _______________, and _______________.

11. The major blood vessels that carry deoxygenated blood to the lungs are the **(a)** _______________. Oxygenated blood is carried away from the lungs by the **(b)** _______________.

12. Your patient is a 70-year-old man with chronic bronchitis and emphysema who experienced an acute onset of shortness of breath while at the grocery store. Describe your ongoing assessment of this patient's head, neck, chest, and abdomen. Be specific when describing the muscle groups that you will inspect to help determine his degree of distress.

____

____

13. The partial pressure of nitrogen = (a) _______________% X atmospheric pressure (b) _______________ mm Hg = (c) _______________ mm Hg. The partial pressure of oxygen (Po_2) = (d) _______________% × atmospheric pressure (e) _______________ mm Hg = (f) _______________ mm Hg.

14. List three physiological factors that can increase the work of breathing.

a. ____

b. ____

c. ____

15. Describe the *structural* aspects of the lung that explain the following:

a. Normal lung expansion:

____

b. Alveolar collapse that occurs because of decreased surfactant in a premature infant:

____

c. Poor ventilation during an asthma attack:

____

16. Each of the diagrams in Fig. 15-1 represents solutions separated by a semipermeable membrane. In each illustration, indicate whether the process of diffusion will cause a net movement of solute particles to the left, right, or not at all.

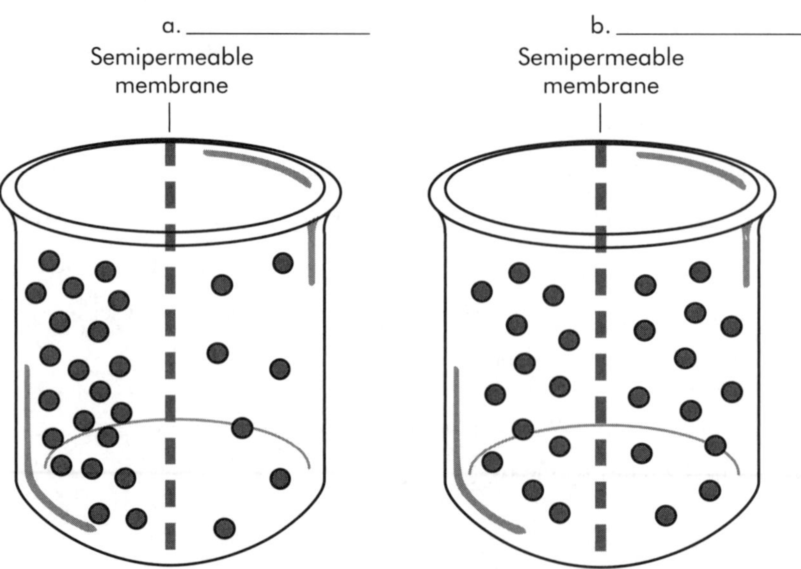

Figure 15-1

17. Complete the missing values for P_{CO_2} and P_{O_2} in the following. Then draw an arrow indicating the direction of movement of each of the gases across the respiratory membrane (toward alveoli or pulmonary capillaries).

Alveolar Gas	Direction of Movement of Gas	Venous Blood (Pulmonary Capillaries)
P_{CO_2} __________ torr		
P_{O_2} __________ torr		

18. Complete the following sentences.

   a. The primary way that oxygen is transported in the blood is by a chemical bond to

   __________________________.

   b. P_{O_2} describes the oxygen level dissolved in blood __________________________.

   c. The amount of carbon dioxide present in the venous blood is influenced by the rate and type of

   __________________________.

   d. Carbon dioxide is transported in the blood in three forms: __________________________,

   __________________________, and __________________________.

19. In one sentence describe the physiological basis for poor blood oxygenation in the following patients:

   a. A 23-year-old woman who is paralyzed completely from Guillain-Barré syndrome:

   ____

   b. A 52-year-old patient with pneumonia:

   ____

   c. An 8-year-old who is having an acute asthma attack:

   ____

   d. A 42-year-old with massive head trauma caused by a motor vehicle crash:

   ____

20. Briefly explain the origin or site of stimulation, location of effect, and action of each of the following mechanisms that control respiration:

Mechanism	Origin of Stimulus	Location of Effect	Action
Inspiratory centers			
Expiratory centers			
Hering-Breuer reflex			
Pneumotaxic center			
Apneustic center			

 Chapter **15** **Airway Management, Respiration, and Artificial Ventilation**

21. For each of the following scenarios, briefly explain why the patient's respirations will increase or decrease or be unchanged.

   a. A 3-year-old loses consciousness from breath-holding following a temper tantrum:

   b. A 34-year-old with a morphine overdose:

   c. A 17-year-old football player with a dislocated shoulder:

   d. A hostage with no apparent injuries who has just been freed:

   e. A student who is sleeping in class:

   f. A patient with chronic obstructive pulmonary disease has fallen. An oxygen level of 15 L/min is being administered by nonrebreather mask:

   g. A lost snow skier who has a core temperature of 84° F (28.9° C):

22. Briefly describe the benefit of the following modified forms of respiration:

   a. Cough:

   b. Sneeze:

   c. Hiccup:

   d. Sigh:

23. For each of the following scenarios, identify the pathological condition or injury you would suspect and list the signs and symptoms the patient may develop.

    a. A 50-year-old man unable to speak after choking on a piece of steak:

    b. A nursing home patient with shortness of breath after "inhaling" some food:

    c. A 17-year-old hockey player who has difficulty speaking after being struck across the neck by a stick:

    d. A 2-year-old with croup:

    e. A 23-year-old who reportedly overdosed, is unconscious, and has vomitus draining from the side of her mouth.

24. You are transporting a patient with severe asthma to a medical center 40 minutes away. What are the advantages of using:

    a. A pulse oximeter in this scenario?

    b. End-tidal CO_2 monitoring in this scenario?

25. For each of the following scenarios, circle the best oxygen-delivery device and explain why you made that selection.

    a. A 76-year-old patient with chronic obstructive pulmonary disease complains of chest pain on the right side and a nosebleed after a fall. Vital signs are normal. **Nasal cannula at 2 L/min oxygen** or **Venturi mask at 24% oxygen?**

    b. A 25-year-old patient involved in a motor vehicle crash has ineffective respirations, cyanosis, and signs of a flail chest segment. **Simple face mask at 8 L/min oxygen** or **bag-valve-mask with reservoir device at 15 L/min oxygen?**

    c. A 45-year-old patient with slight chest pain (SaO_2 on room air is 93%). **Simple face mask at 4 L/min oxygen** or **nasal cannula at 4 L/min oxygen?**

      Chapter **15** **Airway Management, Respiration, and Artificial Ventilation**

d. A 17-year-old patient who sustained a crush injury to the abdomen in a farming accident is pale, with cyanosis around the lips and decreased blood pressure. **Simple mask at 6 L/min oxygen** or **complete non-rebreather mask at 15 L/min oxygen?**

____

26. For each of the following scenarios, choose the airway adjunct from the list that is most appropriate after initial manual airway maneuvers have been used. Explain why you selected your answer.

Oral airway   Nasal airway
Oral endotracheal intubation   Nasal endotracheal intubation
Percutaneous tracheal ventilation   Esophageal–tracheal combitube or King Lt-D airway

a. Your patient is a 17-year-old victim of a snowmobiling accident who struck a concealed barbed wire fence, injuring his neck. The airway is not patent. All attempts to ventilate and to secure the airway, including oral and nasal intubation, are unsuccessful.

____

b. You are called to evaluate a 34-year-old patient who is postictal after a single grand mal seizure. He has snoring respirations and no gag reflex.

____

c. Your patient was pulled from a swimming pool after an unsuccessful dive into the shallow end. He has ineffective shallow respirations and flaccid paralysis of all limbs.

____

d. A 32-year-old woman with a history of diabetes has taken her insulin but has not eaten. She has snoring respirations and can be aroused with painful stimulus.

____

e. A 19-year-old ejected from his all-terrain vehicle has an obviously severe head injury and shallow agonal respirations.

____

f. A 79-year-old is in cardiac arrest of medical origin.

____

27. Describe your actions if you discover the following physical findings after endotracheal intubation of a patient:

a. The carbon dioxide detector fades from purple to yellow as the patient exhales:

____

b. Breath sounds are present bilaterally:

____

218

c. Gurgling is auscultated over the epigastric region during ventilation:

____

d. Breath sounds are diminished significantly over the left lung:

____

e. The patient's color deteriorates, and the abdomen becomes distended:

____

f. The bulb of the esophageal detector device fills in 8 seconds after placement on the end of the endotracheal tube:

____

g. The CO_2 waveform has a sharkfin shape and is 45 mmHg:

____

28. Fill in the blanks with the appropriate airway adjunct(s) from the following list:

Esophageal–tracheal Combitube (ETC)   Oral Endotracheal tube (ETT)
Laryngeal mask airway (LMA)   King LT-D (King)

a. _________________________________ is available in sizes for children and adults.

b. _________________________________ may be used if placed in trachea or esophagus.

c. _________________________________ must visualize the vocal cords to insert.

d. _________________________________ provides best protection against aspiration.

e. _________________________________ requires inflation of two balloons.

f. _________________________________ does not enter the trachea.

29. Briefly describe each step of the orotracheal intubation procedure illustrated in Fig. 15-2.

a. ____

b. ____

c. ____

d. ____

e. ____

f. ____

219

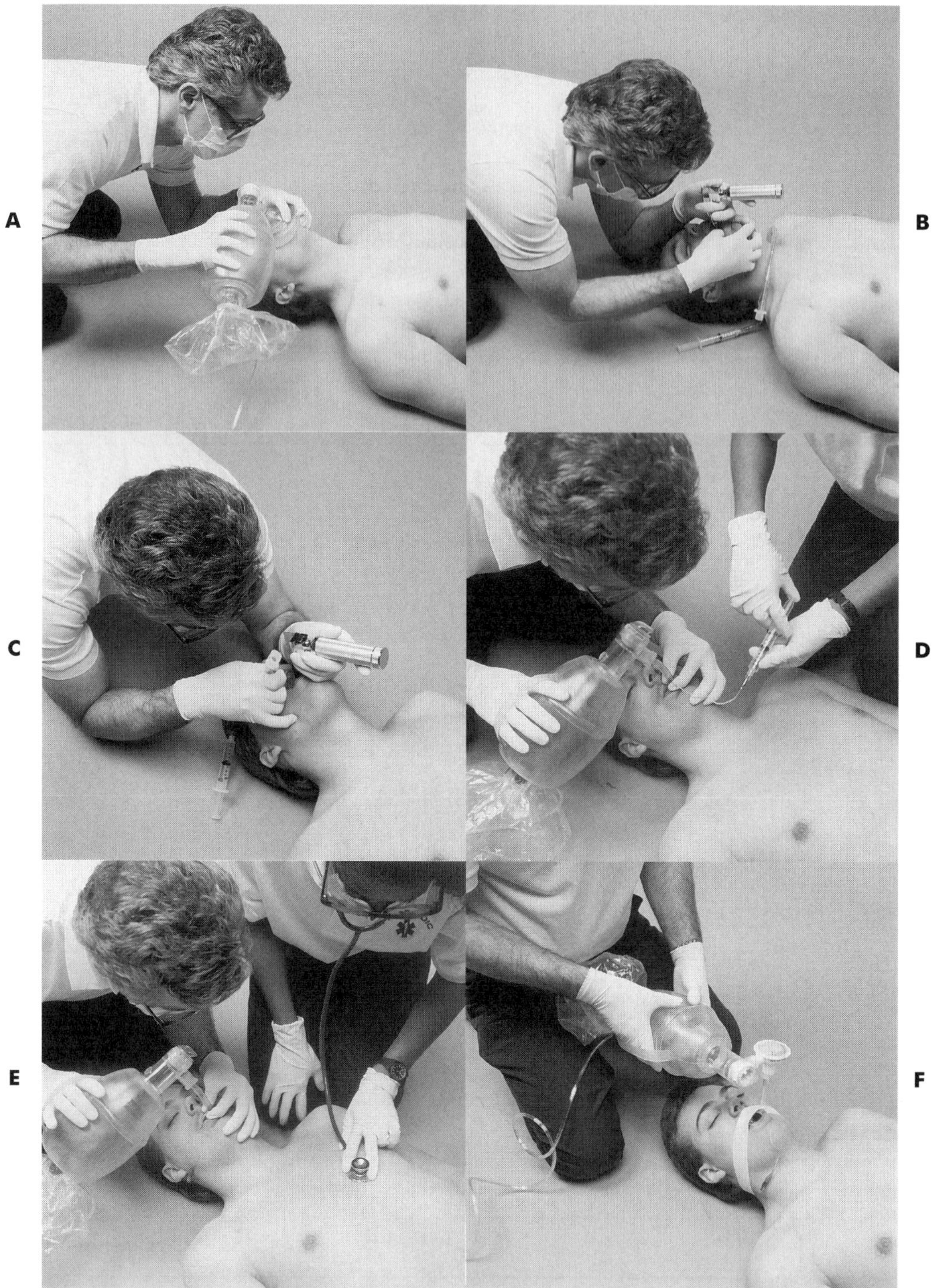

Figure 15-2

30. List one advantage and one disadvantage for each of the following ventilation adjuncts:

Adjunct	Advantage	Disadvantage
a. Mouth to mask		
b. Bag-valve-mask		

31. List three patient situations in which use of tonsil-tip suction is indicated:

    a. ____

    b. ____

    c. ____

32. What precautions should be taken to prevent complications when using a whistle-tip suction device for tracheal suctioning?

____

33. Explain the anatomical basis for the following variations in pediatric airway management:

    a. The oral airway should be inserted only with direct visualization with a tongue blade, never upside down and then rotated:

____

    b. Uncuffed endotracheal tubes are sometimes used for children under 8 years of age:

____

    c. The endotracheal tube may "hang up" in the newborn, necessitating use of the Sellick maneuver to attain successful placement:

____

34. An 86-year-old patient fell down 12 steps. Her chief complaint is rib pain and shortness of breath. On physical examination, you note crepitus and bruising on the lower rib cage. Why is it important to provide rapid, aggressive intervention for this older patient?

____

____

STUDENT SELF-ASSESSMENT

35. What is the term for the transfer of oxygen and carbon dioxide between the peripheral blood capillaries and tissue cells?
    a. External respiration   **c.** Pulmonary ventilation
    b. Internal respiration   **d.** Respiration

36. In what structure must continuous negative pressure be maintained to maintain lung expansion?
    a. Alveoli   **c.** Pleural space
    b. Mediastinum   **d.** Thoracic cage

37. When you arrive at the hospital, blood gasses on your 18-year-old patient indicate that the Po_2 is 70 mm Hg. What does this mean?
    a. Seventy percent of the hemoglobin is filled with oxygen.
    b. The patient is oxygenated adequately.
    c. Less than 3 mL of oxygen is dissolved in 1 L of blood.
    d. The blood sample must have been venous.

Chapter **15** **Airway Management, Respiration, and Artificial Ventilation**

38. Which of the following factors will result in an *increased* energy requirement for breathing?
   a. Loss of pulmonary surfactant
   b. A decrease in airway resistance
   c. An increase in lung compliance
   d. Bronchodilation

39. Which of the following patients is most likely to have a decreased minute volume?
   a. A 17-year-old with deep respirations and signs of hyperventilation
   b. A 20-year-old patient with a head injury with shallow, slow respirations
   c. An alert 45-year-old with a possible myocardial infarction
   d. A 30-year-old in early shock with an increased respiratory rate

40. What does an oxygen saturation reading of 100% mean?
   a. The patient is on 100% oxygen by mask.
   b. The partial pressure of oxygen is 100.
   c. All hemoglobin has converted to oxyhemoglobin.
   d. The blood will not carry any more oxygen.

41. Which of the following conditions causes decreased oxygenation because of increased resistance in the airways?
   a. Asbestosis
   b. Asthma
   c. Poliomyelitis
   d. Tuberculosis

42. Why might the tissues of a patient with anemia not be well oxygenated?
   a. The blood does not reach all tissue to off-load oxygen.
   b. The respiratory drive in the brain is depressed.
   c. The number of red blood cells is insufficient to carry oxygen.
   d. The pulmonary vessels are not well perfused with blood.

43. Respiratory chemoreceptors in the medulla, aortic bodies, and carotid bodies are stimulated by changes in which of the following?
   a. Hemoglobin
   b. Carbon dioxide
   c. Blood volume
   d. Respiratory rate

44. If a person appears to be choking but still can speak and cough, what should the rescuer do?
   a. Deliver five back blows.
   b. Perform the Heimlich maneuver.
   c. Administer five chest thrusts.
   d. Not intervene but just observe.

45. What is the most frequent cause of airway obstruction in the unconscious adult?
   a. Hot dogs
   b. Steak
   c. Tongue
   d. Vomitus

46. You arrive at a private residence, where you find an unconscious 52-year-old man. You open his airway and determine that he is not breathing. His pulse is present. You attempt to ventilate his lungs, but the airflow is blocked. What is your next step?
   a. Assess the pulse.
   b. Reposition the head.
   c. Administer five abdominal thrusts.
   d. Perform a cricothyrotomy.

47. Which of the following represents the *most* effective measure to prevent aspiration of stomach contents?
   a. Elevating the head of the cot 45 degrees
   b. Frequent suctioning of the mouth using a tonsil-tip suction
   c. Inserting an oropharyngeal airway and nasogastric tube
   d. Positioning the patient in the recovery position

48. Your patient attempted suicide by hanging. She is hoarse and has hemoptysis and stridor. What do you suspect?
   a. Laryngeal fracture
   b. Laryngeal spasm
   c. Foreign body obstruction
   d. Tracheal injury

222

49. For which patient is nasopharyngeal airway insertion indicated?
    a. Snoring post-ictal 12-year-oldwith a gag reflex.
    b. 46-year-old in vehicle collision has Battle sign
    c. 24-year-old who was assaulted has epistaxis.
    d. Unresponsive 85-year-old who fell has clear ear drainage

50. To ensure adequate ventilation when combitube airway is used, you must be certain that
    a. The tube passes into the trachea.
    b. The mask seal is tight.
    c. The patient is less than 5 feet tall.
    d. Breath sounds are audible over the gastric area.

51. The King Lt-D airway may be used successfully if the tube is placed in which structure?
    a. The esophagus   c. The right main stem bronchus
    b. The trachea   d. The esophagus or trachea

52. If 30 seconds have elapsed from the last ventilation and tracheal intubation has not been accomplished, what
    should you do?
    a. Remove the tube, hyperventilate, and try again.
    b. Continue if intubation can be done in a few more seconds.
    c. Insert an esophageal obturator airway.
    d. Have another paramedic attempt the skill.

53. Which of the following statements is true regarding percutaneous transtracheal ventilation?
    a. Exhalation time should be shortened in this procedure.
    b. It is a good long-term airway management device.
    c. It minimizes the risk of aspiration.
    d. The high pressures generated may cause pneumothorax.

54. Which of the following is an advantage of the bag-valve-mask device?
    a. It delivers continuous positive airway pressure.
    b. The rescuer can sense the patient's lung compliance.
    c. It is used easily by one rescuer to deliver ventilations.
    d. It eliminates the risk of overpressurization injury.

55. Which of the following indicates a properly placed endotracheal tube?
    a. Misting on the inside of the endotracheal tube
    b. Gurgling is heard during auscultation over the stomach
    c. Esophageal detection bulb refills in 10 seconds
    d. End-tidal CO_2 displays a reading of 20 mmHg

56. Which of the following statements is true regarding endotracheal suctioning?
    a. Preoxygenation for 2 minutes should precede suctioning.
    b. Suction should be applied for a maximum of 30 seconds.
    c. Coughing may cause decreased intracranial pressure.
    d. Suction should be set between 200 and 300 mm Hg.

57. How much oxygen is the patient who is on a nasal cannula at 5 L/min receiving?
    a. 36%   c. 44%
    b. 40%   d. 50%

58. Your patient has been removed from a smoky building and is confused and tachycardic. What is the appropriate
    oxygen delivery device for this person?
    a. Nasal cannula   c. Simple face mask
    b. Nonrebreather mask   d. Venturi mask

    Chapter **15** **Airway Management, Respiration, and Artificial Ventilation**

59. An apneic 18-month-old is rescued from a swimming pool. Which of the following is true for management of the airway and ventilation of this child?
   a. Hyperextend the head to maintain an open airway.
   b. Avoid suctioning the airway to prevent vagal stimulation.
   c. Ventilate at a rate of one breath every 3 to 5 seconds.
   d. Nasopharyngeal airways should not be used in this age.

60. Which complication related to cricothyrotomy will result in the absence of breath sounds when ventilation begins?
   a. Aspiration   **c.** Injury to the vocal cords
   b. False passage   **d.** Perforation of a great vessel

61. You are preparing to insert an oropharyngeal airway in an unresponsive four-year-old male. Which of the following is correct?
   a. If the airway is too long the epiglottis may obstruct the airway.
   b. Insert upside down until it touches the hard palate then rotate.
   c. This will prevent the child from aspiration if he vomits.
   d. It can be safely inserted if the child has a gag reflex.

62. Which of the following is the approximate depth of insertion for an endotracheal tube in an 8-year-old?
   a. 6.0 cm   **c.** 17 cm
   b. 12 cm   **d.** 24 cm

63. At what point do the right and left mainstem bronchi divide from the trachea?
   a. Carina   **c.** Vallecula
   b. Cricoid   **d.** Xiphoid

64. Which airway cartilage prevents aspiration?
   a. Arytenoid   **c.** Cricoid
   b. Corniculate   **d.** Epiglottis

WRAP IT UP

You are dispatched to a school playground for an unconscious person. You arrive with an ALS pumper crew and find a drowsy male who appears to be in his early 20s, lying across a playground bench. He is arousable to voice, but he snores when not stimulated. You open his airway using the head-tilt–chin-lift method, and as you insert a nasal airway, you note some vomitus has dried partially around his mouth. Oxygen saturation readings on room air are 93%, and his lung sounds reveal sonorous wheezes (rhonchi) throughout. His pupils are midpoint and 3 mm and sluggishly react to light. Vital signs are BP 94/58 mm Hg, P 148, R 28 and shallow. You apply oxygen by nonrebreather mask, and the patient quickly is secured onto the stretcher and placed in the ambulance. Your partner shows you some empty pill bottles nearby, and you recognize that he likely has taken some sedatives and antipsychotic drugs. In the ambulance you attach the patient to the ECG monitor, insert a nasogastric tube, set-up automatic BP monitoring, establish an IV, and check blood glucose. As you prepare to depart the scene, the patient's respirations become irregular and slow with apneic pauses. When you attempt to stimulate him, there is no response, and a glance at the monitor reveals a rapidly slowing heart rate and oxygen saturation level. You instruct your partner to set up the intubation equipment as you insert an oral airway and begin to hyperoxygenate with a bag-mask device. When ready, you orally intubate the patient and then verify the correct placement of the tube, secure it, and begin to ventilate using an automatic transport ventilator. His heart rate increases, oxygen saturation levels rise, and his condition remains unchanged for the 10-minute transport to the medical center.

1. Would pulmonary aspiration interfere with the patient's internal or external respiration?

2. What was the likely explanation for this patient's slow irregular respirations?
   a. Anatomical dead space increase   **c.** Decreased intrapulmonary pressure
   b. Central nervous system depression   **d.** Increased atmospheric pressure

3. What actions were taken to reduce the risk of further aspiration?

____

4. Which of the following irregular patterns of breathing was this patient displaying?
   a. Air trapping   **c.** Cheyne-Stokes
   b. Bradypnea   **d.** Kussmaul's

5. Why was the nonrebreather mask chosen as the first oxygen delivery device?

____

6. When the patient's respirations became irregular and slow, what acid-base disturbance most likely was occurring?
   a. Metabolic acidosis
   b. Metabolic alkalosis
   c. Respiratory acidosis
   d. Respiratory alkalosis

7. What measure was taken to correct the acid-base disturbance?

_____________________ *hyperventilation c̄ BVM* _____________________

8. How should the correct size of oral airway have been selected?

____

9. a. Why was suctioning indicated before intubation?

____

____

   b. Should suctioning be performed after intubation? Yes/No. If you answered yes, describe why it would be indicated.

____

____

10. For each of the following methods, describe the finding that suggests tracheal intubation in this patient's situation.

   a. Auscultation over the epigastrium:

____

____

   b. Bilateral auscultation of the lungs:

____

____

   c. Esophageal detector device—syringe:

____

____

    Chapter **15** **Airway Management, Respiration, and Artificial Ventilation**

d. Esophageal detector device—bulb:

____

____

e. Colorimetric end-tidal CO_2 detector:

____

____

f. Digital end-tidal CO_2 detector or capnography:

____

____

g. Oxygen saturation:

____

____

h. Direct laryngoscopic visualization:

____

____

11. What settings should be selected on the automatic transport ventilator?

Rate: ____________/min Volume: ________________mL

CHAPTER 15 ANSWERS

REVIEW QUESTIONS

1. e
(Objective 3)

2. f
(Objective 3)

3. c
(Objective 3)

4. d
(Objective 3)

5. a
(Objective 3)

6. True
(Objective 2)

7. True
(Objective 3)

8. False. The pressure regulator reduces the pressure in the oxygen cylinder to 30 to 70 psi to permit safe administration. The flow meter regulates the amount of oxygen delivered.
(Objective 11)

9. During inspiration, the dome of the diaphragm is flattened when it contracts. This causes an increase in the superior-inferior distance of the chest cavity. The intercostal muscles contract, resulting in an increase in the anteroposterior and lateral diameter of the chest cavity. This increase in the size of the chest cavity results in a pressure drop in the chest approximately 1 mm Hg below atmospheric pressure. This negative pressure causes gas to move into the lungs. During expiration the relaxation of the diaphragm and other breathing muscles results in a decrease in the size of the chest wall and an increase in pressure in the chest approximately 1mm Hg above atmospheric pressure. This positive pressure in the chest forces the gas out of the lungs.
(Objective 3)

10. a. 760 mm Hg; b. intrapulmonic; c. thoracic; d. decrease; e. increase; f. compliance; g. asthma, emphysema, bronchitis, pulmonary edema, and lung cancer.
(Objectives 3 and 4)

11. a. Pulmonary arteries; b. pulmonary veins
(Objective 5)

12. Head: Inspect for cyanosis around lips and "puffing" of the cheeks; neck: inspect for the use of accessory muscles or tracheal tugging; chest: inspect for intercostal muscle use and an increased anteroposterior diameter of the chest, auscultate lung sounds; abdomen: inspect for the use of abdominal muscles when breathing.
(Objective 10)

13. a. 79; b. 760; c. 600.2; d. 21; e. 760; f. 160
(Objective 4)

14. Loss of pulmonary surfactant, increase in airway resistance, and decrease in pulmonary compliance
(Objective 3)

15. a. The lungs are coated with visceral pleura that adhere to the parietal pleura that line the chest wall. In the potential space between these two membranes, negative pressure "holds" the lungs to the chest wall. Disruption of this potential space causes collapse of the lung.
b. Surfactant reduces the surface tension in the alveoli. In other words, surfactant reduces the tendency of the alveolar walls to "stick" together. In the newborn with insufficient surfactant production, extremely high airway pressures must be used to maintain inflation of the alveoli so that effective ventilation can occur.
c. The bronchioles are surrounded by smooth muscle. During an asthma attack, the smooth muscle contracts forcefully and decreases the diameter of the bronchioles, which impairs the exchange of gases.
(Objectives 3 and 16)

16. a. Right; b. not at all
(Objective 6)

17.

Alveolar Gas	Direction Movement of Gas	Venous Blood (Pulmonary Capillaries)
P_{CO_2} *0* torr	←	P_{CO_2} *46* torr
P_{O_2} *100* torr	→	P_{O_2} *40* torr

(Objectives 4 and 6)

     Chapter **15** **Airway Management, Respiration, and Artificial Ventilation**

18. a. Hemoglobin; b. plasma; c. metabolism; d. plasma, blood proteins, and bicarbonate ions.
(Objective 6)

19. a. Loss of function of respiratory muscles prevents ventilation from occurring without mechanical assistance.
b. Compliance of the lungs and surface area for gas exchange will decrease.
c. Resistance in the airways will increase, which will decrease the flow of gases to and from the lungs.
d. The respiratory centers may be damaged, resulting in abnormal or absent breathing. The airway may not be patent.
(Objective 16)

20.

Mechanism	Origin of Stimulus	Location of Effect	Action
Inspiratory centers	Medulla to spinal cord	Send impulses of respiration	Stimulates muscles to phrenic and intercostal nerves
Expiratory centers	Medulla	Send impulses to spinal cord to phrenic and intercostal nerves	Stimulates muscles of respiration to increase force of exhalation
Hering-Breuer reflex	Vagus nerve	Medulla discharges inhibitory impulses	Causes inspiration to cease so lungs do not overinflate
Pneumotaxic center	Pons	Inspiratory center	Inhibits inspiratory center during labored breathing
Apneustic center	Lower pons	Inspiratory center	Baseline stimulation of inspiratory neurons

(Objective 7)

21. a. The respirations increase or resume because of the increased Pco_2, which stimulates the respiratory centers.
b. The respiratory rate decreases as the respiratory centers of the brain are depressed by the morphine.
c. Pain causes an increased respiratory rate.
d. The fear involved in such a situation causes an increased respiratory rate.
e. The respiratory rate slows because of the decreased metabolic rate during sleep.
f. The history of chronic lung disease may mean that the patient is operating on a hypoxic drive. If this is the case, the chemoreceptors will sense an increase in the Po_2 and respond by decreasing the respiratory rate.
g. During hypothermia the metabolic rate decreases, as does the respiratory rate.
(Objective 16)

22. a. The cough reflex is designed to expel foreign matter from the respiratory passages.
b. Sneezing is caused by nasal irritation and also rids the respiratory tract of unwanted irritants.
c. Hiccups serve no known useful purpose but may signal pathological conditions.
d. Sighing provides intermittent hyperinflation of the lungs to help maintain expansion of the alveoli.
(Objective 3)

23. a. Obstructed airway: The patient initially will be apneic, will lose consciousness, and finally will suffer cardiac arrest if untreated.
b. Aspiration of food and possibly gastric juices: Initially the patient may experience a cough, mucus production, decreased breath sounds, or wheezes.
c. Fractured larynx: The patient may experience localized pain, edema, or hemoptysis. Dysphagia and subcutaneous emphysema may be present if airway obstruction is imminent.
d. Croup with potential for laryngeal spasm: The patient may be anxious and have crowing respirations (stridor) because of airway tissue swelling.
e. Decreased level of consciousness may result in partial airway obstruction and aspiration of vomit.
(Objective 8)

24. a. The pulse oximeter permits monitoring of the effectiveness of interventions by observing the oxygen saturation and pulse rate. If the oxygen saturation does not improve, additional interventions may be needed.

b. End-tidal CO_2 will allow you to observe changes in CO_2 that can indicate the patient is worsening (CO_2 levels increase above 45 mmHg) or improving.

(Objective 14)

25. a. Venturi mask at 24% oxygen: A nasal cannula would be ineffective because the patient has a nosebleed.

b. Bag-valve-mask with reservoir device at 15 L/min oxygen: The patient clearly is not ventilating properly and needs ventilatory assistance in addition to the highest flow of oxygen possible.

c. Nasal cannula at 4 L/min oxygen: The simple face mask should never be used with an oxygen flow set at less than 6 L/min.

d. Complete nonrebreather mask at 10 L/min oxygen: The patient is demonstrating signs of shock and decreased oxygenation, so the highest amount of oxygen possible should be administered.

(Objective 11)

26. a. Percutaneous tracheal ventilation: All other less invasive airway maneuvers have been unsuccessful, possibly because of a laryngeal injury. The patient's airway is not patent, so needle access should be attempted.

b. Oral airway: If this is an isolated seizure, the patient's level of consciousness should be improving gradually, and a more invasive airway maneuver probably can be avoided.

c. Nasal intubation: Because of the patient's spontaneous respirations, this would be selected over oral intubation because of the high probability of cervical spine injury.

d. Nasal airway: This should secure the airway quickly while glucose is administered, which should arouse the patient.

e. Oral endotracheal intubation (using manual in-line stabilization of the cervical spine): This would be chosen because of the possibility of cervical spine injury. Nasal intubation would not be an option until basilar skull fracture could be ruled out.

f. Oral intubation: This is the airway of choice in the unconscious apneic patient with no potential for cervical spine injury.

(Objective 13)

27. a. This indicates that the tube is in the correct position. The tube should be secured.

b. The endotracheal tube is in the correct position, so the tube may be secured.

c. If breath sounds are absent, the cuff should be deflated and the tube quickly removed. After hyperventilation of the patient's lungs with a bag-valve-mask and 100% oxygen, another attempt at intubation may be made.

d. The cuff should be deflated and the tube withdrawn 1 to 2 cm. The cuff should be reinflated and correct placement verified by auscultation of breath sounds bilaterally.

e. The tube is probably in the esophagus. Auscultate for breath sounds, and if they are absent or diminished, deflate the cuff and remove the tube immediately. Hyperventilate the patient's lungs with a bag-valve-mask with a reservoir at 100% oxygen.

f. The tube is probably not in the trachea. Placement should be confirmed by auscultation of lung and epigastric sounds and by direct visualization of the vocal cords and use of an end-tidal CO_2 detector.

g. Continue ventilation, the tube is in the trachea, however the waveform shows evidence of bronchospasm so you should consider administering a bronchodilator.

(Objective 14)

28. a. LMA, King, and ETT b. ETC c. ETT d. ETT e. ETC and King f. LMA and King

(Objective 13)

29. a. Hyperventilate the patient's lungs with 100% oxygen for at least 2 minutes.

b. With the laryngoscope in the left hand, insert the blade in the right corner of the mouth, displacing the tongue to the left.

c. Advance the endotracheal tube through the right corner of the mouth and, under direct vision, through the vocal cords.

d. Inflate the cuff with 5 to 8 mL of air, and ventilate the patient's lungs with a mechanical airway device.

e. Confirm endotracheal tube placement by auscultation of the abdomen and chest during ventilation.

f. Secure the endotracheal tube to the patient's head and face, and provide ventilatory support with supplemental oxygen. Continue to monitor correct placement of endotracheal tube using end-tidal CO_2 detection and other methods.

(Objective 13)

Chapter **15** **Airway Management, Respiration, and Artificial Ventilation**

30.

Adjunct	Advantage	Disadvantage
a. Mouth to mask	Easy to apply	Not possible to deliver 100% oxygen
b. Bag-valve-mask	Can give supplemental oxygen Can give 100% oxygen Can vary volume	Mask seal difficult to maintain Frequently requires two persons

(Objective 12)

31. Vomiting with inadequate ability to expel emesis, facial trauma with bleeding in mouth, and epistaxis (nosebleed) where blood is accumulating in the oral cavity.
(Objectives 9 and 13)

32. Place the patient on a cardiac monitor, hyperoxygenate the lungs with 100% oxygen for 5 minutes before the procedure, and apply suction for no longer than 10 seconds.
(Objective 13)

33. a. The tongue is disproportionately large in a child, and the oral airway easily can occlude the airway if it is inserted by rotation.
 b. A child younger than 8 years has a circular narrowing at the level of the cricoid cartilage that serves as a functional cuff.
 c. The vocal cords slope from front to back, necessitating rotation of the tube or performance of the Sellick maneuver to facilitate intubation.
(Objective 15)

34. In many older patients there is increased thoracic rigidity, decreased elastic recoil of the lungs, and diminished Po_2. In addition, the chemoreceptors do not function as well, which results in a decreased ventilatory response because of compromise of the respiratory system. Therefore the patient who experiences a significant chest injury may lack the physiological capability to compensate for the injury and will need aggressive intervention by the paramedic.
(Objective 16)

35. b. External respiration is the transfer of O_2 and CO_2 between the inspired air and pulmonary capillaries. Pulmonary ventilation refers to the movement of air into and out of the lungs. Respiration is the exchange of O_2 and CO_2 between an organism and the environment.
(Objective 2)

36. c. Pressure within the lungs (including the alveolar sacs) drops approximately 1 mm Hg during inspiration to permit the entry of air but is equal to atmospheric pressure at the end of quiet exhalation. The mediastinum does not maintain inflation of the lungs. Integrity of the thoracic cage is necessary to maintain negative pressure within the pleural space.
(Objective 3)

37. c. Only 3 mL of oxgyen can be dissolved in 1 L of blood at the normal arterial Po_2 of 100 mm Hg. Oxygen saturation measures the amount of hemoglobin that is saturated with oxygen. Normal oxygenation for a healthy 18-year-old is indicated by a Po_2 of 80 to 100 or greater. Venous Po_2 is typically about 40 mm Hg.
(Objective 4)

38. a. Without pulmonary surfactant, alveoli tend to collapse, making the work of breathing more difficult. All other factors listed decrease the work of breathing.
(Objective 16)

39. b. Minute volume = Tidal volume × Respiratory rate. Anything that decreases one of these variables without a reciprocal increase in the other decreases the minute volume.
(Objective 16)

40. c. It means that all hemoglobin is saturated with oxygen. When oxygen saturation is 100%, the oxygen is typically between 80% and 100% but may vary under certain pathological conditions.
(Objective 10)

41. b. Oxygenation is impaired in all these examples by different mechanisms.
(Objective 16)

42. c
(Objectives 6 and 16)

43. b
(Objective 7)

44. d. If the patient's physiological signs deteriorate, the rescuer should intervene.
(Objective 8)

45. c
(Objective 8)

46. b. Because the tongue is the most frequent cause of airway obstruction, repositioning the airway may be the only maneuver necessary to permit air exchange.
(Objective 8)

47. d. Suctioning will reduce but not eliminate the risk of aspiration. A nasogastric tube will decrease the risk of aspiration by minimizing the gastric content, but an oropharyngeal airway may stimulate the gag reflex and cause aspiration. The most appropriate position to minimize the risk of aspiration is the left lateral recumbent (recovery) position.
(Objective 9)

48. a. The mechanism of injury and signs are consistent with this life-threatening emergency, which necessitates aggressive airway management.
(Objective 8)

49. a. It is a frequently underused adjunct usually well tolerated by a semiconscious patient with a gag reflex.
(Objective 13)

50. b. The tube should be in the esophagus of a patient more than 5 feet tall, and no sounds should be audible over the gastric area when the patient's lungs are ventilated.
(Objective 13)

51. a. The King LT-D is designed to be placed in the esophagus.
(Objective 13)

52. a. Repeat attempts should be performed after hyperventilation.
(Objective 13)

53. d. Percutaneous transtracheal ventilation is a short-term (less than 45 minutes) airway device used when other measures to secure the airway are unsuccessful. The demand valve does not provide sufficient pressure to ventilate by this method. It offers no protection from aspiration. (Objective 11)

54. b
(Objective 12)

55. d. Misting is not a reliable indicator of tube placement. The esophageal bulb should fill instantly. No sounds should be audible over the epigastrium.
(Objective 12)

  Chapter **15** **Airway Management, Respiration, and Artificial Ventilation**

56. a. Suction should be applied for no longer than 10 seconds. A cough is stimulated frequently and may increase intracranial pressure. Suction should be set between 80 and 120 mm Hg.
(Objective 13)

57. d
(Objective 11)

58. b. A patient with this mechanism and symptoms of hypoxia clearly needs the highest percentage of oxygen available.
(Objective 11)

59. c. Avoid excessive hyperextension of the airway in children. Until you rule out a neck injury this child's head should not be hyperextended. Both suctioning and nasal airways are appropriate in children if indicated.
(Objectives 13 and15)

60. b. If the tube passes into tissue outside of the trachea, ventilation will not be possible. Aspiration, vocal cord injury, and perforation of great vessels also are complications but still may allow delivery of ventilation.
(Objective 13)

61. a. The oropharyngeal airway should be inserted using a tongue-blade in children. It should not be inserted if the child has a gag reflex. An oropharyngeal airway does not protect against aspiration. (Objectives 13 and 15)

62. c. There are two possible methods to calculate approximate depth of ET insertion.
The first is Age/2 + 12 = depth (cm); 8/2 + 12 = 16 cm.
The second is internal diameter of the ET tube x 3 = depth (cm). A 6.0 mm tube x 3 = 18. So the answer 17 is the closest appropriate estimate.
(Objectives 13 and 15)

63. a. The cricoid is a cartilage that encircles the airway. The vallecula is a space that lies behind the epiglottis. The xiphoid is cartilage on the inferior portion of the sternum.
(Objective 1)

64. d. The epiglottis is a flap-like cartilage that prevents entry of foreign substances into the lower airway.
(Objective 1)

WRAP IT UP

1. External respiration is interrupted because the substance aspirated and resulting inflammation of the alveoli impair the passage of oxygen to the pulmonary capillaries.
(Objective 2)

2. b. The drugs the patient ingested are central nervous system depressants that will inhibit the respiratory center in the brain and also impair the protective airway reflexes.
(Objective 7)

3. Suctioning secretions from the airway, nasogastric tube insertion with suction of gastric contents, and endotracheal intubation will help to prevent further aspiration.
(Objective 9)

4. c. Air trapping occurs from chronic obstructive pulmonary disease; bradypnea is a slow regular respiratory pattern; Kussmaul respirations are rapid and deep and occur in diabetic ketoacidosis.
(Objective 10)

5. A non-rebreather mask delivers the highest amount of oxygen.
(Objective 11)

232

6. c. Respiratory acidosis occurs when ventilation is impaired, resulting in decreased oxygen and increased CO_2.
(Objectives 10 and 16)

7. Hyperventilation helps to reverse respiratory acidosis.
(Objective 16)

8. Measure the oropharyngeal airway from the tragus of the ear to the corner of the mouth or the angle of the jaw.
(Objective 13)

9. a. Suctioning vomit from the oropharynx before intubation reduces the risk of aspiration and improves visualization of the vocal cords.
b. After intubation suctioning with a soft whistle-tipped catheter would help to eliminate vomit that previously was aspirated.
(Objectives 9 and 13)

10. a. No sounds heard over epigastrium
b. Breath sounds clearly audible bilaterally
c. Syringe fills freely with air and no stomach contents aspirated
d. Bulb fills with air within 2 seconds and no stomach contents are aspirated
e. Yellow color
f. CO_2 reads 35 to 45 mm Hg
g. Oxygen saturation increases or reads from 93% to 100%
h. Tube directly observed to be passing through vocal cords
(Objective 14)

11. Rate, 11 to 12; volume, 6 to 7 mL/kg
(Objective 12)

 Chapter **15** **Airway Management, Respiration, and Artificial Ventilation**

16 Scene Size-Up

READING ASSIGNMENT

Chapter 16, pages 472-478, in *Mosby's Paramedic Textbook,* ed. 4.

OBJECTIVES

Upon completion of this chapter, the paramedic student will be able to do the following:

1. Describe the purpose of scene size-up.
2. Outline the components of scene size-up.
3. Recognize factors that may contribute to an unsafe scene.
4. Describe scene evaluation techniques.
5. Identify steps in scene management.
6. Outline measures to lower the risks associated with illness or injury on an unsafe scene.
7. Identify additional resources that may be needed to manage multiple patient incidents.

SUMMARY

- Scene size-up is a quick assessment of an emergency scene. It is designed to determine resources needed to manage the scene safely and effectively.
- Dispatch information that assists with scene size-up includes location, type of location, type of situation, possible hazards, and unique issues.
- Special rescue, transport, fire, or other public safety resources may need to be dispatched to help manage the scene.
- Many factors can contribute to an unsafe scene. These may include environmental hazards, hazardous substances, violence, and rescue-related hazards.
- Scene assessment should always begin by asking, "Is the scene safe?" If it is not, identify measures that eliminate or reduce the risk to permit safe entry.
- Perform an initial scene survey. On medical calls, attempt to determine the nature of illness. On trauma calls, gather information related to the mechanism of injury.
- If hazards cannot be corrected, remove the patient from the scene as quickly and safely possible.
- Standard precautions should be used for all patients to minimize the risk of exposure to blood and bloody body fluids.
- Other specialized personal protective equipment may be needed based on the nature of the hazard and the training and role of the paramedic on the scene.
- Multiple patient situations require many resources. Priorities should always be scene safety with protection of the patient and bystanders. Incident command should be established.

REVIEW QUESTIONS

Questions 1 to 3 pertain to the following case study:

You are dispatched from your base on a cold, snowy winter night to a motor vehicle crash with injuries on the highway.

1. After ensuring safety, list five priorities during your scene size-up or assessment on this call.

   a. ____

   b. ____

c. ____

d. ____

e. ____

You find one patient, the driver of a car involved in a single-car collision. His face is covered with blood. He was not restrained and has been ejected about 15 feet from the car. You find him lying motionless in a safe location.

2. What personal protective equipment should you be wearing?

____

3. List at least three factors that indicate this scene may be unsafe.

____

Identify possible diagnoses as you evaluate each element of the scene as described in each of the following statements.

4. a. You are dispatched for an "unresponsive person" on a hot summer day.

____

b. As you approach the scene, you recognize the boarded-up house. You have been there several times for drug-related calls.

____

c. When you are getting your bags out of the ambulance, a woman runs out screaming, "My baby, my baby! He's only 10-months old. Please help him!"

____

d. You are met by the woman's boyfriend when you enter the home. He points you toward a back room. "I told him not to run up those steps," slurs the wobbly man. "I was just taking a little nap and found him there."

____

e. Moving through the house toward the patient, you see a coffee table spilling over with half-empty beer bottles, a bong, and several open pill bottles.

____

f. As you turn the corner, you see a limp infant lying face down at the foot of the steps. You are sweating profusely.

____

g. When you place your hands on either side of his head to hold inline spinal immobilization, you note that his skin is hot and flushed.

____

Questions 5 to 6 pertain to the following case study:

You are dispatched to a home for a call of a patient with "difficulty breathing." Your initial scene assessment reveals several patients with headache and difficulty breathing. You prepare to enter the home.

5. What initial information on this call leads you to believe the scene might be unsafe?

____

6. What factors on this call could contribute to an unsafe scene?

____

7. What measures should be taken to promote your safety on this call?

____

STUDENT SELF-ASSESSMENT

8. You arrive on the scene of a rollover motor vehicle crash involving a small sports car. Which of the following is a component in scene size-up or assessment on this call?
   a. Begin definitive patient care activities.
   b. Contact medical direction with an initial report.
   c. Initiate a mass casualty plan if indicated.
   d. Notify dispatch to send more resources if needed.

9. You are caring for a critically ill patient involved in a two-car motor vehicle collision. You are in the vehicle maintaining your patient's airway. Which measures are needed to reduce your risk of injury as the fire department disentangles the patient from the wreckage?
   a. Don full personal protection, including a self-contained breathing apparatus.
   b. Place a blanket over the patient to prevent glass or metal from impacting them.
   c. Because you are not involved in the rescue, only gloves, a mask, and a gown are needed.
   d. Wear a helmet, turnout coat, steel-toe boots, and leather gloves.

10. As you enter the home of a patient with chest pain, a small dog comes bounding out of the patient's bedroom, barking furiously at you. Which of the following is appropriate?
   a. Because the dog is small, proceed to the patient.
   b. Ask someone to put the dog away before you enter.
   c. Get a leash and tie up the dog out of the way.
   d. Shove the dog to the side with your boot.

11. What is the primary purpose of the scene size-up?
   a. To identify resources needed for safe scene management
   b. To identify the nature and severity of the patient's condition
   c. To recognize the most serious signs and symptoms
   d. To manage all risks present on the scene

12. Which of the following is a component of the scene size-up?
   a. Dispatch information
   b. Patient interventions
   c. Rapid transport
   d. Vital sign assessment

13. What measure should be used to facilitate safe assessment of a potential hazardous materials scene?
   a. Note any abnormal odors.
   b. Assess the patient for burns.
   c. Analyze the liquids on the scene.
   d. Visualize the scene with binoculars.

14. You are treating a patient who has had a suspected stroke. She was found seated out of doors on a very cold night. Which is the most appropriate step to manage the scene?
   a. Apply warm blankets
   b. Move the patient to the ambulance
   c. Infuse warmed intravenous fluids
   d. Cover the patient's head to maintain warmth

15. Your ambulance is first on the scene of a multistory fire at a high rise senior center. Multiple other units have been dispatched and are en route. Which resource should you use immediately that will assist with management of this scene?
   a. Activate the on-call list to call in more personnel.
   b. Call for the hazardous materials team.
   c. Implement the incident command system.
   d. Set up an oxygen cascade to treat multiple inhalation patients.

WRAP IT UP

You are dispatched to respond to a snowmobile collision. On arrival, you find a 17-year-old boy who struck a boating dock submerged under the powdery snow while traveling at a high rate of speed. You don the appropriate protective gear and cautiously evaluate the ice conditions and then with great difficulty approach the patient through the waist-deep snow. He was not wearing a helmet, and you recognize immediately that he has significant head and facial injuries. His eyes are closed, he is not arousable to voice, and his arms and legs extend when you apply painful stimulus. You radio dispatch and request a rescue unit to assist in extricating him across the snowy lake and for a helicopter because it is clear that he will need transport to the regional trauma center, located 70 miles away. As you await the rescue, you apply a cervical collar and secure the patient to the long spine board. You are unable to remove any of his clothing to perform further assessments because of the frigid conditions. You radio the rescue unit on the truck frequency and instruct them to prepare their stokes unit with sled skids and ask them to set up a landing zone on the road for the incoming helicopter. Dispatch updates you that the air unit has a 7-minute estimated time of arrival (ETA), and you ask them to relay your patient's condition, which you continually reevaluate, to the flight crew.
The patient is packaged onto the sled and pulled using a rope and winch to the shore, where the flight crew is waiting. You give them a report and help them move the patient into their aircraft.

1. What type of protective gear would be indicated for this situation?

____

2. Why was it necessary to pause and check ice conditions before proceeding to the patient?

____

3. What is your highest priority in the scene size-up and assessment?
   a. Forming a general impression
   b. Evaluating resources
   c. Initial patient assessment
   d. Scene safety determination

4. Why were resources called for before patient interventions began?

____

REVIEW QUESTIONS

1. a. Determine the mechanism of injury.
   b. Find out the number of persons injured.
   c. Determine the need for rescue or hazardous materials resources and request them from dispatch if needed.
   d. Determine the best access for responders you request.
   e. Secure the area, clearing unnecessary persons from the scene.
   (Objective 2)

2. Goggles, mask, gloves, and possibly a gown
   (Objective 6)

3. The weather is cold, so cold-related injury is possible; the incident is on a highway, which is very high risk; the car is overturned, so there is risk of injury during extrication; and there is evidence the driver may have been intoxicated or had altered mental status at the time of the crash, which increases the risk of patient violence.
   (Objective 3)

4. a. Cardiac or respiratory arrest, diabetic emergency, seizure, stroke, heat-related illness, trauma, or shock
   b. Drug overdose.
   c. SIDS, trauma
   d. Child abuse, trauma
   e. Drug overdose or intoxication
   f. Trauma, cardiac arrest, heat related
   g. Febrile seizure, septic shock, heat-related illness
   (Objective 4)

5. The fact that more than one patient is ill should cause you to suspect an airborne hazard.
   (Objective 2)

6. Poison gases such as carbon monoxide could render this scene unsafe.
   (Objective 3)

7. If the patients are able to walk, have them come outside so you can assess them safely. If fire department personnel with appropriate personal protective equipment are available, have them enter, move the patients out, interrupt the source of the toxic gas (if possible), and ventilate the room to render it safe.
   (Objective 6)

STUDENT SELF-ASSESSMENT

8. d. Patient care activities typically begin after the initial scene size-up. Medical direction should be contacted later. A mass casualty incident is unlikely in this setting.
   (Objective 1)

9. d. You need more than just standard precautions when involved in a vehicle rescue to reduce your risk of injury.
   (Objective 6)

10. b. Even small dogs bite. If possible, ask someone to place the dog in another room behind a closed door.
    (Objective 6)

11. a. EMS often does not have the resource to manage unsafe scenes. Specialty resources such as law enforcement, fire, or rescue should be summoned to mitigate risks identified in the scene size-up.
    (Objective 1)

12. a. Dispatch information will often begin your assessment of the scene.
    (Objective 2)

13. d. Maintain a distance from hazardous materials incidents until safety can be established. Generally, if you can smell the chemical or assess the patient, you are too close.
(Objective 4)

14. b. Moving the patient to the ambulance is a strategy that can assist the paramedic in many unsafe scene situations.
(Objective 5)

15. c. The incident management system will establish an organized framework that you can use to effectively manage this scene.
(Objective 7)

WRAP IT UP

1. If this lake were considered a busy traffic way, a helmet and safety goggles would be indicated. A warm turnout coat with reflective strips, slip-resistant waterproof gloves, and boots with steel insoles and steel toe protection should be worn.
(Objective 6)

2. If the ice were unsafe in any part of the scene, it would be critical to know to prevent injury or death to the rescuers and patient.
(Objective 3)

3. d. Evaluation of scene safety throughout all calls is critical.
(Objective 2)

4. Additional resources often take significant time to deploy. Activating them as early as possible is critical to expedite care and rescue.
(Objective 5)

Chapter **16** **Scene Size-Up**

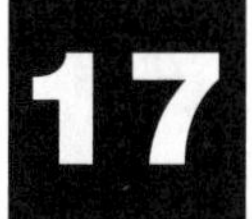 **Therapeutic Communications**

READING ASSIGNMENT

Chapter 17, pages 479-490 in *Mosby's Paramedic Textbook*, ed. 4.

OBJECTIVES

Upon completion of this chapter, the paramedic student will be able to do the following:

1. Define *therapeutic communication.*
2. List the elements of effective therapeutic communication.
3. Identify internal factors that influence effective communication.
4. Identify external factors that influence effective communication.
5. Explain the elements of an effective patient interview.
6. Summarize strategies for gathering appropriate patient information.
7. Discuss methods of assessing the individual's mental status during the patient interview.
8. Describe ways the paramedic can improve communication with a variety of patients. Such patients include (1) those who are unmotivated to talk, (2) hostile patients, (3) children, (4) older adults, (5) hearing-impaired patients, (6) blind patients, (7) patients under the influence of drugs or alcohol, (8) sexually aggressive patients, and (9) patients whose cultural traditions are different from those of the paramedic.
9. Describe methods to communicate in a culturally sensitive manner.

SUMMARY

- Therapeutic communication is a planned act. It is also a professional act. The paramedic, working with the patient, obtains information that is used to meet patient care goals.
- Communication is a dynamic process. It has six elements: the source, encoding, the message, decoding, the receiver, and feedback.
- To effectively communicate with patients, paramedics must genuinely like people. They must be able to empathize with others. They also must have the ability to listen.
- Good communication calls for a favorable physical environment. Factors such as privacy, interruption, eye contact, and personal dress are external influences. These factors can be controlled. This allows the paramedic to better communicate with the patient.
- The patient interview often decides the direction of the physical examination. Good care means that the paramedic sees each patient as an individual. It also means that the patient's needs are met in a caring, concerned, and receptive way.
- Open-ended and closed (direct) questions can be used to get information from the patient. Techniques include resistance, shifting focus, recognizing defense mechanisms, and distraction.
- The first step with any patient is to assess mental status. This can be done by observing the patient's appearance and level of consciousness. The paramedic also can look for normal or abnormal body movements. During normal conversation, the patient should be able to show clear thinking, a normal attention span, and the ability to concentrate on and understand the discussion. The patient's responses to the environment (i.e., affect) should be appropriate to the situation.
- Difficult interviews generally arise from four situations: (1) the patient's condition may affect the ability to speak; (2) the patient may fear talking because of psychological disorders, cultural differences, or age; (3) a cognitive impairment may be present; or (4) the patient may want to deceive the paramedic.
- Paramedics should avoid ethnocentrism and cultural imposition when caring for patients from other cultures.

Match the communication response in column II with the description in column I. Use each response only once.

Column I

1. _______ Making associations or implying a cause

2. _______ Paraphrasing a patient's words

3. _______ Pausing for several moments

4. _______ Reviewing with open-ended questions

5. _______ Having the patient rephrase a word

6. _______ Providing information

7. _______ Refocusing on one aspect of the interview

Column II

a. Clarification
b. Confrontation
c. Empathy
d. Explanation
e. Interpretation
f. Reflection
g. Silence
h. Summary

8. Identify selected elements of the communication process in the following example:

   You tell your 4-year-old patient that you plan to take his temperature. He asks, "Where are you going to take it to?" You clarify that you are going to put a thermometer under his tongue to see whether he has a fever.

   a. Who is the source?

   b. Who did the encoding in the initial message?

   c. Was the decoding effective?

   d. Who was the receiver?

   e. Why was feedback needed?

9. You are caring for a patient who is very emotionally upset. List six actions you can use to convey that you are actively listening to the patient.

   a. ____

   b. ____

   c. ____

   d. ____

   e. ____

   f. ____

10. A patient was assaulted and is found in the midst of a large crowd. How can you control external factors to enable effective communication with this patient?

    ____

    ____

11. Rewrite the following questions into an open-ended format:

    a. Do you feel bad?

    b. Does your chest hurt here?

    c. Did this problem start today?

    d. Are you taking any medicine on a daily basis?

12. Can you identify the problem in each of the following statements if they were made by a paramedic?

    a. I know you can't move your legs right now, but don't worry; everything will be just fine.

    b. You know you won't have this trouble breathing if you quit smoking.

    c. We believe your substernal chest pain may be causing an ischemic area in your myocardium that is going to result in myocardial infarction.

    d. Why didn't you take your blood pressure medicine?

13. You are called to a residence for a woman who fell down the stairs. You begin your assessment and patient management, and by the time you get in the back of the ambulance, you realize that her injuries are not consistent with the mechanism of injury she describes. The patient is reluctant to give you much information, and you strongly suspect domestic violence was the cause of her injuries.

    a. What reasons may this patient have for resistance regarding information?

    b. What statements might you make to begin to talk about this issue?

    c. If she tells you she was beaten up by her husband but doesn't want to leave him or have him arrested, how should you respond?

14. You are called to a college dorm for an "overdose." As you arrive on the scene, the patient is walking toward you.

    a. What is the first step in your mental status examination of this patient?

____

    b. As you begin your conversation with the patient, what observations will you make regarding mental status?

____

15. For each of the following difficult situations, identify three strategies that you may use to attempt to communicate with the patient.

    a. A 72-year-old man has paralysis on the right side. He appears to be awake and alert, but he is not responding to your questions appropriately.

____

    b. You have been called to a jail to care for a patient who has expressed a wish to kill a number of people. He is sitting with his arms folded, and his voice is getting progressively louder.

____

16. Describe your approach when interviewing a 3-year-old child and his father.

____

17. You are caring for a patient in the ambulance who makes inappropriate and sexually suggestive remarks. What should you do?

____

STUDENT SELF-ASSESSMENT

18. Which of the following best describes therapeutic communication?
    a. Verbal and nonverbal behavior that conveys a message
    b. Planned act to communicate and obtain information
    c. Spoken or written words to express ideas or feelings
    d. Decoding and encoding from a messenger to a receiver

19. When a message is put into an understandable format, it is considered which of the following?
    a. Decoded   **c.** Received
    b. Encoded   **d.** Sourced

20. When you try to see the situation from another person's point of view, you are demonstrating which of the following?
    a. Cultural imposition   **c.** Ethnocentrism
    b. Empathy   **d.** Sympathy

21. Which of the following would convey a confident, open attitude during the patient interview in the prehospital setting?
    a. Speaking loudly and quickly
    b. Standing with your arms folded on your chest
    c. Looking into the patient's eyes as the patient speaks
    d. Not invading the patient's personal space

246

22. Which of the following would demonstrate an effective patient communication strategy?
   a. Beginning questions with "How"
   b. Demonstrating personal bias
   c. Interrupting to get to the point
   d. Using medical terminology

23. Which of the following is a normal finding during the mental status examination?
   a. The patient demonstrates long pauses and rapid shifts in conversation.
   b. The patient has an upright posture and is well groomed.
   c. You repeat questions several times before the patient understands you.
   d. The patient is trembling and clenching and unclenching the fists.

24. Which of the following is the most effective method for communicating with a hearing-impaired patient in the prehospital setting?
   a. Lipreading while facing the patient
   b. Sign language
   c. Whatever method the patient prefers
   d. Note writing

25. Which of the following describes an action by a paramedic that could be seen as cultural imposition after you have told them their father died?
   a. You ask them to quiet down because they are wailing and praying loudly.
   b. You do not join in with their ritual prayer ceremony.
   c. You do not allow them to move the patient before the police arrive.
   d. You offend them by placing your arm around the patient's wife.

WRAP IT UP

You are dispatched to a quiet residential neighborhood for an "unknown nature." The local police community officer meets you on the scene and says that he is worried about the resident. The officer has been working with the resident to improve his living conditions. A month ago, he found the 70-year-old patient living without electricity or running water. He was using the nearby creek for toileting, and he used candles to light his home. Currently the patient is living in a nearby community while trying to clean up his home. This morning a sore on his leg began to bleed, and he is unable to control the bleeding. You note a dirty, ulcerated wound that is red and swollen on the patient's lower leg. He tells you that he is diabetic and not to worry, he will take care of it. He then walks over to a dirty basin of water in the yard and begins to clean the wound with a dirty rag.

You take a short history and do a brief physical examination. You determine that the patient needs to be transported for care of his wound. His compliance with his diabetic medicines is questionable, and you are unsure how well his basic nutritional and hygiene needs are being met. The patient adamantly refuses transport; he is afraid he won't ever be able to come home. Your partner begins to argue with him, and the patient becomes progressively more angry and agitated.

1. What message were you trying to encode to the patient?

____

2. What information did he decode from your message?

____

3. What strategy do you think will be most successful for communicating with this patient?
   a. Empathy
   b. Pity
   c. Sympathy
   d. Threats

4. How can you show that you are listening effectively?
  a. Look for weak spots in his arguments that you can debate.
  b. Prepare your answer while you listen so you can respond fast.
  c. Try to ignore the body language and voice tone and just listen to his words.
  d. Summarize the patient's statements to clarify meaning if you are unsure.

5. What are six techniques that you can use from the beginning of the patient interview to improve the chance for an effective patient encounter?

  a. ____

  b. ____

  c. ____

  d. ____

  e. ____

  f. ____

6. Which of the following statements would likely be most effective in this situation?
  a. "Living like this isn't healthy for a human being. You should find somewhere else to live. We need to take you to the hospital to get you to a cleaner place."
  b. "Why are you living in these conditions? Don't you know this isn't healthy?"
  c. "The impaired circulation secondary to your diabetes will prohibit normal mechanisms of healing, leading to possible sepsis. You need immediate medical interventions."
  d. "It looks as though you need some help to heal this wound. Let's take you to the doctor so you can get better quickly and get back to your work here at home."

7. Which of the statements in question 6 appear judgmental?

8. Which of the following would not be helpful in responding to this patient's anger?
  a. "I know you're angry because it seems as if we're telling you what to do. We would just like you to get some care for your wound so you can get home quickly."
  b. You ignore the patient's anger and continue more forcefully with your attempts to make him go to the hospital.
  c. "It seems as though you're angry because you're worried you won't be able to come home if you go to the hospital. Our goal is just the opposite; we know how important your home is to you, and we want you to be healthy so you can stay here."
  d. "You seem really angry; can you tell us why? We'd like to be here to help you solve your problem."
  The patient responds to your partner with a raised voice and tells him he has no business coming on his property and telling him what to do.
  After you calmly sit with the patient for a few minutes and clearly explain your concerns, as well as the actions the hospital may take to get the patient home quickly, he agrees to be transported for care.

CHAPTER 17 ANSWERS

REVIEW QUESTIONS

1. e

2. f

3. g

4. h

5. a

6. d

7. b
(Questions 1–7: Objective 1)

8. a. You (the paramedic) are the source.
b. You did the encoding.
c. No, the patient did not interpret the message in an appropriate manner.
d. The patient was the receiver of the first message.
e. Feedback was needed to clarify the message.
(Objective 2)

9. a. Face the patient when he or she speaks.
b. Maintain eye contact.
c. Avoid crossing your legs or arms.
d. Avoid distracting body movements.
e. Nod in acknowledgment at appropriate times.
f. Lean toward the patient.
(Objective 3)

10. Move the patient into the ambulance as quickly as possible for more privacy. Try to avoid interruptions until the interview is finished.
(Objective 4)

11. a. "How do you feel?"
b. "Describe (or show me) where your chest hurts."
c. "Tell me when this problem began."
d. "What medicines do you take on a daily basis?"
(Objective 5)

12. a. You shouldn't offer false reassurance.
b. Showing disapproval and offering unsolicited advice impair effective communication.
c. Using professional jargon impairs the patient's ability to understand you.
d. "Why" questions may be viewed as accusations.
(Objective 5)

13. a. Her resistance may be related to personal pride, fear of loss of self-esteem, or fear of retribution.
b. Shifting the focus temporarily to her injuries and making statements such as, "I've seen this pattern of injuries before in women who have been hurt by their husbands or boyfriends," may allow her to respond to your comments.
c. Explain that you recognize she is in a dangerous situation and that you are worried about her. Then give her some information about social service agencies that can provide support or help if she changes her mind later. Report your observations to the hospital staff.
(Objective 6)

14. a. Observe the patient's appearance, level of consciousness, and gait. Note how he or she is dressed and groomed. Look for any defensive or aggressive postures.

   b. Talk to the patient to see if he or she is oriented to person, place, and time. Note the quality of speech and the ability to think clearly, maintain a normal attention span, and concentrate on the discussion.
   (Objective 7)

15. a. Consider whether the patient's present illness or a preexisting condition may prevent him from speaking. Tell him you are there to help. Question family members. See whether the patient can nod to answer questions if he is unable to respond verbally.

   b. Make sure you are positioned close to an exit and that law enforcement officers are close by. Try to use normal interviewing techniques. Set limits. Follow protocols for restraint if the patient's behavior becomes violent.
   (Objective 8)

16. Ask the father questions first. Offer a distraction to the child and gradually approach and start talking to him. Speak at eye level in a calm, quiet voice. Use short sentences with concrete explanations.
(Objective 8)

17. Inform the patient of your professional role and the inappropriate nature of the comments. Document the situation; if possible, have another caregiver ride in the patient compartment with you.
(Objective 8)

18. b. Each of the other answers describes communication. Therapeutic communication is a planned, deliberate act that uses specific techniques to build a positive relationship and share information to achieve goals for the patient.
   (Objective 1)

19. b. Decoding involves interpretation of a message.
(Objective 2)

20. b. Cultural imposition means imposing your beliefs or values on people from other cultures. Ethnocentrism is viewing your own life as the most acceptable, the best, or superior to others. Sympathy is the expression of your feelings about another person's predicament.
   (Objective 3)

21. c. Folding your arms may indicate a closed, defensive feeling. Although you need to be aware of a patient's personal space, in the prehospital setting, you need to make close contact on most calls to perform an effective examination.
   (Objective 5)

22. a. Demonstrating personal bias that leads the patient in an unwanted direction can hamper communications. Interruptions occasionally may be necessary if a life-threatening condition exists, but a more appropriate action is to allow the patient to proceed uninterrupted. Excessive use of medical terminology with patients may impair their ability to understand you.
   (Objective 5)

23. b. This observation is just one clue in the examination. All of the other choices reflect possible abnormal mental status exam results.
   (Objective 7)

24. c. The paramedic's abilities (regarding sign language) and the circumstances of the call determine which method can be used. Whenever possible, the method that the patient chooses should be used.
   (Objective 8)

25. a. Cultural rituals for grieving vary. As long as the families practice does not harm anyone or violate any laws, it is appropriate to allow them to continue. It is not an expectation that you join any ritual. If moving the patient could violate your rules until the coroner arrives, you must ask the family to wait. If you know that putting your arm around a family would be considered offensive, that would not be appropriate
   (Objective 9)

250

1. You are trying to encode a message that the patient has a specific medical problem that needs to be cared for in the hospital.
   (Objective 2)

2. The message he has decoded tells him that your efforts to get him to go to the hospital will mean that he may never come home again.
   (Objective 2)

3. a. Telling the patient that you understand his fear and then clarifying the issues may be effective.
   (Objective 2)

4. d. You want him to know that you are listening carefully. You also want to make sure that you understand the meaning of his words.
   (Objective 6)

5. Six strategies you can use are face the patient, maintain eye contact, look attentive (don't cross your arms and legs), avoid distracting movements, nod to acknowledge important points, and lean toward the speaker.

6. d. You should use nonthreatening language and acknowledge the patient's chief concern about getting home.
   (Objective 6)

7. Responses (a) and (b) sound very judgmental k may make the patient even more angry.
   (Objective 6)

8. b. The other answers acknowledge the patient's emotions.
   (Objective 6)

18 History Taking

READING ASSIGNMENT

Chapter 18, pages 491-502, in *Mosby's Paramedic Textbook,* ed. 4.

OBJECTIVES

Upon completion of this chapter, the paramedic student will be able to do the following:

1. Describe the purpose of effective history taking in prehospital patient care.
2. List components of the patient history as defined by the National EMS Education Standards.
3. Outline effective patient interviewing techniques to facilitate history taking.
4. Describe how the paramedic uses clinical reasoning.
5. Outline the process to determine differential diagnoses.
6. Identify strategies to manage special challenges in obtaining a patient history.

SUMMARY

- Obtaining a patient history offers structure to the patient assessment. The history often identifies life threats and sets priorities in patient care.
- Content of the patient history includes date and time, identifying data, source of referral, history, reliability, chief complaint, present illness, past medical history, current health status, and review of body systems.
- Paramedics should ensure patient comfort. Several methods are available to accomplish this. Paramedics should avoid entering the patient's personal space. Sensitivity to the patient's feelings and watching for signs of uneasiness also are important. Paramedics should use appropriate language and ask open-ended and direct questions. Paramedics should use therapeutic communications techniques as well.
- Clinical reasoning requires integrating the patient's history with the physical assessment findings. It also requires knowledge of anatomy, physiology, and pathophysiology to direct appropriate questions to the patient.
- Differential diagnosis is the process of weighing the probability of one disease versus other diseases as accounting for a patient's illness.
- Many challenges can affect history taking. One of these challenges is silent or talkative patients. Another is patients with multiple symptoms. Then there are anxious, angry, or hostile patients. The paramedic also may see intoxication, crying, depression, and sexually attractive or seductive patients. False reassurance is a major issue to consider. Patient may present confusing behaviors and histories. Two other issues are developmental disabilities and communication barriers. With these last two, the issue of talking with family and friends can be complex as well.

REVIEW QUESTIONS

Questions 1 and 2 pertain to the following case study:

You are dispatched to a home to care for a 75-year-old woman who is having chest pain.

1. What additional questions will you need to ask related to her history?

   a. Present illness:

   ____

   b. Significant medical history:

   ____

c. Personal habits and environmental conditions:

____

d. Family history:

____

2. What is her chief complaint?

____

____

3. Your elderly patient fell and has a painful wrist. Discuss any finding in each of the following elements of the SAMPLE history that may explain a reason for her fall.

S. ____

A. ____

M. ____

P. ____

L. ____

E. ____

4. For each of the following patient complaints, list any personal habits and environmental conditions that are important to know during the patient history:

a. A 4-year-old child awakens suddenly with a sore throat, fever, muffled voice, and dysphagia:

____

b. A 25-year-old soldier complains of fever, night sweats, weight loss, and hemoptysis:

____

c. A 40-year-old adult is injured in a motor vehicle collision:

____

d. An 18-year-old woman is complaining of abdominal pain:

____

e. A 72-year-old older adult has slurred speech:

____

f. A 45-year-old person is complaining of depression:

____

g. A 27-year-old person has a heart rate of 50 beats/min:

____

h. A 77-year-old older adult is dirty and has bruises in various stages of healing on the back and arms:

____

i. A 16-year-old young woman is extremely thin and frail looking:

____

5. Describe one technique to use when dealing with each of the following situations during the patient interview:

a. Your elderly patient clearly is distraught and has a lengthy pause in his conversation as he relates a painful story to you:

____

b. The patient begins a long and complex history in much more detail than necessary:

____

c. Within the first 60 seconds of your interview, your patient has related at least five different problems of varying severity:

____

d. The patient is trembling and tearful despite a relatively minor injury:

____

e. The patient asks you to tell her everything will be all right when you know her condition is critical and perhaps even lethal:

____

f. A patient is verbally venting his anger and frustration about his illness:

____

g. The patient strokes your leg in a sexually suggestive manner:

____

h. The patient does not speak or understand your language:

____

6. What is the primary purpose of obtaining a patient history?
   a. To obtain billing information
   b. To detect signs of injury
   c. To establish priorities of patient care
   d. To make the patient comfortable

7. Which of the following is a routine component of the patient history?
   a. Age
   b. Insurance information
   c. Religion
   d. Vital signs

8. Which of the following is true regarding the chief complaint in the patient history?
   a. It is always stated by the patient succinctly and clearly.
   b. It is usually the reason that emergency medical services was called.
   c. It includes significant medical history.
   d. It will remain the same throughout the call.

9. What might be a good question to ask while obtaining the history of present illness for a patient who is experiencing difficulty breathing?
   a. Did it start today?
   b. Is your difficulty breathing pretty bad?
   c. Where is your difficulty breathing?
   d. What makes your breathing better or worse?

10. Your patient is complaining of headache and chest tightness after an exposure to an unknown gas at work. What personal habits should you ask about for this patient?
   a. Exercise
   b. Immunizations
   c. Sleep patterns
   d. Smoking history

11. You plan to administer ketorolac tromethamine (Toradol) to a patient. You will not give it if your patient reports anaphylactic reaction to which drug?
   a. Acetaminophen (Tylenol)
   b. Aspirin
   c. Meperidine (Demerol)
   d. Penicillin

12. For which patient is it most important to determine last oral intake?
   a. A corneal abrasion
   b. A small laceration on the forearm
   c. Dizziness
   d. Shoulder pain

13. Which of the following illnesses is hereditary?
   a. Tonsillitis
   b. Skin cancer
   c. Sickle cell anemia
   d. Tuberculosis

14. Which statement may be most helpful when assessing a patient who is depressed?
   a. "Don't worry; we'll take good care of you."
   b. "Everything will be okay when we get you to the hospital."
   c. "My friend was depressed, and he's just fine now."
   d. "It seems as though you are really sad. I'm here to listen."

15. What is a good approach when you are managing an angry or intoxicated patient who does not pose an immediate danger to him- or herself or the emergency medical services crew?
   a. Physical restraint
   b. Set limits
   c. Threaten
   d. Yell

16. When interviewing a patient who has developmental delays, you should do which of the following?

    a. Clarify answers.   **c.** Omit most questions.

    b. Not ask the patient.   **d.** Speak loudly.

17. When assessing a 4-year-old child who was injured after a long fall, which question would be most appropriate?

    a. On a scale of zero to 10, can you tell me how bad your pain is?

    b. Would you like a shot to help relieve your pain?

    c. Does your pain radiate anywhere?

    d. Can you please point to the place that hurts?

WRAP IT UP

At 0900, you are dispatched to a call for "chest pain." A 45-year-old black woman is complaining of diffuse chest and abdominal pain. She is pale, cool, and diaphoretic. Her husband called you because he was concerned when she said she was too ill to go to work at her law firm, which she has never done before. She is conscious, alert, and oriented and tells you that this began about an hour ago. She is unable specifically to describe the pain but says it is a gnawing sensation sometimes in her chest and left shoulder and other times in the left lower quadrant of her abdomen. She is nauseated as well. Nothing seems to make the pain change in severity (rated as a 5–7), character, or location. She says she is normally healthy and has an insulin pump for her diabetes, which she was diagnosed with at the age of 6 years. She indicates that she has eaten her regular breakfast and had a normal dinner last evening. Just before your arrival, she says her blood sugar was normal for her at this time of day. Her allergies include aspirin and shellfish. She reports no trauma, major surgeries, or hospitalizations since her initial diagnosis of diabetes. She has not traveled recently or had any occupational exposures to anything unusual. She has two teenage children and is premenopausal with irregular periods (last period 5 weeks ago) and uses the rhythm method for birth control. She reports a normal bowel movement this morning. Her parents are both deceased: her father died of an abdominal aneurysm at 48 years of age, and her mother died of a heart attack at 45 years of age. Vital signs are BP 98/58, P 110, and R 24/min; oxygen saturation is 93%; blood glucose 92 mg/dL; and her electrocardiogram shows a sinus tachycardia. Her physical exam reveals some mild tenderness in the abdomen not specifically localized. Peripheral pulses are weak in all extremities. You apply oxygen at 4 L/min by nasal cannula, initiate an IV of normal saline TKO, and begin transport to the hospital while continuing to monitor the patient's vital signs and level of pain.

1. Which of the following illnesses is a possibility based on the history that she has given to you? List the reasons for your response.

Illness	Yes	No	Reasons (Family History, Signs, and Medications)
a. Myocardial infarction			
b. Stroke			
c. Appendicitis			
d. Ectopic pregnancy			
e. Abdominal aortic aneurysm			
f. Urinary tract infection			
g. Gastroenteritis			
h. Hypoglycemia			

2. What could be the significance of neglecting to ask about the following?

    a. Allergies ____

    b. Menstrual history ____

    c. Family history ____

257

3. Why might the patient be reluctant to call 911 with her history and symptoms?

____

____

4. What can you say to the patient if she wants to know what is wrong with her?

____

____

CHAPTER 18 ANSWERS

HISTORY TAKING

1. a. Does anything make the pain better or worse? What does the pain feel like? Show me where the pain is. Does it go anywhere else? On a scale of 1 to 10, with 1 being the least and 10 being the worst, where do you rate your pain? When did you first notice your pain?
   b. How is your health in general? Have you been hospitalized for any major illness or injury? Are you having any other signs or symptoms today (difficulty breathing, nausea, vomiting, dizziness, or palpitations)? Do you have any allergies? What medicines do you take? Have you taken anything today? What significant medical history do you have (heart disease, lung disease, high blood pressure, diabetes)? When did you last eat? Was it anything unusual? What were you doing when you first noticed this pain?
   c. Do you smoke? Do you use alcohol or any other drugs?
   d. Are your parents living? Do (Did) they have any heart disease or other major medical problems?
   (Objective 3)

2. Chest pain
(Objective 2)

3. S—Does the patient have any associated signs or symptoms that may suggest a cardiac or other medical reason for the fall?
   A—Allergies or allergic reactions are unlikely to explain a fall unless the patient becomes hypotensive because of anaphylaxis, loses consciousness, and then falls.
   M—Some daily medicines can cause hypotension (especially orthostatic hypotension) that could lead to a fall. Other sedative, hypnotic, and psychotropic drugs may impair judgment or level of consciousness and predispose a person to a fall. Medications also can suggest preexisting medical conditions such as diabetes, heart disease, or neurological illness that may cause a fall.
   P—Pertinent past medical history may include factors such as heart disease (dysrhythmias); neurological disease (stroke with neurological deficit); diabetes (hypoglycemia); recent surgery; and other conditions that could alter balance, judgment, or consciousness and cause a fall.
   L—If the last meal was not timed correctly and the patient is diabetic or hypoglycemic, a fall could result.
   E—Did the patient have chest pain, visual disturbances, dizziness, palpitations, or any medical reason that could have caused the fall?
   (Objective 3)

4. You should ask about the following:
   a. Immunizations
   b. Tobacco use, alcohol use, screening tests (for tuberculosis), immunizations, home situation, exposure to contagious diseases, travel to other countries
   c. Alcohol or other drugs, use of safety measures (restraint devices)
   d. Diet, exercise, sexual history (possibly physical abuse)
   e. Alcohol and other drugs
   f. Alcohol and other drug use, sleep patterns, home situation, significant other (abuse or violence), sexual history, daily life, patient outlook, and economic condition
   g. Alcohol, drugs, and related substances, exercise and leisure activities

h. Tobacco use, alcohol, other drugs and related substances, diet, home situation and significant other, physical abuse or violence, daily life, housing, and economic condition

i. Tobacco use, alcohol, other drugs and related substances, sleep patterns, diet and exercise, and leisure activities
(Objective 3)

5. a. Remain attentive and listen. Reflect on some of the emotions you sense the patient may be experiencing.

b. Let the patient talk for a few minutes. Summarize his comments.

c. Summarize the comments and ask the patient to select the most pressing ones on which to focus in your examination.

d. Remain calm and caring and reassure the patient.

e. Reassure the patient that you are listening to her fears, that you are there to care for her, and that you understand her condition.

f. Remain calm and set limits about ways he can express his feelings in an appropriate manner. Be alert for signs of escalation so you can maintain the safety of the patient, yourself, and your crew.

g. Be clear that you are in a caring role and you feel the behavior is unacceptable. If it persists, consider trading roles with your partner if appropriate.

h. Determine whether a family member can translate or use a translating resource if available.
(Objective 6)

6. c. The history can provide structure and guidance during the physical examination, during which you hope to find signs of the illness or injury.
(Objective 1)

7. a. Vital signs are part of the physical assessment.
(Objective 2)

8. b. The patient often states the chief complaint but may not be able to do so if he or she is unconscious. Obtain the medical history after the chief complaint. It may change during the call if the patient's condition changes.
(Objective 3)

9. d. "Did the difficulty start today?" is not an open-ended question. A better way to ask about time of onset is, "Tell me when you noticed that you were having trouble breathing." Answer b. also is not an open-ended question. Asking about location is inappropriate with this chief complaint.
(Objective 3)

10. d. Lung function and laboratory values can be affected by smoking and are important information for this patient.
(Objective 3)

11. b. Allergy to other nonsteroidal antiinflammatory drugs also is a contraindication.
(Objective 3)

12. c. Lack of food intake could lead to hypoglycemia and dizziness.
(Objective 3)

13. c.
(Objective 3)

14. d. Offering false reassurances does not benefit the patient.
(Objective 3)

15. b. Establish limits for acceptable behavior.
(Objective 6)

16. a. Use phrases and words that can be understood easily.
(Objective 4)

259

17. d. A child this age will not comprehend a numeric rating scale nor the term "radiate." Children that age will either not want "a shot" or understand what it means.
(Objective 6)

<u>**WRAP IT UP**</u>

1. a. Signs and symptoms of present illness, family history of myocardial infarction at early age, diabetes
   b. Signs and symptoms do not suggest stroke; however, diabetic and family history are strong for vascular disease.
   c. Signs and symptoms vaguely suggest an abdominal condition that may require emergency surgery but may be masked by patient's diabetic history.
   d. Ectopic pregnancy is possible because of her irregular periods, high-risk birth control method, and abdominal pain with radiation to shoulder.
   e. Abdominal aneurysm is a possibility based on family history, race (but male sex would be higher risk), weak pulses, and diabetes.
   f. Urinary tract infection is a high risk in diabetic patients, but you have no report of urinary frequency. Dysuria could be masked by diabetes.
   g. Gastroenteritis: mild abdominal symptoms, nausea but no vomiting, no diarrhea reported
   h. Hypoglycemia: the patient's blood glucose is within the normal range. She does not appear to have other signs or symptoms of hypoglycemia (except tachycardia).
(Objectives 4, 5)

2. a. If myocardial infarction was suspected and aspirin was given without knowledge of the patient's allergy to it, a severe allergic reaction could occur.
   b. If a menstrual history was not obtained, the possibility of pregnancy and ectopic pregnancy might not be considered. The patient could have received radiographs and medications harmful to early fetal development or the possibility of life-threatening ectopic pregnancy might not be considered.
   c. The family history is strongly suggestive of two lethal vascular diseases: myocardial infarction and aortic aneurysm. Without the knowledge of this, certain diagnostic tests could be overlooked and the diagnosis missed.
(Objective 1)

3. The patient may be reluctant to call because of fear or denial of illness.
(Objective 4)

4. Tell her your concerns based on her symptoms, history, and physical findings and explain that further diagnostic tests only available at the hospital will be needed to pinpoint the specific nature of her problem.
(Objective 3)

19 Primary Assessment

Chapter 19, pages 503-511, in *Mosby's Paramedic Textbook,* ed. 4.

OBJECTIVES

Upon completion of this chapter, the paramedic student will be able to do the following:

1. Identify the components of the scene size-up.
2. Identify the priorities in each component of patient assessment.
3. Outline the critical steps in primary patient assessment.
4. Describe findings in the primary assessment that may indicate a life-threatening condition.
5. Discuss interventions for life-threatening conditions that are identified in the primary assessment.
6. Distinguish priorities in the care of the medical versus trauma patient.

SUMMARY

- Sizing up the scene consists of the initial steps performed on every emergency medical services response. These steps help to ensure scene safety. They also provide valuable information to the paramedic.
- Paramedics should ensure they have access to and wear appropriate personal protective equipment to protect against injury or illness related to unsafe scenes and infectious diseases.
- The primary assessment includes the paramedic's general impression of the patient, the assessment for life-threatening conditions, and the identification of priority patients requiring immediate care and transport.
- Assessment of life-threatening conditions entails a systematic evaluation of the patient's level of consciousness, airway, breathing, circulation, and disability. The patient should also be appropriately exposed during the primary assessment to detect life threats.
- Information from the primary survey is used to identify life threats and prioritize patients.
- The paramedic begins resuscitative measures such as airway maintenance, ventilatory assistance, and cardiopulmonary resuscitation immediately after recognizing the life-threatening condition that necessitates each respective maneuver.

REVIEW QUESTIONS

For each of the following primary survey assessment findings, indicate one possible cause and one possible intervention to perform in the primary survey.

Assessment Finding	Possible Cause	Intervention
1. Gurgling respirations		
2. Snoring respirations		
3. Cyanosis and dyspnea		
4. Anxious and pale with no radial pulse		

5. Place a check mark beside each of the following that is an element of the scene size-up.

_________ Identifying the type of situation   _________ Assessing vital signs

_________ Obtaining a history   _________ Identifying the number of patients

_________ Moving bystanders away   _________ Asking for additional assistance

_________ Initiating a mass casualty plan   _________ Opening the airway

_________ Triage   _________ Recognizing risk of danger

6. If the capillary refill is brisk and color returns to the nail bed of a 56-year-old woman in less than 1 second, it is an indicator of good perfusion. True/false? If you said false, explain your answer.

____

7. Stridor is usually resolved by positioning the airway. True/false? If you said false, explain your answer.

____

8. Add a word to each of the following signs or symptoms that would change it to a sign or symptom that indicates a priority patient.

a. _______________ breathing

b. _______________ bleeding

c. _______________ general impression

d. _______________ level of consciousness

9. List four examples of findings in the scene size-up that would lead you to don a mask and eye protection.

____

____

10. What is the primary purpose of the primary survey?
   a. To ensure scene safety
   b. To find and treat life threats
   c. To identify all injuries
   d. To obtain a comprehensive history

11. As you enter the scene, you can hear the patient's audible stridor. Her father is standing over her holding a weapon. What is your priority?
   a. To retreat until the scene is safe
   b. To intervene to treat the stridor
   c. To determine the cause of the stridor
   d. To identify any additional life threats

12. Which of the following is a component of the scene size-up on a multiple vehicle collision?
   a. Begin patient assessment and treat life threats.
   b. Notify the hospital of the number of casualties and the status of each of them.
   c. Assess for vehicles that have placards or are unstable.
   d. Apply oxygen to patients who have difficulty breathing.

13. Which of the following is a step in the primary assessment of an unresponsive patient?
   a. Assess vital signs.
   b. Perform head tilt, chin lift.
   c. Initiate an intravenous line.
   d. Measure blood glucose.

14. As you enter the room, you note that your patient is seated in the tripod position using the accessory muscles to breathe. The skin around his lips is blue. You can tell he is hypoxic from severe respiratory distress. What part of the primary assessment is this?
   a. General impression
   b. Primary assessment
   c. Secondary assessment
   d. Ongoing assessment

15. Which finding in the primary survey would cause you to take immediate action?
   a. Obvious pain when the patient moves
   b. Fruity odor on the patient's breath
   c. Sternal retractions when breathing
   d. Weak, rapid pulse at the radial artery

16. You arrive on a call for a seizure and find a 6-year-old snoring patient who is no longer seizing. She is responsive to painful stimulus. Which intervention has the highest priority?
   a. Administer an antiseizure medicine
   b. Start an intravenous line
   c. Insert a nasopharyngeal airway
   d. Position her in the semi-Fowler position

17. During the initial assessment of a trauma patient, what is the most appropriate method to assess the neurological status?
   a. AVPU
   b. Determination of extraocular muscle function (EOM)
   c. Pupil assessment
   d. Reflex examination

18. Which of the following patient situations represents a life threat identified in the primary assessment of an adult?
   a. Blood pressure in the right arm is much greater than in the left arm.
   b. Heart rate increases by 30 beats/min when the patient stands up.
   c. Stridor is audible.
   d. Temperature is 105.8°F (41°C).

19. You detect that the patient has agonal respirations and a radial pulse during your initial assessment. How should your care and assessment proceed?
   a. Auscultate the chest to determine the proper intervention.
   b. Continue assessment and then manage respiratory failure.
   c. Initiate airway management and ventilation and then proceed.
   d. Treat the respiratory difficulty and transport with no further examination.

20. Your patient was injured when a bomb detonated. She is conscious but lethargic and is breathing 24 times per minute with clear breath sounds and blood spurting from her partially amputated lower leg despite first responders' efforts to apply direct pressure. What is the highest priority intervention for this patient?
   a. Apply oxygen 15 L/min by non-rebreather mask.
   b. Control the bleeding with a tourniquet.
   c. Immobilize on a long spine board.
   d. Rapid transport to the closest trauma center.

21. Which patient is in greatest need of rapid transport to an appropriate medical facility?
   a. Pedestrian struck at low speed with an isolated lower extremity deformity
   b. Collided with a tree while snow skiing and is dyspneic and cyanotic
   c. Stung by a bee and is itching and wheezing with urticaria evident
   d. Found unresponsive, breathing 8 breaths/min with pinpoint pupils

On a hot summer afternoon, you respond for a person who is "unresponsive." The patient's daughter says she has not been able to reach her mother for 2 days. As you enter the kitchen, the heat is intense, but the familiar smell of digested blood fills your nostrils. About 15 prescription bottles are perched around the kitchen sink, and a recycle bin at the door is filled with Scotch bottles. You find the 72-year-old woman at the bottom of four steps in the poorly lit room. Her eyes are closed, and her skin is pale. As you approach the patient and call her name, there is no response. A firm squeeze to her trapezius yields no movement. You heard a faint gurgling noise as her chest rises slightly about eight times per minute. Although you are unable to feel a radial pulse, there is a rapid, irregular, thready pulsation palpable in her carotid artery.

1. What possible illness or injuries would you consider in your differential diagnosis based on your scene size-up?

2. List the findings in the primary assessment that indicate a life threat.

3. Based on the information you have, what interventions should be performed immediately?

4. What additional steps in patient assessment should you perform?

CHAPTER 19 ANSWERS

REVIEW QUESTIONS

Assessment Finding	Possible Cause	Intervention
1. Gurgling respirations	Bleeding from trauma Vomitus	Oropharyngeal suction
2. Snoring respirations	Drug overdose Intoxication Stroke Postictal after seizure Head injury	Narcotic antagonist Manual airway maneuvers Oral or nasopharyngeal airway Position patient
3. Cyanosis and dyspnea	Obstructive airway disease Allergic reaction Chest trauma Neuromuscular disease	Open the airway Administer oxygen Assist ventilation Medicines specific to illness such as bronchodilators
4. Anxious and pale with no radial pulse	Shock related to hypovolemia, anaphylaxis, sepsis, obstructive cause	Airway, oxygen, control obvious external bleeding, administer IV fluids, position, administer appropriate medication

(Objectives 4, 5)

264

5. Identifying the type of situation, identifying the number of patients, moving away bystanders, asking for additional assistance, initiating a mass casualty plan, triage, and recognizing risk of danger are all elements of the scene size-up
(Objective 1)

6. True. If the capillary refill were slow however, it could mean that she has poor peripheral perfusion related to vascular disease or cold and would not be considered reliable.
(Objective 4)

7. False. Stridor indicates airway obstruction. In some cases, positioning the airway can provide temporary relief, but typically, the obstruction should be relieved by addressing the cause. This may include removing a foreign body airway obstruction, medications to treat upper airway swelling, or surgical intervention for traumatic injuries.
(Objective 5)

8. Many answers are possible; a sample is provided.
   a. labored or difficulty or slow or irregular or shallow or absent **breathing**
   b. uncontrolled or internal **bleeding**
   c. poor **general impression**
   d. altered or decreased or diminished **level of consciousness**
(Objective 4 and 6)

9. Examples include imminent delivery, trauma with uncontrolled bleeding, trauma with oral bleeding, vomiting blood, and coughing up blood or violent patient who is spitting
(Objective 1)

STUDENT SELF-ASSESSMENT

10. b. The scene survey is used to determine threats to safety. Other injuries are to be found in the secondary assessment.
(Objective 2)

11. a. Retreat until the scene is made safe and then assess and treat her life threat.
(Objective 2)

12. c. Assessing for unsafe conditions is an element in the scene size-up.
(Objective 1)

13. b. Diagnostic tests are generally done as part of the secondary assessment.
(Objective 3)

14. a. You have not yet spoken to or touched the patient.
(Objective 2)

15. c. Sternal retractions are a sign of severe respiratory distress. Apply oxygen and ventilate if other indicators support this finding.
(Objective 4)

16. c. Snoring indicates a partially obstructed airway. This needs immediate attention.
(Objective 2)

17. a. The other components of the neurological examination are performed later in the assessment.
(Objective 3)

18. c. All other findings are identified later in the examination.
(Objective 4)

19. c. The life threat must be addressed before the examination can proceed.
(Objective 5)

20. b. If bleeding is not controlled, the patient will die.
(Objective 5)

21. b. This patient appears to have significant chest trauma and needs urgent scene care coupled with rapid transport. The first patient appears to have a non–life-threatening injury. The patients in c and d have urgent medical problems and will need transport after treatment on the scene.
(Objective 6)

WRAP IT UP

1. Intoxication, fall, hyperthermia, gastrointestinal bleeding, stroke
(Objective 1)

2. Unresponsive patient; gurgling, slow, shallow respirations; pale skin; no peripheral pulse; rapid, thready, irregular pulse
(Objective 4)

3. Stabilize the spine, manually open the airway, suction the airway, insert an oral or nasal airway, assist ventilation with a bag-mask and 100% oxygen, and prepare for rapid transport.
(Objective 5)

4. Assess breath sounds and measure oxygen saturation (if perfusion permits it), assess the pupils, and expose and inspect for bleeding. In the ambulance, obtain a complete set of vital signs, including temperature; measure blood glucose; monitor ECG; and perform a rapid head-to-toe assessment.
(Objective 3)

20 Secondary Assessment

READING ASSIGNMENT

Chapter 20, pages 512-559, in *Mosby's Paramedic Textbook,* ed. 4.

OBJECTIVES

Upon completion of this chapter, the paramedic student will be able to do the following:

1. Define the purpose of the secondary assessment.
2. Describe physical examination techniques commonly used in the prehospital setting.
3. Describe the examination equipment commonly used in the prehospital setting.
4. Describe the general approach to physical examination.
5. Outline the steps of a comprehensive physical examination.
6. Detail the components of the mental status examination.
7. Distinguish between normal and abnormal findings in the mental status examination.
8. Outline the steps in the general patient survey.
9. Distinguish between normal and abnormal findings in the general patient survey.
10. Describe physical examination techniques used for assessment of specific body regions.
11. Distinguish between normal and abnormal findings when assessing specific body regions.
12. Outline the process of patient reassessment.
13. State modifications to the physical examination that are necessary when assessing children.
14. State modifications to the physical examination that are necessary when assessing older adults.

SUMMARY

- The secondary assessment integrates patient assessment findings with knowledge of epidemiology and pathophysiology to form a filed impression and to identify an appropriate treatment plan.
- The examination techniques commonly used in the physical examination are inspection, palpation, percussion, and auscultation.
- Equipment used during the comprehensive physical examination includes the stethoscope, ophthalmoscope, otoscope, and blood pressure cuff.
- The physical examination is performed in a systematic manner. The exam is a step-by-step process. Emphasis is placed on the patient's present illness and chief complaint.
- The physical examination is a systematic assessment of the body that includes mental status; general survey; vital signs; skin, head, eyes, ears, nose, and throat; chest; abdomen; posterior body; extremities; and neurological examination.
- The first step in any patient care encounter is to note the patient's appearance and behavior. This includes assessing for level of consciousness. This may include assessment of posture, gait, and motor activity; dress, grooming, hygiene, and breath or body odors; facial expression; mood, affect, and relation to person and things; speech and language; thought and perceptions; and memory and attention.
- During the general survey, the paramedic should evaluate the patient for signs of distress, apparent state of health, skin color and obvious lesions, height and build, sexual development, and weight. The paramedic also should assess vital signs.
- The comprehensive physical examination should include an evaluation of the texture and turgor of the skin, hair, and fingernails and toenails.
- Examination of the structures of the head and neck involves inspection, palpation, and auscultation.
- A full knowledge of the structure of the thoracic cage is needed. This knowledge aids in performing a good respiratory and cardiac assessment. Air movement creates turbulence as it passes through the respiratory tree. Air movement produces breath sounds during inhalation and exhalation. In the prehospital setting, the paramedic must examine the heart indirectly. However, the paramedic can obtain details about the size and effectiveness of pumping action through a skilled assessment that includes palpation and auscultation.
- The four quadrants of the abdomen and their contents provide the basis for inspection, auscultation, percussion, and palpation of this body region.

- An examination of the genitalia of either sex can be awkward for the patient and the paramedic. The paramedic should inspect the genitalia for bleeding and signs of trauma (if indicated).
- Examination of the anus is indicated in the presence of rectal bleeding or trauma to the area.
- When examining the upper and lower extremities, the paramedic should direct his or her attention to function. The paramedic also should pay attention to structure.
- Assessment of the spine begins with a visual assessment of the cervical, thoracic, and lumbar curves. The assessment continues with a region-by-region examination for pain, swelling, and range of motion.
- A neurological examination may be organized into five categories: mental status and speech, cranial nerves, motor system, sensory system, and reflexes.
- Reassessment is the ongoing assessment of the patient to determine changes in condition and response to treatment.
- When approaching a pediatric patient, the paramedic should remain calm and confident. The paramedic should observe the child before beginning the physical examination. The paramedic also should make sure to avoid separation of the child and parent. Moreover, the paramedic must establish a rapport with the parents and child and must be honest. One caregiver should be assigned to the child.
- The paramedic should not assume that all older adults have disorders related to aging. Individual differences in knowledge, mental reasoning, experience, and personality influence how these patients respond to examination.

REVIEW QUESTIONS

Match the sign in column II with its definition in column I. Use each answer only once.

Column I

1. _________ Persistent respiratory rate less than 12 breaths/min

2. _________ Normal breath sounds heard over most lung fields

3. _________ Low-pitched, rumbling expiratory sounds

4. _________ Crowing sound associated with upper airway narrowing

5. _________ Crescendo–decrescendo sequence of respirations followed by apnea

6. _________ Irregular respirations interrupted by apneic periods

7. _________ End-inspiratory sounds associated with fluid in the small airways

8. _________ High-pitched airway noise resulting from lower airway narrowing

Column II

a. Biot
b. Bradypnea
c. Cheyne-Stokes
d. Crackles
e. Rhonchi
f. Stridor
g. Vesicular
h. Wheezes

Match the term in column II with the appropriate statement in column I. Use each answer only once.

Column I

9. _________ A child with Down syndrome has slanted openings between the upper and lower eyelids.

10. _________ A patient said the aliens were controlling him.

11. _________ Third-degree burns affect the skin's resiliency.

12. _________ Malnutrition caused the man to be very thin.

13. _________ An older patient staggered when he walked.

14. _________ A paralyzed patient had a persistent erection.

15. _________ A semicircle of blood is seen over the iris.

16. _________ A patient's cirrhosis made him look pregnant.

17. _________ After her stroke, a woman had trouble making the muscles of her mouth form words.

18. _________ An alcoholic's wife told you that the history he gave you was untrue.

Column II

a. Affect
b. Ascites
c. Ataxia
d. Confabulation
e. Delusions
f. Dysarthria
g. Emaciated
h. Hyphema
i. Hypopyon
j. Macula
k. Palpebral fissures
l. Priapism
m. Turgor

19. Describe the correct method of performing each of the following patient assessment techniques.

a. Inspection:

____

b. Palpation:

____

c. Auscultation:

____

20. For each of the following deviations from normal pupil response, list a cause:

Abnormality   **Cause**

a. Dilated/unresponsive ____

b. Constricted/unresponsive ____

c. Unequal/one dilated and unresponsive ____

d. Dull/lackluster ____

21. Your patient is a teenage assault victim who was struck repeatedly on the head with a baseball bat.

a. List the 10 steps in the comprehensive physical examination.

    (1) ____

    (2) ____

    (3) ____

    (4) ____

    (5) ____

    (6) ____

    (7) ____

    (8) ____

    (9) ____

    (10) ____

b. List the components of the mental status examination for this patient.

____

____

____

c. Describe your physical examination of this patient's head and neck, detailing specific examination techniques and the types of normal or abnormal findings you would look for (include ophthalmoscopic and otoscopic examination techniques).

____

____

____

22. You are called to evaluate a patient whose chief complaint is difficulty breathing. Explain your assessment of the thorax.

____

____

23. Your 56-year-old patient has a history of right upper quadrant abdominal pain, malaise, nausea, and vomiting. He is jaundiced and complains of itching. Past history reveals heavy alcohol use. You suspect hepatitis. Describe your physical examination of this patient's abdomen.

____

____

24. You are examining a patient involved in a motor vehicle collision whose automobile was struck on the side. The patient complains of considerable pain in the pelvic area. The primary survey has been completed. The patient's pulse is elevated, but the blood pressure is within normal limits. Describe your examination of this patient's pelvic area.

____

____

25. Your crew arrives at the home of an older patient whose family states that she complained of weakness on one side, stumbled, and fell down five steps. No life-threatening conditions are found in the primary survey, and vital sign assessment reveals a moderately elevated blood pressure and pulse. The patient is slightly confused but cooperative. You suspect a stroke. Describe your assessment of this patient's extremities.

____

____

26. A painter has fallen approximately 20 feet, striking a scaffold rail with his lower back. Primary survey results and vital signs are normal. Outline your physical examination of this patient's back.

____

____

27. Provide the information that is missing in the following table, which outlines examination techniques for cranial nerves.

Cranial Nerve Number	Cranial Nerve Name	Assessment Technique
I		Test smell with ammonia inhalants
II	Optic	
III	Oculomotor	Test EOMs by asking the patient to look up and down, to the left and right, and diagonally up and down to the left and right
VI		
V		
VII	Facial	Note facial symmetry, tics, or abnormal movement; have the patient raise the eyebrows, frown, show the upper and lower teeth, smile, and puff out the cheeks; have the patient close the eyes tightly and resist while you try to open eyelids
VIII		
IX		
X		
XI	Spinal accessory	
XII		

28. List four general guidelines that are helpful when approaching a pediatric patient.

a. ______________________________________

b. ______________________________________

c. ______________________________________

d. ______________________________________

29. Describe two specific developmental differences that influence patient assessment for the children in each of the following age groups.

a. Birth to 6 months:

____

b. 7 months to 3 years:

____

c. 4 to 10 years:

____

d. Adolescence:

____

30. Describe two special considerations and techniques that may be useful when assessing an older patient.

31. Auscultation is the examination technique that involves which of the following?
   a. Listening with a stethoscope
   b. Feeling for masses and assessing for crepitus
   c. Looking for signs of illness
   d. Tapping the body with your finger

32. Which instrument is used to evaluate the retina and macula?
   a. Ophthalmoscope
   b. Otoscope
   c. Penlight
   d. Sphygmomanometer

33. Using an adult blood pressure cuff to evaluate a child's blood pressure can result in which of the following?
   a. False low reading
   b. False high reading
   c. Normal reading
   d. Inability to inflate cuff

34. What is the most important information to guide your physical examination of the patient?
   a. Medications and specific doses
   b. Past medical history
   c. Present illness and chief complaint
   d. Vital signs, including blood pressure

35. Which of the following is a component of the secondary assessment
   a. Chief complaint
   b. History of present illness
   c. Vascular access
   d. Vital signs

36. Which of the following is a component of the mental status examination?
   a. Distal pulses
   b. Pupil reaction
   c. Speech and language
   d. Visual acuity

37. Which of the following is the clearest way to report an altered level of consciousness?
   a. The patient is obtunded.
   b. The patient is semiconscious.
   c. The patient is stuporous.
   d. The patient is unresponsive to pain.

38. Patient memory and attention can be assessed with which of the following?
   a. AVPU method
   b. Digit span
   c. General survey
   d. Glasgow Coma Scale

39. Your patient walks with a limp. What is this known as?
   a. An abnormal gait
   b. Ataxia
   c. Bizarre posture
   d. Cranial nerve palsy

40. What is an odor of acetone on the breath associated with?
   a. Alcohol use
   b. Bowel obstruction
   c. Diabetic conditions
   d. Poor dental hygiene

41. A patient who tells you that he is depressed and suicidal but has an expressionless face may be said to have which condition?

   a. Altered affect   **c.** Altered attention
   b. Altered appearance   **d.** Altered emotion

42. Which sign of distress may be found in a patient who has cardiorespiratory insufficiency, pain, or anxiety?

   a. Bradycardia   **c.** Sweating
   b. Cough   **d.** Wincing

43. Skin color is best assessed by observing the skin on what part of the body?

   a. Arms   **c.** Legs
   b. Face   **d.** Nail beds

44. Which of the following is true regarding oral temperature assessment?

   a. It is used to measure temperature in children older than 1 year of age.
   b. Use it to assess temperature in patients with altered consciousness.
   c. Smoking immediately before assessment can affect the reading.
   d. It is as accurate as oral temperature assessment.

45. What is the proper sequence to examine the abdomen?

   a. Auscultation, inspection, palpation
   b. Inspection, palpation, auscultation
   c. Inspection, auscultation, palpation
   d. Auscultation, palpation, inspection

46. Which of the following findings during examination of the nails is consistent with chronic respiratory or cardiac disease?

   a. Beau lines   **c.** Paronychia
   b. Clubbing   **d.** Terry nails

47. What should you do to verify that vision is present?

   a. Assess bilateral pupil response to light.
   b. Ask the patient to count fingers at a distance.
   c. Lightly touch the cornea with a cotton swab.
   d. Palpate the globe for firmness.

48. To perform an effective otoscopic examination or assess tympanic temperature, you should pull the ear in what direction?

   a. Down and back in adults   **c.** Down and back in infants
   b. Down and forward in adults   **d.** Down and forward in infants

49. What physical finding may be encountered in patients who are pregnant, have leukemia, or are taking phenytoin?

   a. Enlarged gums   **c.** Swollen eyelids
   b. Nasal bleeding   **d.** Tonsillar exudate

50. Chest wall diameter may be increased in patients with what condition?

   a. Heart disease
   b. Implanted cardiac pacemaker
   c. Obstructive pulmonary disease
   d. Rib fractures and pulmonary contusion

51. Which sound may be heard during percussion if hyperinflation caused by pulmonary disease, pneumothorax, or asthma is present?

   a. Dullness   **c.** Resonance
   b. Flatness   **d.** Hyperresonance

52. Which of the following is true regarding assessment of breath sounds?
   a. Normal breath sounds are louder on exhalation.
   b. The stethoscope bell is used to auscultate the lungs.
   c. The patient's mouth should be open.
   d. The patient should be in the supine position.

53. For maximal effectiveness, where should heart sounds be auscultated?
   a. Over the left anterior axillary line
   b. Over the left fifth intercostal space
   c. Over the sternal angle
   d. Over the xiphoid process

54. Simultaneous palpation of the apical and carotid pulses in which each apical beat is not transmitted is known as which of the following?
   a. Mean arterial pressure   c. Pulsus paradoxus
   b. Pulse deficit   d. Pulse pressure

55. Which cause of obstructive shock may present with muffled heart sounds?
   a. Cardiac tamponade   c. Obstructive lung disease
   b. Obesity   d. Myocardial infarction

56. What is a palpable tremor over a blood vessel called?
   a. Bruit   c. Thrill
   b. Murmur   d. Vibration

57. During the vascular examination, the anterior surface of the foot should be palpated to detect which pulse?
   a. Brachial pulse   c. Popliteal pulse
   b. Dorsalis pedis pulse   d. Posterior tibial pulse

58. If a deformity and point tenderness are noted when you examine the pelvis, what condition should you consider?
   a. Appendicitis   c. Ruptured ectopic pregnancy
   b. Internal hemorrhage   d. Spinal cord injury

59. To evaluate motor function in the lower extremities, you should instruct the patient to do what?
   a. Flex and extend the feet and lower and upper legs.
   b. Lift and hold both legs in the air while lying supine.
   c. Move the legs laterally as far as possible bilaterally.
   d. Push the soles of the feet against the paramedic's palms.

60. Which of the following is an example of a test to evaluate gait?
   a. Have the patient hop in place.
   b. Have the patient do the Romberg test.
   c. Have the patient touch each heel to the opposite shin.
   d. Have the patient touch the finger to the nose, alternating hands.

61. Your patient is a 2-year-old toddler in respiratory distress. Level of consciousness, spontaneous movement, respiratory effort, and skin color can be most effectively evaluated when the child is in which position?
   a. Held by the paramedic   c. On the stretcher
   b. Held by the parent   d. Sitting in a chair

62. A young child has an obviously fractured lower leg. Which of the following statements is true regarding the care of this patient?
   a. Communicate only with the child.
   b. Separate the parents from the child.
   c. Establish rapport with the parents.
   d. Tell the parents it could have been worse.

274

63. Which of the following statements is *true* regarding the physical examination of a 2-year-old child?
  a. Abdominal breathing is normal in this age group.
  b. Patient modesty should be a primary concern.
  c. Explanations should be given for each activity.
  d. Separation anxiety will not be a problem.

64. When examining an older patient, what should you do?
  a. Always speak loudly because most of these patients are deaf.
  b. Assume that memory impairment is present.
  c. Anticipate numerous health problems and medications.
  d. Not expect any variation in the examination.

WRAP IT UP

You are called to a small home for a "person fallen." Your patient is an elderly man who fell and is lying naked, trapped between the toilet and the bathtub. He is awake but confused. He has cool skin and some injuries to his head and shoulders from trying to wriggle out of his confined space. His family tells you they couldn't get him on the phone for 24 hours, so they came by this morning to see what was wrong. He is wedged tightly, and you are unable to free him, so a rescue unit is dispatched. Fire personnel bring hand tools and carefully remove the commode without breaking it to avoid making sharp shards of porcelain that may injure your patient. You extricate him onto the backboard after applying a cervical collar and move him to the ambulance. During the rescue, your partner checks around the house, looking for medications, signs of drug or alcohol use, or anything unusual but finds nothing.

The patient's vital signs are BP 100/60, P 112 irregular, and R 20. Oxygen saturation is not detected because the man's extremities are cool, so you administer oxygen by non-rebreather mask at 12 L/min. His temperature is 97.6°F (36.4°C). The patient's pupils are 4 mm, equal, round, and react to light. Inspection of his head reveals abraded areas where he was moving his head to free himself. You palpate no deformities or crepitus of the head or face. He follows commands and can move his eyes in the cardinal fields of gaze. There is no tenderness, swelling, or deformity around the nose or frontal or maxillary sinuses. His lips are pale and cracked, as is his tongue. The trachea is midline, the neck veins are flat, and the patient denies neck pain. However, you do not ask him to move it because of your concern about spinal trauma. Inspection of the chest reveals some redness to the left posterior and lateral aspect in a linear fashion. There is considerable tenderness when those areas are palpated. Respiration excursion seems shallow, and breath sounds are clear but diminished in all fields. Heart sounds are auscultated with the patient supine, and a normal S1 and S2 are audible. Percussion of the abdomen reveals tympany and dullness in the appropriate locations. The patient winces when his abdomen is palpated but does not seem to be able to localize the pain. His liver and spleen are not palpable. His penis is flaccid, and there is no blood at the urinary meatus. His left shoulder has an abraded area that is tender, but no deformity or crepitus is noted. His hands, wrists, and arms appear to have normal range of motion, but the joints seem somewhat enlarged. Examination of the lower extremities is normal. Palpation of the spine is negative. The patient remains confused and unable to tell you what happened but is cooperative. You ask him to smile, and it exaggerates the facial droop that you noticed earlier in your exam. You also detect some slurring of his speech. Evaluation of muscle strength demonstrates some weakness in his right arm and leg. You initiate an IV TKO, determine that his blood glucose is 110 mg/dL, and monitor his vital signs en route to the hospital. He is later diagnosed with a stroke; however, because of his fall and the unknown time of onset, he is not a candidate for fibrinolytic therapy. At the time of follow-up, he is in rehabilitation.

1. What is the purpose of the secondary assessment in this patient?

____

2. Why was a temperature assessment indicated in this patient even though he was found in the house?

____

3. During transport, what should you reassess on this patient?

____

4. Put a ✓ by each area of the cranial nerve examination where an abnormality was detected and fill in the name of the nerve(s) listed.

Cranial Nerve Number	Cranial Nerve Name(s)
I	
II	
II and III	
III, IV, and VI	
V	
VII	
VIII	
IX and X	
XI	
XII	

5. Why were the liver and spleen not palpable?

____

CHAPTER 20 ANSWERS

REVIEW QUESTIONS

1. b

2. g

3. e

4. f

5. c

6. a

7. d

8. h

9. k

10. e

11. m

12. g

13. c

14. l

276

15. h

16. b

17. f

18. d
(Questions 1–18: Objective 11)

19. a. Observe the environment (scene), general patient appearance, and specific body regions to gather data. b. Use the palmar surface of the hands and fingers to feel for texture, mass, fluid, temperature, and crepitus in various body regions. c. Use a stethoscope or the unaided ear to assess sounds generated by the movement of air or gases within the body.
(Objective 2)

20.

Abnormality	Cause
a. Dilated/unresponsive	Cardiac arrest, hypoxia, drug use or misuse
b. Constricted/unresponsive	Injury or disease of the central nervous system, narcotic drug use, use of eye medications
c. Unequal/one dilated	Cerebrovascular accident, direct trauma to the eye, use of eye medications, use of an ocular prosthesis, unilateral brain lesion or swelling
d. Dull/lackluster	Shock or comatose states, dehydration

(Objective 7)

21. a. (1) Mental status; (2) general survey; (3) vital signs; (4) skin; (5) head, eyes, ears, nose, and throat (HEENT); (6) chest; (7) abdomen; (8) posterior body; (9) extremities; (10) neurological examination
(Objective 5)

    b. Assess whether the patient is alert and responsive to touch and verbal and painful stimuli. Assess the patient's general appearance and behavior. Note verbal and motor responses. If the patient is ambulatory when you arrive, note posture, gait, and motor activity. Observe dress and hygiene and note any body odors, such as alcohol. Note facial expression and determine whether it is appropriate for the situation. Is the patient's affect appropriate for the situation? Is the speech understandable and moderately paced? Assess the quality, rate, loudness, and fluency of the patient's speech. Determine whether the patient has organized thoughts. Determine whether the patient is oriented to person, place, and time. Assess remote and recent memory.
(Objective 6)

    c. Inspect for shape and symmetry of the skull and facial bones. Note bleeding, trauma, deformity, or drainage around the face or from the ears or nose. Inspect the mouth for bleeding and loose or missing teeth. Observe for pupil response to light and assess to see whether the patient's vision is intact. Examine the conjunctiva and sclera by asking the patient to look up while both lower eyelids are depressed with the thumbs. Palpate the lower orbital rims to determine structural integrity. Use the ophthalmoscope to check the cornea for lacerations, abrasions, or foreign bodies; to check for hyphema in the anterior chamber; to assess the fundus; to see retinal vessels, the optic nerve, and retina; and to assess the vitreous. Palpate the scalp and face for deformities, swelling, indentations, or bleeding, noting pain or tenderness. Inspect the external ear for signs of bruising, deformity, or discoloration. Look for bleeding in the ear canal. Palpate the bones around the ear to see whether the patient feels discomfort. Look for discoloration on the mastoid process. Assess gross auditory acuity by covering one ear at a time and asking the patient to repeat short test words spoken in soft and loud tones. Pull the auricle up and back to perform the otoscopic examination and look at the eardrum. Before applying the cervical collar but while still maintaining cervical immobilization, inspect to ensure that the trachea is midline and note tracheal tugging or obvious symptoms of trauma. Palpate the anterior and posterior neck, noting pain, deformity, malalignment, or subcutaneous emphysema.
(Objectives 8 and 9)

22. Inspect for chest shape, symmetry, expansion, and the use of accessory muscles. Note the rate, depth, and pattern of respirations. Palpate for tenderness, bulges, depressions, unusual movement, crepitus, and chest expansion. Place both thumbs on the xiphoid process with the palms lying flat on the chest wall and palpate for symmetry. Assess the posterior chest wall by placing the thumbs along the spinous processes at the level of the tenth rib.

Percuss the chest to detect resonance (normal), hyperresonance (hyperinflation), or dullness or flatness (fluid or pulmonary congestion). Auscultate bilaterally (anterior and posterior) with the patient upright if possible and ask the patient to breathe in and out slowly through the open mouth, noting diminished or adventitious sounds. Palpate the apical impulse. Auscultate the heart at the fifth intercostal space to note frequency, intensity, duration, and timing as well as abnormal sounds such as murmurs.
(Objectives 8 and 9)

23. Inspect for symmetry, jaundice, or distension and look for surgical scars. Look for smooth movement of the abdomen during respiration. Auscultate all four quadrants for rumblings. Palpate for tenderness, masses, skin temperature, and rigidity and observe for guarding. Percuss all four quadrants of the abdomen to assess for tympany (normal over the stomach and intestines) and dullness (over organs and solid masses). Percuss the liver by beginning just above the umbilicus in the right midclavicular line in an area of tympany. Continue in an upward direction until the change from tympany to dullness occurs (usually slightly below the costal margin, which indicates the upper border of the liver). During palpation of the liver, the patient should be supine and relaxed. Stand on the patient's right side and place the left hand under the patient in the area of the eleventh and twelfth ribs. Place your right hand on the abdomen, with the fingers pointing toward the patient's head, resting just below the edge of the costal margin. As the patient exhales, press the hand under the patient upward while pushing your right hand gently in and up. If you can feel the liver, it should be firm and nontender. (A healthy adult liver usually cannot be palpated.)
(Objectives 8 and 9)

24. Inspect for obvious trauma, deformity, symmetry, or bleeding, especially from the urethra. Place the hands on each anterior iliac crest and press down and out, noting movement or crepitus. Place the heel of the hand on the symphysis pubis and press down to determine stability. Palpate the femoral pulses.
(Objectives 8 and 9)

25. For each extremity, inspect for position, deformity, and obvious signs of trauma, and compare the right extremity with the left. Palpate for structural integrity. Assess grips; have the patient push and pull the paramedic's hands against force, and have the patient push the feet against the opposing force of the paramedic's hands bilaterally to note muscle strength and tone. Assess distal pulse and sensation in all extremities.
(Objectives 8 and 9)

26. Log roll the patient with cervical immobilization. Inspect the neck for midline position. Inspect the back for signs of injury, swelling, discoloration, and open wounds. Palpate the spine, beginning at the neck and proceeding to the sacrum, noting point tenderness or deformity. Place the palm of your hand over the costovertebral angle and strike the hand with your fist, noting any painful reaction.
(Objectives 8 and 9)

27.

Cranial Nerve Number(s)	Cranial Nerve Name(s)	Assessment Technique
I	Olfactory	Test smell with ammonia inhalants
II	Optic	Test for visual acuity
III	Oculomotor	Inspect the size and shape of the pupils; assess the pupil's response to light
		Test EOMs by asking the patient to look up and down, to the left and right, and diagonally up and down to the left and right
IV	Trochlear	Assess extraocular movement
VI	Abducens	Assess extraocular movement
V	Trigeminal	Ask the patient to clench the teeth while you palpate the temporal and masseter muscles and touch the forehead, cheeks, and jaw to determine sensation

Cranial Nerve Number(s)	Cranial Nerve Name(s)	Assessment Technique
VII	Facial	Note facial symmetry, tics, or abnormal movement; have the patient raise the eyebrows, frown, show the upper and lower teeth, smile, and puff out the cheeks; have the patient close the eyes tightly and resist while you try to open eyelids
VIII	Acoustic	Assess hearing acuity
IX	Glossopharyngeal	See whether the patient can swallow easily and produce saliva and normal voice sounds; ask the patient to hold breath and then assess for slowing of the heart rate; test for gag reflex
X	Vagus	Same as IX
XI	Spinal accessory	Ask the patient to raise and lower the shoulders and turn the head
XII	Hypoglossal	Ask the patient to stick out the tongue and move it in several directions

(Objective 6)

28. Remain calm and confident; do not separate the parents and child unless absolutely necessary; establish rapport with the parents and child; be honest with the child and parents; if possible, assign one caregiver to stay with the child; and observe the patient before the physical examination.
(Objective 13)

29. a. The child is not frightened, the child needs care to maintain body temperature, the child is in constant motion, the child is an abdominal breather, and the paramedic can use the fontanelles to assess overhydration and underhydration. b. Separation anxiety occurs, the child has a fear of strangers, and the paramedic should explain procedures in short sentences. c. The child has a capacity for rational thought, the child can provide a limited history, the paramedic should allow participation in care, the child has a limited understanding of the body, the child fears intrusion into private areas, and the paramedic must explain everything completely. d. The teenager is concerned about body image, and privacy is a major concern. The paramedic should treat the teenager like an adult, and the paramedic must consider sexually transmitted diseases, pregnancy, and drug and alcohol use.
(Objective 13)

30. The patient may have sensory loss that impairs communication, may experience memory loss and confusion, often has numerous health problems that require him or her to take a number of home medications, may have decreased sensory function that can conceal symptoms, and may have fears regarding hospitalization.
(Objective 14)

STUDENT SELF-ASSESSMENT

31. a. Inspection involves looking, palpating involves feeling the body, and selected body areas are tapped during percussion.
(Objective 2)

32. a. The otoscope is used for examining the ears, the penlight can be used to evaluate pupil response, and the sphygmomanometer is used to measure blood pressure.
(Objective 3)

33. a. Blood pressure cuffs that are too wide give a false low reading, and those that are too narrow give a false high reading.
(Objective 3)

34. c. Although all the other information is important, the chief complaint and history of the present illness guide the physical examination and allow the paramedic to focus on key areas.
(Objective 4)

35. d. Chief complaint and history of present illness are historical findings. Vascular access is an intervention.
(Objective 5)

36. c
(Objective 6)

37. d. The other terms are vague and may be interpreted in a variety of ways.
(Objective 7)

38. b. Ask the patient to count from 1 to 10 using only odd numbers. Asking the patient to count by serial sevens or spell a word backward also can be used.
(Objective 7)

39. a. Ataxia is a staggering gait, and postural imbalance is associated with central nervous system lesions. Cranial nerve palsy does not cause a limp.
(Objective 7)

40. c. Diabetic ketoacidosis is associated with an odor of acetone on the breath.
(Objective 9)

41. a
(Objective 7)

42. c. Tachycardia, not bradycardia, is a common trait for all three. Cough is not present with pain or anxiety. Wincing is not associated with cardiorespiratory insufficiency.
(Objective 9)

43. d. This area has less pigmentation, and pallor or cyanosis is easier to see.
(Objective 9)

44. c. Smoking and anything taken orally or inhaled can affect accuracy of this method.
(Objective 8)

45. c. Palpation of the abdomen may create sounds that falsely indicate normal bowel function when none exists.
(Objective 10)

46. b. *Beau lines* are transverse depressions in the nail that inhibit growth and are associated with systemic illness, severe infection, and nail injury. *Paronychia* is an inflammation of the skin at the base of the nail that may result from local infection or trauma. *Terry nails* are transverse white bands that cover the nail except for a narrow zone at the distal tip and are associated with cirrhosis.
(Objective 11)

47. b. Pupil response and corneal touch test the cranial nerves. Palpation of the globe is used to assess for dehydration.
(Objective 10)

48. c. For the adult examination, the auricle should be pulled gently up and back.
(Objective 10)

49. a. This also may be noted if the patient is going through puberty.
(Objective 11)

50. c. This barrel-shaped appearance develops because of air trapping.
(Objective 11)

51. d. Dullness or flatness is heard when fluid is present or pulmonary congestion has occurred. Resonance is usually heard over normal lungs.
(Objective 10)

280

52. c. Normal breath sounds are louder on inspiration. The diaphragm is used to auscultate the lungs. Ideally, the patient should be sitting if the condition permits.
(Objective 11)

53. b. Ideally, the patient should be sitting up and leaning slightly forward or should be in the left lateral recumbent position.
(Objective 10)

54. b. *Mean arterial pressure* is the diastolic pressure plus one third of the pulse pressure. *Pulsus paradoxus* is a fluctuation in the systolic blood pressure with respiration. *Pulse pressure* is the systolic blood pressure minus the diastolic blood pressure.
(Objective 11)

55. a
(Objective 11)

56. c. *Murmurs* are prolonged extra sounds auscultated with a stethoscope. A *bruit* is an abnormal sound audible over the carotid artery or an organ or gland. A *thrill* may feel like a tremor or vibration.
(Objective 11)

57. b. The brachial pulse is on the arm, the popliteal pulse is behind the knee, and the posterior tibial pulse is on the medial aspect of the ankle behind the tibia.
(Objective 10)

58. b. Pelvic fractures are often accompanied by substantial hemorrhage.
(Objective 11)

59. d
(Objective 10)

60. a. Point-to-point movements are evaluated using the heel-to-shin and finger-to-nose tests. Stance and balance are tested with the Romberg test.
(Objective 10)

61. b. Anxiety is usually minimized while the child is in the parent's arms. This can minimize respiratory effort and distress and allow for a more effective assessment.
(Objective 13)

62. c
(Objective 13)

63. c
(Objective 13)

64. c. These numerous illnesses can confuse the clinical picture and complicate the paramedic's examination of the patient.
(Objective 14)

WRAP IT UP

1. You perform the secondary assessment to identify any injuries and to attempt to identify the underlying medical cause of the patient's fall.
(Objective 1)

2. Patients can become hypothermic or hyperthermic in their residence, especially with injury or severe illness.
(Objective 4)

3. Reassess his mental status, vital signs, any response to care, and any trends

4. CN I—not tested—olfactory
   CNs II and III—normal—optic and oculomotor
   CNs III, IV, and VI—normal—oculomotor, trochlear, abducens
   CN V—not tested—trigeminal
   CN VII—abnormal (facial droop)—facial
   CN VIII—not tested—acoustic
   CNs IX and X—not tested—glossopharyngeal and vagus
   CN XI—not tested—spinal accessory
   CN XII—not tested—hypoglossal
   (Objective 7)

5. The liver and spleen should not be palpable in a normal adult.
   (Objective 11)

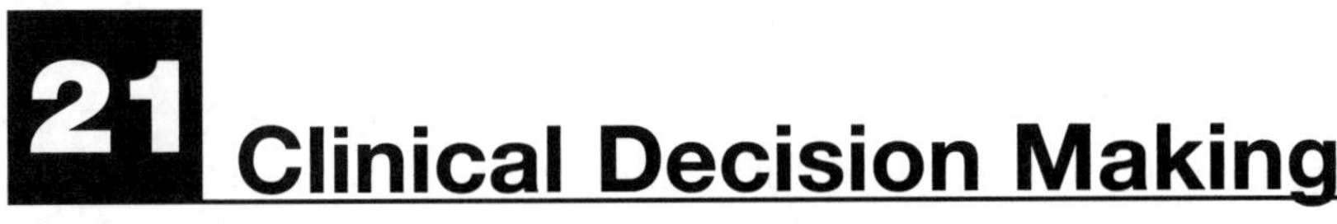

Clinical Decision Making

READING ASSIGNMENT

Chapter 21, pages 560-568, in *Mosby's Paramedic Textbook*, ed. 4.

OBJECTIVES

Upon completion of this chapter, the paramedic student will be able to do the following:

1. List the key elements of paramedic practice.
2. Discuss the limitations of protocols, standing orders, and patient care algorithms.
3. Outline the key components of the critical thinking process for paramedics.
4. Identify elements necessary for an effective critical thinking process.
5. Describe situations that may necessitate the use of the critical thinking process while delivering prehospital patient care.
6. Describe the six elements required for effective clinical decision making in the prehospital setting.

SUMMARY

- The paramedic must be able to do several things at the same time. The paramedic must be able to gather, evaluate, and synthesize information. The paramedic also must be able to develop and implement appropriate patient management plans. The paramedic must apply judgment and exercise independent decision making as well. Lastly, the paramedic must be able to think and work effectively under pressure.
- Protocols, standing orders, and patient care algorithms have several limitations. They may not apply to nonspecific patient complaints that do not fit the model. They also do not address multiple disease etiologies or multiple treatment plans. Moreover, they may promote linear thinking. Clinical decision rules may help determine risk when evaluating patients.
- The critical thinking process includes concept formation, data interpretation, application of principle, evaluation, and reflection on action.
- To reduce the risk of errors in decision making, consciously ask yourself, "Is this the right decision?" Be cautious in error-prone situations. Recognize your biases and use care when making decisions in cases that involve those biases.
- For effective critical thinking, a paramedic must have a solid knowledge base. Paramedics must be able to deal with a large amount of data all at once as well. Paramedics must be able to organize the data, deal with ambiguity, and relate the situation to similar past experience. Paramedics also must be able to reason and construct arguments to support or discount the decision.
- When using assessment-based patient management, paramedics must analyze a patient's problems, determine how to solve them, carry out a plan of action, and evaluate its effectiveness.
- Effective clinical decision making requires the paramedic to read the patient and the scene. The paramedic also must be able to react, reevaluate, and revise the management plan. Then the paramedic must be able to review performance at a run critique.

REVIEW QUESTIONS

1. List the four key elements of paramedic practice described in this chapter.

    a. ____

    b. ____

    c. ____

    d. ____

2. Why is it difficult to follow standard protocols, standing orders, and patient care algorithms in the following situations?

    a. A patient does not speak your language. He appears very ill, is pale and diaphoretic, and has a very slow, irregular heartbeat. He gets very anxious and pulls away when you attempt to establish an intravenous line to give medications.

    b. A patient with chronic obstructive pulmonary disease has signs and symptoms of heart failure and is wheezing.

    c. An elderly patient with severe kyphosis (hunchback posture) has fallen off a ladder but screams in pain when you attempt to immobilize him on the spine board.

    d. A child choked on a toy and is stridorous. Each time you approach to assess her, she begins to cry and has increased distress.

Question 3 pertains to the following case study:

An elderly patient is complaining of chest pain that began 30 minutes ago. She tells you that it began suddenly when she was reading the paper. It is crushing and substernal, rating an "8" on a 0 to 10 scale. It does not radiate, but she feels nauseated and is diaphoretic. She has normal vital signs, clear breath sounds, and no other obvious clinical findings. A 12-lead ECG demonstrates ST segment elevation in leads V_1 and V_2. You and your partner recognize that her presentation is consistent with septal myocardial infarction. You immediately begin oxygen, initiate an intravenous line, and administer nitroglycerin and aspirin. You notify medical direction and transmit the ECG, anticipating the need for cardiac catheterization. You reevaluate her vital signs, breath sounds, and level of pain every 5 minutes during the 15-minute transport to the hospital. During the following shift, your supervisor gives you feedback on the patient's outcome. During the run critique, everyone agrees that the care was good but the scene time was somewhat long. During the ensuing discussion, you identify ways to reduce scene times on future calls.

3. Identify which parts of this scenario demonstrate each of the following phases of the critical thinking process:

    a. Concept formation:

    b. Data interpretation:

    c. Application of principle:

    d. Evaluation:

    e. Reflection on action:

4. List five steps that can help paramedics to think clearly in highly stressful situations.

a. ____

b. ____

c. ____

d. ____

e. ____

5. List the six "Rs" of effective clinical decision making.

a. ____

b. ____

c. ____

d. ____

e. ____

f. ____

6. To practice effectively as a paramedic, you should be able to do which of the following?
a. Gather, evaluate, and synthesize information.
b. Know all current medical techniques.
c. Make diagnoses and provide definitive care.
d. Teach your personal values to patients.

7. Which of the following is an advantage of protocols, standing orders, and patient care protocols?
a. They work well when numerous disease etiologies coexist.
b. They apply to nonspecific patient complaints that do not fit the model.
c. They promote a standardized approach to patient care for classic presentations.
d. They promote linear thinking and cookbook medicine in all situations.

8. You recognize that a patient is hypoglycemic based on the history, physical examination, and blood analysis. What phase of the critical thinking process have you entered when you initiate an intravenous line and administer glucose?
a. Application of principle
b. Concept formation
c. Data interpretation
d. Reflection on action

9. In which of the following situations is a paramedic most likely to use critical thinking skills?
a. The monitor shows ventricular fibrillation.
b. The blood glucose strip reads 40 mg/dL.
c. A patient stops breathing and becomes cyanotic.
d. A trauma patient has severe neck pain but is dyspneic when supine.

10. Which of the following elements needed for effective clinical decision making are you performing when you decide the patient has a tension pneumothorax?
a. React
b. Read the scene
c. Read the patient
d. Review performance at a run critique

You are dispatched to a residence for a seizure at 2300. When you arrive, you find a 2-year-old child who is drowsy but easily arousable. Her mother says she found her shaking in bed. She has a "cold" that began today but is otherwise quite healthy. The child is becoming progressively more awake as you assess her vital signs: P 128; R 28; Sao_2 98%. You are questioning the mother when, moments later, the child seizes again. You move her to the ambulance, and you become concerned when her level of consciousness remains significantly depressed 5 minutes after the seizure, with snoring respirations noted. You insert a nasal airway and administer oxygen as your partner initiates an IV into her left antecubital fossa. You place her on an ECG monitor so you can continuously monitor her heart rate. Her BP is 60/40 mm Hg; you know that's too low for her. Something seems out of place here. After a fluid bolus, her pressure comes up, but she is still very drowsy. You call your report while en route to the pediatric emergency department.

1. What additional measures might you have used to help with your concept formation?

2. Why would it be difficult to follow a standard protocol or algorithm for this child?

3. After interpreting the data you currently have, what are the chief life threats that concern you?

4. How did you react to the data found on this call?

CHAPTER 21 ANSWERS

REVIEW QUESTIONS

1. a. Gather, evaluate, and synthesize information. b. Develop and implement appropriate patient management plans. c. Apply judgment and exercise independent decision making. d. Think and work effectively under pressure. (Objective 1)

2. a. The language barrier makes it impossible to explain properly to the patient what needs to be done, yet you cannot forcibly treat the patient. b. Wheezing caused by chronic obstructive pulmonary disease is treated with a beta agonist such as albuterol; however, treatment for congestive heart failure involves furosemide, nitroglycerin, and morphine. Critical thinking is required to identify subtle findings and point you to the correct

treatment path for this patient. c. The correct treatment for this patient is to place him on a spine board (because of the mechanism of injury and age); however, this increases his pain and perhaps his injury because of his altered anatomy; therefore, critical thinking is required to determine an acceptable compromise to meet this patient's needs. d. Standard of care requires you to perform a patient assessment on this child; however, when you attempt to do this, her condition worsens. You must determine a compromise that will not harm her. (Objectives 2, 5)

3. a. Concept formation occurred when the patient assessment was done. b. Data interpretation included interpretation of the vital signs, physical findings, history, and ECG to determine the likelihood of myocardial infarction. c. Application of principle involved making the interpretation (MI), selecting the appropriate course of care (O_2, intravenous therapy, nitroglycerin, aspirin), and then delivering that care. d. Reassessment of pain, vital signs, and breath sounds constitutes the evaluation phase of the process. e. The run critique provided the opportunity for reflection on action.
(Objective 3)

4. a. Stop and think; b. scan the situation; c. decide and act; d. maintain clear and concise control; e. regularly and clearly reevaluate the patient.
(Objective 4)

5. a. Read the patient; b. read the scene; c. react; d. reevaluate; e. revise the patient management plan; f. review performance at run critique.
(Objective 6)

STUDENT SELF-ASSESSMENT

6. a. Paramedics must know techniques appropriate within their scope of practice that have been approved by medical direction. Paramedics are not expected to make diagnoses. In some cases (e.g., hypoglycemia), paramedics provide definitive care, but in most cases, definitive care is delivered at the hospital. Paramedics must recognize that their personal values may be different from those of the patient.
(Objective 1)

7. c. Each of the other choices represents a possible disadvantage of protocols, standing orders, and patient care protocols.
(Objective 2)

8. a. Concept formation involves the process of gathering elements to determine the "what" of the patient story. Data interpretation occurs when data are gathered and interpreted to form a field impression.
(Objective 3)

9. d. The patient has two concurrent serious problems, and the treatments of these conditions conflict. The paramedic must use critical thinking to resolve the problem.
(Objective 5)

10. a. The determination of life threat is made at the react phase after assessing the elements in b and c. The review occurs after the call.
(Objective 3)

WRAP IT UP

1. Check the environment for any medicines; check her blood glucose level; check her skin temperature; and complete her exam (e.g., pupils, rashes, and so on).
(Objective 3)

2. With no history of this, it is unclear what is causing the seizures. In this case, general measures to ensure airway, breathing, and blood pressure and to manage recurring seizures would be followed.
(Objective 2)

3. Altered level of consciousness; partial airway obstruction; seizures; low blood pressure
(Objective 4)

4. Airway was managed (nasal airway); IV initiated; fluid bolus given; patient monitored; medical direction consulted
(Objective 6)

PART SIX

Chapter 22   Cardiology

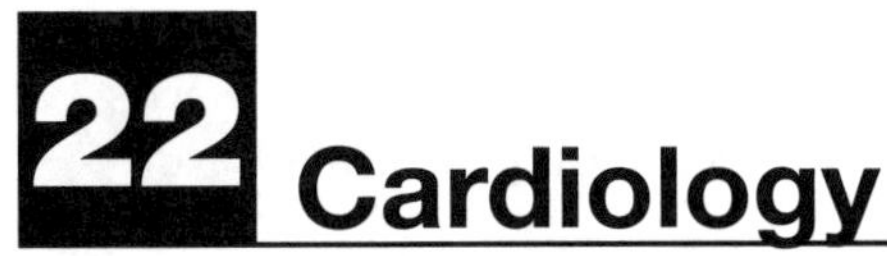

Cardiology

READING ASSIGNMENT

Chapter 22, pages 569-719, in *Mosby's Paramedic Textbook,* ed. 4.

OBJECTIVES

Upon completion of this chapter, the paramedic student will be able to do the following:

 1. Identify risk factors and prevention strategies associated with cardiovascular disease.
 2. Describe the normal anatomy and physiology of the heart.
 3. Discuss electrophysiology as it relates to the normal electrical and mechanical events in the cardiac cycle.
 4. Outline the activity of each component of the electrical conduction system of the heart.
 5. Describe basic monitoring techniques that permit electrocardiogram (ECG) interpretation.
 6. Explain the relationship of the ECG tracing to the electrical activity of the heart.
 7. Describe in sequence the steps in ECG interpretation.
 8. Identify the characteristics of normal sinus rhythm.
 9. When shown an ECG tracing, identify the rhythm, site of origin, possible causes, clinical significance, and prehospital management that is indicated.
10. Outline the appropriate assessment of a patient who may be experiencing a cardiovascular disorder.
11. Describe prehospital assessment and management of patients with selected cardiovascular disorders based on knowledge of the pathophysiology of the illness.
12. Describe the cause and nature of selected congenital cardiovascular defects.
13. List indications, contraindications, and prehospital considerations when using selected cardiac interventions, including basic life support, monitor-defibrillators, defibrillators, implantable cardioverter defibrillators, synchronized cardioversion, and transcutaneous cardiac pacing.
14. List the indications, contraindications, dose, and mechanisms of action for pharmacologic agents used to manage patients with cardiovascular disorders.
15. Identify appropriate actions to take in the prehospital setting to terminate resuscitation.

SUMMARY

- Persons at high risk for cardiovascular disease include those with diabetes, a family history of premature cardiovascular disease, and prior myocardial infarction (MI). Prevention strategies include community educational programs in nutrition, cessation of smoking (smoking prevention for children), and screening for hypertension and high cholesterol.
- The left coronary artery carries about 85% of the blood supply to the myocardium. The right coronary artery carries the rest. The pumping action of the heart is a product of rhythmic, alternate contraction and relaxation of the atria and ventricles. The stroke volume is the amount of blood ejected from each ventricle with one contraction. The stroke volume depends on preload, afterload, and myocardial contractility. Cardiac output is the amount of blood pumped by each ventricle per minute.
- In addition to the intrinsic control of the body in regulating the heart, extrinsic control by the parasympathetic and sympathetic nerves of the autonomic nervous system is a major factor influencing the heart rate, conductivity, and contractility. Sympathetic impulses cause the adrenal medulla to secrete epinephrine and norepinephrine into the blood.
- The major electrolytes that influence cardiac function are calcium, potassium, sodium, and magnesium. The electrical charge (potential difference) between the inside and outside of cells is expressed in millivolts. When the cell is in a resting state, the electrical charge difference is referred to as a resting membrane potential. The specialized sodium–potassium exchange pump actively pumps sodium ions out of the cell. It also pumps potassium ions into the cell. The cell membrane appears to have individual protein-lined channels. These channels allow for passage of a specific ion or group of ions.
- Nerve and muscle cells are capable of producing action potentials. This property is known as excitability. An action potential at any point on the cell membrane stimulates an excitation process. This process is spread down the length of the cell and is conducted across synapses from cell to cell.
- The contraction of cardiac and skeletal muscle is believed to be activated by calcium ions. This results in a binding between myosin and actin myofilaments.

- The conduction system of the heart is composed of two nodes and a conducting bundle. One of the nodes is the sinoatrial (SA) node. The other is the atrioventricular (AV) node.
- Parasympathetic stimulation by the vagus nerve affects primarily the SA and AV node, causing the heart to slow. Sympathetic stimulation increases the heart rate and contractility.
- The electrocardiogram (ECG) represents the electrical activity of the heart. The ECG is generated by depolarization and repolarization of the atria and ventricles.
- Routine monitoring of cardiac rhythm in the prehospital setting usually is obtained in lead II or MCL_1. These are the best leads to monitor for dysrhythmias because they allow visualization of P waves. A 12-lead ECG can be used to help identify changes relative to myocardial ischemia, injury, and infarction; distinguish ventricular tachycardia from supraventricular tachycardia; determine the electrical axis and the presence of fascicular blocks; and determine the presence of bundle branch blocks.
- The normal ECG consists of a P wave, QRS complex, and T wave. The P wave is the first positive deflection on the ECG. The P wave represents atrial depolarization. The P-R interval is the time it takes for an electrical impulse to be conducted through the atria and the AV node up to the instant of ventricular depolarization. The QRS complex represents ventricular depolarization. The ST segment represents the early part of repolarization of the right and left ventricles. The T wave represents repolarization of the ventricular myocardial cells. Repolarization occurs during the last part of ventricular systole. The Q-T interval is the period from the beginning of ventricular depolarization (onset of the QRS complex) until the end of ventricular repolarization or the end of the T wave.
- The steps in ECG analysis include analyzing the QRS complex, P waves, rate, rhythm, and P-R interval.
- Dysrhythmias originating in the SA node include sinus bradycardia, sinus tachycardia, sinus dysrhythmia, and sinus arrest. Most sinus dysrhythmias are the result of increases or decreases in vagal tone.
- Dysrhythmias originating in the atria include a wandering pacemaker, premature atrial complexes, paroxysmal supraventricular tachycardia, atrial flutter, and atrial fibrillation. Common causes of atrial dysrhythmias are ischemia, hypoxia, and atrial dilation caused by congestive heart failure or mitral valve abnormalities.
- When the SA node and the atria cannot generate the electrical impulses needed to begin depolarization because of factors such as hypoxia, ischemia, MI, and drug toxicity, the AV node or the area surrounding the AV node may assume the role of the secondary pacemaker. Dysrhythmias originating in the AV junction include premature junctional contractions, junctional escape complexes or rhythms, and accelerated junctional rhythm.
- Ventricular dysrhythmias pose a threat to life. Ventricular rhythm disturbances generally result from failure of the atria, AV junction, or both to initiate an electrical impulse. They also may result from enhanced automaticity or reentry phenomena in the ventricles. Dysrhythmias originating in the ventricles include ventricular escape complexes or rhythms, premature ventricular complexes, ventricular tachycardia, ventricular fibrillation, asystole, and artificial pacemaker rhythm.
- A 12-lead ECG can be used to help identify changes relative to myocardial ischemia, injury, and infarction; distinguish ventricular tachycardia from supraventricular tachycardia; determine the electrical axis and the presence of fascicular blocks; and determine the presence of bundle branch blocks.
- Partial delays or full interruptions in cardiac electrical conduction are called heart blocks. Causes of heart blocks include AV junctional ischemia, AV junctional necrosis, degenerative disease of the conduction system, and drug toxicity. Dysrhythmias that are disorders of conduction are first-degree AV block, type I second-degree AV block (Wenckebach), type II second-degree AV block, third-degree AV block, disturbances of ventricular conduction, pulseless electrical activity, and preexcitation (Wolff-Parkinson-White) syndrome.
- Common chief complaints of patients with cardiovascular disease include chest pain or discomfort, including shoulder, arm, neck, or jaw pain or discomfort; dyspnea; syncope; and an abnormal heartbeat or palpitations. Paramedics should ask patients suspected of having a cardiovascular disorder whether they take prescription medications, especially cardiac drugs. Paramedics should ask whether patients are being treated for any serious illness as well. They also should ask whether patients have a history of MI, angina, heart failure, hypertension, diabetes, or chronic lung disease. In addition, paramedics should ask whether patients have any allergies or have other risk factors for heart disease.
- After performing the initial assessment of a patient with cardiovascular disease, the paramedic should look for skin color, jugular venous distension, and the presence of edema or other signs of heart disease. The paramedic should listen for lung sounds, heart sounds, and carotid artery bruit. The paramedic should feel for edema, pulses, skin temperature, and moisture
- Atherosclerosis is a disease process characterized by progressive narrowing of the lumen of medium and large arteries. Atherosclerosis has two major effects on blood vessels. First, the disease disrupts the intimal surface. This causes a loss of vessel elasticity and an increase in thrombogenesis. Second, the atheroma reduces the diameter of the vessel lumen. Thus, this decreases the blood supply to tissues.
- Angina pectoris is a symptom of myocardial ischemia. Angina is caused by an imbalance between myocardial oxygen supply and demand. Prehospital management includes placing the patient at rest, administering oxygen, if $SaO_2 < 94\%$ initiating intravenous therapy, administering aspirin, nitroglycerin and possibly morphine, monitoring the patient for dysrhythmias, and transporting the patient for physician evaluation.

292

- Acute MI occurs when a coronary artery is blocked and blood does not reach an area of heart muscle. This results in ischemia, injury, and necrosis to the area of myocardium supplied by the affected artery. Death caused by MI usually results from lethal dysrhythmias (ventricular tachycardia, ventricular fibrillation, and cardiac standstill), pump failure (cardiogenic shock and congestive heart failure), or myocardial tissue rupture (rupture of the ventricle, septum, or papillary muscle). Some patients with acute MI, particularly those in the older age groups, have only symptoms of dyspnea, syncope, or confusion. However, substernal chest pain is usually present in patients with acute MI (70%–90% of patients). ST segment elevation greater than or equal to 1 mV in at least two side-by-side ECG leads indicates an acute MI. However, some patients infarct without ST segment elevation changes. Other conditions also can produce ST segment elevation. Prehospital management of the patient with a suspected MI should include placing the patient at rest; administering oxygen at 4 L/min via nasal cannula if indicated; frequently assessing vital signs and breath sounds; initiating an intravenous line with normal saline or lactated Ringer solution to keep the vein open; monitoring for dysrhythmias; administering medications such as nitroglycerin, morphine, and aspirin; and screening for risk factors for fibrinolytic therapy.
- Left ventricular failure occurs when the left ventricle fails to function as an effective forward pump. This causes a backpressure of blood into the pulmonary circulation. This in turn may lead to pulmonary edema. Emergency management is directed at decreasing the venous return to the heart, improving myocardial contractility, decreasing myocardial oxygen demand, improving ventilation and oxygenation, and rapidly transporting the patient to a medical facility.
- Right ventricular failure occurs when the right ventricle fails as a pump. This causes backpressure of blood into the systemic venous circulation. Right ventricular failure is not usually a medical emergency in itself; that is, unless it is associated with pulmonary edema or hypotension.
- Cardiogenic shock is the most extreme form of pump failure. It usually is caused by extensive MI. Even with aggressive therapy, cardiogenic shock has a mortality rate of 70% or higher. Patients in cardiogenic shock need rapid transport to a medical facility.
- Cardiac tamponade is defined as impaired filling of the heart caused by increased pressure in the pericardial sac.
- Abdominal aortic aneurysms are usually asymptomatic. However, signs and symptoms signal impending or active rupture. If the vessel tears, bleeding initially may be stopped by the retroperitoneal tissues. The patient may be normotensive on the arrival of emergency medical services. If the rupture opens into the peritoneal cavity, however, massive fatal hemorrhage may follow.
- Acute dissection is the most common aortic catastrophe. Any area of the aorta may be involved. However, in 60% to 70% of cases, the site of a dissecting aneurysm is in the ascending aorta just beyond the takeoff of the left subclavian artery. The signs and symptoms depend on the site of the intimal tear and on the extent of dissection. The goals of managing suspected aortic dissection in the prehospital setting are relief of pain and immediate transport to a medical facility.
- Acute arterial occlusion is a sudden blockage of arterial flow. Occlusion most commonly is caused by trauma, an embolus, or thrombosis. The most common sites of embolic occlusion are the abdominal aorta, common femoral artery, popliteal artery, carotid artery, brachial artery, and mesenteric artery. The location of ischemic pain is related to the site of occlusion.
- Noncritical peripheral vascular conditions include varicose veins, superficial thrombophlebitis, and acute deep vein thrombosis. Of these conditions, deep vein thrombosis is the only one that can cause a life-threatening problem. This problem is pulmonary embolus.
- Hypertension often is defined by a resting blood pressure that is consistently greater than 140/90 mm Hg. Chronic hypertension has an adverse effect on the heart and blood vessels. It requires the heart to perform more work than normal. This leads to hypertrophy of the cardiac muscle and left ventricular failure. Conditions associated with chronic, uncontrolled hypertension are cerebral hemorrhage and stroke, MI, and renal failure.
- Hypertensive emergencies are conditions in which a blood pressure increase leads to significant, irreversible end-organ damage within hours if not treated. The organs most likely to be at risk are the brain, heart, and kidneys. As a rule, the diagnosis is based on altered end-organ function and the rate of the rise in blood pressure, not on the level of blood pressure.
- Valvular heart disease may occur as the result of infection or be related to heart disease. When one or more of these valves become narrowed, hardened, or thickened (stenotic), the valves do not open or close completely. As a result, blood does not flow with proper force or direction.
- Infectious heart disease includes endocarditis, pericarditis and myocarditis. Complications can be severe and may include heart failure.
- Cardiomyopathy is alteration or weakness of the heart muscle. It can cause heart failure or sudden death.
- Basic cardiac life support helps to maintain the circulation and respiration of victims of cardiac arrest. Basic life support is continued until advanced cardiac life support is available. Two mechanisms are thought to be responsible for blood flow during cardiopulmonary resuscitation. One is direct compression of the heart between the sternum and the spine. This increases pressure within the ventricles to provide a small but critical amount of blood flow to the lungs and body organs. The second one is increased intrathoracic pressure transmitted to all intrathoracic

vascular structures. This creates an intrathoracic-to-extrathoracic pressure gradient. This gradient causes blood to flow out of the thorax. A number of mechanical devices provide external chest compression. Others provide chest compression with ventilation in the cardiac arrest patient.

- Cardiac monitor-defibrillators are classified as manual or automated external defibrillators. Defibrillation is the delivery of electrical current through the chest wall. Its purpose is to terminate ventricular fibrillation and certain other nonperfusing rhythms.
- Implantable cardioverter defibrillators work by monitoring the patient's cardiac rhythm. When a monitored ventricular rate exceeds the preprogrammed rate, the implantable cardioverter defibrillator delivers a shock of about 6 to 30 J through the patches. This is an attempt to restore a normal sinus rhythm.
- Synchronized cardioversion is designed to deliver a shock about 10 msec after the peak of the R wave of the cardiac cycle. (Thus, the device avoids the relative refractory period.) Synchronization may reduce the amount of energy needed to end the dysrhythmia. It also may decrease the chances of causing another dysrhythmia.
- Transcutaneous cardiac pacing is an effective emergency therapy for bradycardia, complete heart block, and suppression of some malignant ventricular dysrhythmias. Proper electrode placement is important for effective external pacing.
- It is becoming more and more evident that patients who cannot be resuscitated in the prehospital setting rarely survive. This is the case even if they are resuscitated temporarily in the emergency department. Cessation of resuscitative efforts in the prehospital setting should follow system-specific criteria established by medical direction.

REVIEW QUESTIONS

Match each term in Column II with its definition in Column I. Use each answer only once.

Column I

1. _________ Heart rate × Stroke volume

2. _________ Volume available for ventricles to pump each contraction

3. _________ Peripheral vascular resistance produces this pressure

4. _________ Ventricular relaxation

5. _________ Cardiac output x peripheral vascular resistance

6. _________ Increased myocardial contractility in response to increased preload

7. _________ Ventricular ejection per heartbeat

Column II

a. Afterload
b. Blood pressure
c. Cardiac output
d. Contractility
e. Diastole
f. Preload
g. Starling law
h. Stroke volume
i. Systole

8. Identify a prevention strategy for each of the following risk factors for cardiovascular disease and a community resource where you can refer the patient to assist with modification of this risk factor.

Risk Factor	Prevention Strategy	Resource
a. Smoking		
b. Hypercholesterolemia		
c. Obesity		
d. Sedentary lifestyle		

9. Explain how the sympathetic and parasympathetic divisions of the autonomic nervous system influence cardiac function in the following areas.

	Sympathetic	Parasympathetic
a. Heart rate		
b. Myocardial contractility		
c. Lungs		
d. Blood vessels (peripheral)		

10. Name the two adrenal hormones and describe the effects of each on the cardiovascular system.

Name	Function
a.	
b.	

11. Fill in the blanks in the following sentences about electrophysiology:

Within the body, separated charged particles with opposite charges have a **(a)** _______________ force of attraction that gives them **(b)** _______________ energy. This energy is released when the cell membrane becomes **(c)** _______________ to the charged particles and allows the charges to come together. The electrical charge between the inside and outside of cells is the **(d)** _______________ difference and is measured in **(e)** _______________. Although there is a relatively equal number of positively and negatively charged ions inside and outside the cell, the intracellular area has a **(f)** _______________ charge because of the **(g)** _______________ charged proteins that cannot move outside the cell. The electrical charge difference in the resting state has the potential to do work and is known as the resting membrane **(h)** _______________ (RMP). During this phase, the inside of the cell is electrically **(i)** _______________ relative to the outside of the cell (approximately **[j]** _______________ mV). The RMP results primarily from the difference between the intracellular and extracellular **(k)** _______________ ion level. Because of the chemical gradient (more of these ions inside than outside of the cell), the **(l)** _______________ would move out of the cell in an attempt to achieve equilibrium. However, these ions remain in the cell because of the negative intracellular charge generated by the **(m).** _______________ In the RMP, sodium will not rush into the cell because the cell membrane is not **(n)** _______________ to sodium. The ability of nerve and muscle cells to produce action potentials is known as **(o)** _______________. If this action potential results in a decreased charge difference across the cell membrane, the RMP becomes less negative, and this is called **(p)** _______________. If a stimulus is strong enough to cause depolarization of a cell membrane to a level called the **(q)** _______________, a chain reaction of permeability changes cause an **(r)** _______________ to spread over the entire cell membrane. Action potentials have two phases: a **(s)** _______________ phase and a **(t)** _______________ phase. During an action potential, the sodium ions rush into the cell, and RMP becomes **(u)** _______________ on the inside and **(v)** _______________ on the outside of the cell membrane. This occurs during the **(w)** _______________ phase. The repolarization phase results from potassium leakage outside the cell and the return of the cell membrane to its normal resting **(x)** _______________ state.

12. Answer the following questions regarding the five phases of the cardiac action potential:

a. During phase 0 (rapid depolarization), what causes the inside of the cell to become positive?

____

b. What is the membrane potential during phase 1 (early rapid repolarization)?

____

c. How is the membrane potential held at 0 during phase 2 (plateau phase)?

____

d. What happens to the membrane potential of the cell during phase 3 (terminal phase of rapid repolarization)?

____

e. How is the balance of sodium and potassium restored during phase 4?

____

f. Why can cardiac pacemaker cells depolarize without an external stimulus to initiate an action potential?

____

INTRODUCTION TO ELECTROCARDIOGRAM MONITORING

13. Circle the correct response in each of the following statements:
The electrocardiogram tracing represents an amplified view of the myocardial **(a)** action potentials/contractions. If the voltage displayed is positive, the electrocardiogram tracing will display a(n) **(b)** upward/downward/isoelectric deflection. Cardiac pacemaker cells spontaneously can generate impulses, a property known as **(c)** automaticity/conductivity. This rhythmic activity occurs because these cells do not have a stable **(d)** action potential/resting membrane potential.

14. Label Fig. 22-1 illustrating the cardiac conduction system.

a. ____

b. ____

c. ____

d. ____

e. ____

f. ____

g. ____

h. ____

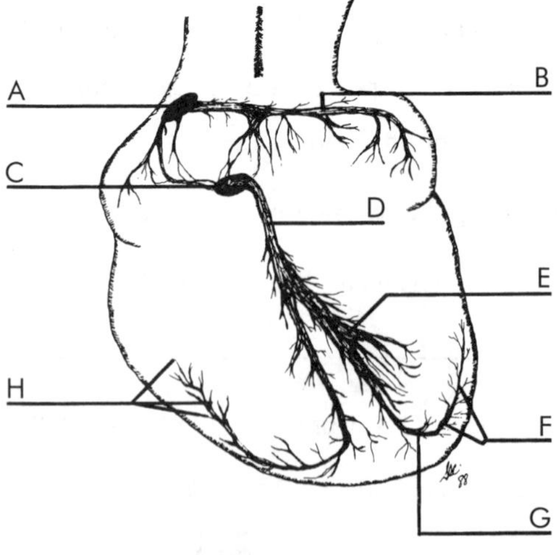

Figure 22-1

15. The sinoatrial node is the dominant pacemaker. If it fails to fire, what will happen?

____

16. Briefly describe the mechanism for ectopic impulse formation by each of the following mechanisms:

    a. Enhanced automaticity:

____

    b. Reentry:

____

ASSESSMENT OF THE PATIENT WITH CARDIAC DISEASE

17. A 62-year-old woman complains of chest pain. What questions should you ask using the OPQRST mnemonic to determine the nature and severity of her pain?

    O. ____

    P. ____

    Q. ____

    R. ____

    S. ____

    T. ____

18. List three chief complaints that may lead you to believe a patient has a cardiovascular problem.

    a. ____

    b. ____

    c. ____

19. An older man experiences a syncopal episode at a local gym. List at least two questions you should ask in an attempt to determine the nature of his syncopal episode.

    a. ____

    b. ____

20. A 34-year-old woman walks into your ambulance base complaining of a fluttering sensation in her chest. What will your history and physical examination include to determine the cause of this sensation?

____

____

Questions 21 to 23 pertain to the following case study:

An 87-year-old woman calls you to her home and complains of weakness and nausea. On arrival, you find her seated on the commode. She is pale, cool, and diaphoretic. Her blood pressure is 70 mm Hg by palpation, and her electrocardiogram is shown in Fig. 22-2.

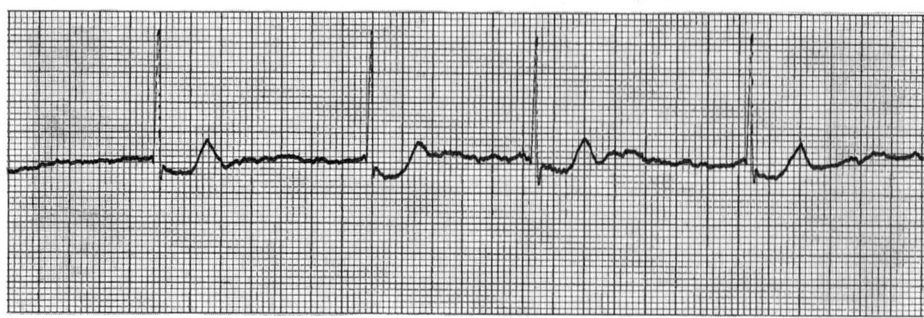

Figure 22-2

21. What information from this patient's medical history will be important to elicit at this time?

22. What is your interpretation of her electrocardiogram?

23. She tells you that she is taking digoxin, diltiazem, potassium, and furosemide. Could any of her home medicines be playing a role in her problem? If yes, which ones and why?

24. An older man is found unresponsive and bradycardic in a local park. A caretaker states that he complained of chest pain before collapsing. No one is available to give you any information regarding his history. Briefly outline specific findings you may encounter in your patient assessment if he has a history of cardiac problems.

25. Place the positive (+) and negative (−) and electrodes for the four leads shown in Fig. 22-3.

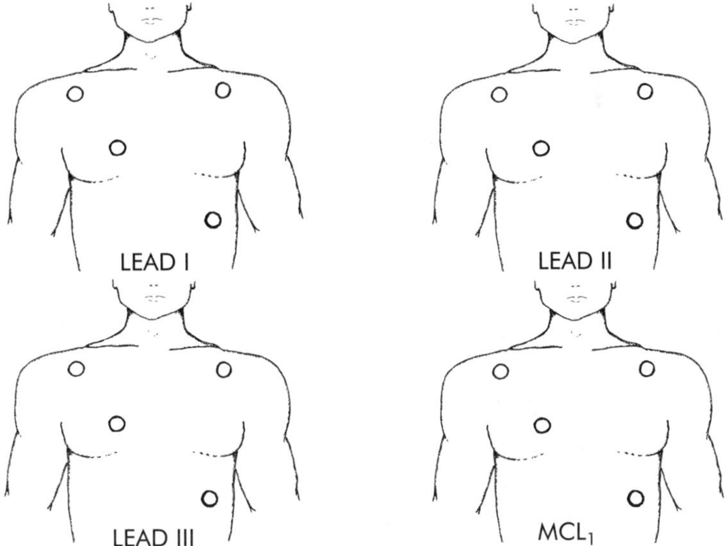

Figure 22-3

26. Describe the location of each of the 10 electrodes needed to record a 12-lead electrocardiogram.

a. _______________________   f. _______________________

b. _______________________   g. _______________________

c. _______________________   h. _______________________

d. _______________________   i. _______________________

e. _______________________   j. _______________________

27. List six problems that may interfere with a clear electrocardiogram recording. For each problem, discuss a possible solution.

a. _______________________   d. _______________________

b. _______________________   e. _______________________

c. _______________________   f. _______________________

28. Label Fig. 22-4 with the appropriate measurement intervals

a. _______ mm

b. _______ second

c. _______ second

d. _______ second

e. _______ second

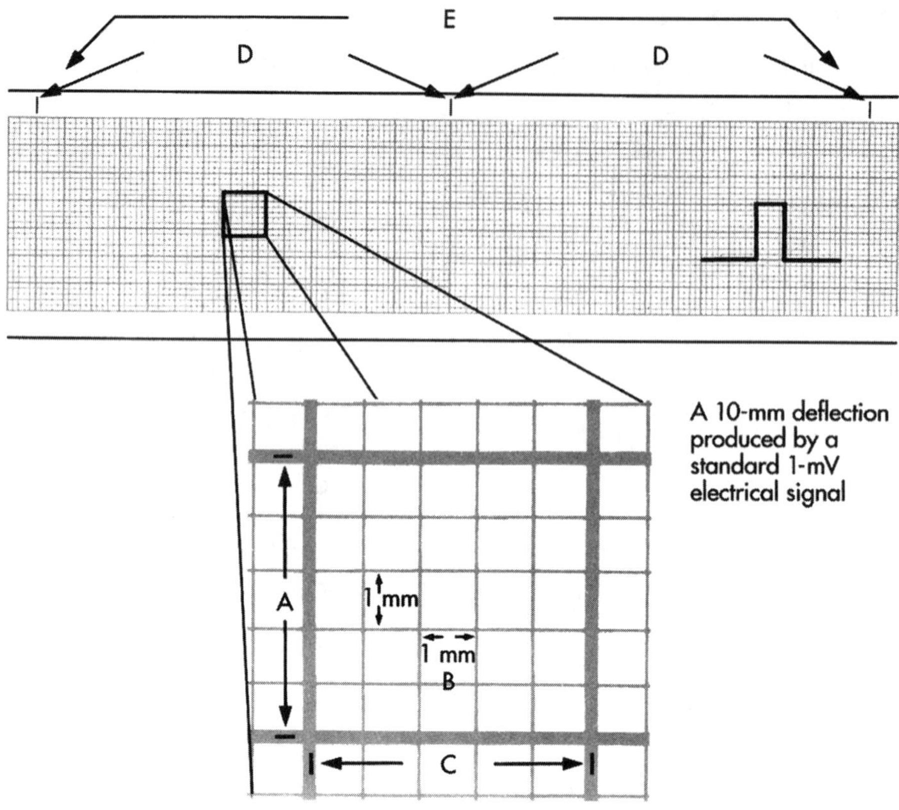

Figure 22-4

29. Label the sample electrocardiogram tracing in Fig. 22-5.

a. _______________________________

b. _______________________________

c. _______________________________

d. _______________________________

e. _______________________________

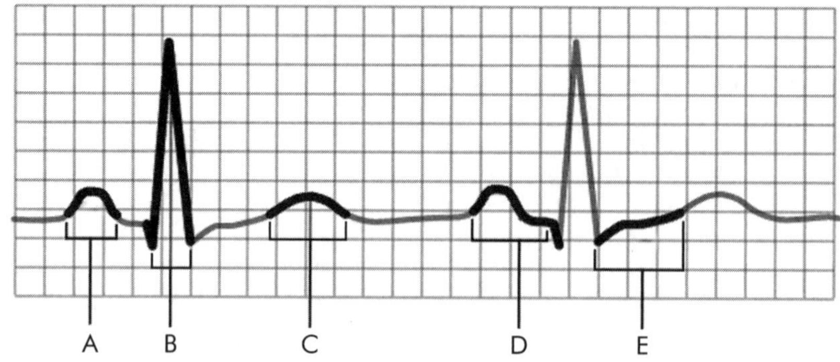

Figure 22-5

30. List five causes of artifact.

    a. _______________________________________

    b. _______________________________________

    c. _______________________________________

    d. _______________________________________

    e. _______________________________________

ELECTROCARDIOGRAM INTERPRETATION

31. List the five steps in electrocardiogram analysis.

    a. _______________________________________

    b. _______________________________________

    c. _______________________________________

    d. _______________________________________

    e. _______________________________________

32. Calculate the rate of the electrocardiogram in Fig. 22-6 using four different methods, describing the steps you use in each method.

    a. _______________________________________

    b. _______________________________________

    c. _______________________________________

    d. _______________________________________

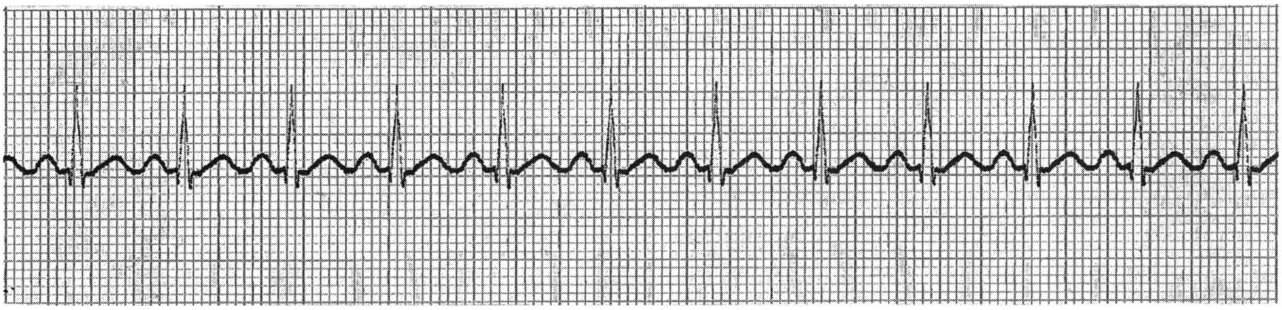

Figure 22-6

33. If the rate in question 32 is within normal limits, can we assume the patient is stable? Explain your answer.

____

34. Which method of calculation would be most accurate if the rhythm in question 32 was

    a. Regular?

____

b. Irregularly irregular?

____

35. What criterion must be met when analyzing the electrocardiogram rhythm to determine that the rhythm is regular?

____

36. What analysis can be made about conduction in each of the following examples?

    a. The QRS complex width is less than or equal to 0.12 second.

____

    b. The QRS complex width is greater than 0.12 second.

____

37. List the four criteria that must be evaluated when analyzing the P waves.

    a. ____

    b. ____

    c. ____

    d. ____

38. Briefly describe the significance of each of the following P-R interval findings.

    a. P-R interval of 0.08 second:

____

    b. P-R interval of 0.16 second:

____

____

    c. P-R interval of 0.24 second:

____

39. Analyze the electrocardiogram rhythm strip in Fig. 22-7 using the five steps described in question 31 and give your interpretation.

    a. Step 1:

____

    b. Step 2:

____

c. Step 3:

____

d. Step 4:

____

e. Step 5:

____

Interpretation:

____

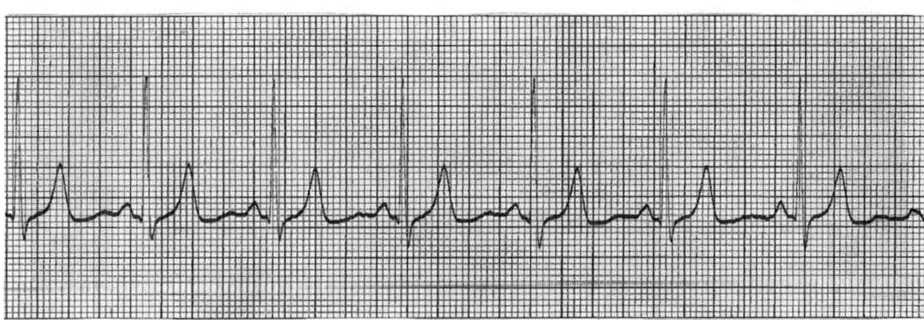

Figure 22-7

INTRODUCTION TO DYSRHYTHMIAS

40. When a dysrhythmia is noted on the monitor, what factors must be considered to determine whether any intervention is necessary?

____

41. Dysrhythmias originating in the sinoatrial node frequently result from increases or decreases in

a. ____

Electrocardiographic features common to all sinoatrial node dysrhythmias are

b. QRS complex.

____

c. P waves (lead II).

____

d. P-R interval.

____

42. List two causes of each bradycardic and tachycardic dysrhythmia that originates in the sinus node.

a. Sinus bradycardia:

____

b. Sinus tachycardia:

____

Complete the missing information on Flashcards 1 to 4 at the end of the text.

43. Complete Flashcard 1 (Fig. 22-8): sinus bradycardia.

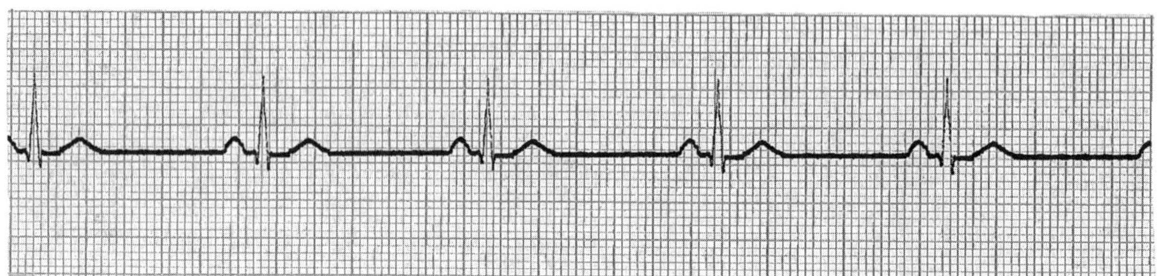

Figure 22-8

44. Complete Flashcard 2 (Fig. 22-9): sinus tachycardia.

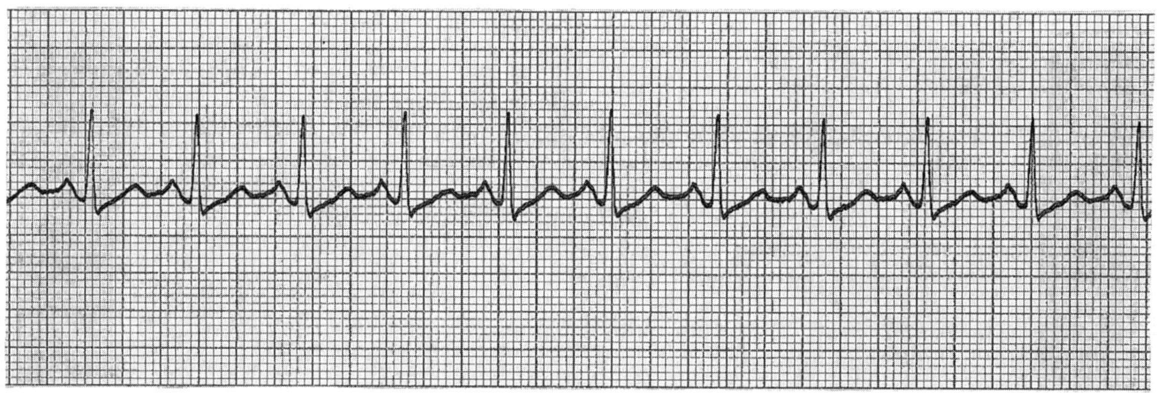

Figure 22-9

45. Complete Flashcard 3 (Fig. 22-10): sinus dysrhythmia.

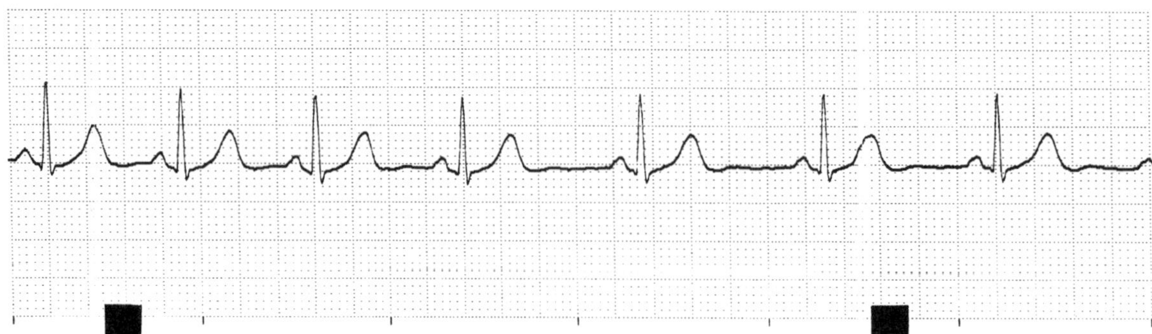

Figure 22-10

Chapter **22** **Cardiology**

46. Complete Flashcard 4 (Fig. 22-11): sinus arrest.

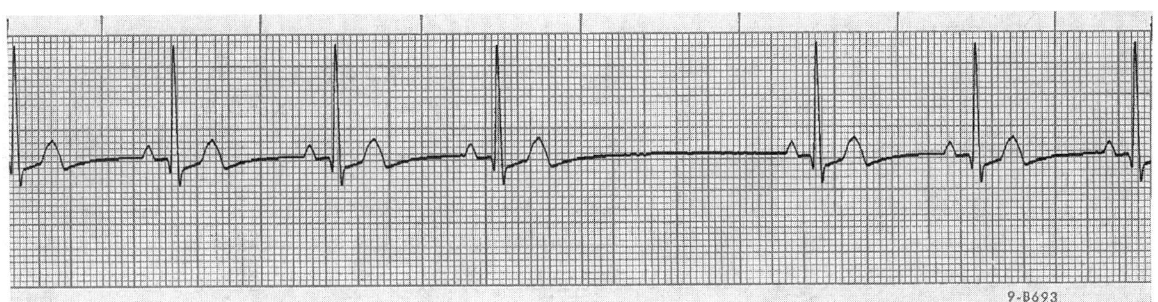

Figure 22-11

47. Atrial dysrhythmias originate in the **(a)** ______ of the **(b)** ______ or in the **(c)** ______ pathways.

48. Common features of atrial dysrhythmias are

    a. QRS complex.

    ____

    b. P waves (if present).

    ____

    c. P-R intervals.

    ____

49. List four causes of dysrhythmias that originate in the atria.

    a. ____

    b. ____

    c. ____

    d. ____

Complete the missing information on Flashcards 5 to 9 showing dysrhythmias originating in the atria.

50. Complete Flashcard 5 (Fig. 22-12): wandering atrial pacemaker.

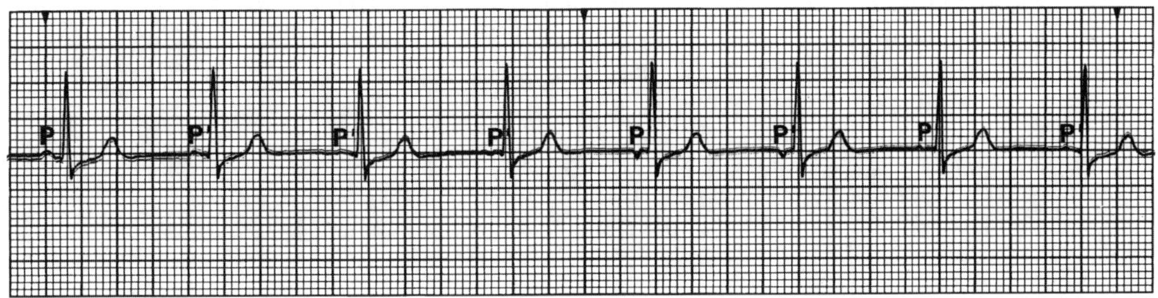

Figure 22-12

51. Complete Flashcard 6 (Fig. 22-13): premature atrial contraction.

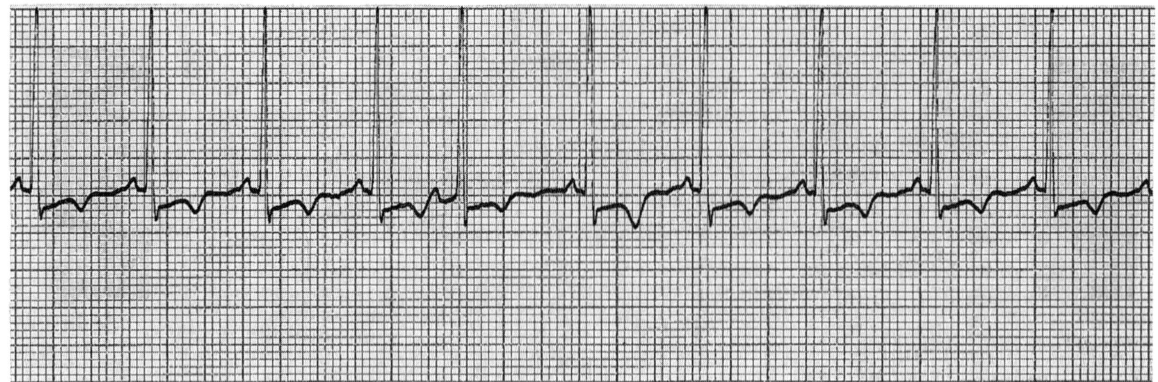

Figure 22-13

52. Complete Flashcard 7 (Fig. 22-14): supraventricular tachycardia.

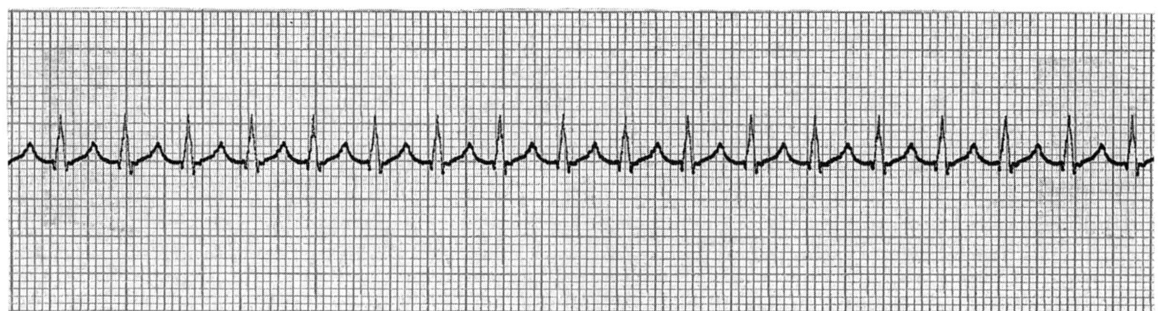

Figure 22-14

53. Complete Flashcard 8 (Fig. 22-15): atrial flutter with 3:1 conduction.

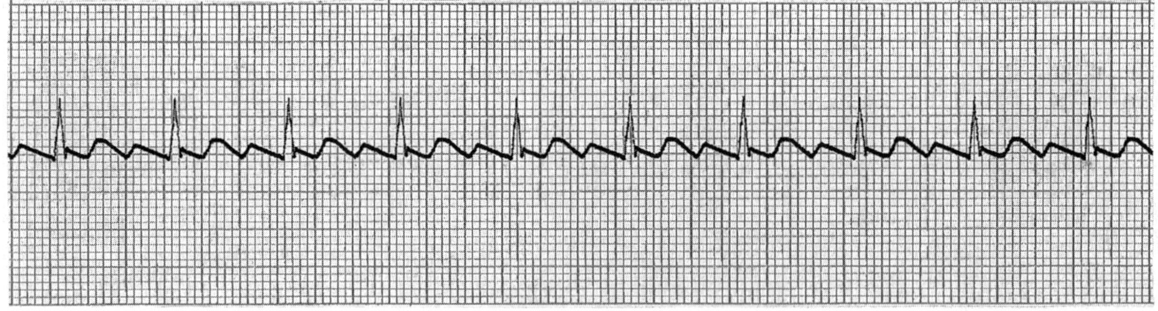

Figure 22-15

54. Complete Flashcard 9 (Fig. 22-16): atrial fibrillation.

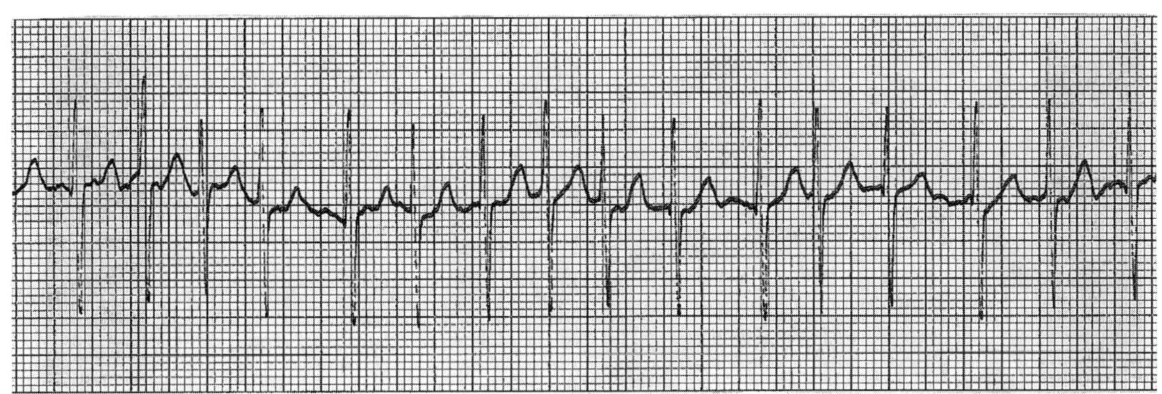

Figure 22-16

55. Rhythms that start in the atrioventricular node or junction are called (a) _______ rhythms. These rhythms share the following common features:

a. QRS complex:

____

b. P waves:

____

c. P-R interval:

____

56. List four causes of dysrhythmias that start in the atrioventricular junction.

a. ____

b. ____

c. ____

d. ____

Complete the missing information on Flashcards 10 to 12 showing dysrhythmias originating in the atrioventricular junction.

57. Complete Flashcard 10 (Fig. 22-17): sinus rhythm (borderline bradycardia) with two premature junctional contractions.

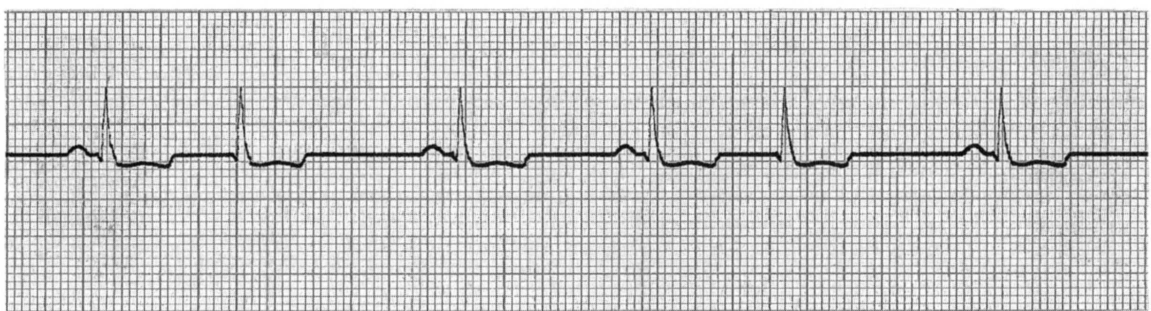

Figure 22-17

58. Complete Flashcard 11 (Fig. 22-18): junctional escape rhythm.

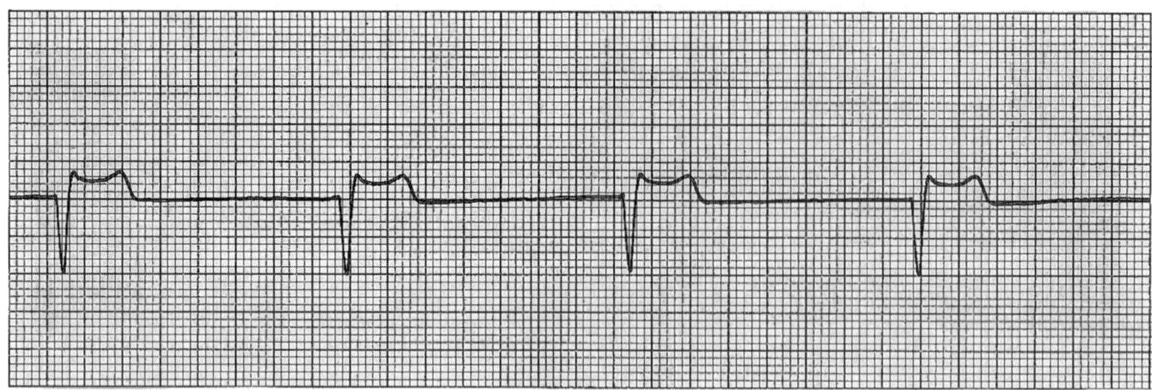

Figure 22-18

59. Complete Flashcard 12 (Fig. 22-19): accelerated junctional rhythm.

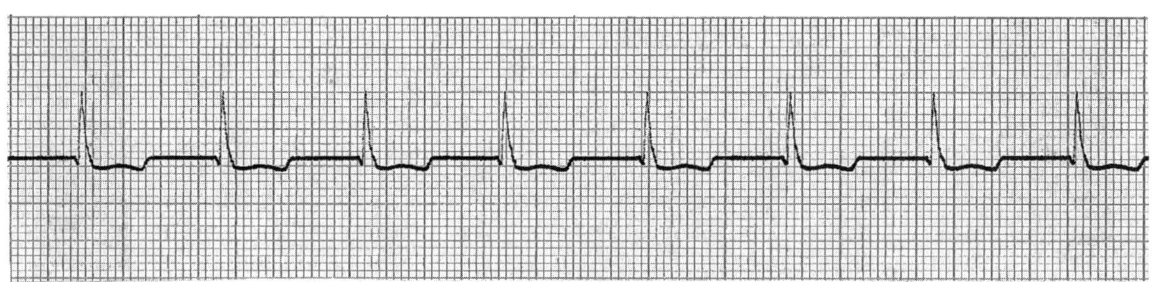

Figure 22-19

60. Rhythms originating from the ventricle have an intrinsic rate of **(a)** _________________ to _________________ but can be accelerated at rates up to **(b)** _________________ or tachycardic at rates greater than **(c)** _________________.

61. List five causes of dysrhythmias that originate in the ventricles.

   a. ____

   b. ____

   c. ____

   d. ____

   e. ____

62. Identify five steps that can be used when evaluating a 12-lead electrocardiogram to distinguish between wide-complex tachycardias of ventricular versus supraventricular origin.

   a. ____

   b. ____

   c. ____

308

d. ____

e. ____

Complete the missing information on Flashcards 13 to 18 showing dysrhythmias originating in the ventricles.

63. Complete Flashcard 13 (Fig. 22-20): ventricular escape rhythm.

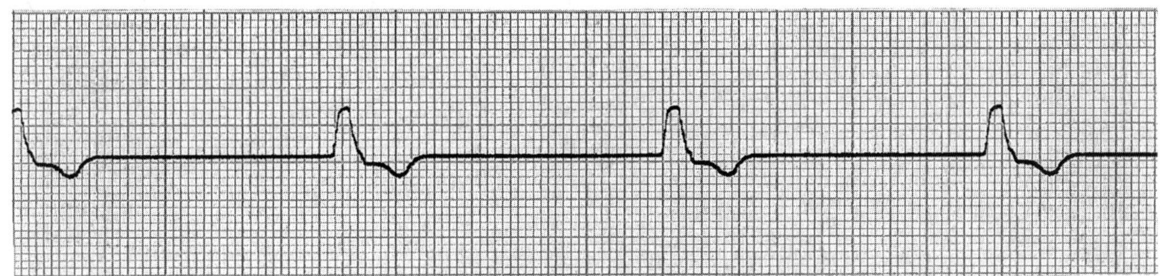

Figure 22-20

64. Complete Flashcard 14 (Fig. 22-21): normal sinus rhythm with one premature ventricular contraction.

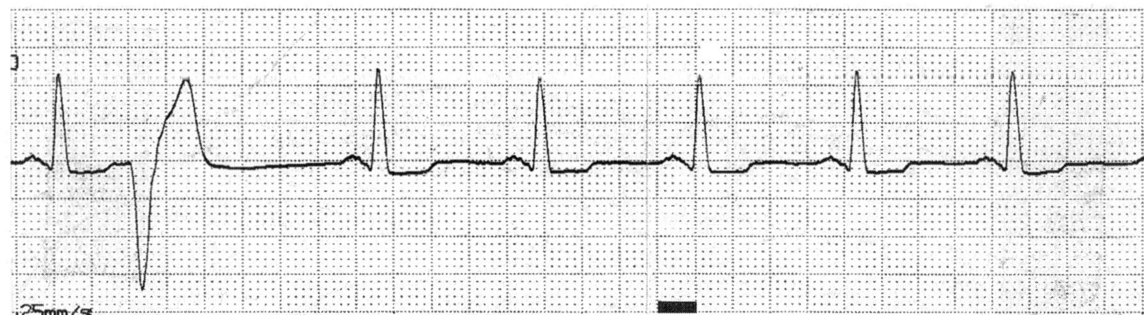

Figure 22-21

65. Complete Flashcard 15 (Fig. 22-22): monomorphic ventricular tachycardia.

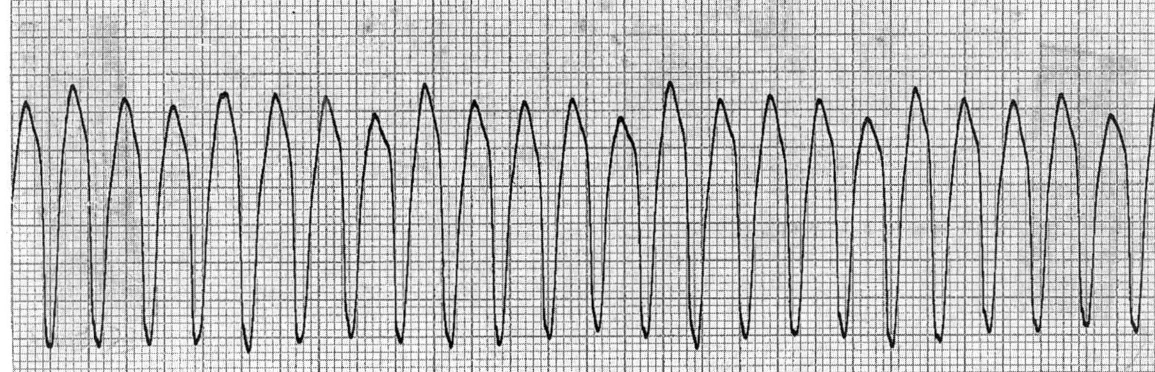

Figure 22-22

66. Complete Flashcard 16 (Fig. 22-23): ventricular fibrillation.

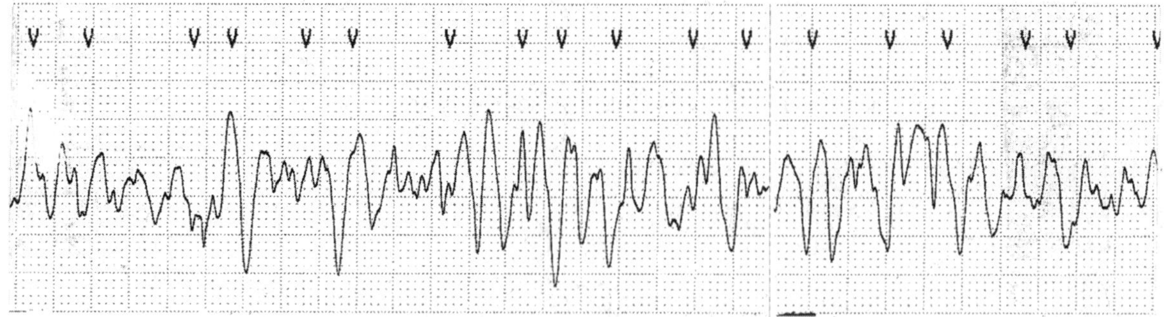

Figure 22-23

67. Complete Flashcard 17 (Fig. 22-24): asystole.

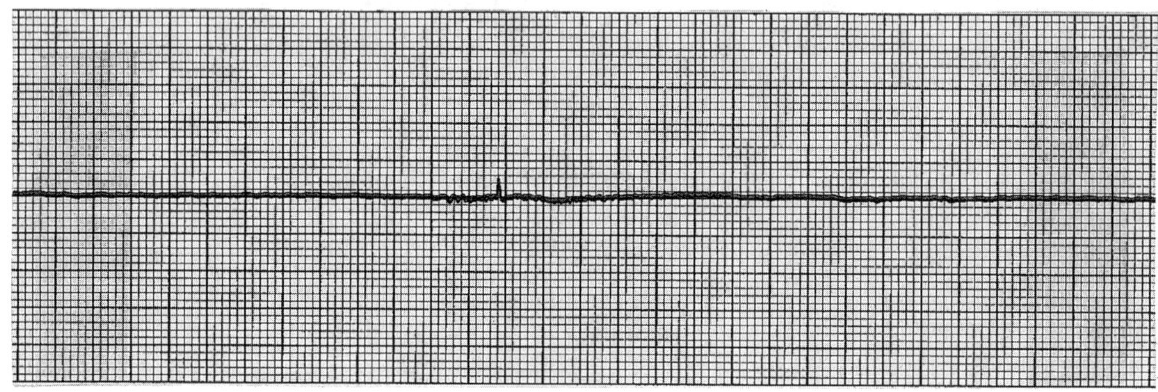

Figure 22-24

68. Complete Flashcard 18 (Fig. 22-25): ventricular paced rhythm.

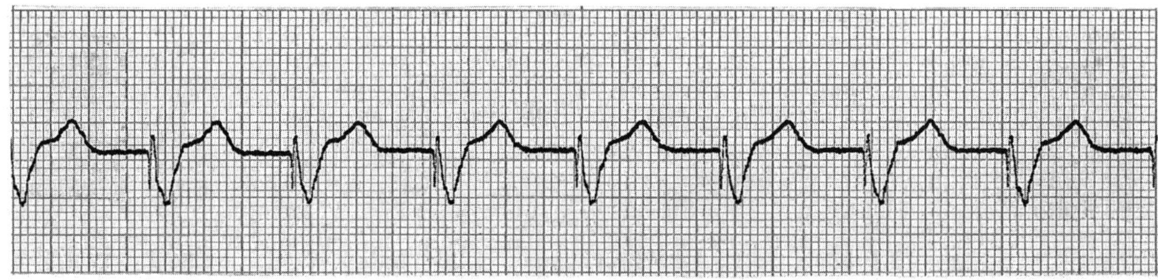

Figure 22-25

69. Delays or interruptions in cardiac electrical conduction are called **(a)** _________________. They may be caused by disease of the **(b)** _________________.

70. List five causes of dysrhythmias caused by delays in cardiac electrical conduction.

   a. ____

   b. ____

   c. ____

d. ____

e. ____

Complete the missing information on Flashcards 19 to 22 showing dysrhythmias originating from conduction disorders.

71. Complete Flashcard 19 (Fig. 22-26): sinus rhythm with first-degree atrioventricular block.

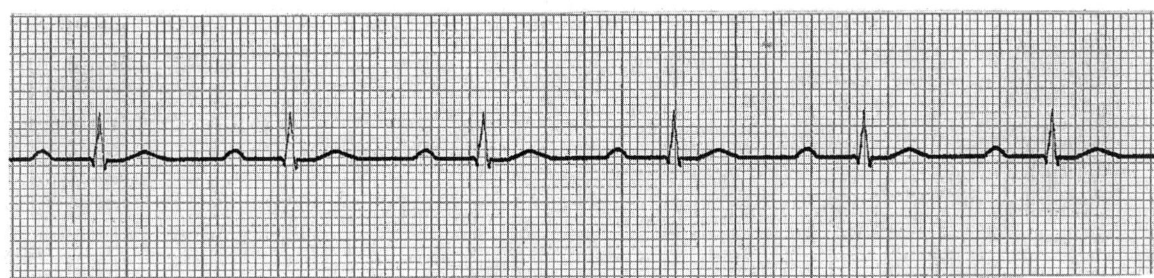

Figure 22-26

72. Complete Flashcard 20 (Fig. 22-27): second-degree atrioventricular block (Mobitz type I or Wenckebach).

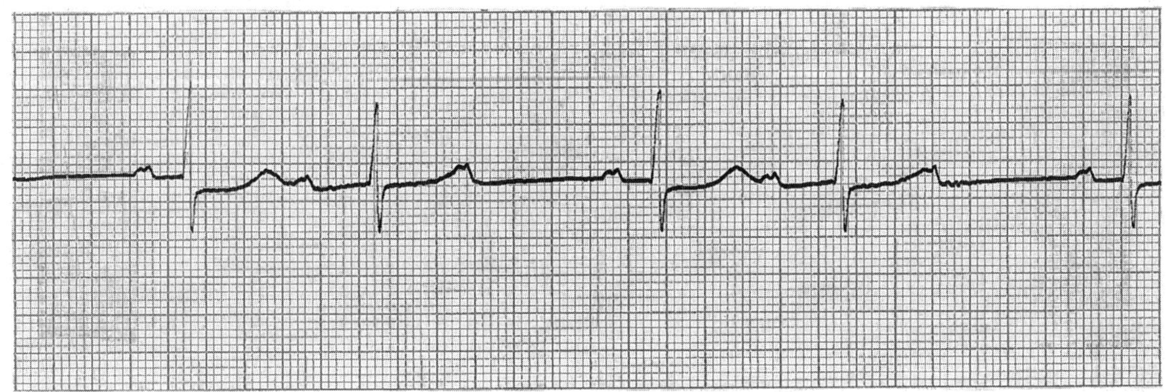

Figure 22-27

73. Complete Flashcard 21 (Fig. 22-28): second-degree atrioventricular block (Mobitz type II).

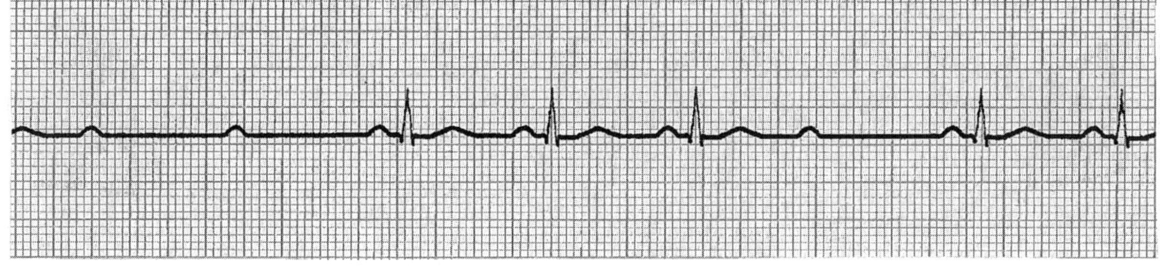

Figure 22-28

74. Complete Flashcard 22 (Fig. 22-29): third-degree (complete) atrioventricular block.

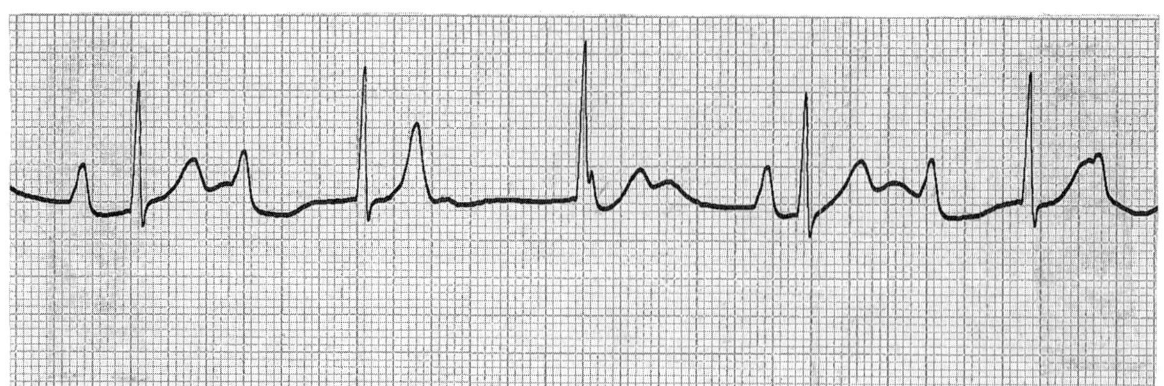

Figure 22-29

75. List the characteristics to identify the following:
   a. Right bundle branch block _____
   b. Left bundle branch block _____
   c. Anterior hemiblock _____
   d. Posterior hemiblock _____

76. Identify patients at risk for developing complete heart block if they are given procainamide, digoxin, verapamil, or diltiazem:

   a. ____

   b. ____

   c. ____

77. An approximately 50-year-old man is found unconscious in a parking lot downtown. He is pulseless and apneic. The attendant is certain he has been there less than 5 minutes but does not know what happened. The patient's electrocardiogram is shown in Fig. 22-30.

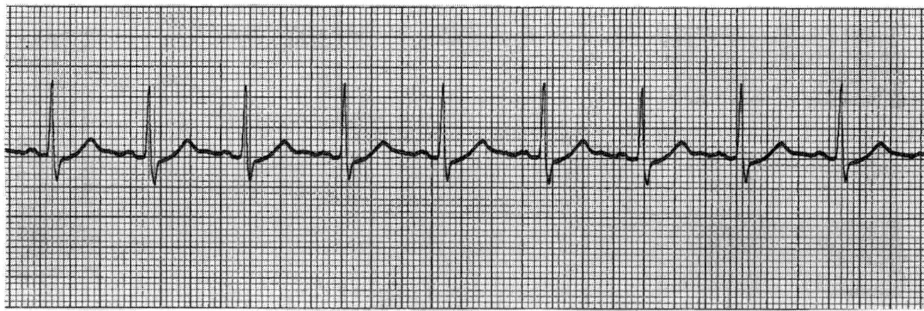

Figure 22-30

   a. You identify the rhythm as

   ____

   b. Outline the appropriate interventions for this patient based on current treatment guidelines by the American Heart Association.

   ____

78. Outline the electrocardiogram features characteristic of Wolff-Parkinson-White syndrome.

a. QRS complex:

____

b. P-R interval:

____

79. Why is it clinically important to recognize a patient with a history of Wolff-Parkinson-White syndrome?

____

____

SPECIFIC CARDIOVASCULAR DISEASES

80. Explain the pathophysiology of atherosclerotic effects on blood vessels.

____

____

81. List two triggers that may initiate an anginal attack in a susceptible patient:

a. ____

b. ____

82. Describe the following features of angina:

a. Duration:

____

b. Relieved by:

____

83. How can a paramedic distinguish between unstable angina and myocardial infarction in the prehospital environment?

____

84. Briefly outline the sequence of pathophysiological events that occur from the time that a clot forms until cardiac tissue dies in acute myocardial infarction.

____

____

85. Complete the information regarding myocardial infarction that is missing in the following table:

Area of Heart Injured or Infarcted	Coronary Vessel Involved Most Often	Leads with	Leads with visible ST Segment Changes
Anterior			
Lateral			
Septal			
Inferior			

86. How much ST segment elevation must be present to be clinically significant?

____

87. List six conditions other than myocardial infarction that can cause ST segment elevation.

    a. ____

    b. ____

    c. ____

    d. ____

    e. ____

    f. ____

88. List the five-step analysis described in this text for infarct recognition.

    a. ____

    b. ____

    c. ____

    d. ____

    e. ____

89. Identify four complications resulting from myocardial infarction.

    a. ____

    b. ____

    c. ____

    d. ____

Questions 90 to 94 pertain to the following case study:

A 57-year-old, 80-kg man with a history of untreated hypertension complains of crushing midsternal chest pain that began 2 hours ago. He takes no medicines but admits to smoking two packs of cigarettes per day. His blood pressure is 162/102 mm Hg, and his SaO_2 is 92%. His electrocardiogram strip is shown in Fig. 22-31.

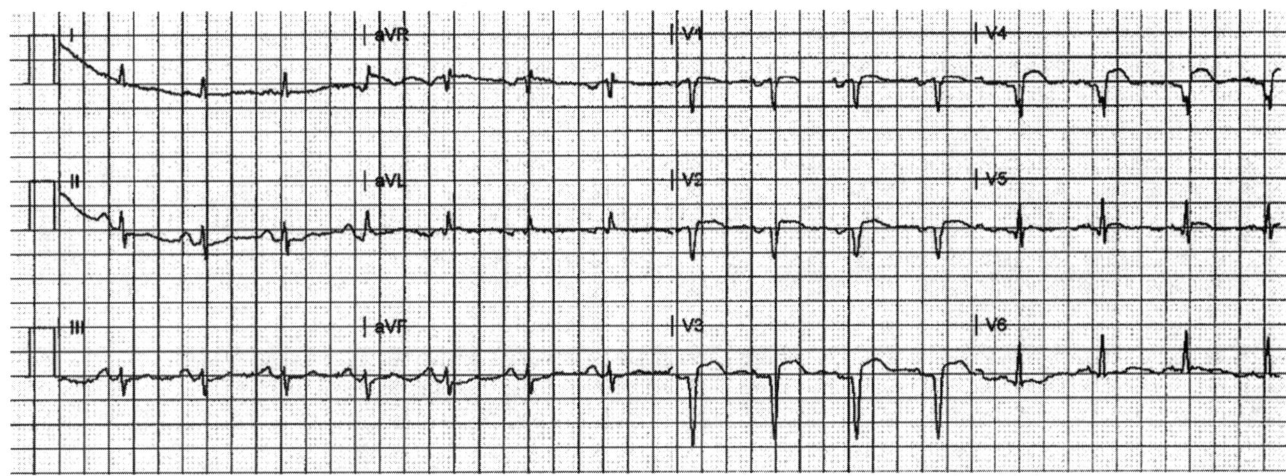

Figure 22-31

90. What other associated signs or symptoms may be present if the patient is experiencing a myocardial infarction?

91. What is your interpretation of his electrocardiogram?

92. Describe general treatment measures you will use for this patient.

93. List three drugs (excluding oxygen) with the appropriate dosage to administer to this patient.

    a. ____

    b. ____

    c. ____

94. You transmit the 12-lead electrocardiogram to the hospital and are asked to determine whether the patient meets inclusion or exclusion criteria for fibrinolytic therapy.

    a. List four inclusion criteria:

    b. List 10 contraindications to fibrinolytic administration.

c. Aside from the contraindications above, what three high-risk criteria suggest that this patient would benefit from PCI?

95. Interpret each of the following 12-lead electrocardiograms.

a. Fig. 22-32:

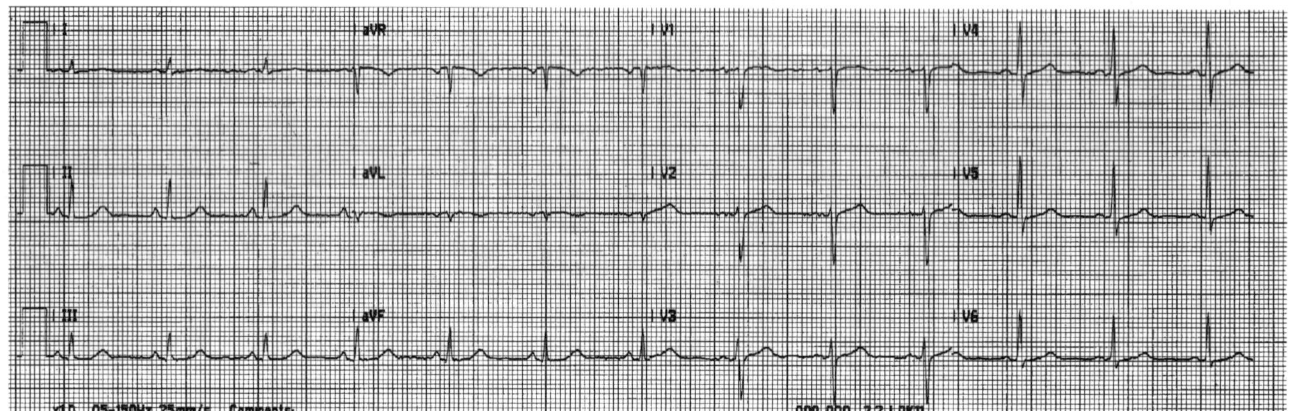

Figure 22-32

b. Fig. 22-33:

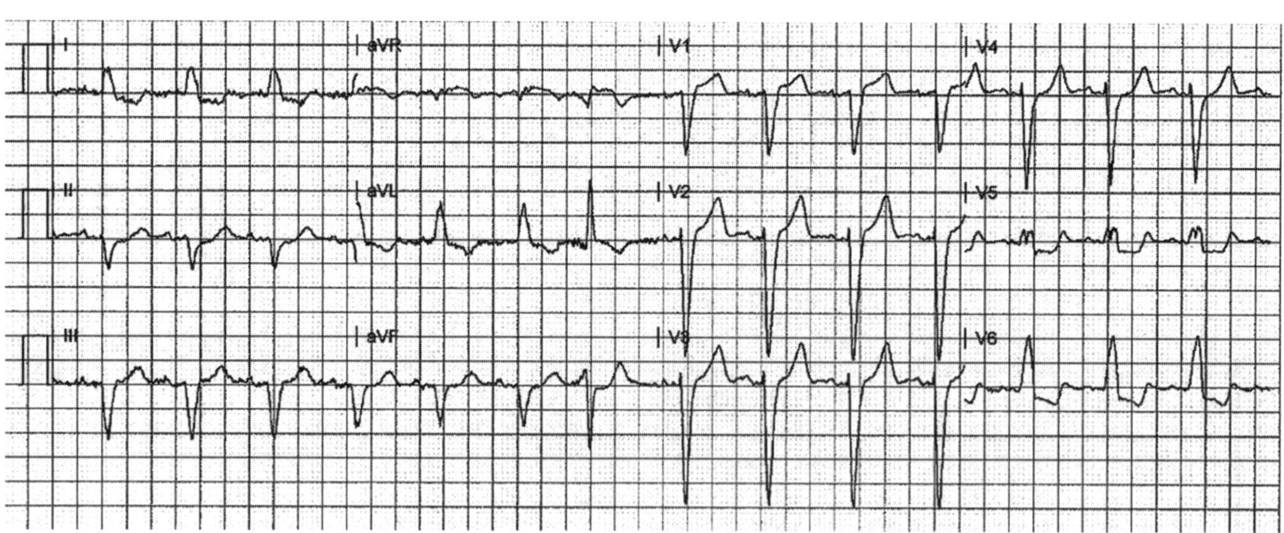

Figure 22-33

c. Fig. 22-34:

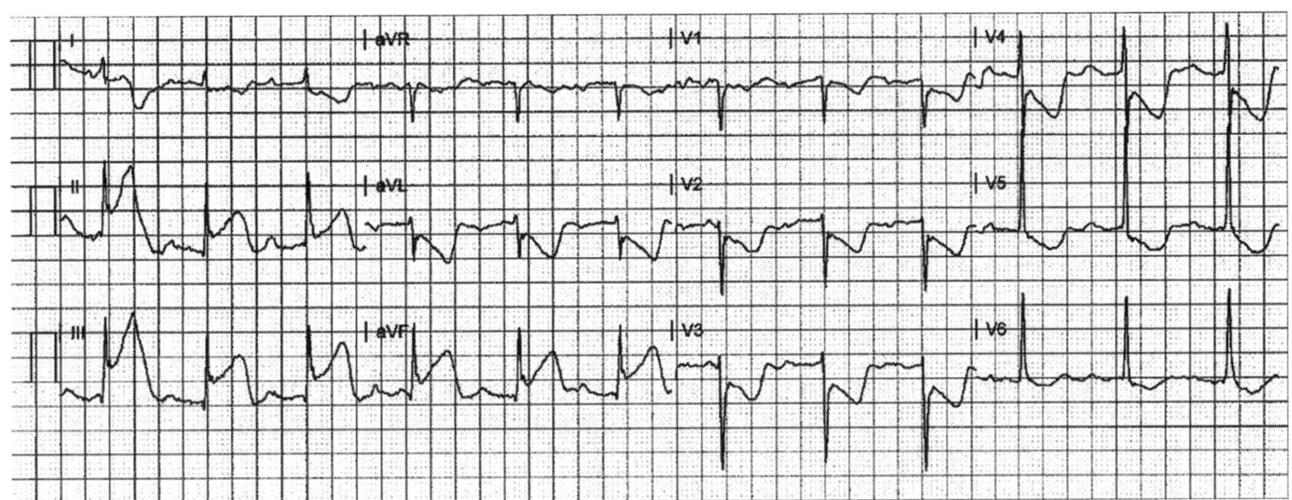

Figure 22-34

d. Fig. 22-35:

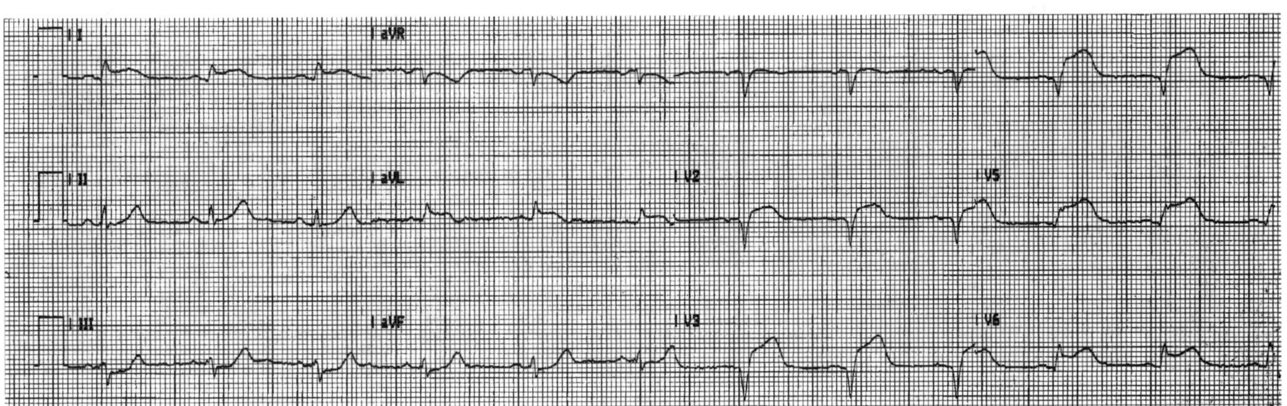

Figure 22-35

Questions 96 to 100 pertain to the following case study:

An 80-kg patient who had a syncopal episode and chest pain has the following electrocardiogram (Fig. 22-36).

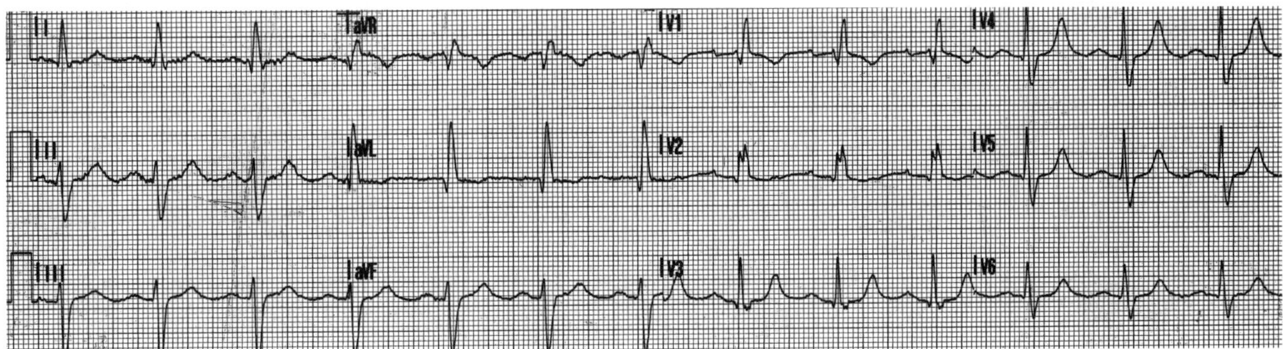

Figure 22-36

96. What is the axis of this electrocardiogram? _______________________________________

97. The QRS complex duration is 0.134 second. Draw a triangle that begins at the J point in lead V_1 and, working backward, ends at the first QRS deflection that is encountered. Does the triangle point up or down?

____

98. Based on your determination of axis, the QRS duration, and the triangle you drew, identify the two blocks that are present in this electrocardiogram.

____

99. What is the significance of these blocks?

____

100. Based on the patient's chief complaint and your electrocardiogram findings, what interventions would you perform in addition to routine cardiac care?

____

Questions 101 to 105 pertain to the following case study:

A 72-year-old, 70-kg woman calls you to her home and complains of a sudden onset of severe dyspnea without chest pain. You find her anxious, sitting upright, with diaphoretic skin and circumoral cyanosis. Her only home medicine is a diuretic. Vital signs are blood pressure, 170/106 mm Hg; pulse, 124 beats/min; and respirations, 28 breaths/min and labored. Rales are audible to the level of the scapulae. SaO_2 is 86%. Her electrocardiogram is shown in Fig. 22-37.

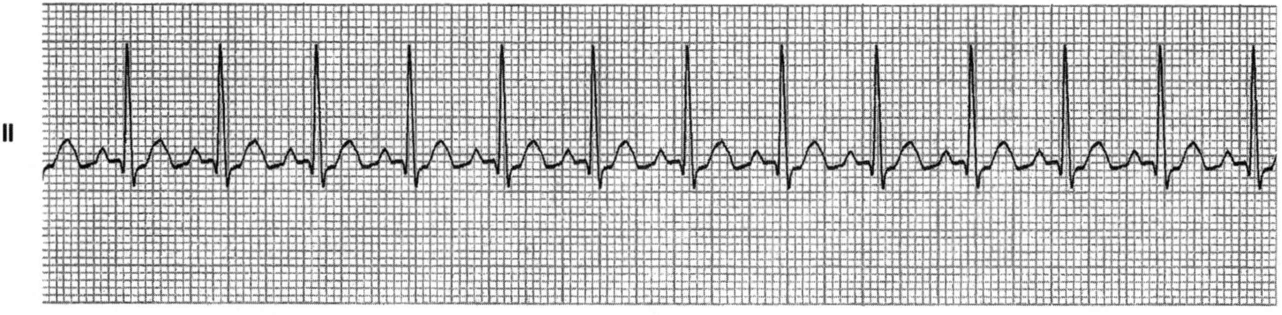

Figure 22-37

101. What medical condition or conditions do you suspect?

____

102. What other physical findings would help confirm this diagnosis?

____

103. What nonpharmacologic intervention should you perform as soon as possible?

____

Chapter **22** **Cardiology**

104. You wish to administer other pharmacologic agents to improve her oxygenation. List three drugs that you would consider, and give the correct dose and desired effect of each.

a. ____

b. ____

c. ____

105. Describe how the treatment plan would change if her blood pressure was 82/50 mm Hg but her other signs and symptoms remain the same?

106. List causes and signs and symptoms of right ventricular failure.

a. Causes:

____

b. Signs and symptoms:

____

Questions 107 to 110 pertain to the following case study:

You are evaluating a 67-year-old man who has a history of two myocardial infarctions. His wife states he had chest pain that began 4 hours ago but that he refused to let her call emergency medical services and then passed out. He is conscious but confused and is pale and diaphoretic. His blood pressure is 80/50 mm Hg, his respiratory rate is 20 breaths/min, his SaO_2 is 90%, and his breath sounds are clear. His only home medicine is nitroglycerin paste, which he has on his left chest. This patient's electrocardiogram is shown in Fig. 22-38.

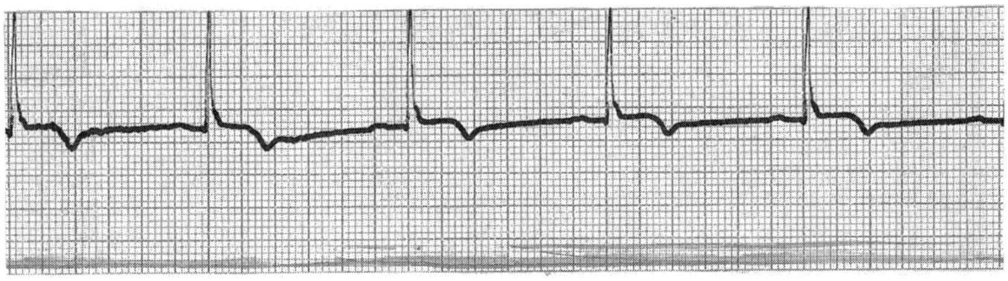

Figure 22-38

107. What is your interpretation of his electrocardiogram?

____

108. What drug and dosage will you administer in consultation with medical direction to correct this dysrhythmia?

____

After administering the first dose of this drug, the heart rate accelerates to 70 beats/min; however, the patient's other physical findings remain unchanged.

109. What do you suspect this patient is suffering from?

____

110. List critical interventions, including drug therapy, that you should use, assuming that your estimated time of arrival to the hospital is 30 minutes.

Questions 111 to 114 pertain to the following case study:

A 70-year-old man experiences a sudden onset of a "tearing" abdominal pain at the area of the umbilicus that radiates to his back. He is pale and complains of the urge to defecate. His only history is hypertension, for which he takes captopril. Vital signs are blood pressure, 106/70 mm Hg; pulse, 100 beats/min; and respirations, 20 breaths/min. On physical examination, you auscultate a bruit over the periumbilical area.

111. What illness do you suspect?

---

112. Should you palpate this patient's abdomen?

113. Should you allow this patient to go to the toilet and defecate?

114. Briefly outline your management of this patient.

Questions 115 to 117 pertain to the following case study:

An older man complains of a severe "ripping" pain between his scapulae that extends down to his legs. He is pale and diaphoretic and has the following vital signs: blood pressure 170/110 mm Hg in the right arm and 130/80 mm Hg in the left arm.

115. What medical emergency do you suspect?

---

116. Describe other physical findings that may confirm your suspicions.

---

117. Outline your management of this patient in the prehospital phase.

---

118. Differentiate between the following characteristics of embolic arterial occlusion and thrombotic arterial occlusion.

	Embolic	Thrombotic
Causes:		
Onset:		
Signs and symptoms:		

119. An older woman calls you to her home because she bumped her leg and a varicose vein is bleeding. What care should be rendered to this patient?

____

120. List three signs or symptoms of acute deep vein thrombosis.

   a. ____

   b. ____

   c. ____

Questions 121 to 124 pertain to the following case study:

A 60-year-old man complains of a severe headache, blurred vision, and vomiting. He states that he has a history of hypertension but has not been taking his medicine because the cost is too high. His vital signs are blood pressure, 190/128 mm Hg; pulse, 88 beats/min; and respirations, 20 breaths/min.

121. What medical emergency do you suspect?

____

122. If this man is not treated promptly, what other signs and symptoms may result?

____

123. Outline general management principles for this patient.

____

124. If your transport time is delayed, list one drug (with the appropriate dose) that medical direction may order to lower this patient's blood pressure.

____

TECHNIQUES OF MANAGING CARDIAC EMERGENCIES

125. You are at a friend's home playing tennis. After retrieving the ball, you turn around see that your friend has collapsed on the court. Outline the steps you must take from this moment until emergency medical services arrives if your friend has had a cardiac arrest. (Assume that no one else is nearby to help.)

____

____

____

126. A basic life support unit is caring for a patient who is in cardiac arrest when your advanced life support unit arrives on the scene. An automated external defibrillator without a display is attached to the patient, and five shocks already have been delivered.

   a. When should you defibrillate this patient if you determine that ventricular fibrillation is present?

____

   b. If a rescuer is in contact with the patient when the automated external defibrillator fires, will an injury occur?

____

You arrive on the scene to care for a patient who is pulseless and apneic. A bystander is performing CPR when you arrive. The monitor displays the rhythm shown in Fig. 22-39.

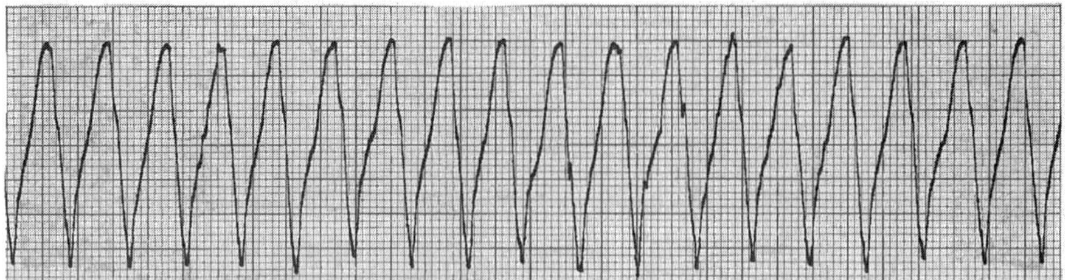

Figure 22-39

127. What is your interpretation of the electrocardiogram?

____

128. What is your first intervention after rhythm determination and verification of pulselessness?

____

129. List two factors that will improve the success rate of this treatment.

    a. ____

    b. ____

130. List the steps in performing this intervention.

____

____

____

____

131. You are at the home of a patient whose wife states that he was experiencing severe chest pain. Moments after you hook up the patient to your monitor, he loses consciousness, and the rhythm shown in Fig. 22-40 is displayed. Blood pressure is 60 mm Hg by palpation, and ventilations are adequate. Another paramedic applies oxygen by non-rebreather mask at 12 L/min. State the appropriate therapy for this patient up to and including administration of the first drug.

____

____

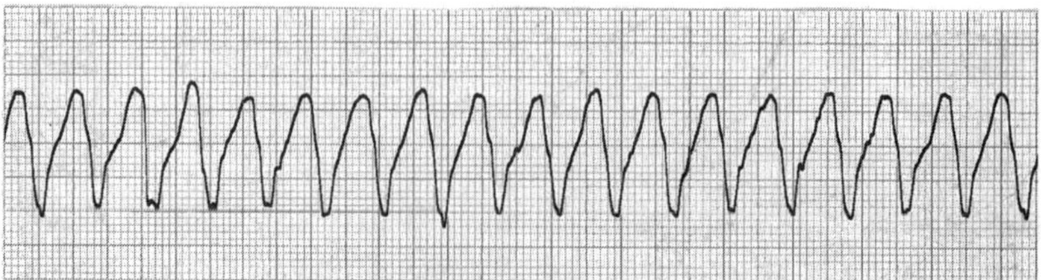

Figure 22-40

322

132. What is the advantage of synchronized cardioversion?

____

133. Briefly outline the steps in synchronized cardioversion that are different from unsynchronized cardioversion.

____

____

134. An unresponsive 69-year-old patient has a blood pressure of 76/50 mm Hg. The ECG is shown in Fig. 22-41.

    a. What is your interpretation of the electrocardiogram?

____

    b. Assuming that IV access is not obtainable, and no drugs are readily available, list the steps you would take to initiate transcutaneous pacing on this patient.

____

____

____

____

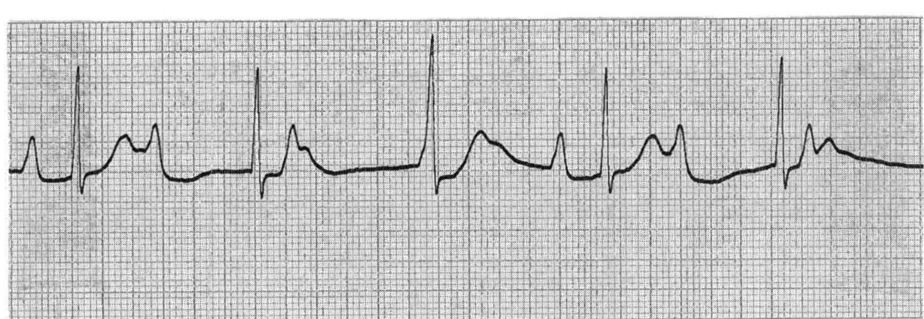

Figure 22-41

135. An older man is found unresponsive, apneic, and pulseless in the busy bathroom of a shopping mall. A quick examination reveals the monitor pattern shown in Fig. 22-42.

    a. What is your interpretation of the rhythm?

____

    b. What drugs (with appropriate doses) should be administered?

____

    c. What causes for this arrest should you consider?

____

323

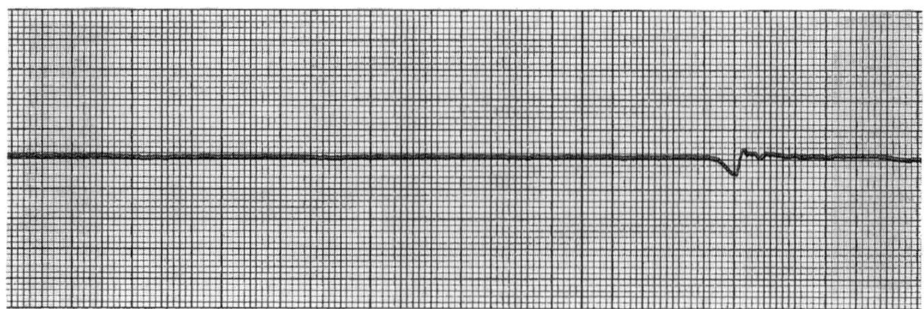

Figure 22-42

136. You are en route to the hospital with a 55-year-old man who you suspect is having an acute myocardial infarction. Suddenly, the patient gasps and becomes pulseless and apneic. As you look at the monitor, you note the electrocardiogram shown in Fig. 22-43.

    a. What is the rhythm?

    b. What single treatment modality is most likely to restore circulation in this patient?

    c. List the appropriate drugs (in the proper order) with correct doses that may be given to this patient if the answer in (b) is unsuccessful.

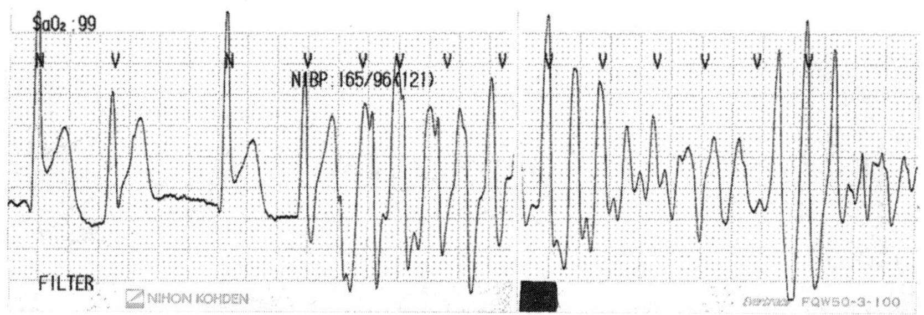

Figure 22-43

137. For each of the following situations, state whether criteria to stop resuscitation have been met. Explain your decision. Assume the patient is now in asystole.

    a. The patient is 94 years old and was found in asystolic arrest, having last been seen 30 minutes previously. You have intubated the patient and gave epinephrine twice.

b. A 65-year-old patient collapses outside a mall. You have been resuscitating for 20 minutes, although you have not been able to intubate. You have administered epinephrine (three doses). It is a snowy day.

____

c. A 16-year-old person is in full arrest after falling from a fourth-floor balcony. You initially got back a sinus rhythm with a pulse, but now asystole is on the monitor. The patient was intubated en route, and you have two large-bore intravenous lines infusing wide open and have given three doses of epinephrine.

____

____

d. A 70-year-old person is in asystole. You have intubated and given epinephrine (three doses) with no success. You elect to terminate resuscitation, but the family is objecting strongly.

____

____

STUDENT SELF-ASSESSMENT

138. Your patient is experiencing chest pain. He is 75 years of age; says his last cholesterol test result was 300 mg/dL; and takes Glucophage (metformin), Accupril, and indapamide. How many risk factors for cardiovascular disease did you identify in this patient?
  a. Two   **c.** Four
  b. Three   **d.** Five

139. Blood pressure is equal to which of the following?
  a. Heart rate × Stroke volume × Cardiac output
  b. Stroke volume × Peripheral vascular resistance
  c. Heart rate × Stroke volume × Peripheral vascular resistance
  d. Heart rate × Contractility × Stroke volume

140. Your patient is experiencing signs of a large infarct affecting the anterior portion of the left ventricle. Which coronary vessel most likely is involved?
  a. Circumflex artery   **c.** Left anterior descending
  b. Coronary sinus   **d.** Right coronary artery

141. Which valve separates the left atrium from the left ventricle?
  a. Aortic   **c.** Pulmonic
  b. Mitral   **d.** Tricuspid

142. The magnetic force that occurs when particles with opposite charges are separated across the cell membrane is known as which of the following?
  a. Action potential   **c.** Millivolts
  b. Depolarization   **d.** Potential energy

143. Which ions are critical to maintain the normal resting membrane potential?
  a. Chloride   **c.** Sodium
  b. Phosphate   **d.** Sulfate

144. Which drugs may affect the threshold level of cardiac conduction cells?
  a. Atropine **c.** Nitroglycerin
  b. Morphine   **d.** Verapamil

325

145. Which phase of the cardiac action potential represents depolarization?

    a. Phase 1   **c.** Phase 3

    b. Phase 2   **d.** Phase 4

146. What is the purpose of the absolute refractory period in the heart?

    a. To allow electrolyte balance to be restored

    b. To initiate the next action potential

    c. To permit the muscle to relax so the heart can fill

    d. To stretch the cardiac fibers for more forceful contraction

147. Which are the smallest divisions of the His bundles?

    a. Anterior-superior fascicles

    b. Posterior-inferior fascicles

    c. Right and left bundle branches

    d. Purkinje fibers

148. Why do pacemaker cells fire repeatedly without external stimulation?

    a. Cerebral biorhythms cause intrinsic stimulation.

    b. Epinephrine initiates the action potential in regular cycles.

    c. Sympathetic nervous system causes hormonal stimulation.

    d. They have an unstable resting membrane potential.

149. Why is there a conduction delay in the atrioventricular node of the normal cardiac cycle?

    a. So ectopic rhythms do not have a chance to enter the cycle

    b. So simultaneous contraction of the atria can occur

    c. To allow for contraction of the atria before ventricular contraction

    d. To permit refilling of the coronary arteries before atrial systole

150. Which of the following may cause a decrease in sinoatrial node discharge, resulting in a decreased heart rate?

    a. Acetylcholine   **c.** Norepinephrine

    b. Epinephrine   **d.** Parasympatholytic effects

151. Mechanisms that produce dysrhythmias following reentry include which of the following?

    a. Atropine administration   **c.** Hypercapnia

    b. Digitalis toxicity   **d.** Hyperkalemia

152. Which of the following signs or symptoms would be atypical for a coronary event?

    a. Abdominal discomfort   **c.** Jaw pain

    b. Dyspnea   **d.** Syncope

153. Dyspnea associated with myocardial infarction usually is related to which of the following?

    a. Chronic obstructive pulmonary disease

    b. Drug administration

    c. Hypercarbia

    d. Pulmonary congestion

154. Syncope should be assumed to be caused by a dysrhythmia if which of the following is associated with it?

    a. Nausea preceded the event.

    b. The patient is older.

    c. The patient has a history of diabetes.

    d. It occurred when the patient was standing.

155. When evaluating a patient for jugular venous distension, the paramedic should do which of the following?

    a. Raise the head of the bed 90 degrees.

    b. Raise the head of the bed 45 degrees.

    c. Put the patient in the supine position.

    d. Have the patient stand with assistance.

326

156. Why may it be helpful to find the point of maximum impulse on the patient's chest?
   a. For appropriate defibrillation or pacing patch placement
   b. For assessment of strength of myocardial contractions
   c. To identify a point to auscultate the mitral valve
   d. To place electrodes for monitoring a 12-lead electrocardiogram

157. What does the electrocardiogram tracing assess?
   a. Cardiac output
   b. Electrical conduction
   c. Myocardial contractility
   d. Stroke volume

158. Which of the following represents a bipolar lead?
   a. aV_F
   b. aV_R
   c. Lead II
   d. V_1

159. In lead II, the positive electrode is located on the left lower extremity. During normal conduction, which way should the QRS complex deflect?
   a. Biphasic
   b. Downward
   c. Isoelectric
   d. Upward

160. You are looking at leads II, III, and aV_F. What part of the heart can you "view" in those leads?
   a. Anterior
   b. Inferior
   c. Lateral
   d. Septum

161. Modified chest leads mimic the view that can be obtained by looking at which of the following?
   a. Augmented leads
   b. Limb leads
   c. Posterior leads
   d. V leads

162. Where should the positive electrode be placed for MCL_1?
   a. Below the lateral end of the left clavicle
   b. Below the lateral end of the right clavicle
   c. Fourth intercostal space to the right of the sternum
   d. Left axillary line at the level of the fifth intercostal space

163. Why are leads II and MCL_1 preferred for routine monitoring for dysrhythmias?
   a. P waves can be visualized easily.
   b. The tallest QRS complex can be seen.
   c. Rates are calculated more easily.
   d. ST segment elevation or depression can be viewed.

164. Which precordial leads are septal leads?
   a. aV_L
   b. V_1 and V_2
   c. V_3 and V_4
   d. V_5 and V_6

165. What represents the absence of electrical activity in the heart on the electrocardiogram strip?
   a. Isoelectric line
   b. P wave
   c. QRS complex
   d. ST segment

166. What is the normal duration of the QRS complex?
   a. 0.04 to 0.08 second
   b. 0.08 to 0.10 second
   c. 0.12 to 0.14 second
   d. 0.14 to 0.16 second

167. During what point does the absolute refractory period occur in the heart?
   a. P wave
   b. P-R interval
   c. Q-T interval
   d. T wave

168. To assess abnormal QRS width accurately, the paramedic should do which of the following?
   a. Determine the J point and measure back from it.
   b. Identify the lead with the widest QRS complex and then measure it.
   c. Measure from the end of the P wave to the end of the S wave.
   d. Measure from R-R wave from left to right.

169. There are 10 small boxes between the R waves on the electrocardiogram tracing. What is the heart rate?
   a. 6 beats/min   **c.** 60 beats/min
   b. 30 beats/min   **d.** 150 beats/min

170. Identify the electrocardiogram tracing in Fig. 22-44.
   a. Normal sinus rhythm
   b. Sinus rhythm with first-degree atrioventricular block
   c. Second-degree heart block type II
   d. Ventricular demand pacer with capture

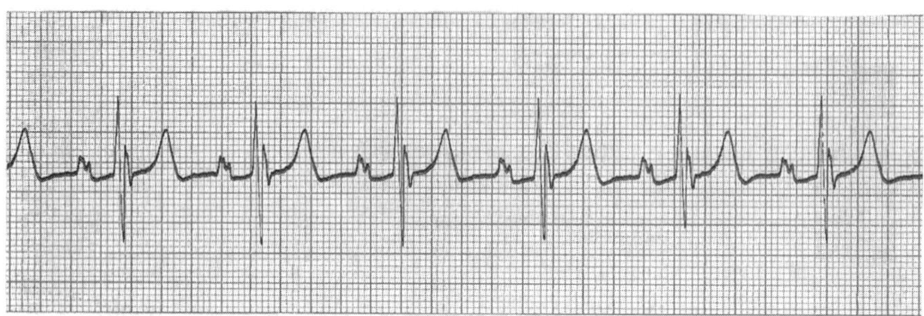

Figure 22-44

171. Identify the electrocardiogram tracing in Fig. 22-45.
   a. Accelerated idioventricular rhythm
   b. Junctional tachycardia
   c. Ventricular pacemaker
   d. Ventricular tachycardia

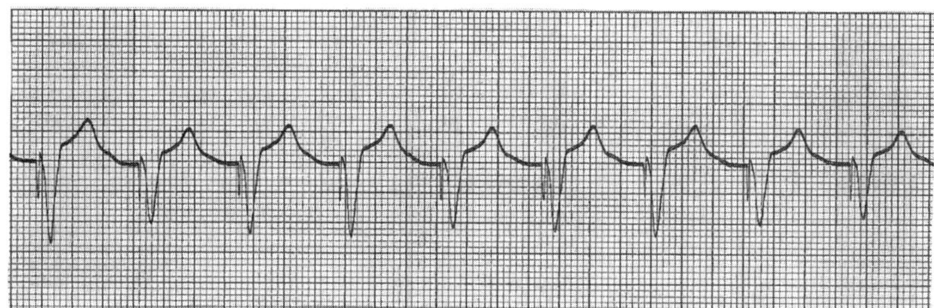

Figure 22-45

172. Identify the electrocardiogram tracing in Fig. 22-46.
   a. Multifocal premature ventricular contractions
   b. Couplet of premature ventricular contractions
   c. Ventricular bigeminy
   d. Ventricular escape rhythm

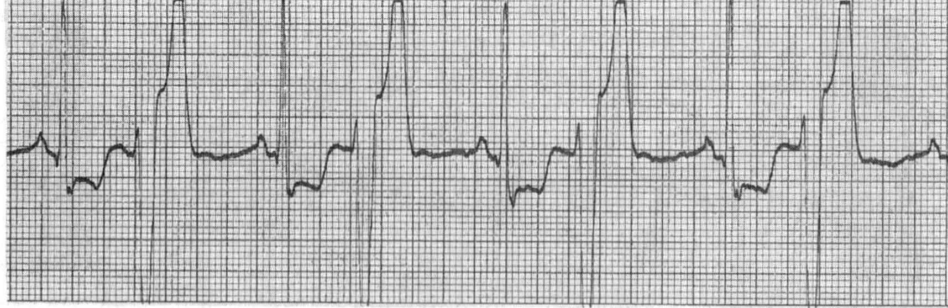

Figure 22-46

173. Identify the electrocardiogram tracing in Fig. 22-47.
  a. Second-degree atrioventricular block type I
  b. Second-degree atrioventricular block type II
  c. Sinus arrest
  d. Sinus arrhythmia

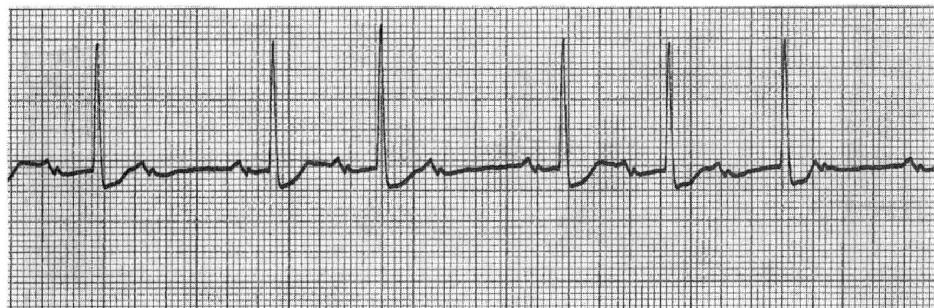

Figure 22-47

174. Identify the electrocardiogram tracing in Fig. 22-48.
  a. Atrial fibrillation
  b. Atrial flutter
  c. Junctional tachycardia
  d. Third-degree atrioventricular block

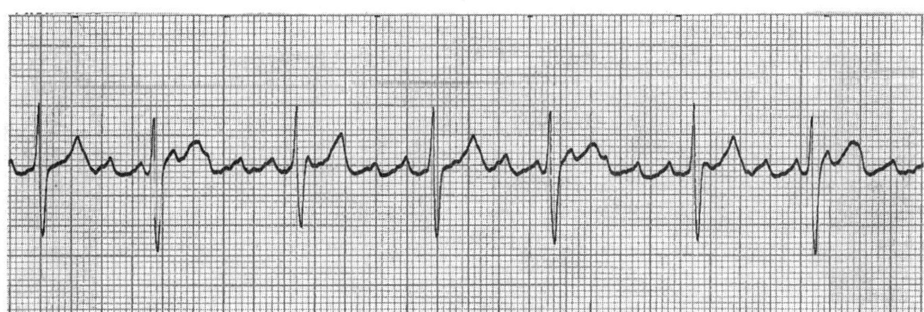

Figure 22-48

175. Identify the electrocardiogram tracing in Fig. 22-49.
  a. Atrial fibrillation **c.** Atrial tachycardia
  b. Atrial flutter   **d.** Sinus tachycardia

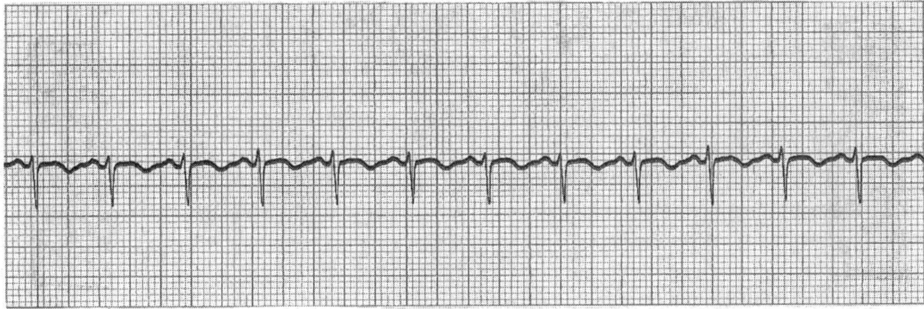

Figure 22-49

176. Identify the electrocardiogram tracing in Fig. 22-50.
  a. Accelerated junctional rhythm followed by pacemaker
  b. Junctional rhythm followed by pacemaker
  c. Junctional rhythm followed by idioventricular
  d. Second-degree atrioventricular block type II followed by idioventricular

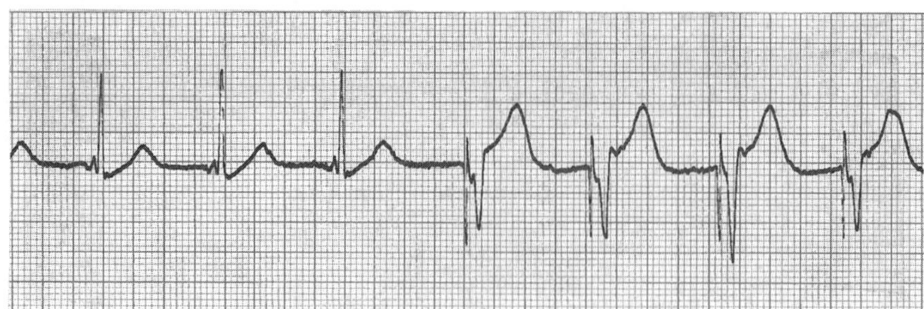

Figure 22-50

177. You are treating a 60-year-old woman with atrial fibrillation at a rate of 168 beats/min. Her blood pressure is 80 mm Hg by palpation, and she feels faint. Which of the following interventions is appropriate?
   a. Adenosine 6 mg via rapid intravenous administration
   b. Verapamil 2.5 mg intravenously over 2 minutes
   c. Procainamide 30 mg/min intravenously
   d. Synchronized biphasic cardioversion at 120 J

178. Which of the following is an ectopic rhythm?
   a. Atrial tachycardia
   b. Junctional tachycardia
   c. Normal sinus rhythm
   d. Sinus bradycardia

179. Which of the following is a cause of sinus bradycardia?
   a. Digoxin
   b. Albuterol
   c. Atropine
   d. Cocaine

180. What is the most common cause of decreased cardiac output in atrial fibrillation or atrial flutter?
   a. Decreased ventricular contractility
   b. Development of blood clots
   c. Inadequate atrial filling
   d. Loss of atrial kick

181. What can atrial fibrillation cause?
   a. Congestive heart failure
   b. Pericarditis
   c. Rheumatic heart disease
   d. Vagal stimulation

182. If your patient has accelerated junctional rhythm, what medical history should you inquire about that is associated specifically with this rhythm?
   a. Chronic obstructive pulmonary disease
   b. Diabetes
   c. Marijuana use
   d. Treatment with digoxin

183. Which of the following mechanisms may cause ventricular dysrhythmias?
   a. Enhanced automaticity
   b. Reentry phenomena
   c. Enhanced automaticity and reentry phenomena
   d. Neither enhanced automaticity nor reentry phenomena

184. Premature ventricular contractions that occur every second complex are known as which of the following?
   a. Bigeminy
   b. Couplets
   c. Idioventricular
   d. Multifocal

185. Your patient has a wide-complex tachycardia. Which of the following electrocardiogram findings would indicate ventricular tachycardia?
    a. All precordial leads (V leads) have a positive deflection.
    b. Negative QRS deflection with a single peak in MCL_1 and MCL_6.
    c. Positive QRS complex in leads I, II, and III.
    d. RS interval is less than 0.10 second in any V lead.

186. What type of pacemaker fires only when the patient's own heart rate drops below a predetermined rate?
    a. Asynchronous
    b. Demand
    c. Dual chamber
    d. Fixed rate

187. What rhythm occurs when a complete block develops at or below the atrioventricular node?
    a. Bundle branch block
    b. Fascicular block
    c. Second-degree atrioventricular block type II
    d. Third-degree atrioventricular block

188. Which of the following is true regarding left bundle branch block?
    a. It produces an initial R wave in V_1 instead of the normal small Q wave.
    b. There is a shallow, narrow QS pattern, and the QRS complex is less than 0.12 second.
    c. There is an RSR prime pattern seen in V_1 with a QRS complex greater than 0.12 second.
    d. The fibers that usually fire the interventricular septum are blocked.

189. Which of the following has the greatest potential to deteriorate into complete heart block?
    a. Anterior hemiblock
    b. Bifascicular block
    c. Posterior hemiblock
    d. Right bundle branch block

190. Your patient has a history of Wolff-Parkinson-White syndrome. You note a rapid wide-complex atrial fibrillation. Which drug is appropriate for this patient?
    a. Adenosine
    b. Amiodarone
    c. Diltiazem
    d. Magnesium

191. What distinguishes unstable angina from stable angina?
    a. It is caused by atherosclerotic disease of the coronary arteries.
    b. The pain lasts 1 to 5 minutes and is relieved by oxygen or nitroglycerin.
    c. The pain changes in its onset, frequency, duration, or quality.
    d. It is precipitated by physical exertion or emotional stress.

192. Death from myocardial infarction is most commonly the result of which of the following?
    a. Dysrhythmias
    b. Low blood pressure
    c. Pulmonary embolism
    d. Cardiac rupture

193. What should you administer to a stable patient with acute ST segment elevation myocardial infarction of the right ventricle?
    a. Aspirin 324 mg chew and swallow
    b. Lactated Ringer solution at 500 mL/hr intravenously
    c. Oxygen 15 L/min by non-rebreather mask
    d. Nitroglycerin 0.4 mg sublingual

194. For which of the following ECG findings would you notify the hospital to alert the cardiac catheterization team and cardiologist?
    a. Pathological Q waves
    b. Peaked tented T waves
    c. Right axis deviation
    d. ST segment elevation

195. What is the primary reason nitroglycerin is administered to patients with pulmonary edema?
    a. It reduces preload and afterload.
    b. It increases the Starling reflex.
    c. It improves coronary blood flow.
    d. It relieves chest pain.

196. When a patient has right ventricular heart failure, where does blood back up?
   a. Aorta
   b. Pulmonary arteries
   c. Pulmonary veins
   d. Venae cavae

197. What is the primary cause of poor perfusion in cardiogenic shock?
   a. Decreased blood volume
   b. Decreased venous capacitance
   c. Decreased capillary permeability
   d. Decreased stroke volume

198. Your patient has a history of cancer and is having chest pain and tachycardia. What early sign may indicate the development of cardiac tamponade?
   a. Decreased systolic pressure
   b. Jugular venous distension
   c. Pericardial friction rub
   d. Tracheal deviation

199. Which is the most common presentation of dissection of the thoracic aorta?
   a. Chest heaviness of slow onset
   b. Intense back pain with sudden onset
   c. Neck pain that began suddenly
   d. Substernal dull pain that increased gradually

200. Acute arterial occlusion may result in which of the following?
   a. Absent distal pulses
   b. Hypertension
   c. Pulmonary congestion
   d. Torsades de pointes

201. You suspect that your patient has an arterial occlusion affecting the lower leg. Which of the following treatment measures would be appropriate?
   a. Initiate intravenous fluid therapy and administer a fluid challenge.
   b. Massage the affected extremity to encourage circulation.
   c. Immobilize the affected extremity and protect it from injury.
   d. Administer 40 mg of furosemide intravenously to flush out the embolus.

202. What accounts for risk of left ventricular failure associated with chronic, uncontrolled hypertension?
   a. Accelerated atherosclerosis
   b. Increased afterload
   c. Increased blood volume
   d. Polycythemia vera

203. According to the American Heart Association, what ratio of compressions and ventilations should be performed in the patient in cardiac arrest?
   a. 2:15
   b. 15:2
   c. 2:30
   d. 30:2

204. You work at a service that uses biphasic defibrillation. Which of the following is true regarding this device?
   a. Higher defibrillation doses are needed.
   b. It compensates for chest impedance.
   c. The batteries are larger.
   d. The energy flows in one direction.

205. What principle should be followed when placing patches on the chest for defibrillation?
   a. Anterior-posterior placement may be used for patches.
   b. Never reverse the polarity, or defibrillation will not occur.
   c. Place one patch over the sternum directly over the heart.
   d. Use pediatric patches for children up to 8 years of age.

206. What should you consider when caring for a patient who has an implantable cardioverter defibrillator?
   a. Apply a magnet to the chest to activate these devices if the patient is unresponsive.
   b. If the first defibrillation attempt is unsuccessful, paddle placement should be changed.
   c. Three shocks should be delivered before CPR.
   d. Touching the patient during implantable cardioverter defibrillator defibrillation is dangerous.

332

207. Which statement is true regarding synchronized cardioversion?
- **a.** It is faster than unsynchronized cardioversion.
- **b.** It is not as safe as unsynchronized cardioversion.
- **c.** It is indicated for pulseless ventricular tachycardia.
- **d.** It is indicated for unstable paroxysmal supraventricular tachycardia.

208. When attempting to initiate transcutaneous pacing on a conscious patient, set the current at which of the following?
- **a.** 70 to 80 per minute and increased until the patient is stable
- **b.** 50 mA and increase until capture occurs
- **c.** 70 to 80 per minute and decrease until the patient becomes unstable
- **d.** Maximum mA and decrease until capture is lost

209. Which of the following drugs blocks parasympathetic stimulation?
- **a.** Amiodarone
- **b.** Atropine
- **c.** Lidocaine
- **d.** Magnesium

210. Your patient has ST segment elevation in leads II and aVL. His BP drops to 70 mm Hg after a dose of nitroglycerin. What should you do first?
- **a.** Administer dopamine 2 to 20 mcg/kg /min.
- **b.** Infuse a normal saline fluid bolus.
- **c.** Place him in the Trendelenburg position.
- **d.** Perform a right-sided 12-lead ECG.

211. Which of the following is an action of morphine sulfate?
- **a.** Dilation of peripheral vasculature
- **b.** Increase in cardiac preload
- **c.** Causes amnesia
- **d.** Bronchodilation

212. Which of the following is true of digoxin?
- **a.** It increases the force of ventricular contraction.
- **b.** It is used to treat bradycardia.
- **c.** It causes decreased cardiac output.
- **d.** It increases impulse conduction through the atrioventricular node.

213. Which drug enhances action of the beta receptors?
- **a.** Amyl nitrite
- **b.** Atropine
- **c.** Epinephrine
- **d.** Labetolol

214. A 60-year-old, 100-kg woman has a blood pressure of 80/50 mm Hg. The electrocardiogram is shown in Fig. 22-51. Which of the following is appropriate to correct this?
- **a.** Atropine 0.5 mg intravenously
- **b.** Dopamine 2 to 20 mg/kg/min
- **c.** Epinephrine 2 to 10 mcg/kg/min
- **d.** Synchronized cardioversion

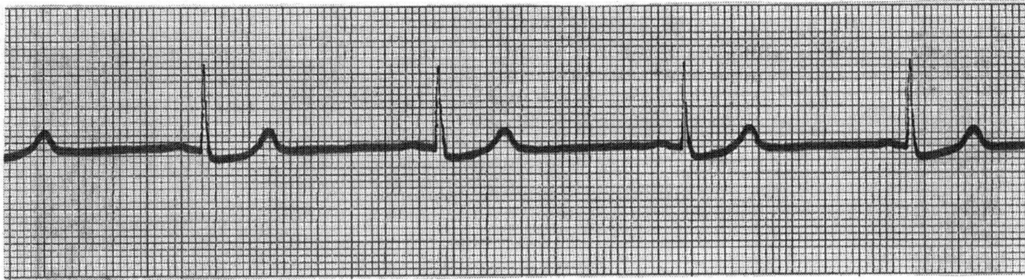

Figure 22-51

215. Which criteria should be considered to determine whether to terminate resuscitation of a patient?
   a. Livor or rigor mortis
   b. Older adult patient
   c. Quality of life judgments
   d. Time of collapse before EMS arrival

216. Which type of rhythm is atrial fibrillation?
   a. Atrial ventricular nodal reentry tachycardia
   b. Atrial ventricular reentry tachycardia
   c. Electrical mechanical dissociation
   d. Escape rhythm

217. By which mechanism are impedance threshold devices (ITD) thought to be helpful?
   a. Enhance blood flow to the brain
   b. Increase sinus node firing
   c. Suppress ventricular dysrhythmias
   d. Improve oxygen diffusion in lungs

218. What is the chief advantage of mechanical CPR devices?
   a. Compress the chest harder than human rescuers
   b. Depress the heart in more precise location
   c. Minimize interruptions in chest compressions
   d. Time compressions to correspond to cardiac cycle

219. What alteration in patient assessment must be considered for a patient with a left ventricular assist device?
   a. Patient assessment should not vary from those without the device.
   b. Pulses may or may not be palpated depending on underlying cardiac output.
   c. Capillary refill should be expected to be prolonged if the device is working properly.
   d. The patient will not lose consciousness if ventricular fibrillation develops.

WRAP IT UP

"4027 respond to a cardiac arrest, 1425 Humes, 4027 …": the dispatcher's familiar voice jolts you awake from a nap. As you respond, you are updated that CPR instructions are in progress. You hear the local fire department announce their arrival at the scene when you are about 10 blocks away, and as you walk into the house, you can hear a mechanical voice say, "Deliver shock now." As the firefighter presses the button on the AED, the patient's lifeless body jolts, and a firefighter immediately resumes chest compressions. Two minutes later, after connecting the patient to your monitor-defibrillator, you note the presence of an organized rhythm. "Resume chest compressions," you say as you rethink your strategy. In 2 minutes, you quickly check breathing and pulse and are surprised to feel weak, slow pulsations under your fingers at the carotid artery. "Begin ventilations," you instruct the firefighter at the patient's head, and she begins to ventilate the patient with a bag. You note a bradycardic rhythm that appears to be increasing at a fairly rapid rate. "He's breathing!" the firefighter ventilating the patient exclaims. The patient begins to cough and push away the bag from his face. Vital signs are BP 100/70 mm Hg, P 88, R 18, SaO_2 95%. You calm the patient, apply oxygen, and start an IV. The patient's wife says her 55-year-old husband was complaining of indigestion for about an hour before he collapsed. He is normally healthy and takes no medications, so he would not let her take him to the emergency department (ED). After the patient is secured in the ambulance, you perform a 12-lead electrocardiogram. You note 4-mm ST segment elevation in leads V_1 to V_4. The patient is awake but slightly confused and rubbing his chest. You give him aspirin and nitroglycerin after obtaining another BP at 116/84 mm Hg. His ED stay is brief; the cardiologist whisks him to the cardiac catheter laboratory, where balloon angiography is performed. As you enter your times in the computer, you note that the initial fire department unit arrived 4 minutes after the 911 call was placed. They delivered the shock 90 seconds later. You meet the patient 1 month later at the grocery store with his four children; he is ready to return to work and is emotional as he gives you his thanks.

1. Place a check mark beside the elements of the chain of survival that were present on this call.
   a. _____ Early recognition of the emergency
   b. _____ Activation of 911
   c. _____ Early cardiopulmonary resuscitation
   d. _____ Early defibrillation
   e. _____ Early advanced care
   f. _____ Rapid interventional cardiology

334

2. What rhythm(s) was the patient in when the fire department arrived?

____

3. What antidysrhythmic drug(s) could you have administered if he remained in this rhythm?

____

4. What walls of the heart are damaged, based on the12-lead electrocardiogram findings?

____

5. What coronary blood vessels are likely occluded?

____

6. What complication, aside from dysrhythmia would you expect if he had not had angioplasty to open the occluded coronary blood vessels?

____

7. Which element of this patient's situation would be a relative contraindication to fibrinolytic therapy?
   a. Cardiopulmonary resuscitation less than 10 minutes
   b. Suspected aortic dissection
   c. Terminal illness
   d. Uncontrolled hypertension

8. At what rate and volume should the firefighter ventilate after the patient's pulse returns?
   Rate _______ Vol _______

CHAPTER 22 ANSWERS

REVIEW QUESTIONS

1. c
   (Objective 2)

2. f
   (Objective 2)

3. a
   (Objective 2)

4. e
   (Objective 2)

5. b
   (Objective 2)

6. g
   (Objective 2)

7. h
   (Objective 2)

8.

Risk Factor	Prevention Strategy	Resource
a. Smoking	Quit smoking with use of medications, hypnosis, behavior modification, health clinic	Private physician, American Heart Association, cancer association, alternative nicotine products
b. Hypercholesterolemia	Diet modification, drugs	Private physician, health clinic, heart association
c. Obesity	Diet, exercise	Private physician exercise, community health clinic, dietitian, American Heart Association
d. Sedentary lifestyle	Exercise program, leisure activities	Private physician, local hospital

(Objective 1)

9.

	Sympathetic	Parasympathetic
a. Heart rate	Increase	Decrease
b. Myocardial	Increase	No effect contractility
c. Lungs	Beta-bronchiolar dilation	Constriction
d. Blood vessels (peripheral)	Constriction	No effect

(Objective 2)

10. a. Epinephrine: increased heart rate, contractility, bronchiolar dilation, and blood vessel constriction in skin, kidneys, gastrointestinal tract, and viscera
b. Norepinephrine: peripheral vasoconstriction
(Objective 2)

11. a. Magnetic
b. Potential
c. Permeable
d. Potential
e. Millivolts
f. Negative
g. Negatively
h. Potential
i. Negative
j. −70 to −90
k. Potassium
l. Potassium
m. Proteins
n. Permeable
o. Excitability
p. Depolarization
q. Threshold potential
r. Action potential
s. Depolarization
t. Repolarization
u. Positive
v. Negative
w. Depolarization
x. Membrane potential
(Objective 3)

12. a. Sodium rushes into the cell through the fast sodium channels.

    b. The membrane potential drops to approximately 0.

    c. The slow calcium channels allow calcium to enter the cell while potassium continues to leave, maintaining the membrane potential of 0.

    d. The membrane potential returns to $-90\,mV$.

    e. The sodium pump allows the exchange of sodium and potassium to their proper compartments.

    f. During phase 4, cardiac pacemaker cells slowly depolarize from their most negative membrane potential to a level at which threshold is reached and phase 0 begins. Nonpacemaker cells maintain a stable resting membrane potential and do not depolarize unless stimulated by a sufficiently strong stimulus.

(Objective 3)

13. a. Action potentials; b. upward; c. automaticity; d. resting membrane potential

(Objective 3)

14. a. Sinoatrial node; b. intranodal pathways; c. atrioventricular node; d. common bundle of His; e. left posterior bundle branch; f. Purkinje fibers; g. left anterior bundle branch; h. right bundle branch

(Objective 2)

15. The next pacemaker (atrioventricular node) should take over and fire.

(Objective 4)

16. a. Acceleration of phase 4 depolarization so cells reach their threshold prematurely (may result from digoxin toxicity, increased catecholamine levels, hypoxia, hypercapnia, myocardial ischemia, infarction, increased venous return, hypokalemia, hypocalcemia, heating or cooling of the heart, or atropine administration)

    b. Reactivation of tissue by a returning impulse

(Objective 4)

17. O— Onset. What were you doing when the pain began?

    P— Is there anything that makes the pain better or worse?

    Q— What does the pain feel like? (Is it sharp, dull, crushing, or squeezing?)

    R— Where is the pain? Does it go anywhere else?

    S— On a scale of 1 to 10, with 1 being no pain and 10 being the worst pain you have ever had, describe your pain.

    T— When did you first feel the pain?

(Objective 11)

18. Chest pain, dyspnea, syncope, and palpitations

(Objective 11)

19. How did you feel before you passed out? What were you doing when you passed out? What position were you in before you passed out (i.e., lying down, sitting, or standing)? How long were you unconscious? Do you have a history of heart disease or other significant medical history? What medicines do you take? Do you feel unusual in any other way? How has your health been over the past several days?

(Objective 11)

20. Pulse rate and regularity, electrocardiogram, vital signs, circumstances of occurrence, duration, associated symptoms, previous history of palpitations, medical history, and daily medicines

(Objective 11)

21. Major medical illnesses, home medicines, and similar previous episodes

(Objective 11)

22. Atrial fibrillation with a slow ventricular response

(Objective 10)

23. Yes. Digoxin (Lanoxin) or calcium channel blocker (Cardizem) toxicity can cause this presentation. Digitalis toxicity is more likely in a patient who also is taking a diuretic (furosemide).

(Objective 11)

24. Neck: jugular venous distension. Chest: implanted pacemaker generator, median sternotomy scar, lung sounds (crackles), heart sounds (S_3 gallop), and pulse deficit. Abdomen: generator for automatic implantable cardioverter defibrillator visible. Extremities: edema and ulceration. Back: sacral edema. Medical alert tags or medical information in wallet.
(Objective 11)

25.

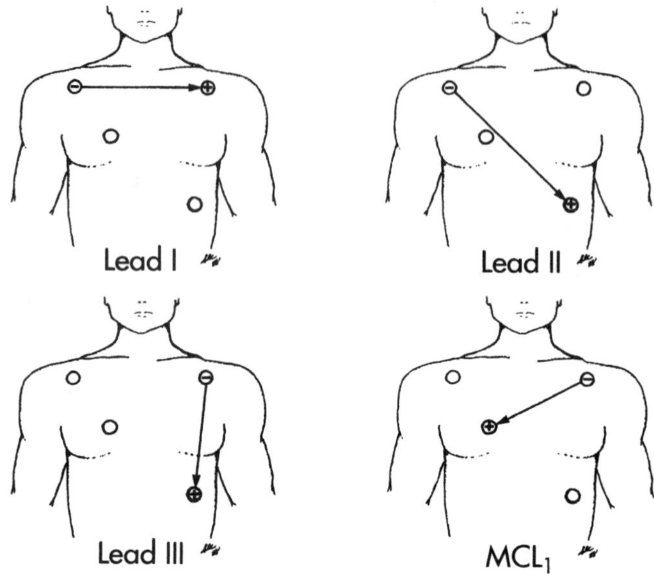

(Objective 5)

26. a. Right arm (right anterior forearm)
b. Left arm (left anterior forearm)
c. Right leg (right lower leg)
d. Left lower leg (left leg)
e. V_1, fourth intercostal space to the right of the sternum
f. V_2, fourth intercostal space to the left of the sternum
g. V_4, fifth intercostal space, midclavicular line
h. V_3, between V_2 and V_4
i. V_5, anterior axillary line in a straight line with V_4
j. V_6, midaxillary line, level with V_4 and V_5 (In women, V_4 to V_6 should be placed under the left breast.)
(Objective 5)

27. a. Excessive body hair: Shave.
b. Diaphoresis: Dry the area and apply tincture of benzoin.
c. Poor electrode placement: Reapply correctly.
d. 60-cycle interference: Run monitor on batteries.
e. Poor cable connections: Recheck all connections.
f. Close proximity to electrical motors
(Objective 5)

28. a. 5; b. 0.04; c. 0.20; d. d3; e. 6
(Objective 5)

29. a. P wave; b. QRS complex; c. T wave; d. P-R interval; e. ST segment
(Objective 8)

30. Muscle tremor, AC (60-cycle interference), loose electrodes, patient movement, loss of electrode contact, and external chest compression
(Objective 6)

31. Analyze the QRS complex; analyze the P waves; analyze the rate; analyze the rhythm; analyze the P-R interval.
(Objective 7)

32. a. Triplicate method (120 beats/min): Find the R wave on the dark line, count 300-150-100-75 for each next dark
   line until the next R wave. The R wave falls between 100 and 150. Estimate rate to be 120 beats/min.
   b. R-R method: 300 ÷ Number of large boxes between R waves = 300 ÷ (almost) 3 = 100 beats/min
   c. R-R method: 1500 ÷ Number of small boxes between R waves = 1500 ÷ 13 = 115 beats/min
   d. 6-second method: Number of R waves in a 6-second strip × 10 = 12 × 10 = 120 beats/min
   (Objective 7)

33. No, this reveals only the rate, not the perfusion status (and the rate is faster than normal for an adult).
   (Objective 7)

34. a. R-R method (1500 ÷ Number of small boxes between the R waves) or triplicate method (but only if R waves
   both fall on dark lines)
   b. The 6-second method is the most accurate and quick estimate for irregular rhythm.
   (Objective 7)

35. The R-R distance should be equal when measured left to right across an electrocardiogram strip (it can vary no
   greater than 0.16 second).
   (Objective 7)

36. a. Conduction through the ventricles is normal.
   b. Conduction through the ventricles is delayed and may follow an abnormal pathway.
   (Objective 6)

37. Are they regular? Is there a P wave in front of each QRS complex? Are they upright or inverted? Do they all look
   the same?
   (Objective 7)

38. a. Electrical impulse that progressed from the atria to the ventricles through pathways other than the
   atrioventricular node of the bundle of His
   b. Normal conduction from the sinoatrial node through the atrioventricular node
   c. Delay in conduction of impulse through the atrioventricular node or bundle of His
   (Objective 6)

39. a. QRS complex: 0.08 sec (normal is less than 0.12 sec)
   b. P waves: regular, one for each QRS complex, upright, all the same
   c. Rate: 75 beats/min (triplicate method)
   d. Rhythm: regular (R-R intervals equal)
   e. P-R interval: 0.14 sec. Interpretation: normal sinus rhythm
   (Objectives 7 and 8)

40. Patient history, chief complaint, and physical findings
   (Objective 10)

41. a. Parasympathetic stimulation
   b. QRS complex less than 0.12 sec (unless a conduction delay is present)
   c. P waves (regular, preceding each QRS complex, upright, similar)
   d. P-R interval: 0.12 to 0.20 sec
   (Objective 9, 10)

42. a. Sinus node disease, increased parasympathetic vagal tone, hypothermia, hypoxia, and drug effects (digitalis,
   propranolol, verapamil)
   b. Exercise, fever, anxiety, ingestion of stimulants, smoking, hypovolemia, anemia, congestive heart failure,
   and excessive administration of atropine or vagolytic or sympathomimetic drugs (cocaine, phencyclidine,
   epinephrine, isoproterenol)
   (Objective 10)

43. QRS complex: 0.08 second. P waves: present, upright, similar. Rate: 50 beats/min. Rhythm: regular. P-R interval: 0.16 second. Interpretation: sinus bradycardia. Distinguishing features: all features of normal sinus rhythm except that rate is less than 60 beats/min. Treatment: stable—observe; unstable—atropine 0.5 to 1.0 mg every 3 to 5 minutes to a maximum dose of less than 2.5 mg (0.03 to 0.04 mg/kg), transcutaneous pacing, dopamine 5 to 20 mcg/kg/min, epinephrine 2 to 10 mcg/min, isoproterenol 2 to 10 mcg/min
(Objective 10)

44. QRS complex: 0.06 second. P waves: present, upright, similar. Rate: 110 beats/min. Rhythm: regular. P-R interval: 0.16 second. Interpretation: sinus tachycardia. Distinguishing features: all features of normal sinus rhythm except that rate is greater than 100 beats/min. Treatment: stable—none; unstable—seek and treat underlying cause
(Objective 9, 10)

45. QRS complex: 0.08 second; P waves: present, upright, similar. Rate: 70 beats/min. Rhythm: irregular. P-R interval: 0.12 second. Interpretation: sinus dysrhythmia. Distinguishing features: all features of normal sinus rhythm but irregular rhythm that varies in cycles. Treatment: none
(Objective 10)

46. QRS complex: 0.08 second. P waves: normal, upright. Rate: 50 beats/min. Rhythm: irregular. P-R interval: 0.16 second. Interpretation: sinus arrest. Distinguishing features: normal sinus rhythm until the sinoatrial node fails to fire. Treatment: stable—observe; unstable—atropine and transcutaneous pacing
(Objective 10)

47. a. Tissues; b. atria; c. internodal
(Objective 10)

48. a. QRS complex: normal
b. P waves (if present): different from normal sinus P waves
c. P-R interval: abnormal, shortened, or prolonged
(Objective 10)

49. Stress, overexertion, tobacco, caffeine, Wolff-Parkinson-White syndrome, digoxin toxicity, hypoxia, chronic obstructive pulmonary disease, congestive heart failure, damage to sinoatrial node, rheumatic heart disease, and atherosclerotic heart disease
(Objectives 9, 10)

50. QRS complex: 0.06 second. P waves: changes from beat to beat. Rate: 75 beats/min. Rhythm: regular. P-R interval: variable. Interpretation: wandering atrial pacemaker. Distinguishing features: typically slightly irregular P wave shapes and variable P-R interval. Treatment: stable—monitor; unstable after bradycardia—treat as bradycardia
(Objective 10)

51. QRS complex: 0.06 second. P waves: present, upright. Rate: 100 beats/min. Rhythm: regular interrupted by premature beats. P-R interval: 0.10 second (premature atrial contraction 0.16 second). Interpretation: normal sinus rhythm with one premature atrial contraction. Distinguishing features: extra beat occurring earlier than next expected sinus beat; premature atrial contraction has features of sinus beat except that P-R interval may be different. Treatment: none
(Objective 10)

52. QRS complex: 0.06 second. P waves: unable to determine, may be hidden in T wave. Rate: 180 beats/min. Rhythm: regular. P-R interval: unable to determine. Interpretation: supraventricular tachycardia. Distinguishing features: rate greater than 150 beats/min, with complexes originating in the atria (QRS complex is <0.12 second unless a conduction defect is present.) Treatment: stable—oxygen, intravenous line, 12-lead electrocardiogram, consideration of vagal maneuvers, adenosine (6 mg, 12 mg, 12 mg rapid intravenous push at 1- to 2-minute intervals), diltiazem or verapamil or beta-blockers, consider digoxin (Class IIb); unstable—synchronized cardioversion at 50, 100, 200, 300, and 360 J
(Objective 10)

53. QRS complex: 0.06 second. P waves: f-R waves. Rate: 100 beats/min. Rhythm: regular. P-R interval: none. F-R interval: may vary. Interpretation: atrial flutter with 3:1 conduction. Distinguishing features: flutter waves. Treatment: stable—(usually no treatment prehospital); with tachycardic rate—diltiazem or verapamil or beta-blockers or digoxin to control rate; if impaired cardiac function is present—diltiazem or amiodarone or digoxin; unstable—synchronized cardioversion at 50, 100, 200, 300, and 360 J
(Objective 10)

54. QRS complex: 0.06 second. P waves: none. Rate: 160 beats/min. Rhythm: irregularly irregular. P-R interval: none. Interpretation: atrial fibrillation. Distinguishing features: irregularly irregular, no P waves, fibrillation waves. Treatment: calcium channel or beta-blocker; impaired cardiac function—diltiazem or amiodarone; acute and associated with serious signs or symptoms—synchronized cardioversion at 100, 200, 300, and 360 J
(Objective 10)

55. a. junctional (nodal); b. normal; c. may occur before, during, or after QRS complex or may be absent; inverted in lead II; d. often less than 0.12 second
(Objective 9,10)

56. Increased vagal tone on sinoatrial node, pathologic slowing of sinoatrial discharge, complete atrioventricular block, digitalis toxicity, damage to the atrioventricular junction, inferior wall myocardial infarction, and rheumatic fever
(Objective 9)

57. QRS complex: 0.08 second. P waves: present, upright, similar in underlying rhythm, absent in premature beats. Rate: 60 beats/min. Rhythm: irregular. P-R interval: 0.16 second (underlying rhythm), none in premature beats. Interpretation: sinus rhythm (borderline bradycardia) with two premature junctional contractions. Distinguishing features: premature beats occurring earlier than next expected sinus beat, lack of P waves, QRS complex within normal limits. Treatment: monitor patient and treat bradycardia if present and symptomatic.
(Objective 10)

58. QRS complex: 0.08 second. P waves: absent. Rate: 40 beats/min. Rhythm: regular. P-R interval: none. Interpretation: junctional escape rhythm. Distinguishing features: rate 40 to 60 beats/min, inverted P waves if present (may occur before, during [absent], or after QRS complex). Treatment: stable—monitor; unstable—atropine 0.5 to 1.0 mg every 5 minutes to total dose of 2.5 mg (0.03–0.04 mg/kg), transcutaneous pacing, dopamine 5 to 20 mcg/kg/min, epinephrine 2 to 10 mcg/min, and isoproterenol 2 to 10 mcg/min
(Objective 10)

59. QRS complex: 0.08 second. P waves: absent. Rate: 80 beats/min. Rhythm: regular. P-R interval: none. Interpretation: accelerated junctional rhythm. Distinguishing features: rate 60 to 100 beats/min, inverted P waves in lead II if present (may be absent or occur before, during, or after QRS complex). Treatment: monitor.
(Objective 10)

60. a. 20, 40; b. 100 beats/min; c. 100 beats/min
(Objective 9)

61. Failure of higher pacemakers, heart block, myocardial ischemia, hypoxia, acid–base or electrolyte imbalance, congestive heart failure, increased catecholamine levels, use of stimulants, medicine toxicity (digitalis, tricyclic antidepressant overdose), sympathomimetic drugs, cardiac trauma, and electrical injury
(Objective 9)

62. If unstable, all rhythms need cardioversion. If stable, the following:
a. Assess leads I, II, III, MCL$_1$ (V$_1$), and MCL$_6$ (V$_6$) to determine axis deviation. If the QRS complex is negative in leads I, II, and III (extreme right axis or "no-man's land") and positive in MCL$_1$ (V$_1$), the rhythm is ventricular tachycardia; if not,
b. Assess the QRS deflection in MCL$_1$ (V$_1$) and MCL$_6$ (V$_6$). Positive QRS deflections with a single peak, a taller left rabbit ear, or an RS complex with a fat r wave or slurred s wave in MCL$_1$ (V$_1$) indicates ventricular tachycardia. A negative QS complex, a negative rS complex, or any wide Q wave in MCL$_6$ (V$_6$) also indicates ventricular tachycardia.
c. If right axis deviation is present (negative QRS complex in lead I; positive QRS complex in leads II and III) and the QRS complex is negative in MCL$_1$ (V$_1$), it indicates ventricular tachycardia.

d. If all precordial (V) leads are positive or negative (precordial concordance), it indicates ventricular tachycardia.
e. If the RS interval is greater than 0.10 second in any V lead, it indicates ventricular tachycardia.
(Objective 9,10)

63. QRS complex: 0.16 second. P waves: absent. Rate: 40 beats/min. Rhythm: regular. P-R interval: none. Interpretation: ventricular escape rhythm. Distinguishing features: rate 20 to 40 beats/min, absent P waves, QRS complex greater than 0.12 second. Treatment: oxygen, transcutaneous pacing, dopamine 5 to 20 mcg/kg/min, epinephrine 2 to 10 mcg/min, and isoproterenol 2 to 10 mcg/min
(Objective 10)

64. QRS complex: underlying rhythm 0.10 second. Premature beat: 0.16 second. P wave: present, upright (except premature beat). Rate: 75 beats/min. Rhythm: regular interrupted by premature beats. P-R interval: 0.16 second (underlying rhythm). None: premature beat. Interpretation: normal sinus rhythm with one premature ventricular contraction. Distinguishing features: ectopic beat occurs earlier than next expected sinus beat, wide bizarre QRS complex with T wave deflection opposite QRS complex, no P waves, compensatory pause. Treatment: in the presence of hemodynamically compromising premature ventricular contractions—oxygen, lidocaine 1.0 to 1.5 mg/kg repeated at 0.5- to 0.75-mg/kg doses to a maximum of 3 mg/kg
(Objective 10)

65. QRS complex: 0.20 second. P waves: absent. Rate: 230 beats/min. Rhythm: regular. P-R interval: none. Interpretation: monomorphic ventricular tachycardia. Distinguishing features: rate greater than 100 beats/min (usually >150 beats/min), regular, no P waves, QRS complex equal to or greater than 0.12 second. Treatment: stable—oxygen, procainamide or sotalol or amiodarone or lidocaine; impaired cardiac function—amiodarone or lidocaine; unstable—synchronized cardioversion at 100, 200, 300, and 360 J; or unconsciousness, hypotension, or pulmonary edema—defibrillate at 100, 200, 300, and 360 J or equivalent biphasic energy; pulseless—treat as ventricular fibrillation
(Objective 10)

66. QRS complex: none. P waves: none. Rate: none. Rhythm: none, chaotic. P-R interval: none. Interpretation: ventricular fibrillation. Distinguishing features: no organized rhythm, chaotic fibrillatory waves. Treatment: rapid defibrillation at 200, 300, and 360 J or equivalent biphasic energy, cardiopulmonary resuscitation, intubation, epinephrine or vasopressin, amiodarone or lidocaine, magnesium sulfate, and procainamide; consider sodium bicarbonate
(Objective 10)

67. QRS complex: none. P waves: none. Rate: none. Rhythm: none. P-R interval: none. Interpretation: asystole. Distinguishing features: isoelectric rhythm. Treatment: cardiopulmonary resuscitation, transcutaneous pacing, epinephrine, atropine, and consideration of underlying cause
(Objective 10)

68. QRS complex: 0.16 second. P waves: absent. Rate: 80 beats/min. Rhythm: regular. P-R interval: none. Interpretation: ventricular paced rhythm. Distinguishing features: pacemaker spike followed by wide-complex ventricular beat. Treatment: none
(Objective 10)

69. a. Heart blocks; b. conduction system
(Objective 9)

70. Myocardial ischemia, acute myocardial infarction, increased parasympathetic tone, drug toxicity (digitalis, propranolol, verapamil), and electrolyte imbalance
(Objective 9)

71. QRS complex: 0.06 second. P waves: present, upright. Rate: 60 beats/min. Rhythm: regular. P-R interval: 0.32 second. Interpretation: sinus rhythm with first-degree atrioventricular block. Distinguishing features: P-R interval greater than 0.20 second. Treatment: observe
(Objective 10)

72. QRS complex: 0.08 second. P waves: present, upright, more P waves than QRS complexes. Rate: 60 beats/min. Rhythm: irregular. P-R interval: progressively longer until one is not conducted. Distinguishing features: more P waves than QRS complexes, progressively lengthens P-R interval until a QRS complex is dropped. Interpretation:

second-degree atrioventricular block (Mobitz type I or Wenckebach). Treatment: asymptomatic—observe; if bradycardic with hemodynamic compromise—oxygen, atropine, transcutaneous pacing, dopamine, epinephrine, and isoproterenol
(Objective 10)

73. QRS complex: 0.06 second. P waves: present, upright, more P waves than QRS complexes. Rate: 50 beats/min. Rhythm: irregular. P-R interval: 0.16 second for conducted P waves. Interpretation: second-degree atrioventricular block (Mobitz type II). Treatment: stable—transport for transvenous pacemaker insertion; unstable—oxygen, transcutaneous pacing, dopamine, epinephrine, and isoproterenol
(Objective 10)

74. QRS complex: 0.08 second. P waves: present, upright. Rate: 50 beats/min. Rhythm: regular. P-R interval: no relationship between P waves and QRS complexes. Interpretation: third-degree (complete) atrioventricular block. Distinguishing features: R-R interval usually regular, more P waves than QRS complexes, no relationship between P waves and QRS complex. Treatment: stable—monitor and transport for transvenous pacemaker insertion; unstable—oxygen, transcutaneous pacing, atropine 0.5 to 1.0 mg (maximum dose, 0.04 mg/kg), dopamine 5 to 20 mcg/kg/min, epinephrine 2 to 10 mcg/min, and isoproterenol 2 to 10 mcg/min
(Objective 10)

75. a. QRS complex equal to or greater than 0.12 second. QRS complexes produced by supraventricular activity. RSR prime pattern. In V_1, line drawn backward from the J point into the QRS makes a triangle pointing up.
    b. QRS complex less than 0.12 second. QRS complexes produced by supraventricular activity. QS pattern. In V_1, line drawn backward from J point into the QRS makes a triangle pointing down
    c. QRS complex less than 0.12 second. QRS complexes produced by supraventricular activity and pathological left axis deviation. A small Q wave followed by a tall R wave in lead I, and a small R wave followed by a deep S wave in lead III
    d. Right axis deviation with a normal QRS complex
    (Objective 9)

76. a. Any patient with type II atrioventricular block
    b. Any patient with evidence of disease of both bundle branches
    c. Any patient with two or more blocks of any kind
    (Objective 9)

77. a. Pulseless electrical activity (the patient has a rhythm but no perfusing pulse)
    b. If the patient is unresponsive and not breathing, begin 30 chest compressions followed by two breaths. Establish intravenous or intraosseous access, and give epinephrine 1.0 mg every 3 to 5 minutes or one dose of vasopressin 40 u IV/10 to replace the first or second dose of epinephrine; consider advanced airway; consider causes (hypovolemia, pulmonary embolus, acidosis, trauma, tension pneumothorax, cardiac tamponade, hypoxia, hypothermia, hypoglycemia, hypokalemia or hyperkalemia, massive myocardial infarction, drug overdose) and treat if causes are found.
    (Objective 10)

78. a. QRS normal or wide. Delta wave and onset of QRS complex are slurred or notched
    b. P-R interval is usually less than 0.12 second.
    (Objective 9)

79. Patients with Wolff-Parkinson-White syndrome are susceptible to paroxysmal supraventricular tachycardias. Verapamil is contraindicated because it may cause rapid atrial to ventricular conduction and lead to ventricular fibrillation and sudden death.
    (Objective 9)

80. Atherosclerosis is a process that progressively narrows the lumens of medium and large arteries. Thick, hard atherosclerotic plaques called atheromata form, especially in areas of turbulent blood flow. The plaques are thought to be an endothelial cell response to chronic mechanical or chemical injury. The response includes platelet adhesion and aggregation and proliferation and migration of smooth muscle cells from the media into the intima. Eventually, the atheromata become fibrotic and calcified and partially or totally obstruct the involved arteries. The two major effects are (1) disruption of the intimal surface, causing a loss of vessel elasticity and an increase in thrombogenesis and (2) a reduction in the diameter of the vessel lumen with resulting decreased blood supply to tissues.
    (Objective 12)

81. a. Physical exertion; b. emotional stress
(Objective 12)

82. a. Angina typically lasts 1 to 5 minutes but may last as long as 15 minutes.
b. Relieved by rest, nitroglycerin, or oxygen
(Objective 12)

83. Unless 12-lead electrocardiogram interpretation is available, it is impossible to distinguish between these two
conditions in the field. Even a negative 12-lead electrocardiogram does not exclude acute myocardial infarction. Serial
cardiac enzyme tests and electrocardiograms and other tests such as echocardiograms and stress tests may be needed.
Both patients should be managed as though they are having a myocardial infarction (excluding thrombolytic therapy).
(Objective 12)

84. Atherosclerotic plaque forms in coronary artery; plaque ruptures; platelets adhere to it, and then thrombus forms
on the plaque; as thrombus enlarges, it occludes the coronary artery. (Other causes are coronary vasospasm,
coronary embolism, severe hypoxia, hemorrhage into diseased arterial wall, and shock.)
(Objective 12)

85.

Area of Heart Injured or Infarcted	Coronary Vessel Involved Most Often	Leads with Visible ST Segment Changes
Anterior	Left coronary	V_3, V_4
Lateral	Left coronary	V_5, V_6, I, aV_L
Septal	Left coronary	V_1, V_2
Inferior	Right coronary	II, III, aV_F

(Objective 12)

86. a. 0.1 mV in at least two contiguous precordial leads or two or more limb leads.
(Objective 12)

87. Left bundle branch block, some ventricular rhythms, left ventricular hypertrophy, pericarditis, ventricular
aneurysm, and early repolarization
(Objective 12)

88. a. Identify rate and rhythm; b. Identify the area of infarct; c. Consider miscellaneous conditions; d. Assess the
patient's clinical presentation; e. Recognize the infarction and initiate treatment.
(Objective 12)

89. Lethal dysrhythmias, congestive heart failure, pulmonary edema, cardiogenic shock, and myocardial tissue rupture.
(Objective 12)

90. Nausea; vomiting; diaphoresis; radiation of pain to the neck, jaw, left arm, or back; palpitations; dyspnea;
pulmonary edema; hypotension; and a sense of impending doom
(Objective 12)

91. ST segment elevation in leads V_2, V_3, and V_4. Possible acute anterior myocardial infarction.
(Objective 12)

92. Minimize physical activity, monitor electrocardiogram and oxygen saturation (if pulse oximetry is available),
assess vital signs frequently (including lung sounds for crackles), and establish an intravenous line to keep the
vein open with normal saline or lactated Ringer solution.
(Objective 12)

93. Aspirin 160 to 325 mg chewed; nitroglycerin 0.4 mg sublingually, repeated two times; morphine sulfate 2 to 4 mg
intravenously titrated to relieve pain
(Objective 12)

344

94. a. Patient is alert and able to give informed consent; chest pain or symptoms of acute myocardial infarction
for at least 15 minutes and less than 12 hours; electrocardiogram changes consistent with an ST segment
elevation myocardial infarction or new LBBB; chest pain and electrocardiogram changes that persist after the
administration of sublingual nitroglycerin
b. SBP >180 mm Hg; DBP >110 mm Hg; right vs. left arm systolic BP difference >15 mm Hg; structural CNS
disease; CHI within 3 months; major trauma, surgery, GI/GU bleed within <6 weeks; takes blood thinners or
has bleeding problems; CPR >10 min; pregnancy; advanced diseases of the liver or kidney or advanced cancer
(Objective 12)
c. HR >100 beats/min and BP <100 mm Hg; pulmonary edema (rales); or signs of shock (cool, clammy)

95. a. Normal axis; no ST segment elevation, depression; normal 12-lead electrocardiogram
b. QRS 0.14 second; pathologic left axis deviation; left bundle branch block; cannot detect ST segment
elevation in the presence of left bundle branch block
c. Normal axis; ST segment elevation leads II, III, aV_F; ST segment depression in leads aV_L, V_2, V_3, V_4, V_5;
possible inferior myocardial infarction
d. Normal axis; ST segment elevation leads I, aV_L, V_2, V_3, V_4, V_5, V_6; extensive anterior myocardial infarction
(Objective 12)

96. There is a pathologic left axis deviation; QRS is upright in lead I and down in leads II and III
(Objective 12)

97. The triangle should point upward.
(Objective 6)

98. The patient has a left anterior hemiblock (pathologic left axis deviation) and a right bundle branch block
(QRS >0.12 sec and upward triangle).
(Objective 6)

99. The presence of more than one block is known as bifascicular block and is associated with a high risk of
advancement to complete heart block and increased mortality in the presence of myocardial infarction. This
patient's symptoms suggest the potential for myocardial infarction.
(Objective 6)

100. The potential for serious rhythm deterioration should be anticipated. Prophylactic application of defibrillation
or pacing pads in this setting may be indicated based on local protocol.
(Objective 12)

101. Left ventricular failure leading to pulmonary edema and possible myocardial infarction
(Objective 12)

102. Pulmonary edema: orthopnea and frothy, blood-tinged sputum. Myocardial infarction: chest pain, radiation of
pain, nausea, and vomiting
(Objective 12)

103. Apply continuous positive airway pressure (CPAP)
(Objective 12)

104.

Drug	Dose	Desired Effect
a. Furosemide	0.5–1.0 mg/kg intravenously	Venodilation and diuresis
b. Morphine	2–4 mg intravenously	Venodilation, decreased myocardial work, and decreased anxiety
c. Nitroglycerin	0.4 mg sublingually	Peripheral vasodilation and decreased preload and afterload

(Objectives 12 and 14)

Chapter **22** **Cardiology**

105. Continuous positive airway pressure, nitroglycerin, morphine, and furosemide would be contraindicated if she were hypotensive. Consider treatment with dopamine 2 to 20 mcg/kg/min. Rapid transport is indicated as cardiogenic shock is complicated to manage and has a high mortality.
(Objective 12)

106. a. Left ventricular failure, pulmonary embolism, right ventricle infarct, chronic hypertension, chronic obstructive pulmonary disease, and valvular disease
b. Jugular venous distension, tachycardia, enlarged liver or spleen, peripheral and sacral edema, and ascites
(Objective 12)

107. Sinus bradycardia
(Objective 10)

108. Administer oxygen by non-rebreather mask and give atropine 0.5 mg intravenously
(Objectives 10 and 13)

109. Cardiogenic shock
(Objective 11)

110. High-flow oxygen by non-rebreather mask (his SaO_2 was 90%); supine position (if tolerated); intravenous therapy with normal saline; dopamine infusion via intravenous piggyback 2 to 20 mcg/kg/min (remove nitroglycerin paste and wipe chest with gauze); obtain 12-lead ECG and monitor electrocardiogram for dysrhythmias.
(Objective 12)

111. Expanding or ruptured abdominal aortic aneurysm
(Objective 12)

112. Palpation in this situation could cause a bulging aneurysm to rupture. If medical direction advises palpation, it should be done gently.
(Objective 12)

113. No. Increased intraabdominal pressure could cause rupture of the aneurysm.
(Objective 12)

114. Administer oxygen, transport rapidly, initiate two large-bore intravenous lines en route and infuse normal saline or lactated Ringer solution to keep the vein open unless the patient's condition deteriorates.
(Objective 12)

115. Dissecting thoracic aortic aneurysm
(Objective 12)

116. Unequal peripheral pulses, neurologic deficit, or signs of pericardial tamponade
(Objective 12)

117. Minimize movement and anxiety, administer high-concentration oxygen, initiate a 14- or 16-gauge intravenous line in the arm with good pulses (higher blood pressure) to keep the vein open, administer pain medication in consultation with medical direction, and monitor vital signs and the electrocardiogram frequently.
(Objective 12)

　　

118.

	Embolic	**Thrombotic**
Causes	Clot breaks loose and travels to narrow area in blood vessel	Clot develops at narrow spot in blood vessel
Onset	Rapid	Gradual
Signs and symptoms	Pulseless extremity pain; decreased motor and sensory function; pallor; cool skin temperature distal to the occlusion; decreased capillary refill; possible shock	Pain in hips, lower limbs, buttocks, leg, and abdomen (depends on the affected artery); pain; delayed motor and sensory function; pallor; decreased skin temperature distal to the occlusion; decreased capillary refill; possible shock

(Objective 12)

119. Control bleeding with direct pressure. The bleeding may be persistent and require hospital management.
(Objective 12)

120. Pain, edema, warmth, erythema, tenderness, and a palpable cord
(Objective 12)

121. Hypertensive encephalopathy
(Objective 12)

122. Aphasia, hemiparesis, transient blindness, seizures, stupor, coma, and death
(Objective 12)

123. Calm the patient, apply oxygen, and insert an intravenous line to keep the vein open; monitor electrocardiogram; and transport rapidly.
(Objective 12)

124. Nitroglycerin paste; labetalol 10 to 20 mg intravenously over 1 to 2 minutes
(Objective 14)

125. Determine unresponsiveness and look for absence of breathing; leave the patient to call for help or get an AED if no one else is available; if you cannot feel a carotid pulse within 10 seconds, begin cardiopulmonary resuscitation until help arrives (30 compressions: two ventilations).
(Objective 13)

126. a. Two minutes from the previous shock. During CPR, establish an intravenous or intraosseous line and administer epinephrine 1 mg (1:10,000) IV.
b. Yes. It is possible for an electric shock resulting in injury or death.
(Objective 13)

127. Ventricular tachycardia (monomorphic)
(Objective 9)

128. Defibrillate (biphasic, 120–200 J; monophasic, 360 J) and then resume chest compressions immediately.
(Objective 13)

129. Amount of time patient has been in pulseless ventricular tachycardia, quality of bystander CPR, and proper patch or paddle placement
(Objective 13)

130. Apply conductive gel on the patient's chest (or hands-off defibrillation patches); turn on power (there is a separate power source for the defibrillator and monitor with some monitors); select correct energy level; place paddles (or patches) in an appropriate position on the patient's chest; charge the defibrillator; call "clear" and

visually check to ensure that no one is in contact with the patient or cot; lean firmly on the paddles (if used) with 20 to 25 lb of pressure; discharge both paddle buttons simultaneously (or depress discharge button on monitor for hands-off defibrillator). Resume chest compressions immediately after shock is delivered. (Objective 13)

131. Synchronized cardioversion at 100, 200, 300, and 360 J (or equivalent biphasic). (Objective 13)

132. It is synchronized with the patient's heartbeat so there is less risk of firing on the relative refractory period and causing ventricular fibrillation. (Objective 13)

133. Depress the synchronize button before each synchronized shock. If paddles are used, hold the paddles firmly on the chest after activation until they discharge. Ensure monitor is marking QRS complexes. (Objective 13)

134. a. Third-degree atrioventricular block
b. Apply oxygen and apply the pacing and monitoring pads; ensure adequate upright R wave on monitor; select pacing mode; select pacing rate at 80 beats/min; set current at 50 mA and slowly increase until capture is observed; reassess the patient's vital signs (use right arm for blood pressure); and document and obtain rhythm strips.
(Objective 13)

135. a. Asystole; b. epinephrine 1.0 mg every 3 to 5 minutes (may substitute vasopressin 40 units for first or second dose). c. Pulmonary embolus, acidosis, tension pneumothorax, cardiac tamponade, hypoxia, hypovolemia, hypothermia, hypo- or hyperkalemia, hypoglycemia, myocardial infarction, or drug overdose (PATCHMD).
(Objectives 9, 13, and 14)

136. a. Ventricular fibrillation; b. defibrillation; c. epinephrine 1.0 mg every 3 to 5 minutes or 1 dose vasopressin 40 U (to replace first or second epinephrine dose) intravenous bolus, amiodarone 300 mg intravenous bolus.
(Objectives 9, 13, and 14)

137. a. Stop resuscitation if your protocols allow. The patient is older than 18 years and unresponsive to treatment.
b. Do not stop resuscitation. The patient is older than 18 years. The patient may be hypothermic. Transport and continue resuscitation.
c. Do not stop resuscitation. The patient is younger than 18 years and has sustained trauma, and you were able to get back a perfusing pulse during the resuscitation.
d. Consult with medical direction before you stop resuscitation. The patient has met criteria for resuscitation; however, the family objects strongly, so medical oversight may advise that efforts should continue.
(Objective 15)

138. d. His identified risk factors are male sex, age, hypercholesterolemia, diabetes, and hypertension (Accupril is an angiotensin-converting enzyme inhibitor, and indapamide is a diuretic).
(Objective 1)

139. c. Blood pressure = Cardiac output × Peripheral vascular resistance
(Objective 1)

140. c. The circumflex supplies the lateral and posterior portions of the left ventricle and part of the right ventricle. The right coronary artery and the left anterior descending supply most of the right atrium and ventricle and the inferior aspect of the left ventricle.
(Objective 2)

141. b. The aortic valve separates the aorta and left ventricle, the pulmonic valve separates the pulmonary arteries and right ventricle, and the tricuspid valve separates the right atrium and right ventricle.
(Objective 2)

142. d. The electrical charge is the potential difference and is measured in millivolts. Depolarization (electrical conduction) occurs when sodium rushes into the cell, altering the electrical balance.
(Objective 3)

143. c. Potassium is also essential.
(Objective 3)

144. d. Calcium channel blockers selectively block the slow channel and alter the threshold level.
(Objective 3)

145. a. Phase 0 is the rapid depolarization phase, phase 1 is the early rapid depolarization phase, phase 2 is the plateau phase, phase 3 is the terminal phase of rapid repolarization, and phase 4 is the period between action potentials.
(Objective 3)

146. c. This allows complete relaxation of the cardiac muscle before another contraction can be initiated.
(Objective 3)

147. d. The His bundle divides into the right and left bundle branches. The left bundle divides into the anterior and posterior fascicles. A third fascicle of the left bundle branch that innervates the interventricular septum and the base of the heart also has been identified. The bundle branches subdivide and become Purkinje fibers.
(Objective 4)

148. d. The resting membrane potential gradually decreases with time until it reaches a critical threshold, at which time depolarization results.
(Objective 4)

149. c. This pause allows the atria to finish contraction and empty before ventricular contraction occurs.
(Objective 4)

150. a. Acetylcholine causes the cell membrane of the sinoatrial node to become hyperpolarized, causing a delay in reaching threshold, and therefore it decreases the heart rate. All other answers increase heart rate.
(Objective 4)

151. d. The other answers represent causes of dysrhythmias that result from enhanced automaticity.
(Objective 4)

152. a. Mental status change, abdominal or gastrointestinal complaints, or vague complaints of ill-being may be presenting symptoms in an older adult patient with a coronary event.
(Objective 5)

153. d. If the heart is unable to pump effectively, blood will back up into the lungs, causing decreased diffusion of gases in the lungs and dyspnea.
(Objective 5)

154. b. Younger patients may experience syncope because of increased vagal tone. Nausea or syncope when standing does not predict the incidence of dysrhythmias.
(Objective 5)

155. b
(Objective 5)

156. c. Peripheral pulses and perfusion would be used to assess strength of myocardial contractions. Placement of patches usually is performed using ribs and gross anatomy.
(Objective 5)

157. b. The electrocardiogram does not measure mechanical events.
(Objective 7)

Chapter **22** **Cardiology**

158. c. The others are unipolar leads (a single positive electrode and a reference point).
(Objective 6)

159. d. If the depolarization moves toward a positive electrode, the tracing should show an upward deflection.
(Objective 6)

160. b. These leads all look up onto the inferior portion of the heart.
(Objective 6)

161. d. These leads may help distinguish between supraventricular tachycardia with aberration and ventricular tachycardia and can help diagnose bundle branch blocks.
(Objective 6)

162. c. The negative lead is placed at the lateral end of the left clavicle. The positive lead for MCL_6 is placed on the left axillary line at the level of the fifth intercostal space.
(Objective 6)

163. a. Many dysrhythmias involve abnormalities of the P wave.
(Objective 6)

164. b. V_3 and V_4 are anterior leads, and V_5 and V_6 are lateral precordial leads.
(Objective 6)

165. a. This is used as the baseline.
(Objective 6)

166. b
(Objective 8)

167. c. The relative refractory period is from the peak of the T wave onward.
(Objective 6)

168. b. In some leads, part of the QRS complex is blended with the baseline and is difficult to measure.
(Objective 9)

169. d. $1500 \div 10 = 150$ beats/min
(Objective 7)

170. b
(Objective 10)

171. c
(Objective 10)

172. c
(Objective 10)

173. a
(Objective 10)

174. b
(Objective 10)

175. d
(Objective 10)

176. a

(Objective 10)

177. d. Adenosine is not indicated for atrial fibrillation, and verapamil is not indicated when a patient has hypotension. The patient needs electrical cardioversion because her condition is unstable. Procainamide is indicated for ventricular dysrhythmias.

(Objective 10)

178. a. It originates from tissue other than an intrinsic pacemaker.

(Objective 10)

179. a. Albuterol and cocaine cause tachycardia. Atropine is used to treat bradycardia.

(Objective 10)

180. d. The atria cannot contract to empty. This decreases the blood flow to the ventricles and the cardiac output.

(Objective 10)

181. a

(Objective 10)

182. d. It also is associated with excessive catecholamine administration, damage to the atrioventricular junction, inferior wall myocardial infarction, and rheumatic fever.

(Objective 11)

183. c. Other causes include failure of higher pacemakers to initiate impulses.

(Objective 10)

184. a. Couplets are two premature ventricular contractions in a row. An idioventricular rhythm originates in the ventricles and supersedes the underlying rhythm. Multifocal premature ventricular contractions have varied appearance depending on their site of origination.

(Objective 9)

185. a. Precordial concordance with all positive or all negative deflection in the V leads indicates ventricular tachycardia.

(Objective 9)

186. b. Asynchronous (fixed rate) pacemakers stimulate the heart at a set rate regardless of the action of the heart. A dual chamber pacemaker stimulates the atria and the ventricles.

(Objective 13)

187. d. Bundle branch block occurs when one of the bundles of His is blocked. Second-degree atrioventricular block type II is an intermittent block.

(Objective 9)

188. d. It yields an initial Q wave in MCL_1 (V_1) instead of the normal small R wave. There will be a deep QS pattern that is at least 0.12 second.

(Objective 9)

189. b. The blockage of two of the three pathways for ventricular conduction (right bundle branch block with anterior or posterior hemiblock, and left bundle branch block) poses the greatest risk.

(Objective 9)

190. d. Diltiazem may cause rapid atrial to ventricular conduction down the accessory pathway and may lead to ventricular fibrillation and sudden death.

(Objective 14)

191. c. Both have the same cause.
(Objective 12)

192. a. Hypotension caused by pump failure and cardiac rupture can occur but is much less common than lethal dysrhythmias.
(Objective 12)

193. a. A fluid challenge may be given to a patient who is hypotensive; however, in the normotensive patient, intravenous fluids should be infused to keep the vein open. Nitroglycerin is contraindicated in right ventricular infarction. Oxygen by nasal cannula is administered if the patient's SaO_2 is less than 94%.
(Objective 12)

194. d. Generally, STEMI teams are activated only when there is ST segment elevation. Q waves indicate myocardial damage that is often not acute. Peaked T waves may represent an ECG change associated with hyperkalemia. Right axis deviation indicates a hemi-block.
(Objective 10)

195. a. The vasodilation from nitroglycerin decreases preload and afterload and decreases the workload on the left ventricle.
(Objectives 12 and 14)

196. d. Signs include jugular venous distension and peripheral edema.
(Objective 12)

197. d. The left ventricle cannot pump effectively, so stroke volume decreases.
(Objective 12)

198. b. Decreased systolic pressure is a later sign. Muffled heart sounds are associated with this. Tracheal deviation is seen in tension pneumothorax.
(Objective 12)

199. b. The pain often is described as ripping or tearing and is high intensity.
(Objective 12)

200. a
(Objective 12)

201. c
(Objective 12)

202. b. The increased afterload makes it harder for the left ventricle to eject blood. Enhanced atherosclerosis associated with hypertension increases the patient's risk for myocardial infarction, stroke, and renal failure.
(Objective 12)

203. d. The goal is to "push hard and push fast" when performing CPR.
(Objective 13)

204. b. Lower energy levels may be used. Energy flow is bidirectional. Battery size is not affected.
(Objective 13)

205. b. Anterior-posterior placement is not practical for paddle use. Avoid placing the patch or paddle over the sternum because bone is a poor conductor of electricity. Pediatric paddles are indicated for children younger than 1 year of age.
(Objective 13)

206. b. The implantable cardioverter defibrillator sequence includes up to five shocks in 2 minutes. There is no danger in touching the patients. Strong magnets may inactivate the device.
(Objective 13)

207. d
(Objective 13)

208. b
(Objective 15)

209. b
(Objective 14)

210. b. Inferior wall infarcts often occur with right ventricular infarcts. These make the heart preload dependent. Administer the fluid and then obtain a right-sided ECG.
(Objective 12)

211. a. Morphine will decrease the preload. It is contraindicated in patients with head injury. It does not cause bronchodilation.
(Objective 14)

212. a
(Objective 14)

213. c
(Objective 14)

214. c. The correct dose of dopamine is 2 to 20 mcg/kg/min; for epinephrine, it is 2 to 10 mcg/min (not mcg/kg/min).
(Objective 14)

215. a. None of the other criteria should be used alone to evaluate whether resuscitation should be stopped.
(Objective 15)

216. a. Rhythms such as Wolff-Parkinson-White are AVRT rhythms. Electrical mechanical dissociation is the presence of electrical heart activity without mechanical activity. An escape rhythm originates from a pacemaker site such as the atrioventricular node or the ventricles.
(Objectives 6, 9)

217. a. The ITD enhances blood flow but does not affect oxygenation or myocardial electrical activity.
(Objective 13)

218. c. Human compressions can decrease over time as fatigue sets in. Mechanical devices must be positioned carefully or they can compress ineffectively.
(Objective 13)

219. b. If the patient's underlying stroke volume is low, a pulse may not be palpable. Normal signs of circulation such as capillary refill should be present if the pump is functioning properly. Ventricular fibrillation will cause unconsciousness because of lack of cardiac output.
(Objective 13)

1. a, b, c, d, e, f
   (Objective 12)

2. Ventricular fibrillation and ventricular tachycardia are the only two rhythms that will advise a shock on an automated external defibrillator.
   (Objective 13)

3. Amiodarone is preferred.
   (Objective 14)

4. ST segment elevation in leads V_1 to V_4 would indicate septal and anterior myocardial infarction.
   (Objective 9)

5. Left coronary
   (Objective 2)

6. a. The other risk factors mentioned would be absolute contraindications.
   (Objective 14)

7. 10 to 12 breaths/min; 6 to 7 mL/kg volume
   (Objective 13)

Diseases of the Eyes, Ears, Nose, and Throat

READING ASSIGNMENT

Chapter 23, pages 721-739, in *Mosby's Paramedic Textbook,* ed. 4.

OBJECTIVES

Upon completion of this chapter, the paramedic student will be able to do the following:

1. Label a diagram of the eye.
2. Describe the pathophysiology, signs and symptoms, and specific management techniques for each of the following disorders of the eye: conjunctivitis, corneal abrasion, foreign body, inflammation (chalazion and hordeolum), glaucoma, iritis, papilledema, retinal detachment, central retinal artery occlusion, and orbital cellulitis.
3. Label a diagram of the ear.
4. Describe the pathophysiology, signs and symptoms, and specific management techniques for each of the following conditions that affect the ear: foreign body, impacted cerumen, labyrinthitis, Meniere disease, otitis media, and perforated tympanic membrane.
5. Label a diagram of the nose.
6. Describe the pathophysiology, signs and symptoms, and specific management techniques for each of the following conditions that affect the nose: epistaxis, foreign body, rhinitis, and sinusitis.
7. Label a diagram of the oropharynx.
8. Describe the pathophysiology, signs and symptoms, and specific management techniques for each of the following conditions that affect the oropharynx and throat: toothache and dental abscess, Ludwig angina, epiglottitis, laryngitis, tracheitis, oral candidiasis, peritonsillar abscess, pharyngitis, tonsillitis, and temporomandibular joint disorders.

SUMMARY

- The eye is composed of its primary vision structures and accessory structures that protect, lubricate, move, and aid in their function. Cranial nerves control vision, pupil constriction, and movement of the eyes. Consider nervous system disease if these functions are impaired.
- Conjunctivitis is inflammation or infection of the eye sometimes called pink eye. Infectious conjunctivitis is contagious.
- A corneal abrasion is a scrape or scratch of the cornea. It is very painful and may cause tearing, redness, and blurred vision. Patch the eye and administer a topical ophthalmic anesthetic if permitted by protocol.
- Foreign bodies in the eye are very painful and cause pain and tearing. Irrigation of the eye may be indicated to remove small foreign bodies.
- Two types of eyelid inflammation are chalazion (obstructed oil gland) and hordeolum (sty).
- Glaucoma is caused by an increase in intraocular pressure related to excess aqueous humor. This results in pressure on the optic nerve and can lead to blindness if untreated. Signs and symptoms include a loss of peripheral vision, pain, headache, vomiting, and blurred vision.
- Iritis is inflammation of the iris. It can cause blindness if untreated.
- Papilledema is swelling of the optic disc caused by an increase in intracranial pressure (ICP). The increased ICP may be related to illness or injury.
- The retina is the eye structure central to vision. Tears, breaks, and defects in the retina cause retinal detachment. Without treatment, retinal detachment leads to blindness. Signs and symptoms include increase in floaters, light flashes in the eye, or the appearance of a curtain over the field of vision.
- Central retinal artery occlusion occurs when blood supply to the retina is blocked. If circulation is not reestablished within 60 to 90 minutes, permanent loss of vision occurs. Onset is marked by sudden, painless loss of vision or the sense that a shade has been pulled down over the eye.
- Orbital cellulitis is an infectious of the tissue around the eye that can lead to serious complications that include blindness, sepsis, and meningitis. Signs and symptoms include fever, pain and swelling of the eyelids, eye pain,

decreased vision, bulging eyes, malaise, and impaired eye movement. Immediate treatment with intravenous antibiotics is essential.

■ When excess ear wax (cerumen) accumulates in the ear it can cause earache, hearing loss, tinnitus, itching, odor, or discharge. Removal of the wax usually resolves the symptoms.
■ Swelling of the inner ear causes labyrinthitis. This causes vertigo and tinnitus.
■ Meniere disease causes vertigo, tinnitus, and hearing loss. This can lead to nausea and vomiting. Stroke can cause similar symptoms and should be ruled out.
■ Otitis media is an infection or inflammation of the inner ear. In addition to earache, it can produce a number of signs and symptoms.
■ Infection or trauma can cause perforation of the tympanic membrane. This can result in brief pain, hearing loss, and drainage from the affected ear.
■ Epistaxis is bleeding from the structures of the nose or nasopharynx. Attempt to control epistaxis by positioning the patient upright, leaning forward. Apply direct pressure on the nose until bleeding is controlled. Treat for shock if indicated.
■ It is common for children to place foreign bodies in their noses. Transport for physician examination and removal.
■ Rhinitis is a runny nose. Common causes are infection, allergy, and foreign body in the nose.
■ Sinusitis is inflammation of sinuses and nasal passages. Signs and symptoms include cough; fever; halitosis; nasal congestion; headache; and pressure sensation over the eyes, nose, or cheek.
■ Toothache is frequently caused by tooth decay, abscess, cracked tooth, an exposed root, or gum disease. Transport for definitive care and pain management.
■ Ludwig angina is cellulitis of the tissues under the tongue. It can cause rapid tissue swelling and airway obstruction. Signs and symptoms include dyspnea, confusion, fever, neck pain, redness or swelling, weakness, or drooling. Urgent transport is needed.
■ Epiglottitis is inflammation of the epiglottis caused by bacterial infection. It can lead to airway obstruction. Signs and symptoms include sore throat, high fever, drooling, and a muffled voice. Airway obstruction is possible. Perform minimal interventions unless airway obstruction occurs.
■ Laryngitis is a hoarse voice and swollen lymph nodes associated with inflamed vocal cords.
■ Tracheitis is a bacterial infection of the upper airway and subglottic trachea. It can cause respiratory failure and arrest. Be prepared to manage the airway and ventilate if needed.
■ Oral candidiasis is a yeast fungal infection of the mouth. It covers the tongue and mucous membranes with a thick cream-colored coating.

REVIEW QUESTIONS

1. Label the following diagram of the eye.

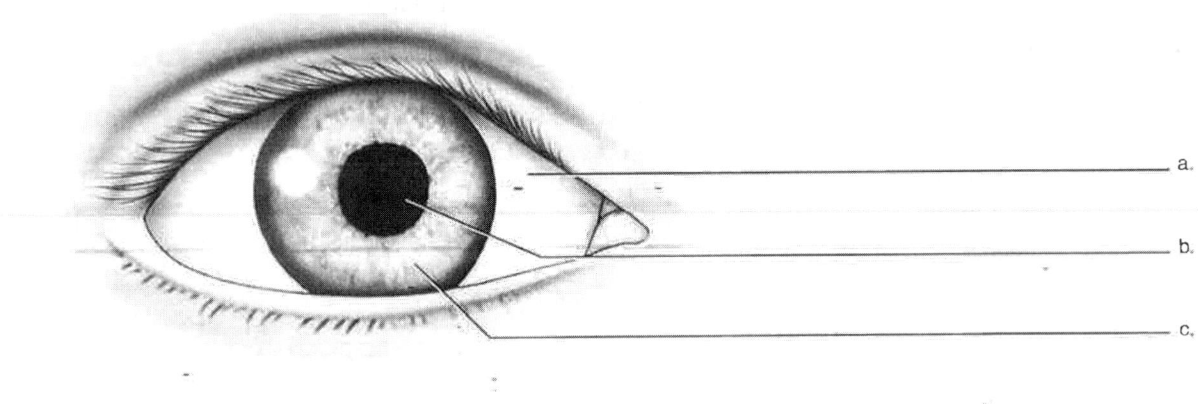

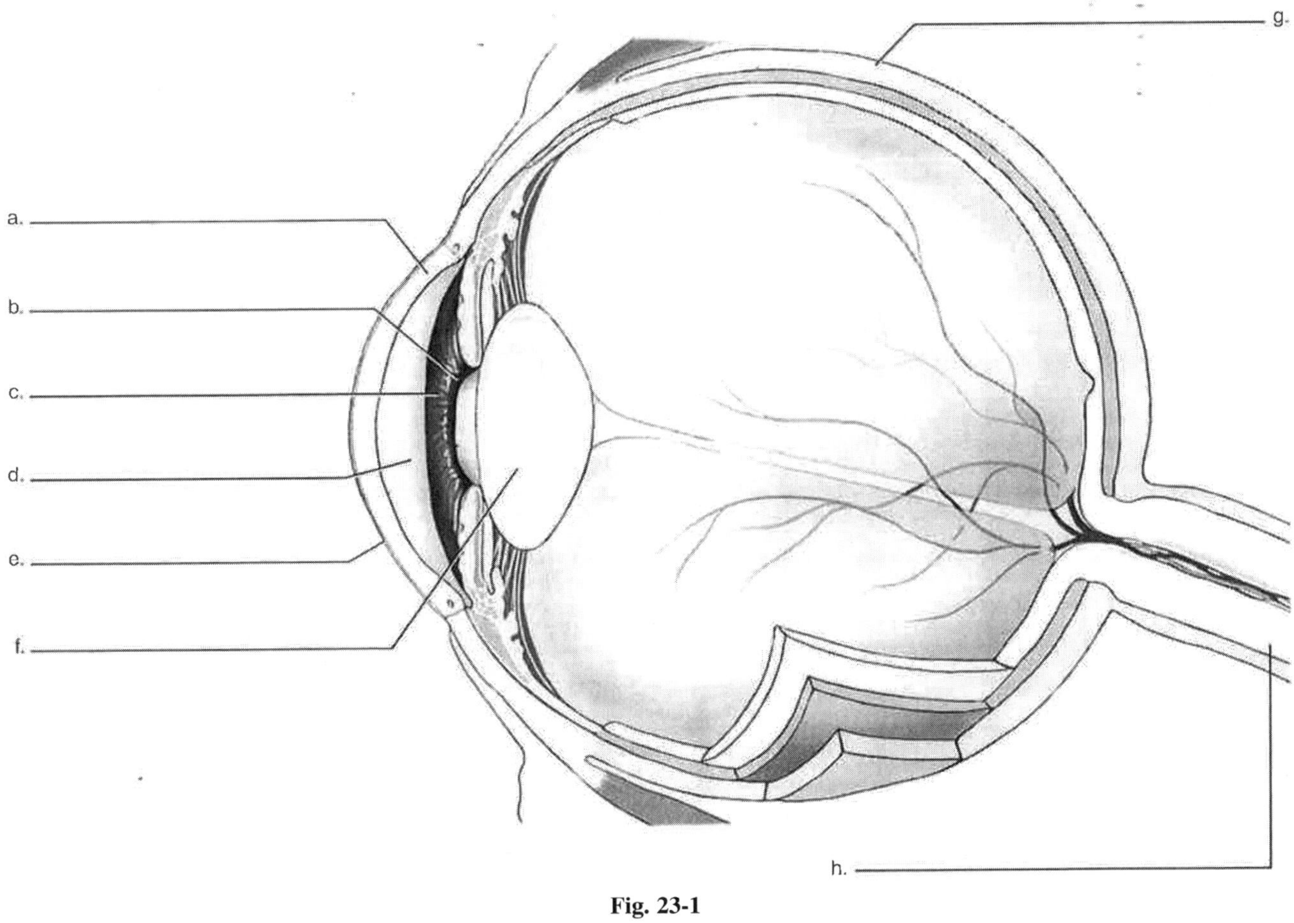

Fig. 23-1

Match the disease of the eye from column II with its description in column I. Use each answer only once.

Column I

2. _________ Sudden, often unilateral, painless blindness

3. _________ Commonly called a sty.

4. _________ Cornea of eye is scraped causing severe pain

5. _________ Increased eye pressure that can damage the optic nerve

6. _________ Infection around eye that can lead to sepsis or blindness

7. _________ Inflamed membrane that lines the eye.

8. _________ Light sensitive tissue of eye is pulled out of position.

9. _________ Blocked oil gland on the eyelid.

10. _________ Swelling of optic disc caused by increased intracranial pressure.

11. _________ Inflammation also called anterior uveitis.

Column II

a. Conjunctivitis
b. Corneal abrasion
c. Foreign body
d. Chalazion
e. Glaucoma
f. Hordeolum
g. Iritis
h. Papilledema
i. Retinal detachment
j. Central retinal artery occlusion
k. Orbital cellulitis

12. Label the following diagram of the ear.

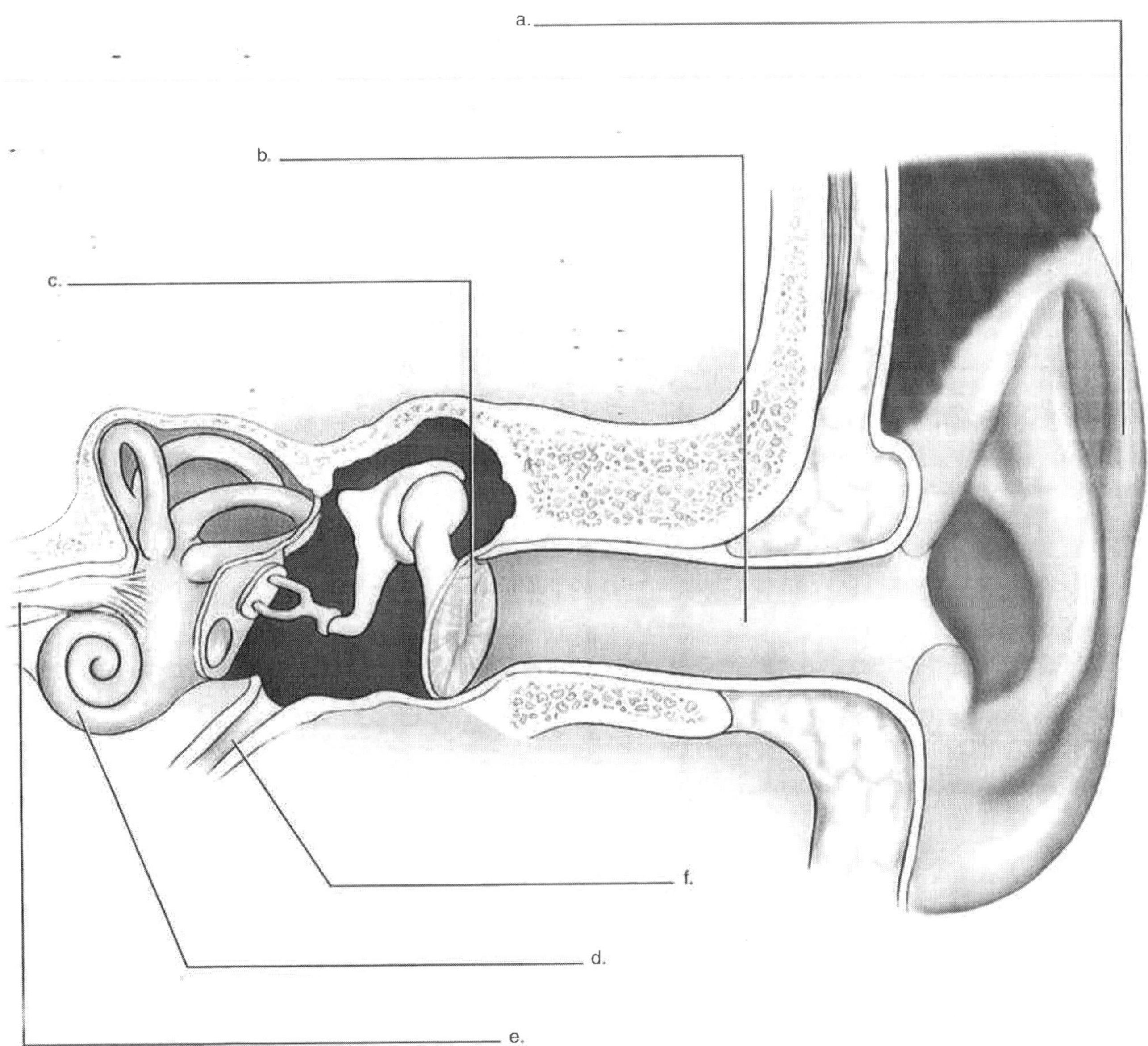

Fig. 23-2

Match signs or symptoms from Column II with each of the injuries or diseases of the ear listed in Column I. You may use the terms in Colum II more than once.

Column I

13. _______ Foreign body

14. _______ Impacted cerumen

15. _______ Labyrinthitis

16. _______ Meniere disease

17. _______ Otitis media

18. _______ Perforated tympanic membrane

Column II

a. Bleeding
b. Fever
c. Hearing loss
d. Odor
e. Pain
f. Purulent drainage
g. Tinnitus
h. Vertigo

19. Label a diagram of the oral cavity.

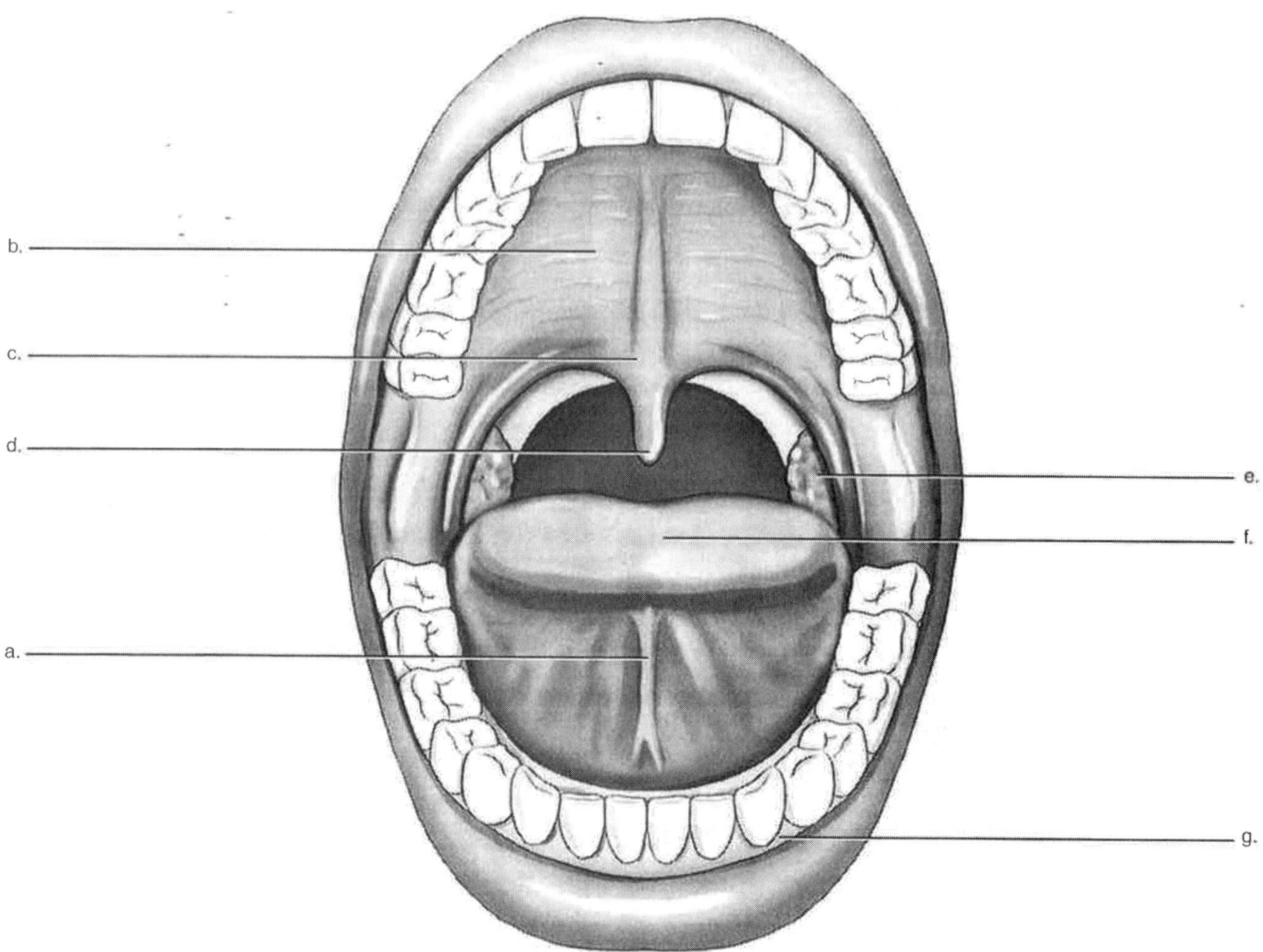

Fig. 23-3

20. Place a check mark beside each condition of the oropharynx and throat that creates a high risk for complete airway obstruction.

    a. _______ Dental abscess
    b. _______ Epiglottitis
    c. _______ Laryngitis
    d. _______ Ludwig angina
    e. _______ Oral candidiasis
    f. _______ Peritonsillar abscess
    g. _______ Pharyngitis
    h. _______ Temporomandibular joint disorders
    i. _______ Tracheitis

STUDENT SELF-ASSESSMENT

21. You are transporting a patient with conjunctivitis who has thick green discharge from the eye. Which of the following is indicated?

    a. Eye protection   **c.** Prophylaxis with antibiotics
    b. Full face protection   **d.** Standard precautions

22. Which sign or symptom is most strongly associated with corneal abrasion?

    a. Blood in the anterior chamber   **c.** Purulent drainage
    b. Loss of vision in the affected eye   **d.** Tearing

362

23. What should the patient with a hordeolum who is refusing transport be advised to do?
   a. Apply warm compresses.
   b. Puncture the infected area.
   c. Scrub the area with iodine.
   d. Treat fever with ibuprofen.

24. What is usually the first sign of glaucoma?
   a. Elevated blood pressure
   b. Fever and headache
   c. Loss of peripheral vision
   d. Purulent drainage

25. What is the patient with iritis likely to complain of?
   a. Sudden, painless loss of vision
   b. Intermittent high fever
   c. Photophobia
   d. Nausea and vomiting

26. Which of the following patients is likely to have papilledema?
   a. A 6-month-old infant who was shaken violently by a caregiver
   b. A 22-year-old person who failed to wear safety glasses while welding
   c. A 14-year-old girl who impaled a fish hook in her eye
   d. A 76-year-old person who has atrial fibrillation with a rapid heart rate

27. A 42-year-old patient with type 1 diabetes complains of a sudden onset of "floaters" in his eye and wishes to refuse transport after you determine his blood glucose is 86 mg/dL. What should you tell him?
   a. This is a common phenomenon in patients whose diabetes is difficult to control.
   b. He has an optical emergency and needs to be transported immediately.
   c. He should check his blood glucose often and call again if his vision does not improve.
   d. That he should schedule an appointment with an ophthalmologist within 1 week.

28. Which vision emergency is characterized by sudden, painless loss of vision in one eye?
   a. Central retinal artery occlusion
   b. Glaucoma
   c. Papilledema
   d. Retinal detachment

29. A patient who has a sty has progressive redness in the tissues around the eye with a purple eyelid and has shaking chills. What should you suspect?
   a. Corneal abrasion
   b. Unrelated illness
   c. Bacterial periorbital cellulitis
   d. Unreported traumatic injury

30. A 72-year-old man had sudden onset of a staggering gait. He complains of ringing in his ears feels the room is spinning. He has vomited twice. Which of the following do you suspect?
   a. Cerumen impaction
   b. Meniere disease
   c. Otitis media
   d. Perforated tympanic membrane

31. Your patient is a 2-year-old toddler with a 4-day history of fever, irritability, and pulling at his ears. Today he was noted to have blood and pus draining from the affected ear. What does this likely mean?
   a. You should irrigate the ear canal with warm normal saline.
   b. The child is developing labyrinthitis.
   c. He will develop permanent hearing loss.
   d. His eardrum perforated and will likely heal spontaneously.

32. Which structure divides the nose medially?
   a. External meatus
   b. Nares
   c. Septum
   d. Sinuses

33. How should a conscious patient with epistaxis be positioned?
   a. Fowler
   b. Prone
   c. Modified Trendelenburg
   d. Supine

34. What is your chief concern when transporting a patient with Ludwig angina?
   a. Acute coronary event
   b. Airway obstruction
   c. Sepsis
   d. Stroke

35. Which of the following is true regarding tracheitis?
    a. It is usually caused by a virus.
    b. Swelling occurs at the carina.
    c. Expiratory stridor may be present.
    d. Expect to see it in young adults.

36. A 34-year-old man has a fever and weakness. There is a thick cream-colored coating on his tongue. What underlying condition should you expect?
    a. Human immunodeficiency viral infection
    b. Chronic rheumatoid arthritis
    c. Acute renal failure
    d. Gastroenteritis treated with Pepto-Bismol

37. Your patient complains of sore throat and fever. Which additional sign may be present if this patient has peritonsillar abscess?
    a. Clenched jaw
    b. Crepitus
    c. Intercostal retraction
    d. Expiratory wheeze

38. What sign or symptom might you find in a patient with a temporomandibular joint problem?
    a. Chills or fever
    b. Inability to close the mouth
    c. Purulent drainage
    d. Subcutaneous emphysema

39. Which structure separates the nasal cavity from the oral cavity?
    a. Frontal bone
    b. Maxilla
    c. Palate
    d. Uvula

WRAP IT UP

At 0300, you are dispatched for a patient with "fever." Your patient is a 48-year-old man who you know. He has a history of alcoholism and diabetes, and you transported him 2 weeks prior after he sustained facial trauma in a fight. He is seated leaning forward. As you begin to speak to him, you notice his voice is muffled, and he is slightly confused. He is dabbing the corners of his mouth with a paper towel and spits often into an empty beer can. He is complaining of pain in his mouth, right ear, and neck. His vital signs are BP 94/58 mmHg, P 128, R 28, T 102.6°F (39.2°C), SaO_2 94%, and BGL 180 mg/dL. His tongue appears slightly swollen, and the tissue under it is hard. His neck is also swollen, and the lymph nodes are enlarged.

1. What are your priorities for his care?

____

____

2. Which assessment finding has you most concerned about his airway?

____

____

3. What additional sign would indicate the condition of his airway is deteriorating?

____

____

4. What condition(s) should you suspect are causing his illness? Justify your decision.

____

____

REVIEW QUESTIONS

1. a. Cornea
   b. Pupil
   c. Iris
   d. Aqueous humor
   e. Conjunctiva
   f. Lens
   g. Sclera
   h. Optic nerve
   (Objective 1)

2. j

3. f

4. b

5. e

6. k

7. a

8. i

9. d

10. h

11. g
    (Questions 2–11, Objective 2)

12. a. Pinna
    b. Auditory canal
    c. Ear drum
    d. Cochlea
    e. Auditory nerve
    f. Eustachian tube
    (Objective 3)

13. a, c, d, e, f
    (Objective 4)

14. c, d, e, g
    (Objective 4)

15. c, g, h
    (Objective 4)

16. c, e, g, h
    (Objective 4)

17. b, c, e
    (Objective 4)

18. a, c
(Objective 4)

19. a. frenulum
   b. hard palate
   c. soft palate
   d. Uvula
   e. Tonsil
   f. tongue
   g. gingiva
(Objective 7)

20. b, d, i
(Objective 8)

STUDENT SELF-ASSESSMENT

21. d. The stretcher should be cleaned following this and every patient.
(Objective 2)

22. d. The patient also experiences pain, a sensation of foreign body in the eye, blurred vision, and spasm of the muscles around the eye.
(Objective 2)

23. a. The area may be scrubbed gently with mild soap. The pustule should not be squeezed. If the patient develops fever, he or she should be advised to see a physician immediately.
(Objective 2)

24. c. If the increase in intraocular pressure is sudden, the patient may have eye pain, headache, vomiting, and blurred vision.
(Objective 2)

25. c. Other signs and symptoms include reddened eye, ocular or periorbital pain, and blurred or cloudy vision.
(Objective 2)

26. a. Papilledema signals an increase in the intracranial pressure.
(Objective 2)

27. b. Patients with diabetes are at high risk for retinal detachment. A sudden increase in the number of floaters is a common sign. Urgent evaluation is essential to preserve vision.
(Objective 2)

28. a. This is an emergency. The patient has the best change for a good outcome if treated within 60 to 90 minutes after the onset of symptoms.
(Objective 2)

29. c. This patient needs urgent care to reduce the risk of blindness, hearing loss, meningitis, and sepsis.
(Objective 2)

30. b. The severity and sudden onset of this man's signs and symptoms point to Meniere disease. He should also be evaluated for stroke. Posterior stroke can produce similar findings.
(Objective 4)

31. d. The child should be evaluated by a physician. Most eardrum perforations heal spontaneously.
(Objective 4)

32. c. The septum is composed of cartilage and bone and forms the center of the nose.
(Objective 5)

33. a. Sit the patient upright and squeeze the nose firmly.
(Objective 6)

34. b. The swelling can obstruct the patient's airway.
(Objective 8)

35. c. It is usually bacterial and occurs most often in children 2 to 5 years of age.
(Objective 8)

36. a. Newborns and patients on antibiotics or inhaled corticosteroids are also high risk for candidiasis. Pepto-Bismol can produce a black coating on the tongue.
(Objective 8)

37. a. Trismus is a common finding in patients with peritonsillar abscesses. The patient may also have difficulty swallowing.
(Objective 8)

38. b. The patient may have many other signs or symptoms, including pain and vision or hearing problems.
(Objective 8)

39. c. The hard and soft palate prevent food and liquids from entering the nasopharynx.
(Objective 5)

WRAP IT UP

1. Suction his airway if needed, administer oxygen by a non-rebreather mask, establish an intravenous line, and transport rapidly to the closest appropriate facility.
(Objective 8)

2. The fact that he is drooling indicates substantial swelling in the upper airway.
(Objective 8)

3. If he develops severe dyspnea with stridor, it would signal impending airway obstruction.
(Objective 8)

4. This is most likely Ludwig angina. He is at risk because of diabetes and alcoholism; his fever and infection follow trauma to the mouth; he has fever, pain in the mouth, neck, and ear; he has swelling of the tongue and induration under it. Other less likely possibilities include peritonsillar abscess or epiglottitis.
(Objective 8)

Chapter **23** **Diseases of the Eyes, Ears, Nose, and Throat**

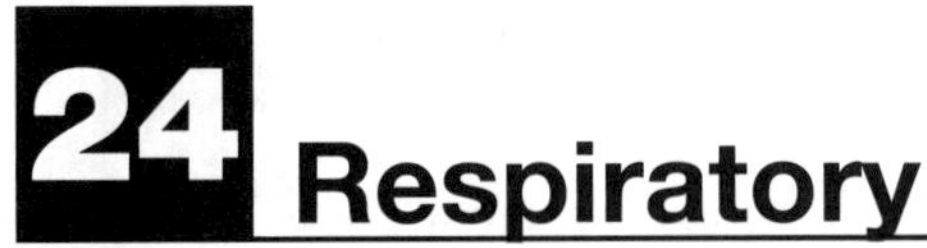

Respiratory

READING ASSIGNMENT

Chapter 24, pages 740-763, in *Mosby's Paramedic Textbook*, ed. 4.

OBJECTIVES

Upon completion of this chapter, the paramedic student will be able to do the following:

1. Distinguish the pathophysiology of respiratory emergencies related to ventilation, diffusion, and perfusion.
2. Outline the assessment process for the patient who has a respiratory emergency.
3. Describe the causes, complications, signs and symptoms, and prehospital management of patients diagnosed with obstructive airway disease, pneumonia, adult respiratory distress syndrome, pulmonary thromboembolism, upper respiratory infection, spontaneous pneumothorax, hyperventilation syndrome, and lung cancer.

SUMMARY

- Diseases responsible for respiratory emergencies include those related to ventilation, diffusion, and perfusion. Ventilation moves air into and out of the lungs. Diffusion is the process of gas exchange. Perfusion is circulation of blood through the tissues.
- Patients should be assessed for chief complaint, signs and symptoms of respiratory distress, and past medical history. The physical examination should determine vital signs, indicators of increased work of breathing, breath sounds, and peripheral edema or cyanosis. Capnometry, oximetry, and peak flow measurements supplement the physical examination findings.
- Obstructive airway disease is a triad of distinct diseases that often coexist. These are chronic bronchitis, emphysema, and asthma. The main goal of prehospital care for these patients is the correction of hypoxemia through improved air flow.
- Chronic bronchitis is characterized by inflammatory changes and excessive mucus production in the alveoli. These patients often have low blood oxygen levels and excess carbon dioxide levels.
- Emphysema causes abnormal enlargement of air spaces beyond the terminal bronchioles and destruction and collapse of the alveoli.
- Asthma, or reactive airway disease, is characterized by reversible airflow obstruction caused by bronchial smooth muscle contraction; hypersecretion of mucus, resulting in bronchial plugging; and inflammatory changes in the bronchial walls. The typical patient with asthma is in obvious distress. Respirations are rapid and loud. Treatment focuses on bronchodilation, hydration, and reducing inflammation.
- Pneumonia is a group of specific infections (bacterial, viral, or fungal). These infections cause an acute inflammatory process of the respiratory bronchioles and the alveoli. Pneumonia usually manifests with classic signs and symptoms. These include a productive cough and associated fever that produces "shaking chills." Prehospital care of patients with pneumonia includes airway support, oxygen administration, ventilatory assistance as needed, intravenous (IV) fluids, cardiac monitoring, and transport.
- Adult respiratory distress syndrome (ARDS) is a fulminant form of respiratory failure. It is characterized by acute lung inflammation and diffuse alveolar-capillary injury. It develops as a complication of illness or injury. In ARDS, the lungs are wet and heavy, congested, hemorrhagic, and stiff, with decreased perfusion capacity across alveolar membranes. Treatment includes airway and ventilatory support.
- Positive end-expiratory pressure (PEEP) maintains pressure at the end of exhalation. Adding PEEP in the respiratory circuit keeps alveoli open and pushes fluid from the alveoli back in the interstitium or capillaries. Continuous positive airway pressure (CPAP) maintains constant airway pressure throughout the entire respiratory cycle. CPAP improves diffusion and helps reexpand collapsed alveoli. Biphasic positive airway pressure delivers variable airway pressure throughout the respiratory cycle.
- Pulmonary thromboembolism is a blockage of a pulmonary artery by a clot or other foreign material. When one or more pulmonary arteries are blocked by an embolism, a section of lung is ventilated but hypoperfused. Hypotension, shock, and death can occur. Prehospital care is mainly supportive and includes oxygen administration, IV access, and transport for definitive care.

- Upper respiratory infections (URIs) affect the nose, throat, sinuses, and larynx. Signs and symptoms of a URI include sore throat, fever, chills, headache, cervical adenopathy, and an erythematous pharynx. Prehospital care is based on the patient's symptoms.
- A primary spontaneous pneumothorax usually results when a subpleural bleb ruptures. This allows air to enter the pleural space from within the lung. Signs and symptoms include shortness of breath and chest pain that often are sudden in onset, pallor, diaphoresis, and tachypnea. Prehospital care is based on the patient's symptoms and degree of distress.
- Hyperventilation syndrome is abnormally deep or rapid breathing. This type of breathing results in an excessive loss of carbon dioxide. If the syndrome clearly is caused by anxiety, prehospital care is mainly supportive (i.e., calming measures and reassurance). The paramedic may suspect that the syndrome is a result of illness or drug ingestion. If this is the case, care may include oxygen administration and airway and ventilatory support.
- Lung cancer is an expression of the uncontrolled growth of abnormal cells. As the disease progresses, signs and symptoms may include cough, hemoptysis, dyspnea, hoarseness, and dysphagia. Prehospital management includes airway, ventilatory, and circulatory support.

REVIEW QUESTIONS

Match the description in column I with the correct noninfectious pulmonary disease in column II. Use each answer only once.

Column I

1. ________ Chronic production of excessive mucus, hypoxia, and inflammation of bronchi

2. ________ Pulmonary edema secondary to trauma, inhaled toxins, or metabolic disorders

3. ________ Condition caused by a rupture of a bleb in the lung

4. ________ Impaired oxygenation resulting from blockage of a pulmonary artery by a clot

5. ________ Bronchiolar smooth muscle spasm and excess mucus production caused by allergy

6. ________ Bacterial, viral, or fungal lung infection

7. ________ Uncontrolled abnormal cell growth in the lung

8. ________ Chronic disease that results in a decrease in the alveolar membrane surface area and polycythemia

Column II

a. Adult respiratory distress syndrome
b. Asthma
c. Chronic bronchitis
d. Emphysema
e. Lung cancer
f. Hyperventilation syndrome
g. Pneumonia
h. Pulmonary thromboembolism
i. Spontaneous pneumothorax

9. For each case below, identify whether the respiratory problem is related to ventilation, diffusion, or perfusion or is a combination of two or more of these factors.
   a. Your person is found unconscious with a plastic bag over her head.
   b. A 26-year-old person is found semiconscious with a respiratory rate of 8 breaths/min. Track marks are found on the arms and legs and under the tongue.
   c. An elderly woman with a history of congestive heart failure is acutely dyspneic and cyanotic. She has crackles throughout her lungs and coughs up frothy, bloody sputum.
   d. A woman has experienced vaginal bleeding for 2 weeks. She has profound fatigue and shortness of breath.
   e. A 56-year-old person is choking in a restaurant.
   f. Your patient delivered a baby yesterday and has severe chest pain and dyspnea and an Sao_2 of 89% on room air.
   g. An 88-year-old person has a large flail segment of the right chest and is hypoxic.

Questions 10 to 12 pertain to the following case study:

You are dispatched to a call for "difficulty breathing." Dispatch tells you en route that the first responders report that the patient is in moderate respiratory distress.

10. What conditions come to mind en route to this call?

____

11. What findings in your initial assessment would indicate life-threatening respiratory distress?

____

12. What information should be gathered during the focused history and physical examination of this patient?

____

____

13. Differentiate between chronic bronchitis and emphysema by completing the following table.

Disease	Chronic Bronchitis	Emphysema
Mechanics of ventilation		
Oxygenation		
Skin color		
Physical build		
Mucus production		

Your 65-year-old patient has a history of chronic bronchitis and emphysema. She states that she has become acutely short of breath today and cannot complete a sentence without gasping for air. Auscultation of her lungs reveals inspiratory and expiratory wheezes.

14. How much oxygen should you administer to this patient? _______________________________________

15. Name a drug other than oxygen that may be administered to alleviate this patient's dyspnea if not contraindicated by the history or physical findings.

____

16. Describe any additional patient care to be given en route to the hospital.

____

____

Questions 17 to 22 pertain to the following case study:

A 19-year-old man became acutely short of breath during a soccer game. He states that he has a history of asthma. On examination, you note inspiratory and expiratory wheezes throughout the lung fields. Vital signs are BP, 130/80 mm Hg; pulse, 136 beats/min; and respirations, 30 breaths/min. You also note a pulsus paradoxus of 30 mm Hg.

17. Describe the pathophysiologic changes in the lungs that cause the patient's signs and symptoms.

____

18. Why would you perform a peak expiratory flow rate measurement on this patient?

19. Other than oxygen, what drug can be administered to treat this patient? Include the correct dose and route.

20. Describe how you will reassess the patient after the medication has been administered and what you will find if the patient's condition is improving.

21. If therapy is unsuccessful and the patient continues to deteriorate despite aggressive medication therapy, what condition might exist?

22. What additional treatment measures will you use?

23. You respond to a call for difficulty breathing. Your assessment reveals that the patient is wheezing. List one pathologic cause of wheezes for each of the following:

a. Upper airway obstruction:

b. Lower airway obstruction:

c. Trauma:

d. Alveolar pathology:

e. Interstitial space pathology:

Questions 24 to 26 pertain to the following case study:

A physician calls 9-1-1 to have you transport a patient with a diagnosis of pneumonia from her office to the hospital.

24. List four types of pneumonia.

a.

b.

c. ____

d. ____

25. What signs and symptoms may be present if this patient has bacterial pneumonia?

____

26. Describe the prehospital care of patients with known or suspected pneumonia.

____

____

27. You are transporting a 56-year-old man from a rural hospital to a trauma center 70 miles away. He was involved in a head-on motor vehicle collision 24 hours ago. He has been diagnosed with bilateral pulmonary contusions and two fractured ribs. Early in his care, he received a large volume of normal saline intravenously. He has been increasingly short of breath, was intubated before your arrival, and is very difficult to ventilate. Paralytic drugs and sedatives were administered immediately before your departure.

    a. What problem do you suspect?

____

    b. Describe the measures you will use during transport to assess and care for this patient.

____

28. List eight factors that increase the risk of pulmonary emboli.

    a. ____

    b. ____

    c. ____

    d. ____

    e. ____

    f. ____

    g. ____

    h. ____

29. List at least 10 possible signs and symptoms of pulmonary embolism.

____

____

30. List common characteristics of a patient who develops spontaneous pneumothorax.

____

31. What is an extrinsic factor associated with the development or exacerbation of respiratory disease?
    a. Cardiac or circulatory pathologies
    b. Smoking
    c. Genetic predisposition
    d. Stress

32. What factor is essential for normal ventilation to occur?
    a. Adequate blood volume
    b. Functional diaphragm and intercostal muscles
    c. Interstitial space that is not filled with fluid
    d. Pulmonary capillaries that are not occluded

33. Your patient has a chronic respiratory illness; she called you complaining of difficulty breathing. What is usually the most reliable indicator of the severity of the patient's present condition?
    a. One- or two-word dyspnea
    b. Pallor and diaphoresis
    c. Patient's description of severity
    d. Tachycardia

34. Which physical finding indicates chronic hypoxemia?
    a. Accessory muscle use
    b. Carpopedal spasm
    c. Clubbing
    d. Pursed-lip breathing

35. How can you distinguish chronic bronchitis from both emphysema and asthma?
    a. Cough
    b. Excessive mucus production
    c. Resistance to air flow
    d. Wheezing

36. Which physical finding is evidence of chronic emphysema on physical examination?
    a. Decreased anterior-posterior chest diameter
    b. Decreased capillary refill in the nail beds
    c. Diminished breath sounds throughout the lungs
    d. Decreased diastolic blood pressure

37. Pulmonary hypertension can lead to which of the following?
    a. Pulmonary edema
    b. Pulmonary embolism
    c. Renal failure
    d. Right heart failure

38. What contributes to the signs and symptoms of an acute asthma attack?
    a. Bronchial muscle dilation
    b. Bronchial inflammation
    c. Decreased dead air space
    d. Pulmonary hypertension

39. Which physical finding is the most serious when found in an asthma patient who appears to be having acute respiratory distress?
    a. Expiratory wheezing
    b. Inspiratory wheezing
    c. Silent chest and prolonged expiration
    d. Wheezing audible without a stethoscope

40. Pharmacologic therapy to treat wheezing in patients with bronchitis or asthma usually includes which of the following?
    a. Albuterol
    b. Aminophylline
    c. Epinephrine
    d. Isoproterenol

41. Which finding may signal impending respiratory failure in a 20-year-old patient with asthma?
    a. End-tidal CO_2 of 50 mm Hg
    b. SaO_2 of 94%
    c. Heart rate of 108 beats/min
    d. Glasgow Coma Scale score of 15

374

42. What is the most effective preventive measure for bacterial pneumonia?
    a. Antibiotic therapy
    b. Patient positioning
    c. Strict isolation measures
    d. Vaccination

43. Which is the greatest risk factor for aspiration pneumonia?
    a. Patients older than 80 years of age
    b. Diagnosis of influenza
    c. Glasgow Coma Scale score is 12
    d. Premature birth

44. Which of the following is true about adult respiratory distress syndrome regardless of the cause?
    a. Death always occurs as a result of this complication.
    b. Disseminated intravascular coagulation always occurs.
    c. Pneumonia is a secondary complication.
    d. Pulmonary edema will result.

45. The blood pressure of a 72-year-old patient on continuous positive airway pressure (CPAP) drops to 80/50 mm Hg. What action should you take first?
    a. Administer a fluid bolus
    b. Begin a dopamine drip
    c. Discontinue CPAP
    d. Intubate the trachea

46. What are the signs and symptoms of pulmonary embolus primarily related to?
    a. The patient's age
    b. The cause of the embolus
    c. The origin of the embolus
    d. The size of the embolus

47. What is the most important action the paramedic can take to prevent the spread of upper respiratory infections?
    a. Obtain the appropriate immunizations.
    b. Place a mask on the patient during transport.
    c. Practice good hand washing techniques.
    d. Wear a mask and goggles during patient care.

48. Which of the following is associated with the development of spontaneous pneumothorax?
    a. Asthma
    b. Free-base cocaine use
    c. IV drug abuse
    d. Thromboembolus

49. Which of the following is a cause of hyperventilation?
    a. Aspirin overdose
    b. Narcotic overdose
    c. Hypoglycemia
    d. Hypothermia

50. Exposure to what substance is the most common risk factor for lung cancer?
    a. Cigarette smoke
    b. Asbestos
    c. Coal products
    d. Ionizing radiation

WRAP IT UP

You know as you respond to a call for "difficulty breathing" that your patient is likely quite ill because the dispatcher has a pumper running the call with you. The patient is a 74-year-old man with a history of asthma and chronic bronchitis. He is leaning forward in a tripod position using pursed-lip breathing, his neck muscles strain with each breath, and he is able to say only two or three words at a time. His son tells you that his dad hasn't been feeling well all week. Today he became much worse, developing a fever and coughing up green sputum flecked with blood. His home medicines include ipratropium (Atrovent), beclomethasone (Beclovent), Advair, Singulair, and albuterol.

The patient's skin is gray and wet, his radial pulse is rapid, and an initial oxygen saturation reading is 84% on room air. His lungs sound wet and noisy, with wheezes throughout but somewhat diminished in the left base, so you apply a nebulizer mask with albuterol 2.5 mg and set the oxygen at 7 L/min. In the ambulance, the ECG monitor shows sinus tachycardia at 120/min, the Sao_2 is 94% and BP is 164/90 mm Hg, his skin is now dry, and he is speaking a bit more clearly. You start an IV, administer methylprednisolone (125 mg IV), and administer oxygen by nasal cannula at 4 L/min. The patient is admitted with a diagnosis of left lower R lobe pneumonia. He returns home in 4 days.

1. Which of the following was likely the primary problem for this patient's acute hypoxia?
   a. Inadequate diffusion between alveoli and pulmonary capillaries
   b. Inadequate perfusion of blood through the pulmonary capillary bed
   c. Inadequate ventilation in and out of the lungs
   d. a and b
   e. a and c

2. Put a ✓ beside the signs or symptoms of life-threatening respiratory distress that this patient displayed.
   a. _____ Altered mental status   e. _____ One- or two-word dyspnea
   b. _____ Severe cyanosis   f. _____ Tachycardia
   c. _____ Absent breath sounds   g. _____ Pallor or diaphoresis
   d. _____ Audible stridor   h. _____ Accessory muscle use

3. Based on this patient's reported history, what would you anticipate?
   a. He normally produces very little sputum.
   b. A thin, pink appearance would be normal for him.
   c. Lung tissue is scarred and susceptible to infection.
   d. In the absence of disease, the PO_2 is normal.

4. Explain your rationale for administration of

   a. Albuterol

   ____

   b. Methylprednisolone

   ____

5. Why might levalbuterol be a better choice for this patient? _______________________________

6. Which is true about pneumonia?
   a. It is always caused by a bacterial infection.
   b. Fever is always present.
   c. Antibiotic treatment always cures it.
   d. Inflammation of the alveoli interferes with gas exchange.

CHAPTER 24 ANSWERS

REVIEW QUESTIONS

1. c

2. a

3. i

4. h

5. b

6. g

7. e

8. d

(Questions 1–8, Objective 3)

9. a. This is a problem with diffusion because insufficient oxygen is available to diffuse across the alveolar membrane into the capillaries.

b. This represents a problem with ventilation. The drugs may have depressed the central nervous system, causing slower, shallower breathing.

c. This is likely to be related to a problem with diffusion from the fluid that has leaked into the interstitial spaces and with perfusion because the left side of the heart is not functioning well.

d. These symptoms are likely related to anemia, which causes a problem with perfusion so oxygen cannot be carried to the tissues.

e. Airway obstruction creates a problem with ventilation.

f. These signs and symptoms suggest pulmonary embolism, which creates a problem with perfusion.

g. Flail chest is often accompanied by pulmonary contusion. This would create a problem with ventilation because of the mechanical disruption and diffusion related to the fluid in the pulmonary spaces.

(Objective 1)

10. Asthma, chronic obstructive pulmonary disease, heart failure, pulmonary edema, pulmonary embolism, bronchiolitis (infants), foreign body aspiration, toxic inhalation, pneumonia, spontaneous pneumothorax, hyperventilation syndrome, and lung cancer are some of the conditions that may present with this chief complaint. (Objective 3)

11. Signs and symptoms that indicate a life threat include alterations in mental status, severe cyanosis, absent breath sounds, audible stridor, one- or two-word dyspnea, tachycardia, pallor and diaphoresis, cardiac dysrhythmias, a pulse rate over 130 beats/min, poor, floppy muscle tone, and the presence of retractions or the use of accessory muscles. (Objective 2)

12. You should ask about the patient's chief complaint and determine whether he or she has any chest pain, productive or nonproductive cough, hemoptysis, wheezing, or signs of respiratory infection (e.g., fever or increased sputum production). Inquire about the patient's medical history, especially with regard to similar problems and the individual's perceived severity of this episode. Obtain a medication history and ask whether the patient has ever needed intubation to manage this type of illness. The physical examination should begin by noting your general impression of the patient. Note the patient's position, mentation, ability to speak, respiratory effort, and skin color. Observe the heart rate for tachycardia or bradycardia. Note any abnormal respiratory patterns. Assess the face and neck for pursed-lip breathing and use of accessory muscles. Evaluate the neck for jugular venous distension. Inspect the chest for injury, indicators of chronic disease, accessory muscle use, and chest symmetry. Auscultate the lungs for abnormal breath sounds. Assess the extremities for peripheral cyanosis, clubbing of the fingers, and carpopedal spasm. (Objective 2)

13.

Disease	Chronic Bronchitis	Emphysema
Mechanics of ventilation	Inflammation of airways and congestion with mucus; retain CO_2	Resistance to airflow, especially on exhalation
Oxygenation	Hypoxia	Decreased
Skin color	Cyanotic	Normal unless ill
Physical build	"Bloated"; may be related to right heart failure	Barrel chest; thin
Mucus production	Chronic production of large amount of sputum	Not excessive unless ill

(Objective 3)

14. Oxygen should be administered initially at 2 L/min if the patient is not in respiratory failure. If rapid improvement does not occur, the flow of oxygen should be increased while the paramedic carefully monitors the patient. If the patient's condition is critical, intubation and assisted ventilation may be necessary.
(Objective 3)

15. Albuterol, levalbuterol
(Objective 3)

16. Transport the patient in a position of comfort; apply continuous positive airway pressure if indicated by protocol; instruct the patient to use pursed-lip breathing and to minimize physical activity to conserve energy for breathing; calmly reassure and care for the patient and provide a cool environment for transport.
(Objective 3)

17. An acute asthma attack is marked by reversible airflow obstruction caused by bronchial smooth muscle contraction; hypersecretion of mucus, causing bronchial plugging; and inflammatory changes in the bronchial walls. Increased work of breathing increases negative pressure in chest, which affects blood pressure.
(Objective 3)

18. Measurement of the peak expiratory flow rate can aid in the determination of the severity of an asthma attack, as well as the evaluation of the effectiveness of treatment in reversing airway obstruction.
(Objective 2)

19. Albuterol, 0.5 mL (2.5 mg) or (levalbuterol 0.63–1.25 mg) in 2.5 mL of normal saline by nebulizer at 6 to 7 L/min O_2.
(Objective 3)

20. Ask the patient if his breathing is easier. Observe the patient for decreased anxiety, changes in level of consciousness, and the ability to converse more easily. Note the degree of respiratory distress by observing the patient's position, use of accessory muscles, and respiratory rate. Monitor vital signs (the pulse and respiratory rate should decrease, and pulsus paradoxus should drop below 20 mm Hg). As the patient improves, the inspiratory and then expiratory wheezes should disappear.
(Objective 2)

21. Status asthmaticus
(Objective 3)

22. Make sure that oxygen is at 100% and humidified, increase the fluid rate to hydrate the patient, administer other medications (e.g., methylprednisolone, hydrocortisone) as ordered by medical direction, expedite transport, monitor the patient closely for signs of respiratory failure, and prepare to intubate if necessary. If intubation is indicated, follow local medical protocols, which may include sedation (ketamine, benzodiazepine, or barbiturates); paralyze the patient; intubate; confirm endotracheal tube placement; ventilate at 6 to 10 breaths/min and use smaller tidal volumes (6–8 mL/kg); and use shorter inspiratory time and longer expiratory time.
(Objective 3)

23. a. Upper airway obstruction: foreign body, epiglottitis;
    b. lower airway obstruction: asthma, airway edema;
    c. trauma: inhalation injury, adult respiratory distress syndrome (ARDS) secondary to pulmonary contusion;
    d. alveolar pathology: chronic obstructive pulmonary disease (COPD), lung cancer, inhalation injury;
    e. interstitial space pathology: pulmonary edema, near drowning
(Objective 3)

24. Viral, bacterial, mycoplasmal, and aspiration
(Objective 3)

25. Signs and symptoms of bacterial pneumonia include shaking chills, tachypnea, tachycardia, cough with sputum (rust colored, hemoptysis, yellow, green, or gray), malaise, anorexia, flank or back pain, vomiting, fever, wheezing, fine crackles, dyspnea, and sore throat
(Objective 3)

378

26. Care includes airway support, oxygen administration, ventilatory assistance, IV fluids, cardiac and oxygen saturation monitoring, and transportation. If wheezing is present, bronchodilator therapy may be used. (Objective 3)

27. a. Adult respiratory distress syndrome; b. Monitor the rise and fall of the chest to determine the effectiveness of ventilation; note any difficulty or increasing pressure necessary to ventilate the patient; frequently assess vital signs, observing for an increased heart rate; monitor the electrocardiogram, end-tidal CO_2, and oxygen saturation by pulse oximetry; observe for cyanosis. Ventilate with high-flow oxygen; ventilate with positive end-expiratory pressure using a Boehringer valve if trained and authorized by medical direction; and administer steroids and diuretics if ordered by medical direction. (Objective 3)

28. Extended travel; prolonged bed rest; obesity; older adulthood; burns; varicose veins; surgery of the thorax, abdomen, pelvis, and legs; pelvic or leg fractures; malignancy; use of birth control pills; congenital or acquired coagulopathies; pregnancy; chronic obstructive pulmonary disease; congestive heart failure; sickle cell anemia; cancer; atrial fibrillation; myocardial infarction; previous pulmonary embolism; deep vein thrombosis; infection; diabetes mellitus; and multiple trauma (Objective 3)

29. Dyspnea, cough, hemoptysis, pain, anxiety, syncope, hypotension, diaphoresis, increased respiratory rate, increased heart rate, fever, distended neck veins, chest splinting, pleuritic chest pain, pleural friction rub, crackles, right bundle branch block, and wheezes (localized) (Objective 3)

30. This typically occurs in tall, thin men between the ages of 20 and 40 years. It may also be found in patients with COPD; patients with acquired immunodeficiency syndrome (AIDS) who have pneumonia; and drug abusers who deeply inhale free-base cocaine, marijuana, or inhalants such as glue or solvents. (Objective 3)

STUDENT SELF-ASSESSMENT

31. b. Cardiac, genetic, and stress factors are all intrinsic factors. (Objective 1)

32. b. Adequate blood volume and patent pulmonary capillaries are related to perfusion. Normal interstitial space affects diffusion. (Objective 1)

33. c. All of the answers represent findings that indicate respiratory distress; however, in a patient with chronic respiratory illness, the patient's reported level of distress is often the best indication of the severity of the condition. (Objective 2)

34. c. This sign takes a long time to develop. Acutely hypoxic patients may use accessory muscles or pursed-lip breathing in an attempt to improve ventilation. Carpopedal spasm is seen secondary to hypocapnia. (Objective 2)

35. b. All will have wheezing and cough when acutely ill. Resistance to airflow is seen in all three conditions, although less so in emphysema. (Objective 3)

36. c. The patient is more likely to be tachycardic than bradycardic. Capillary refill is an indicator of perfusion (flow) rather than oxygenation. (Objective 3)

37. d. Right-heart failure can develop secondary to pulmonary hypertension (cor pulmonale). The right side of the heart increasingly is forced to pump harder to overcome the excess pressure in the pulmonary arteries. Eventually, it cannot force the blood through, and fluid backs up to the venous side of the system. (Objective 3)

38. b. Bronchial dilation and excessive thick mucus production also contribute to asthma's signs and symptoms.
(Objective 3)

39. c. Expiratory wheezing indicates narrowing of the smaller airways. As the larger airways become obstructed, inspiratory wheezing becomes audible. When the obstruction becomes so severe that almost no airflow is present, the chest is silent, with diminished breath sounds and no wheezes.
(Objective 3)

40. a. Albuterol is a beta-2 agonist that causes relatively few side effects. Although all the other drugs also cause bronchodilation, they are rarely used because of their high incidence of side effects.
(Objective 3)

41. a. Increasing CO_2 levels mean that ventilation is decreasing. Mild hypoxia or tachycardia are found in respiratory distress. A GCS score of 15 is normal.
(Objective 3)

42. d. The vaccine is 80% to 90% effective in the prevention of pneumonia caused by the pneumococcus bacillus.
(Objective 3)

43. c. Altered level of consciousness may impair the gag reflex or the patient's ability to handle secretions.
(Objective 3)

44. d. Not all patients die, although the mortality rate is high (>65%). Disseminated intravascular coagulation may occur in some but not all patients.
(Objective 3)

45. c. Continuous positive airway pressure (CPAP) can decrease venous return and reduce the blood pressure. Other interventions may be indicated after the CPAP is removed based on the patient's underlying condition.
(Objective 3)

46. d. The size and location of the embolus determine whether mild signs and symptoms or sudden death occurs.
(Objective 3)

47. c. Most upper respiratory infections have no identifiable cause. Good hand washing is an important action for preventing their spread.
(Objective 3)

48. b. Other risk factors for spontaneous pneumothorax include patients with emphysema; people with AIDS who develop pneumonia; and healthy tall, thin men between the ages of 20 and 40 years.
(Objective 3)

49. a. An aspirin overdose can cause metabolic acidosis with an increased rate and depth of respiration to compensate. Narcotic overdose is associated with respiratory depression. Respirations may slow in hypothermia.
(Objective 3)

50. a. Heavy smokers have a 25 times greater risk of developing lung cancer than nonsmokers.
(Objective 3)

WRAP IT UP

1. e. Mucus production and inflammation of the alveoli impair ventilation and diffusion.
(Objective 1)

2. b, e, f, g, h
(Objective 2)

3. c. Patients with chronic bronchitis tend to be overweight and have persistent hypoxia and chronic excessive mucus production.
(Objective 2)

4. a. Albuterol is a bronchodilator that relaxes bronchiolar smooth muscle, enlarging the airway passages and allowing better exchange of gases in the lungs.

   b. Methylprednisolone is a steroid that reduces swelling and inflammation in the lung tissues, permitting better airflow and diffusion.
(Objective 3)

5. Levalbuterol is less likely to increase the heart rate than albuterol. Because this is an elderly patient who is already tachycardic (HR, 120 beats/min), it would be the drug of choice (if available).
(Objective 3)

6. d. Pneumonia can be caused by bacterial, viral, or fungal infections. Not all of these organisms are susceptible to antibiotics. Fever may not be present, especially in immunocompromised patients.
(Objective 3)

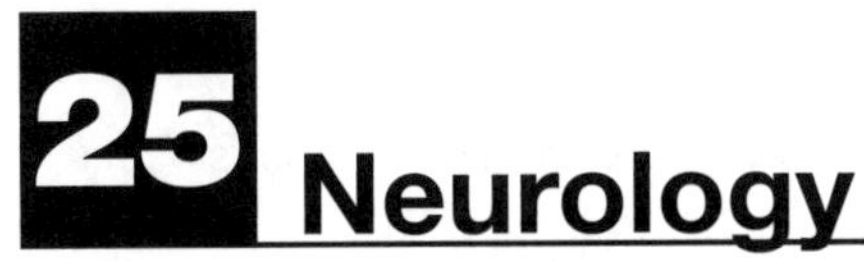

Neurology

READING ASSIGNMENT

Chapter 25, pages 764-799, in *Mosby's Paramedic Textbook*, ed. 4.

OBJECTIVES

Upon completion of this chapter, the paramedic student will be able to do the following:

1. Describe the anatomy and physiology of the nervous system.
2. Outline pathophysiologic changes in the nervous system that may alter the cerebral perfusion pressure.
3. Describe the assessment of a patient with a nervous system disorder.
4. Describe the pathophysiology, signs and symptoms, and specific management techniques for each of the following neurologic disorders: coma, stroke and intracranial hemorrhage, seizure disorders, headaches, brain neoplasm and brain abscess, and degenerative neurologic diseases.

SUMMARY

- The human body's ability to maintain a state of balance, or *homeostasis,* results from the nervous system's regulatory and coordinating activities. The vertebral arteries and the internal carotid arteries supply blood to the brain.
- Neurologic emergencies are a consequence of structural changes or damage, circulatory changes, or alterations in intracranial pressure that affect cerebral blood flow.
- Cerebral blood flow depends on cerebral perfusion pressure (CPP). CPP decreases when mean arterial pressure (MAP) drops or when intracranial pressure increases. CPP = MAP – ICP
- The primary survey begins by determining the patient's level of consciousness and by ensuring an open and patent airway. Key elements of the physical examination that may provide clues to the nature of the neurologic emergency include the patient history and the history of the event, vital signs, and respiratory patterns.
- The neurologic exam may include assessment of AVPU, Glasgow Coma Scale, posturing or paralysis, reflexes, pupil size and response, and extraocular movements.
- *Coma* is an abnormally deep state of unconsciousness. The patient cannot be aroused from this state by external stimuli. In general, two mechanisms produce coma: structural lesions and toxic-metabolic states.
- *Stroke* is a sudden interruption in blood flow to the brain that results in a neurologic deficit. Strokes can be classified as ischemic strokes or hemorrhagic strokes. Use a stroke scale to assess for the presence of stroke. Rapid transport to a stroke resource center (if available) is indicated.
- A *seizure* is a brief alteration in behavior or consciousness. It is caused by abnormal electrical activity of one or more groups of neurons in the brain. In the prehospital setting, determining the cause of a seizure is not as important as other measures. These include managing the complications and recognizing whether the seizure is reversible with therapy (e.g., it is caused by hypoglycemia).
- The four fairly common types of headaches are tension headaches, migraines, cluster headaches, and sinus headaches.
- A central nervous system tumor, or *neoplasm,* is a mass in the cranial cavity or spinal cord. This mass can be either malignant or benign. Heredity may play a role in the development of brain tumors. They also are associated with several risk factors. These include exposure to radiation, tobacco use, dietary habits, some viruses, and the use of some medications.
- A *brain abscess* is a buildup of purulent material (pus) surrounded by a capsule within the brain. It develops from a bacterial infection. The infection often starts in the nasal cavity, middle ear, or mastoid bone.
- Dementia is a slow, progressive loss of awareness of time and place. Alzheimer disease is the most common cause of dementia. Picks disease is another type of dementia. It is associated with language disturbance.
- Huntington disease causes degeneration of neurons in the brain. This causes uncontrolled movements and intellectual and emotional impairment.
- Creutzfeldt-Jakob disease is characterized by rapid progression of dementia.
- Muscular dystrophy is an inherited muscle disorder. The cause is unknown. The disease is marked by a slow but progressive degeneration of muscle fibers.

383

- Damage to the white matter of the brain in multiple sclerosis may lead to fatigue, vertigo, clumsiness, unsteady gait, slurred speech, blurred or double vision, and facial numbness or pain.
- Guillain-Barré syndrome is an autoimmune disorder that causes muscle weakness that progresses to paralysis that includes the muscles of respiration.
- The term *dystonia* refers to local or diffuse changes in muscle tone. These may cause painful muscle spasms, unusually fixed postures, and strange movement patterns.
- Parkinson disease usually begins as a slight tremor in one hand, arm, or leg. In the later stages, the disease affects both sides of the body, causing stiffness, weakness, and trembling of the muscles.
- The term *central pain syndrome* refers to infection or disease of the trigeminal nerve. This causes intense pain of the face.
- Acoustic neuroma is a noncancerous tumor that affects the eighth cranial nerve. It impairs balance and hearing.
- Glossopharyngeal neuralgia is an irritation of cranial nerve IX that causes pain in the nose, ear, and throat.
- Hemifacial spasm results in involuntary contractions of muscles on one side of the face.
- *Bell palsy* is paralysis of the facial muscles. It is caused by inflammation of the seventh cranial nerve. The condition is usually one sided and temporary. It often develops suddenly.
- Amyotrophic lateral sclerosis is also called *Lou Gehrig disease*. It is one of a group of rare nervous system disorders. In these disorders, the nerves that control muscular activity degenerate in the brain and spinal cord.
- Peripheral neuropathies usually arise from damage to or irritation of either the axons or their myelin sheaths. This slows or fully blocks the passage of electrical signals.
- The term *myoclonus* refers to rapid and uncontrollable muscle contractions or spasms. These occur at rest or during movement.
- *Spina bifida* is a congenital defect in which part of one or more vertebrae fails to develop completely. This leaves a portion of the spinal cord exposed.
- Polio is caused by a virus. The severity of the disease can range from unapparent infection, to a febrile illness without neurologic aftereffects, to aseptic meningitis, and finally to paralytic disease and possibly death.

REVIEW QUESTIONS

For each of the causes in column I, identify the appropriate general cause of coma in column II. Each answer may be used more than once.

Column I

1. ________ The patient's blood pressure rose suddenly to 240/140 mm Hg.

2. ________ The patient's chronic bronchitis is much worse.

3. ________ The patient has missed dialysis for 1 week.

4. ________ The patient's blood alcohol level is 400 mg/dL.

5. ________ The patient's glucose level is 30 mg/dL.

6. ________ The teenage patient has meningitis.

Column II

a. Cardiovascular system
b. Drugs
c. Infectious
d. Metabolic system
e. Respiratory system
f. Structural cause

Match the illness in column II with the description in column I. Use each illness only once.

Column I

7. ________ Blurred vision and unsteady gait

8. ________ Severe muscle spasms because of torticollis

9. ________ Burning sensation in the feet because of diabetes

10. ________ Viral illness causing respiratory paralysis

11. ________ Muscle trembling because of a decrease in dopamine

12. ________ Male genetic disorder that causes muscle wasting

13. ________ Intense facial pain activated by a trigger point

Column II

a. Amyotrophic lateral sclerosis
b. Bell palsy
c. Central pain syndrome
d. Dystonia
e. Multiple sclerosis
f. Muscular dystrophy
g. Myoclonus
h. Parkinson disease
i. Peripheral neuropathy
j. Polio
k. Spina bifida

14. _________ Central nervous system degeneration in
patients older than age 50 years that leads
to severe muscle deterioration

15. _________ Temporary facial paralysis caused by
inflammation

16. _________ Genetic defect that leaves the spinal cord
exposed

17. Complete the following sentences.

The cells of the nervous system that protect the neurons are called **(a)** _______________ _______________

_______________. Each neuron has three main parts. The area that contains the nucleus is the **(b)**

_______________; one or more branching projections that receive impulses are known as the **(c)** _______________;

and a single, elongated projection that transmits impulses is called the **(d)** _______________. In the peripheral

nervous system, bundles of axons and their sheaths are called **(e)** _______________. Neurons are classified by the
direction in which they transmit impulses. The neurons that transmit impulses to the spinal cord and brain from

the body are **(f)** _______________ neurons. Neurons that transmit impulses away from the brain to muscle and

glandular tissue are **(g)** _______________ neurons. Neurons that conduct impulses from sensory neurons directly

to motor neurons are **(h)** _______________. In its resting state, the charge inside the neuron is **(i)** _______________,

and the charge outside the neuron is **(j)** _______________. When the neuron is stimulated while the outside is

positively charged, **(k)** _______________ ions rush into the cell and begin a wave of **(l)** _______________ that

travels down the cell. Myelinated axons have interruptions in the myelin sheaths, called **(m)** _______________,

_______________ that cause the action potential to be conducted more **(n)** _______________ than unmyelinated

axons. The space between the nerve endings of two adjacent neurons is known as a(n) **(o)** _______________.

Impulses are transmitted across these spaces by neurotransmitters such as **(p)** _______________, _______________,

and _______________.

18. List the basic anatomic components of a reflex.

____

19. Name the two paired arteries that supply blood to the brain.

a. Posterior: ____

b. Anterior: ____

20. State whether the following factors will _increase_, _decrease_, or _not change_ the cerebral blood flow.

a. Intracranial pressure of 30 mm Hg: _______________________________________

b. Mean arterial pressure of 40 mm Hg: ______________________________________

c. Expanding tumor in the brain: ____

d. Hypovolemic shock: ____

21. List at least two causes of coma for each of the following six general classifications.

    a. Structural:

____

    b. Metabolic:

____

    c. Drug induced:

____

    d. Cardiovascular:

____

    e. Respiratory:

____

    f. Infectious:

____

22. A patient has a neurologic disorder. He opens his eyes and speaks when you call his name but does not know what day it is. He is moving all extremities normally.

    a. List six specific questions you should ask the family to elicit the nature of the neurologic problem.

____

____

    b. What vital sign findings would suggest increased intracranial pressure?

____

    c. Using the AVPU assessment, describe the patient's level of consciousness.

____

    d. What is his score on the Glasgow Coma Scale?

____

    e. How will you assess this patient's eyes?

____

23. State whether the following symptoms of coma are most likely to be found in structural or toxic-metabolic coma.

    a. Asymmetric neurologic findings: ____

    b. Slow onset: ____

    c. Unilateral fixed and dilated pupil: ____

Chapter **25** **Neurology**

24. A 65-year-old woman was found unresponsive by her neighbors. She has snoring respirations at a rate of 8 breaths/min, and you easily place an oral airway. Carotid and radial pulses are present and rapid. Blood pressure is 110/70 mm Hg. She flexes to painful stimuli, no history is available, and her blood glucose level is 60 mg/dL. Outline your assessment and management of this patient, including the appropriate dose and route of administration of any drugs you would give.

____

____

____

Questions 25 to 29 refer to the following case study:

An elderly African American man is lying on the sofa. His family states, "He hasn't been acting right." He is awake and confused, with slurred speech. He follows commands appropriately. When you ask him to smile, he has an apparent facial droop on the right. Ongoing assessment reveals weakness in the left arm and leg. His vital signs are BP, 160/108 mm Hg; P, 72 beats/min; and R, 16 breaths/min and regular. His Sao_2 is 95%, and his blood glucose level is 94 mg/dL. He has no allergies, and his medications include hydrochlorothiazide, nitroglycerin, and insulin. His family states that a similar incident occurred yesterday and lasted about 5 minutes after he took a walk. He smokes one pack of cigarettes a day.

25. List eight risk factors for stroke that you can identify for this patient and note whether each is modifiable or nonmodifiable.

Risk Factor	Modifiable (Yes or No)
a.	
b.	
c.	
d.	
e.	
f.	
g.	
h.	

26. List at least six signs or symptoms of cerebrovascular accident that are common to embolic and thrombotic strokes. (Place a star beside the ones experienced by this patient.)

____

____

27. List the physical findings that would indicate the probability of stroke for this patient based on

a. The Cincinnati stroke scale: ____

____

b. The Los Angeles Prehospital Stroke Screen: _________________________________

____

387

Chapter **25** **Neurology**

28. List the seven *D*s of stroke management.

D ____

D ____

D ____

D ____

D ____

D ____

D ____

29. Outline your prehospital care of this patient.

____

____

____

30. Although patients may have diverse presentations, describe the typical progression of signs and symptoms of hemorrhagic stroke.

____

____

31. List five causes of seizures:

a. ____

b. ____

c. ____

d. ____

e. ____

32. State the type of seizure for each of the following signs and symptoms.

a. Numbness of the body or unusual visual, auditory, or taste symptoms:

____

b. Brief loss of consciousness in a child (without loss of posture) that lasts less than 15 seconds:

____

c. Partial seizure activity that spreads in an orderly fashion to the surrounding areas:

____

d. Preceding aura followed by loss of consciousness and tonic-clonic motor activity followed by a postictal state:

____

e. Aura followed by automatisms such as lip smacking and chewing, during which time the patient is amnesic:

____

33. What history should be obtained from the family of a patient who has had a grand mal seizure?

____

34. List two findings that suggest that the seizure is hysterical rather than grand mal.

a. ____

b. ____

35. State whether each of the following characteristics is more suggestive of seizure or syncope:

a. It starts in a standing position:

____

b. It is preceded by lightheadedness:

____

c. The patient remains unconscious for minutes to hours:

____

d. Tachycardia occurs:

____

36. List two anticonvulsants (with the appropriate doses) that may be given to an adult patient having a seizure.

a. ____

b. ____

37. Identify the type of headache (tension, migraine, cluster, or sinus) typically associated with each of the following case presentations.

a. You are dispatched at 0100 to care for a patient who is complaining of a severe headache that woke him. He says the pain is most intense around his left eye, and you note that his eyes are tearing and his nose is

running._____________________________

b. Your partner is recovering from an upper respiratory infection and complaining of a headache that affects her forehead and upper face. She describes an intense pressure sensation that increases when she bends over.

____

c. Your patient is complaining of a dull, throbbing headache that started a week ago and will not stop.

____

d. A 24-year-old woman is complaining of a severe headache that began as an intense throbbing on the right side of her head and is now generalized. She has vomited three times. She indicates a history of this and takes a beta-blocker._________________

STUDENT SELF-ASSESSMENT

38. Which blood vessel or vessels supply the front lobes of the brain?
   a. Anterior cerebral arteries   **c.** Posterior cerebral arteries
   b. Midline basilar artery   **d.** Right and left vertebral arteries

39. An important function of the circle of Willis is to maintain blood supply to the brain if which of the following occurs?
   a. The patient becomes hypoxic because of shock.
   b. The patient has a large hemorrhagic stroke.
   c. Intracranial pressure increases suddenly.
   d. The vertebral or internal carotid arteries are blocked.

40. Which of these factors will cause a decrease in the cerebral blood flow?
   a. Blood pressure of 70/50 mm Hg
   b. Intracranial pressure of 15 mm Hg
   c. Decreased levels of intraocular fluid
   d. Body temperature of 102°F (38.9°C)

41. Which respiratory pattern associated with neurologic or endocrine disorders requires immediate assisted ventilation?
   a. Ataxic respirations
   b. Hyperpnea
   c. Neurogenic hyperventilation
   d. Kussmaul respirations

42. What is posturing caused by structural impairment of the subcortical regions of the brain called?
   a. Extension rigidity   **c.** Dysconjugate gaze
   b. Flexion rigidity   **d.** Flaccidity

43. Your comatose patient's pupils are 2 mm and round and reactive to light. What does this suggest?
   a. Barbiturate overdose   **c.** Opiate overdose
   b. Medullary injury   **d.** Temporal herniation

44. How should you manage a postictal patient with a known seizure disorder who initially aroused to pain and then began to moan and move spontaneously?
   a. Administration of naloxone (2 mg IV)
   b. Administration of diazepam (5 mg IV)
   c. Intravenous fluid therapy with normal saline (100 mL/hr)
   d. Lateral recumbent positioning of the patient

45. Which 35-year-old patient is at highest risk of ischemic stroke?
   a. Cigarette smoker
   b. Obese person with asthma
   c. Person with hypertension and sickle cell disease
   d. Person with a known cerebral aneurysm

46. Which of the following findings would indicate a high probability of stroke based on the Cincinnati prehospital stroke scale?
   a. The patient has the worst headache ever felt.
   b. The patient cannot speak clearly to you.
   c. The patient experiences a new onset of seizures.
   d. The patient complains of double vision.

390

47. Your patient has continuous, rapid muscle jerking that the family says is related to his neuromuscular disease. What are these movements called?
   a. Dystonia
   b. Atrophy
   c. Myoclonus
   d. Palsy

48. Which characteristic is associated with Pick disease?
   a. Aphasia
   b. Rapid onset
   c. Staggering gait
   d. Weak grips

49. Why does a patient with acoustic neuroma lose hearing?
   a. Cancer blocks the ear canal
   b. Compression of cranial nerve VIII
   c. Cochlear infection
   d. Cerumen impaction

50. A 52-year-old man has Huntington disease. What is a likely cause of impaired oxygenation?
   a. Aspiration of fluids
   b. Apnea secondary to seizure
   c. Degeneration of alveoli
   d. Constriction of chest muscles

51. What alteration in pulmonary function would you anticipate as the signs and symptoms of Guillain- Barré syndrome progress?
   a. Decreased minute volume
   b. Decreased end-tidal CO_2
   c. Increased tidal volume
   d. Increased dead air space

WRAP IT UP

You respond to a call for "seizures." When you arrive, you find a 72-year-old man who opens his eyes to pain, pushes your hand away when you apply nail bed pressure, calls out cuss words, then quickly appears to sleep again and has snoring respirations. You insert a nasal airway and administer oxygen by mask while you continue your examination. His wife explains that he was in the bathroom having a bowel movement when she heard a noise, and when she got to him, his limbs jerked rhythmically for several minutes, and then he "passed out." She says that he had been complaining of a headache this morning. He takes furosemide and enalapril. As you continue your examination, the patient becomes progressively more awake. His vital signs are BP, 192/98 mm Hg; P, 96 beats/min; R, 20 breaths/min; Sao_2, 99% (on oxygen); blood glucose, 99 mg/dL; pupils 4 mm, equal, and reactive to light. You initiate an IV of normal saline TKO and, seeing no traumatic injury on your exam, move the patient to your stretcher. In the ambulance, you place the patient on an ECG monitor and observe a normal sinus rhythm. You transport him 4 minutes to the closest hospital, continuously monitoring his neurologic status and vital signs, which have not changed. As you move him to the emergency department cot, he experiences another seizure with tonic-clonic movements; his breathing then becomes ataxic, his pupils become fixed and dilated, he is unresponsive to painful stimulus, and his heart rate drops quickly until his ventilations are assisted. CT scan reveals a large hemorrhagic stroke, and the patient dies within 6 hours of arrival at the hospital.

1. What were the patient's Glasgow Coma Scale values

   a. Initially: ____

   b. After his seizure in the ED: ____

2. Were any signs of increased intracranial pressure present

   a. When you arrived: ____

   b. After the patient had his second seizure: ____

3. If the patient had continued to have a seizure, list two drugs (and their appropriate dose) that could have been administered.

    a. ____

    b. ____

4. Explain some possible causes of the patient's condition that you tried to rule out as you initially assessed the patient.

____

____

5. Identify at least four risk factors for stroke that you have determined this patient had.

____

____

6. Place a ✓ beside the signs or symptoms of stroke that this patient showed.

a. _______ Aphasia			**h.** _______ Headache
b. _______ Ataxia			**i.** _______ Hemiparesis
c. _______ Confusion			**j.** _______ Incontinence
d. _______ Coma			**k.** _______ Monocular blindness
e. _______ Diplopia			**l.** _______ Numbness
f. _______ Dizziness			**m.** _______ Seizure
g. _______ Dysarthria			

7. What leads you to believe that this patient had a hemorrhagic rather than an ischemic stroke?

____

8. Which is true of this patient's Cincinnati or Los Angeles Prehospital Stroke Screen?
    a. Both demonstrate a high probability of stroke.
    b. Both confirm the presence of stoke.
    c. Neither can be performed on this patient.
    d. Only the LAPSS demonstrates stroke in this case.

CHAPTER 25 ANSWERS

REVIEW QUESTIONS

1. a

2. e

3. d

4. b

5. d

6. c

7. e

8. d

9. i

10. j

11. h

12. f

13. c

14. a

15. b

16. k
(Questions 1-16, Objective 4)

17. a. Neuroglia; b. cell body; c. dendrites; d. axon; e. white matter; f. sensory; g. motor; h. interneurons; i. negative; j. positive; k. sodium; l. depolarization; m. nodes of Ranvier; n. quickly; o. synapse; p. norepinephrine, epinephrine, and dopamine.
(Objective 1)

18. Sensory receptor, sensory neuron, interneurons, motor neuron, and effector organ
(Objective 1)

19. a. Vertebral arteries; b. internal carotid arteries
(Objective 1)

20. a. Decrease; b. decrease; c. decrease; d. decrease
(Objective 2)

21. a. Intracranial bleeding, head trauma, brain tumor, or another space-occupying lesion; b. anoxia, hypoglycemia, diabetic ketoacidosis, thiamine deficiency, kidney and liver failure, and postictal phase of a seizure; c. barbiturates, narcotics, hallucinogenics, depressants, and alcohol; d. hypertensive encephalopathy, shock, dysrhythmias, and stroke; e. chronic obstructive pulmonary disease and toxic inhalation; f. meningitis and sepsis
(Objective 4)

22. a. Why did you call EMS? What happened during the course of this situation? Does the patient have any medical problems, such as heart or lung disease, neurologic illness, diabetes, or high blood pressure? Does the patient have a history of drug or alcohol abuse or stroke? Has this ever happened to him before? Do you know if he has had any injuries recently?
b. Increased blood pressure, decreased pulse, widened pulse pressure, slow or irregular respiratory rate
c. He is responsive to verbal stimuli.
d. GCS score = 13
e. Assess the pupils for shape, size, equality, and response to light. Assess the patient's extraocular movements by asking him to follow your finger movements with his eyes (to the extreme left, up and down, to the extreme right, up and down).
(Objective 3)

23. a. Structural; b. toxic-metabolic; c. structural
(Objective 4)

24. Secure the airway and ventilate with 100% oxygen (with inline immobilization of the spine if indicated). Assess the carotid and radial pulses. Assess vital signs, oxygen saturation, breath sounds, ECG, and pupil response. Scan the body for obvious trauma. Draw a blood sample while initiating an IV with 0.9% normal saline. Because the blood glucose level is less than 80 mg/dL, administer thiamine (100 mg IV), reassess, administer 25 g of $D_{50}W$ IV, and reassess. (If the blood glucose level had been normal, you would have administered naloxone [Narcan] [2 mg IV] and reassessed.) If no improvement occurs and the patient has no gag reflex, she should be intubated (and tube placement verified). Perform ongoing assessment and transport.
(Objectives 3, 4)

25.	Risk Factor	Modifiable (Yes or No)
	a. Age (elderly)	No
	b. Race (African American)	No
	c. Gender (male)	No
	d. Hypertension	Yes
	e. Heart disease (nitroglycerin)	Yes
	f. Diabetes (insulin)	Yes
	g. Transient ischemic attacks	Yes
	h. Smoking	Yes

(Objective 4)

26. Confusion* or coma, dysarthria*, aphasia, facial droop* or facial numbness, hemiparesis* or hemiplegia, convulsions, incontinence, diplopia, headache, dizziness, ataxia, monocular blindness, or vertigo
(Objective 4)

27. a. Facial droop, arm drift, and slurred speech; b. Patient is older than age 45 years, has no history of seizures, symptom duration is longer than 24 hours, patient is not a wheelchair user, blood glucose is normal, and the patient has obvious asymmetry of smile and arm strength.
(Objective 4)

28. Detection, dispatch, delivery (to a stroke center), door (appropriate hospital for rapid treatment of stroke), data (include CT scan), decision (appropriateness of fibrinolytic therapy), drug.
(Objective 4)

29. Make sure that his airway remains patent. Try to determine the time of onset. Administer supplemental oxygen if his Sao_2 drops below 94% or his condition worsens. Monitor vital signs and ECG. Elevate the head of the stretcher 15 degrees. Initiate IV LR or NS at 50 mL/hr. Protect the affected extremities. Maintain normal temperature. Notify and transport quickly to the closest stroke center. Control seizures, if present, with benzodiazepines. Comfort and reassure the patient and family.
(Objective 4)

30. Hemorrhagic stroke commonly occurs during stress or exertion. It starts abruptly and often begins with a headache, nausea, vomiting, and progressive deterioration of neurologic status. The patient may rapidly lose consciousness or have a seizure.
(Objective 4)

31. Stroke, head trauma, toxins, hypoxia, hypoglycemia, infection, metabolic abnormalities, brain tumor, vascular disorders, eclampsia, and drug overdose
(Objective 4)

32. a. Simple sensory seizure (partial seizure); b. petit mal (generalized seizure); c. jacksonian seizure (partial seizure); d. grand mal seizure (generalized seizure); e. complex partial seizures (partial seizure).
(Objective 4)

33. History of seizures, including frequency and medication compliance; description of seizure (length, features, incontinence, tongue biting); history of head trauma; fever, headache, or nuchal rigidity before seizure; medical history, including diabetes, cardiovascular disease, and stroke
(Objective 4)

34. With a hysterical seizure, the following do not occur: trauma to the tongue, incontinence, and response to conventional therapy. A hysterical seizure may stop with a sharp command or sternal rub.
(Objective 4)

35. a. Syncope; b. syncope; c. seizure; d. seizure
(Objective 4)

36. Lorazepam (1 to 2 mg IV) or diazepam (5 to 10 mg IV) every 15 minutes as necessary
(Objective 4)

37. a. Cluster headache; b. sinus headache; c. tension headache; d. migraine headache.
(Objective 4)

STUDENT SELF-ASSESSMENT

38. a. The internal carotid arteries give rise to the anterior cerebral arteries. The vertebral arteries supply the cerebellum and unite to form the basilar artery.
(Objective 1)

39. d. The circle of Willis would not protect against a large cerebral bleed, systemic hypoxia, or increased ICP. It can help to maintain blood flow if a clot exists in the vertebral or carotid arteries.
(Objective 1)

40. a. This will decrease CPP. CPP does not usually decrease until the ICP exceeds 22 mm Hg (the body compensates to that level). Fluid in the eye has no influence on CPP. Metabolic rate will increase, but CPP is not affected by a temperature of 102°F (38.9°C).
(Objective 2)

41. a. Ataxic respirations are slow, shallow, and irregular. Assist ventilation with a bag-mask immediately.
(Objective 4)

42. a. Flexion posturing occurs with impairment of the cortical regions of the brain. Flaccidity is usually caused by brain stem or cord dysfunction. Dysconjugate gaze is not a posture but an abnormal eye movement.
(Objective 3)

43. c. Barbiturate overdose and medullary injury are more likely to present with dilated pupils. Temporal herniation causes a unilateral dilated pupil.
(Objective 3)

44. d. Airway maintenance is critical. Drug administration would be indicated only if the seizure recurs.
(Objective 4)

45. c. Hypertension and sickle cell disease are independent predictors of stroke. Asthma is not a risk factor, but obesity is. An aneurysm is a risk factor for hemorrhagic stroke.
(Objective 4)

46. b. The three components of the stroke scale are facial droop, arm drift, and speech disturbances. All other choices are possible signs or symptoms of stroke but are not included in the stroke scale.
(Objective 4)

47. c. *Dystonia* refers to an alteration in muscle tone that can cause painful spasms, fixed postures, or strange movement patterns. *Inanition* refers to starvation or failure to thrive. *Palsy* is weakness.
(Objective 4)

48. a. Dementia and speech disorders are associated with Pick disease.
(Objective 4)

49. b. This is a noncancerous tumor that compresses the vestibular portion of the eighth cranial nerve.
(Objective 4)

50. a. Huntington disease causes uncontrolled movements, dementia, and difficulty swallowing.
(Objective 4)

51. a. As the respiratory muscles become paralyzed, the tidal volume decreases as does the minute volume, causing an increase in end-tidal CO_2. Dead air space is not affected.
(Objective 4)

1. a. 10; b. 3 (no response to pain)
   (Objective 3)

2. Altered level of consciousness; hospital: decreasing level of consciousness, bradycardia, fixed and dilated pupils, ataxic breathing
   (Objective 3)

3. Lorazepam (Ativan), 1 to 4 mg IV given slowly; or diazepam (Valium), 5 mg over 2 minutes
   (Objective 4)

4. Intracranial bleeding, head trauma, brain tumor, anoxia, hypoglycemia, seizure disorder, drug overdose, poisoning, hypertensive encephalopathy, dysrhythmia, stroke, meningitis
   (Objective 3)

5. High blood pressure, age, male gender
   (Objective 4)

6. d, h, m
   (Objective 4)

7. Symptoms developed abruptly, occurred during exertion (using the toilet), seizure ensued, as did progressive and rapid deterioration
   (Objective 4)

8. c. The patient is unconscious and unable to be evaluated using either scale.
   (Objective 3)

26 Endocrinology

READING ASSIGNMENT

Chapter 26, pages 800-823, in *Mosby's Paramedic Textbook,* ed. 4.

OBJECTIVES

Upon completion of this chapter, the paramedic student will be able to do the following:

1. Describe how hormones secreted from endocrine glands help the body to maintain homeostasis.
2. Describe the anatomy and physiology of the pancreas and how its hormones maintain normal glucose metabolism.
3. Discuss pathophysiology as a basis for key signs and symptoms, patient assessment, and patient management for diabetes and diabetic emergencies of hypoglycemia, diabetic ketoacidosis, and hyperosmolar hyperglycemic nonketotic syndrome.
4. Discuss pathophysiology as a basis for key signs and symptoms, patient assessment, and patient management for disorders of the thyroid gland.
5. Discuss pathophysiology as a basis for key signs and symptoms, patient assessment, and patient management of emergencies related to Cushing syndrome and Addison disease.

SUMMARY

- The endocrine system consists of ductless glands and tissues. These glands and tissues produce and secrete hormones. Endocrine glands secrete their hormones directly into the bloodstream. They exert a regulatory effect on various metabolic functions. All hormones operate within feedback systems. (These are either positive or negative.) These systems work to maintain an optimal internal environment.
- The pancreatic islets are composed of beta cells, alpha cells, and other cells. The beta cells secrete insulin. The alpha cells secrete glucagon. The other cells are of questionable function. The chief functions of insulin are to increase glucose transport into cells, increase glucose metabolism by cells, increase the liver glycogen level, and decrease the blood glucose concentration toward normal. Glucagon has two major effects: (1) increase blood glucose levels by stimulating the liver to release glucose stores from glycogen and other glucose storage sites (glycogenolysis) and (2) stimulate gluconeogenesis through the breakdown of fats and fatty acids, thereby maintaining a normal blood glucose level.
- Diabetes mellitus is characterized by a deficiency of insulin or an inability of the body to respond to insulin. Diabetes generally is classified as type 1 or type 2. People with 1 diabetes have inadequate insulin production. Treatment for type 1 consists of insulin administration, exercise, and diet regulation. Type 2 diabetes is caused by cellular resistance to insulin and ultimately decreased insulin production. Most patients with type 2 diabetes require oral hypoglycemic medications, exercise, and dietary regulation to control the illness. Some require insulin administration.
- Hypoglycemia is a syndrome related to blood glucose levels below 70 mg/dL. A diabetic patient with behavioral changes or unconsciousness should be treated for hypoglycemia. This condition is a true emergency. It requires immediate administration of glucose to prevent permanent brain damage or death.
- Diabetic ketoacidosis (DKA) results from an absence of or a resistance to insulin. The signs and symptoms of DKA are related to hypovolemia. They usually are slow in onset.
- Hyperosmolar hyperglycemic nonketotic syndrome is a life-threatening emergency. It often occurs in older patients with type 2 diabetes. It also frequently occurs in people with undiagnosed diabetes. The hyperglycemia produces a hyperosmolar state. This causes osmotic diuresis, dehydration, and electrolyte imbalances.
- Important components of the patient history in the assessment of patients with diabetes include the onset of symptoms, food intake, insulin or oral hypoglycemic use, alcohol or other drug consumption, predisposing factors, and any associated symptoms.
- Any patient with a glucose reading below 70 mg/dL (varies by protocol) and signs and symptoms consistent with hypoglycemia generally should be given dextrose.
- Thyrotoxicosis is any toxic condition that results from overactivity of the thyroid gland.

- Thyroid storm is a life-threatening condition resulting from an overactive thyroid gland. Thyroid hormones play a key role in controlling body metabolism. They are essential in children for normal physical growth and development.
- Myxedema is a condition that results from a thyroid hormone deficiency. Myxedema coma is a rare illness. In addition to myxedema, it is characterized by hypothermia and mental obtundation. It is a medical emergency.
- Cushing syndrome is caused by an abnormally high circulating level of corticosteroid hormones. These are produced naturally by the adrenal glands.
- Addison disease is a rare but life-threatening disorder. It is caused by a deficiency of the corticosteroid hormones cortisol and aldosterone. These are normally produced by the adrenal cortex.

REVIEW QUESTIONS

Match the signs or symptoms in column II with the appropriate diabetic emergencies in column I. Each answer may be used more than once.

Column I

1. _____ Diabetic ketoacidosis

2. _____ Hyperosmolar hyperglycemic nonketotic coma

3. _____ Hypoglycemia

Column II

a. Abdominal pain
b. Coma
c. Cool, clammy skin
d. Fruity breath odor
e. Kussmaul respirations
f. Polyuria
g. Psychotic behavior
h. Seizures
i. Tachycardia
j. Warm, dry skin
k. Vomiting

4. Name the hormone secreted from each of these cells in the pancreas.

   a. Alpha cells: ________________________________

   b. Beta cells: ________________________________

   c. Delta cells: ________________________________

5. When food is ingested, it is broken down into smaller units and used or stored. Name the breakdown products and storage sites for the following food types.

Food	Breakdown Products	Storage
a. Carbohydrates		
b. Proteins		
c. Fats		

6. a. How is excess glucose stored in the liver?

   ____

   b. How are glucose stores released from the liver?

   ____

7. Briefly explain the role of glucagon in the metabolism of food.

   ____

8. Why does a patient develop cerebral signs and symptoms of hypoglycemia rapidly?

____

9. List at least three signs or symptoms that might lead you to suspect that a patient has undetected type 1 diabetes.

____

____

____

10. List at least three medical illnesses associated with long-term diabetes.

____

____

____

11. You arrive on the scene of a suspected diabetic emergency. You find a 35-year-old man whose wife says he took his insulin 2 hours ago and has not eaten. He arouses only to pain and has noisy, snoring respirations. He has no other medical history. Outline the steps in your patient management.

____

____

____

____

Questions 12 to 16 refer to the following case study:

A 20-year-old patient with diabetes complains of difficulty breathing. The patient states that he has had the flu for 2 days. His respiratory rate is 40 breaths/min, and his breath has a very sweet odor. You auscultate his lungs, and his breath sounds are clear bilaterally.

12. What do you suspect?

____

13. What other specific questions will you ask about the history of this patient's illness?

____

____

14. What specific findings will you be looking for during your physical assessment of the patient?

____

You perform a blood glucose analysis, and your machine reads "high." The patient appears dehydrated.

399

Chapter **26** **Endocrinology**

15. What interventions should you perform for this patient in the prehospital setting?

____

16. Should you be concerned about rapid transport for this patient? Why?

____

17. List six factors that predispose a patient to the development of hyperosmolar hyperglycemic nonketotic coma.

a. ____

b. ____

c. ____

d. ____

e. ____

f. ____

18. Complete the missing information for each endocrine disorder in the table below.

Disorder	Endocrine Gland and Hormone Affected	Hormone Excess or Shortage?	Signs and Symptoms	Life Threat?
Graves disease				
Thyroid storm				
Myxedema				
Cushing syndrome				
Addison disease				

STUDENT SELF-ASSESSMENT

19. How do hormones achieve their desired actions?
  a. They travel by ducts to the specific organ to be stimulated.
  b. They stimulate nerves to send messages to their target tissue.
  c. They trigger cell-specific receptors to initiate specific functions.
  d. They activate the organ adjacent to the gland that produces them.

20. What is the primary action of insulin?
  a. To reduce the glucose needs of the cells
  b. To increase blood glucose levels
  c. To transport glucose into the cells
  d. To manufacture amino acids

21. Which of the following is an oral hypoglycemic agent given to lower blood glucose?
  a. Avalide　　　　　　　**c.** Insulin
  b. Glucagon　　　　　　**d.** Glimepiride

22. Which is a characteristic of type 2 diabetes?
  a. It is the most serious form of diabetes.
  b. Cells develop resistance to insulin.
  c. It has a sudden onset of symptoms.
  d. It results from weight loss.

400

23. What is the breakdown of glucose stores in the liver called?
   a. Glucagon
   b. Glucosuria
   c. Gluconeogenesis
   d. Glycogenolysis

24. Which action is indicated first when you are unable to establish intravenous access in a 30-year-old patient with diabetes who cannot swallow, with a blood glucose of 40 mg/dL and a Glasgow Coma Scale score of 14?
   a. Initiate intraosseous access.
   b. Administer glucagon.
   c. Place glucose paste in the buccal space.
   d. Reassess the blood glucose level.

25. When giving $D_{50}W$ to a person with diabetes who is also known to have alcoholism, what should you administer?
   a. Glucagon
   b. Half the usual dose
   c. Insulin
   d. Thiamine

26. What is an advantage of glucagon over $D_{50}W$?
   a. Faster acting
   b. Less expensive
   c. Given IM
   d. More effective

27. What is the correct dose of glucagon for a hypoglycemic adult?
   a. 0.5 to 1 mg IM
   b. 1 to 2 mg IM
   c. 12.5 g IV
   d. 25 g IV

28. Which of the following signs or symptoms would be unlikely in a patient who is in a hyperosmolar hyperglycemic nonketotic coma?
   a. Altered level of consciousness
   b. Dry mucous membranes
   c. Fruity breath odor
   d. Thirst

29. An anxious patient complains of abdominal pain and difficulty breathing. Her vital signs are BP, 80/50 mm Hg; P, 136 beats/min; and R, 24 breaths/min. You note basilar rales in her lungs. What endocrine condition may cause this presentation?
   a. Cushing syndrome
   b. Graves disease
   c. Myxedema
   d. Thyroid storm

30. Your patient is a 60-year-old man with type 2 diabetes who takes glyburide/metformin (Glucovance). He is difficult to arouse and has a blood glucose of 28 mg/dL. Which of the following is true regarding his case?
   a. This may be a rare case of metabolic alkalosis.
   b. Hypoglycemia is common in patients who take oral agents.
   c. If you treat him with $D_{50}W$, his blood glucose will not drop again.
   d. Ask if he has recently started any new medicine and consult medical direction.

31. Why is it advisable that a patient with diabetes type 2 who has a hypoglycemic episode be transported to the hospital even if the blood glucose and the patient's level of consciousness return to normal?
   a. There is a high incidence of rhythm disturbance.
   b. The patient is at risk for sudden cardiac death.
   c. The onset and duration of oral agents varies so hypoglycemia may recur.
   d. It indicates that the patient was not compliant with his or her medication.

At 1400 on a warm summer day, you respond for a "diabetic sick case." When you arrive, you find a 21-year-old patient with type 1 diabetes who is pale, cool, and diaphoretic; she responds to painful stimuli only by telling you to go away. Her husband tells you that she is 8 weeks pregnant, and she hasn't been feeling well for a couple of days because of her "morning sickness." He says her insulin is off schedule, and her sugars have been "all over the place." Her vital signs are BP, 100/70 mm Hg; P, 120 beats/min; and R, 20 breaths/min. You start an IV and simultaneously obtain a blood glucose level, which is 34 mg/dL. Minutes after 25 g of $D_{50}W$ has been administered IV, the patient awakens and is embarrassed about the situation. She refuses further treatment and transport; you contact medical direction, which recommends that she call her endocrinologist for an appointment immediately.

1. Which is true about type 1 diabetes?
   a. It results from a pituitary abnormality.
   b. Its symptoms occur when glucagon production decreases.
   c. It occurs when the cells lose their ability to absorb glucose.
   d. It results from inadequate pancreatic production of insulin.

2. Which hormone is responsible for the initial shakiness, tachycardia, and dry mouth felt by people with diabetes who are hypoglycemic?
   a. Adrenocorticotrophic hormone
   b. Epinephrine
   c. Glucagon
   d. Vasopressin

3. Put a ✓ beside the signs or symptoms this patient had that could indicate hypoglycemia. Put an × beside those that could indicate diabetic ketoacidosis (hyperglycemia).
   a. _______ Altered level of consciousness   d. _______ Tachycardia
   b. _______ Cool skin   e. _______ Sweaty
   c. _______ Hypotension

4. How would your patient care have changed if
   a. The patient had been alert, and oriented.

   ____

   ____

   b. Her blood glucose had been 434 mg/dL.

   ____

   ____

   c. Your blood glucose monitor had not functioned.

   ____

   ____

Chapter **26** **Endocrinology**

REVIEW QUESTIONS

1. a, b, d, e, f, i, j, k

2. b, f, h, i, j

3. b, c, g, i, j
(Questions 1–3, Objective 3)

4. a. Glucagon; b. insulin; c. somatostatin
(Objective 2)

5.

Food	Breakdown Products	Storage
a. Carbohydrates	Glucose	Liver and muscles (excess converted to fat)
b. Proteins	Amino acids	Small amounts in cytoplasm of all cells
c. Fats	Fatty acids, glycerol	Liver and fat cells

(Objective 2)

6. a. Glucose is stored in the liver as glycogen. b. As the blood sugar begins to drop, glucagon is released from the pancreas and stimulates the breakdown of glycogen to glucose.
(Objective 2)

7. Glucagon breaks down glycogen and stimulates gluconeogenesis (the formation of glucose from amino acids).
(Objective 2)

8. Glucose cannot be stored in the brain; therefore, when blood sugar drops, no reserves exist. The brain cannot use fats or proteins for energy.
(Objective 3)

9. New onset of diabetes is associated with increased fluid intake (polydipsia), increased urine output (polyuria), dizziness, blurred vision, and rapid weight loss.
(Objective 3)

10. Long-term complications of diabetes include blindness, kidney disease, peripheral neuropathy, autonomic neuropathy, peripheral vascular disease, heart disease, and stroke.
(Objective 3)

11. Assess and protect the airway; place a nasal or oral airway and suction if necessary; evaluate breathing, assist if necessary, and administer oxygen; assess pulse; evaluate vital signs; determine blood glucose level; start an IV in the antecubital space; if the blood glucose is less than 80 mg/dL, administer $D_{50}W$ (25 g IV) and reassess the patient.
(Objective 3)

12. Diabetic ketoacidosis or a pulmonary problem.
(Objective 3)

13. Have you had any vomiting or diarrhea? If yes, how much? When did you last eat? What medications do you take, and when did you last take them (especially insulin)? How much have you been urinating? Do you feel dizzy when you stand up? Have you lost any weight? Are you thirsty, and have you been drinking a lot of fluids? Do you have any abdominal pain?
(Objective 3)

14. As you perform your total patient assessment, you should check to see if the patient has warm, dry skin; dry mucous membranes; tachycardia; postural hypotension; fruity breath odor; or a decreased level of consciousness. (Objective 3)

15. Oxygen should be administered and the patient monitored for dysrhythmias. An IV of 0.9% normal saline should be initiated. Medical direction likely will advise infusion at a rapid rate, often 250 mL/hr or more. (Objective 3)

16. Transport rapidly because definitive treatment includes administration of insulin, which is not usually available on EMS units. (Objective 3)

17. Type 2 diabetes; advanced age; preexisting cardiac or renal disease; inadequate insulin secretion or action; increased insulin requirements (stress, infection, trauma, burns, myocardial infarction); medications such as thiazide diuretics, glucocorticoids, phenytoin, sympathomimetics, propranolol, and immunosuppressants; and parenteral or enteral feedings (Objective 17)

18.

Disorder	Endocrine Gland and Hormone Affected	Hormone Excess or Shortage?	Signs and Symptoms	Potentially Life Threatening?
Graves disease	Thyroid hormone	Excess	Enlarged thyroid, swollen neck, protruding eyes	Yes if it progresses to thyroid storm
Thyroid storm	Thyroid hormone	Excess	Tachycardia, heart failure, dysrhythmias, shock, hyperthermia, restlessness, agitation, abdominal pain, coma	Yes
Myxedema	Thyroid hormone	Shortage	Hoarse voice, fatigue, weight gain, cold intolerance, depression, dry skin, hair loss, infertility, constipation, heavy menses	Not unless it progresses to myxedema coma
Cushing syndrome	Adrenal cortex (corticosteroid hormones)	Excess	Round, red face; obese trunk; wasted limbs; acne; purple stretch marks; increased facial and body hair; hump on neck; weight gain; hypertension; psychiatric disturbance; insomnia; diabetes	No
Addison disease	Adrenal cortex (cortisol, aldosterone)	Shortage	Weakness, weight loss, anorexia, hyperpigmented skin, hypotension, hyponatremia, hyperkalemia, gastrointestinal disturbances	Usually not unless a rapid, acute onset occurs

(Objectives 4, 5)

19. c. Hormones travel through the blood and may trigger a receptor site in only one organ or throughout the body, depending on the hormone.
(Objective 1)

20. c. Insulin increases glucose transport into cells, increases glucose metabolism by cells, increases liver glycogen levels, and decreases the blood glucose concentration.
(Objective 2)

21. d. Avalide is an antihypertensive agent. Glucagon is given to increase blood glucose. Insulin lowers blood glucose but is not given orally.
(Objective 3)

22. b. Most patients with type 2 diabetes can control the disease with diet and oral hypoglycemic agents. This disease has a slow onset and does not often cause life-threatening emergencies.
(Objective 3)

23. d. Glucagon is a pancreatic hormone. Glucosuria is urine that contains glucose. Gluconeogenesis is the formation of glucose from the breakdown of fats and fatty acids.
(Objective 2)

24. b. If the patient does not respond to the glucagon, intraosseous access should be established, and intravenous $D_{50}W$ should be administered. The patient may aspirate if you administer oral glucose.
(Objective 3)

25. d. Thiamine promotes the uptake of glucose in the brain.
(Objective 3)

26. c. When an IV cannot be established in a patient with hypoglycemia, glucagon may be given IM. Glucagon is slower, more expensive, and less effective than $D_{50}W$.
(Objective 3)

27. a. 0.5 to 1 mg IM
(Objective 3)

28. c. No ketogenesis occurs with HHNK; therefore, no acetone (fruity) breath odor is noted, as it is in hyperglycemia.
(Objective 3)

29. d. These conditions are caused by adrenergic hyperactivity.
(Objective 4)

30. d. If the patient who takes an oral agent becomes hypoglycemic, use standard treatment for hypoglycemia. Then, try to identify a cause—it may be a recent addition of a new drug (especially antibiotics). Contact medical direction.
(Objective 3)

31. c. Refusal of care after a hypoglycemic episode is high risk for patients with type 2 diabetes. Strongly encourage the patient to be transported to further evaluation.
(Objective 3)

1. d. Type 1 diabetes is characterized by inadequate production of insulin by the pancreas.
   (Objective 3)

2. b. The body releases epinephrine in an attempt to stimulate the release of sugar stored in the liver.
   (Objective 3)

3. Hypoglycemia: a, b, c, d, e; hyperglycemia: a, c, d
   (Objective 3)

4. a. Oral glucose or foods high in simple sugars (e.g., sweetened orange juice) could have been given.
   b. A high blood glucose level would have indicated diabetic ketoacidosis. Oxygenation and rapid administration of lactated Ringer solution would have been indicated along with careful monitoring of the patient (including ECG). Administration of sodium bicarbonate would usually also be ordered in that situation.
   c. If no blood glucose value could be obtained, then based on the patient history and presenting signs and symptoms, $D_{50}W$ would be given and the patient's response monitored. (If the EMS blood glucose monitor is not working, the patient's monitor could be used.)
   (Objective 3)

27 Immune System Disorders

Chapter 27, pages 824-842, in *Mosby's Paramedic Textbook*, ed. 4.

OBJECTIVES

Upon completion of this chapter, the paramedic student will be able to do the following:

1. Outline the structure of the immune system.
2. Describe the antigen–antibody response.
3. Distinguish between natural and acquired immunity.
4. Differentiate between a normal immune response and an allergic reaction.
5. Distinguish between the four types of hypersensitivity reaction.
6. Describe signs and symptoms and management of local allergic reactions based on an understanding of the pathophysiology associated with this condition.
7. Identify allergens associated with anaphylaxis.
8. Describe the pathophysiology, signs and symptoms, and management of nonsystemic allergic reaction.
9. Describe the pathophysiology, signs and symptoms, and management of anaphylaxis.
10. Define autoimmune disease.
11. Describe the pathophysiology, signs and symptoms, and prehospital considerations for patients who have collagen vascular diseases such as systemic lupus erythematous and scleroderma.
12. Identify major complications associated with organ transplant.
13. List infections associated with organ transplant.
14. Outline characteristics of organ rejection.
15. Recognize side effects associated with antirejection medications.

SUMMARY

- The immune system is designed to prevent foreign substances from entering the body. If that fails, this system should launch an attack to find and destroy these foreign substances.
- Organs of the immune system include the spleen, tonsils, adenoids, lymph nodes, and thymus.
- Lymphocytes are the primary units of the immune system. There are B lymphocytes and T lymphocytes. B lymphocytes produce antibodies. This is called humoral immunity. T lymphocytes provide immune protection with three types of cells. Killer T cells attack invading organisms, helper T cells encourage B-cell antibody production, and suppressor T cells regulate the immune response so it does not attack the body. T cells provide cell-mediated immunity.
- Natural immunity is present at birth. It is not antigen specific. Acquired immunity develops after exposure to specific antigens.
- Local allergic reactions do not produce life-threatening signs and are treated with antihistamines such as diphenhydramine.
- Anaphylaxis is an immediate, systemic, and life-threatening reaction.
- Antigens are substance that trigger antibody formation.
- Antibodies bind to the antigen that produced them. Antibodies aid in neutralizing the antigen and removing it from the body.
- Allergic reaction is an increased physiologic response to an antigen after a previous exposure to the same antigen. Localized allergic reactions do not affect the entire body.
- Anaphylaxis is the most extreme form of allergic reaction. Rapid recognition and aggressive therapy are needed for patient survival.
- Anaphylaxis is a form of type I hypersensitivity reaction.
- Localized allergic reactions affect the skin, nasal passages, or eyes, not the lungs or cardiovascular system. They are treated with an antihistamine such as diphenhydramine.
- Almost any substance can cause anaphylaxis. The risk of anaphylaxis increases with the frequency of exposure.
- Chemical substances released by basophils and mast cells cause signs and symptoms of anaphylaxis. These chemicals include histamine, leukotrienes, and other substances.
- Symptoms of anaphylaxis may include a sudden onset of hives, angioedema, pruritus; sneezing, and coughing; airway obstruction; wheezing; hypotension or vascular collapse; chest pain; nausea, vomiting, or diarrhea; and weakness, headache, syncope, seizures, or coma.

- Determine if the patient has used an epinephrine autoinjector or taken diphenhydramine before arrival.
- Treatment of anaphylaxis includes administration of epinephrine and, if the patient is hypotensive, 1 to 2 L of normal saline. Additional interventions may include antihistamines, inhaled beta agonists, corticosteroids, glucagon, and vasopressors.
- Autoimmune disease occurs when the body's immune system attacks normal body cells, causing harm.
- Collagen vascular disease is also called connective tissue disease.
- Systemic lupus erythematosus, or lupus, is a disease of young women that can damage many organs. It often causes a butterfly rash on the nose and cheeks. Severe damage to the gastrointestinal (GI) organs, kidneys, lungs, and central nervous system are possible.
- Scleroderma means hard skin. It is caused by increased collagen production. Systemic scleroderma may cause Raynaud phenomenon and dysfunction of the esophagus, GI tract, kidneys, heart, and lungs.
- Solid organ transplants include kidney, liver, pancreas, heart, and lung.
- Infection, rejection, and drug toxicity are the key complications after organ transplant.
- Infections may include community-acquired bacterial or viral diseases, opportunistic infections, and others. Normal signs and symptoms of infection may be masked by the immunosuppressive therapy.
- When the body recognizes the transplanted tissue as "nonself," it begins to reject it. Rejection may be hyperacute (within minutes), acute (within 1 week), or chronic (more than 1 week).
- Immunosuppressive drugs have many side effects. Three drug groups known to cause many adverse effects include cyclosporine, azathioprine, and corticosteroids.

REVIEW QUESTIONS

1. Indicate whether each of the following statements refers to B lymphocytes or T lymphocytes.

   a. Produce antibodies __B__

   b. Protects the body from its own defense __T__

   c. Play a role in humoral immunity __B__

   d. Attack organisms with "killer" cells __T__

2. Complete the following sentences.
   Antigens can enter the body by four routes: (a) _______________, (b) _______________,
   (c) _______________, or (d) _______________. The allergic reaction is initiated when a circulating
   (e) _antibodies_ combines with a specific antigen, causing (f) _hypersensitivity_ reaction or to antibodies
   bound to (g) _mast cells_ or (h) _basophils_.

3. List agents in each of the following groups that can cause anaphylaxis.

   a. Drugs: ____

   b. Insects: ____

   c. Foods: ____

   d. Other: ____

4. List the signs and symptoms associated with each of the following chemical mediators released from basophils and mast cells in an anaphylactic reaction.

   a. Histamines: ____

   ____

   b. Leukotrienes: ____

   ____

c. Eosinophil chemotactic factor: ____

____

5. You are called to a church picnic to care for a 30-year-old woman. Her skin is very red, and she has wheezing and dyspnea. After a careful assessment, you determine that she is having an anaphylactic reaction.

   a. What other illness or injury may produce these symptoms? _______________________

   ____

   b. List two home medicines that may influence your care of this patient. _______________

   ____

Questions 6 to 8 refer to the following case study:

You are at a Chinese restaurant caring for a 25-year-old patient experiencing an anaphylactic reaction. His lips are swollen, and he is in acute respiratory distress with wheezing and has a blood pressure of 90/70 mm Hg.

6. What are some causative agents that may be found at this restaurant that could trigger this man's anaphylaxis?

7. After a rapid primary survey and vital sign assessment, you determine that immediate pharmacologic therapy is indicated. Identify two drugs, with the appropriate dose and route, that may be indicated for this patient.

   a. ____________________________________   _______________________________________

   b. ____

8. Describe other signs or symptoms that this patient may have.

   ____

   ____

9. You arrive at a dental office, where you find a 35-year-old woman who rapidly developed hives, angioedema, and stridor after an injection of a local anesthetic. She is unconscious and has labored, stridorous respirations; no radial pulse; and a rapid, irregular, barely palpable carotid pulse. No medicines have been administered to treat her. Describe your priorities of care for this patient, including the appropriate drugs, doses, and routes.

   ____

   ____

A 37-year-old woman had a kidney transplant 6 months ago from an anonymous donor. She had developed end-stage renal disease related to lupus erythematosus. She is complaining of weakness, flank pain, and swelling. Her vital signs are BP 160/108 mm Hg, P 128 beats/min, R 20 breaths/min, SaO_2 95% on room air, T 101.4°F (38.6°C). Her home medicines include prednisone, mycophenolate mofetil (CellCept), and valganciclovir (Valcyte).

10. **a.** Was this an allograft or isograft procedure? _______________

    b. What are you considering in his differential diagnosis? _________________________________

    c. For each medication she is taking, list an indication and one possible adverse effect that could be causing her signs or symptoms. _________________________________

   Chapter **27** **Immune System Disorders**

11. Which organ, if surgically removed after trauma, has the greatest impact on the immune system?
  a. Kidney
  b. Liver
  c. Lung
  d. Spleen

12. Which of the following is an example of natural immunity?
  a. Breast milk transmission of IgA antibodies
  b. Kupffer cells in the lobes of the liver
  c. Immunity after infection with chicken pox
  d. Vaccination with hepatitis B vaccine

13. What is the term used for any substance that causes the formation of antibodies in the body?
  a. Anaphylactic
  b. Antigen
  c. Basophil
  d. Mast cell

14. Which immunoglobulin (antibody) is responsible for anaphylaxis?
  a. IgA
  b. IgE
  c. IgG
  d. IgM

15. Which of the following is a sign or symptom of a type IV (localized) allergic reaction?
  a. Angioedema
  b. Hoarseness
  c. Vomiting
  d. Wheezing

16. Your 20-year-old patient has hives, normal vital signs, and clear breath sounds. He complains of severe itching. Which treatment is indicated first in this situation?
  a. Diphenhydramine (Benadryl), 25 mg IM
  b. Epinephrine (Adrenalin), 0.3 mg (1:1000) IM
  c. Normal saline, 200 mL IV infusion
  d. Oxygen 4 lpm by nasal cannula

17. What term is used for mediators that cause blood vessels to dilate?
  a. Chemotactic substances
  b. Leukotactic substances
  c. Opsonins
  d. Vasoactive substances

18. Which of the following is a common cause of anaphylaxis?
  a. Acetaminophen
  b. Diphenhydramine
  c. Grapes
  d. Peanuts

19. What is the most likely cause of death in anaphylaxis?
  a. Upper airway obstruction
  b. Hypoxia resulting from bronchospasm
  c. Hypotension resulting from fluid leakage
  d. Vasogenic shock caused by histamines

20. Which skin sign is most likely with anaphylaxis?
  a. Petechiae
  b. Pallor
  c. Rhinorrhea
  d. Urticaria

21. Diphenhydramine is considered which of the following?
  a. Anticholinergic
  b. Antihistamine
  c. Bronchodilator
  d. Sedative–hypnotic

22. Which of the following is a potential complication of IV epinephrine?
  a. Dysrhythmias
  b. Myocardial ischemia
  c. Seizures
  d. Vomiting
  e. All of the above

23. Which is true of an autoimmune disease?
    a. The immune system is weakened.
    b. The immune system attacks body tissue.
    c. This disease is prevented by vaccination.
    d. This disease is activated by killer T cells.

24. A 23-year-old patient tells you she has "lupus." She is weak and dyspneic. Which complication of this disease is likely to explain her symptoms?
    a. Anemia
    b. Chronic obstructive pulmonary disease
    c. Dysrhythmias
    d. Pulmonary emboli

25. Which patient's signs and symptoms are characteristic of early scleroderma?
    a. A 24-year-old woman who has a butterfly-shaped rash on her face
    b. A 36-year-old man who has severe joint pain when he awakens
    c. A 38-year-old woman whose fingers are cold and white and then turn blue
    d. A 73-year-old man who has a barrel-shaped chest

26. Your patient had a lung transplant 3 years ago. Why is she at increased risk for cancer?
    a. Anemia
    b. Foreign antigens
    c. Hyperplasia in new lung
    d. Immunosuppression

27. A 22-year-old patient has a sudden onset of angioedema, urticaria, pruritus and bronchospasm. What type of hypersensitivity reaction is this?
    a. Type I   c. Type III
    b. Type II   d. Type IV

WRAP IT UP

You are dispatched for a "person down." You find the patient in the cafeteria, lying unconscious. Coworkers tell you that she complained of itching and said, "That bee just stung me." She then complained of difficulty breathing, and after a 9-1-1 call was made, she became unconscious. You ask about any known allergies, and no one seems to know. They tell you she was at her doctor's office this morning for a vaccination, and when the police officer on the scene looks through her purse, he shows you aspirin, ibuprofen, and penicillin tablets. The remnants of her partly eaten lunch are on the table: fried shrimp; deviled eggs; fruit salad with strawberries, mangoes, and a sesame honey dressing; peanut butter crackers; and a glass of milk. Her skin is flushed red, and she has raised welts on her arm; her eyes and lips appear swollen; and her breathing is stridorous. Her vital signs are BP, 76 mm Hg by palpation; P, 134 beats/min; R, 24 breaths/min; and Sao$_2$, 88%. You administer oxygen by non-rebreather mask; at the same time, your partner draws up 0.1 mg of epinephrine and administers it IV over 5 minutes. You start an IV of normal saline and give a fluid bolus; you then administer diphenhydramine (25 mg slow IV) followed by methylprednisolone (125 mg IV). The stridor has now subsided, but you hear some persistent wheezing in the lungs, and the woman's vital signs are now BP, 104/60 mm Hg; P, 120 beats/min; R, 20 breaths/min; and Sao$_2$, 98%. You administer an albuterol updraft for the persistent wheezing and continue to monitor her condition, which has improved dramatically by the time you arrive at the hospital. She is discharged with a prescription and instructions for an EpiPen and is told to purchase a bracelet or necklace to alert first responders to her severe allergic condition.

1. Which of the following describes the internal mechanisms responsible for this patient's life-threatening condition?
    a. IgE antibodies react to a foreign antigen, triggering the release of histamines, leukotrienes, and other chemicals.
    b. IgM antibodies initiate a type IV allergic reaction, which triggers a life-threatening release of kinins.
    c. IgG antibodies trigger the release of antigens, which stimulate the eosinophil chemotactic factor of anaphylaxis.
    d. Immunoglobulins begin a process of cellular destruction in the lymphatic system that causes anaphylaxis.

2. List the possible causes of anaphylaxis that you observed on this patient call.

3. Put a ✔ beside the signs or symptoms of anaphylaxis that were observed in this patient.

a. _____ Hoarseness

b. __✓__ Stridor

c. __✓__ Laryngeal edema

d. _____ Rhinorrhea

e. __✓__ Bronchospasm

f. _____ Increased mucus production

g. _____ Accessory muscle use

h. __✓__ Wheezing

i. _____ Decreased breath sounds

j. __✓__ Tachycardia

k. __✓__ Hypotension

l. _____ Dysrhythmia

m. _____ Chest tightness

n. _____ Nausea

o. _____ Vomiting

p. _____ Abdominal cramps

q. _____ Diarrhea

r. _____ Anxiety

s. _____ Dizziness

t. __✓__ Syncope

u. _____ Weakness

v. _____ Headache

w. _____ Seizure

x. __✓__ Coma

y. __✓__ Angioedema

z. __✓__ Urticaria

aa. __✓__ Pruritus

bb. __✓__ Erythema

cc. __✓__ Edema

dd. _____ Tearing of the eyes

4. Explain your rationale for each of the following interventions that were performed for this patient.

a. Oxygen administration: ____

____

b. Epinephrine administration: ____

____

c. Normal saline fluid bolus: ____

____

d. Diphenhydramine administration: ____

____

e. Steroid administration: ____

____

f. Albuterol administration: ____

____

REVIEW QUESTIONS

1. B cells; T cells; B cells; T cells
(Objective 1)

2. a. Injection; b. ingestion; c. inhalation; d. absorption; e. antibody; f. hypersensitivity; g. mast cells; h. basophils
(Objective 2)

3. a. Antibiotics (especially penicillin and other beta lactams), local anesthetics, cephalosporins, chemotherapeutics, aspirin, nonsteroidal antiinflammatory agents, opiates, muscle relaxants, IV contrast agents, vaccines, and insulin; b. wasps, bees, and fire ants; c. peanuts, tree-grown nuts, soybeans, cod, halibut, shellfish, egg white, strawberries, food additives, wheat and buckwheat, sesame and sunflower seeds, cotton seed, milk, and mango; d. latex
(Objective 7)

4. a. Histamine release may result in decreased blood pressure, increased gastrointestinal secretions, rhinorrhea, tearing, flushing, urticaria, and angioedema. b. Leukotrienes cause wheezing, which may precipitate chest pain (resulting from coronary vasoconstriction) and enhance the hypotensive effects of histamine. c. Eosinophil chemotactic factor can produce fever, chills, bronchospasm, and pulmonary vasoconstriction.
(Objective 9)

5. a. These same respiratory signs and symptoms could be caused by asthma, upper airway obstruction, pulmonary edema, or toxic inhalation. b. If the patient takes a beta-blocker (e.g., atenolol, propranolol), it could interfere with the action of epinephrine. If the patient has already self-administered epinephrine (EpiPen, AnaPen), determine the time it was administered and whether symptoms have improved or worsened since administration.
(Objective 9)

6. Foods such as crab, shrimp, nuts, egg, and food additives are known to cause anaphylaxis.
(Objective 7)

7. a. Epinephrine, 0.3 to 0.5 mg (1:1000) IM; b. diphenhydramine (Benadryl), 25 to 50 mg IM or IV, and then albuterol (Proventil, Ventolin) updraft.
(Objective 9)

8. He may also have stridor, hoarseness, tachypnea, tachycardia, agitation, headache, seizures, decreasing level of consciousness, angioedema, tearing, swelling of the tongue, urticaria, pruritus, sneezing, coughing, tracheal tugging, intercostal retractions, decreased breath sounds, dysrhythmias, chest tightness, nausea, vomiting, and diarrhea
(Objective 9)

9. Secure the airway, ventilate with 100% oxygen, and intubate. Initiate normal saline IV therapy with a large-bore catheter into the antecubital space, infuse fluid rapidly, and administer epinephrine (0.1 mg [1:10,000] IV) over 5 minutes (try to do this simultaneously with airway management if resources permit). Administer IM if any delay in vascular access. If necessary, administer diphenhydramine (25–50 mg IM or slow IV) as a second-line drug. Reevaluate the need to administer a second dose of epinephrine if the patient has not responded. Consider giving methylprednisolone. Administer inhaled albuterol if wheezing is present.
(Objective 9)

10. a. This is an allograft procedure. Isografts transplants involve an identical twin donor.
    b. Consider organ rejection and infection.
    c. Prednisone is a steroid used to decrease the risk of inflammation; it can cause edema. Mycophenolate mofetil (CellCept) is an antirejection drug; it can cause urinary tract infection, hypertension, and edema. Valganciclovir (Valcyte) is an antiviral drug that can cause fever.
(Objectives 12, 13, 14, and 15)

11. d. The spleen is an organ of the immune system.
(Objective 1)

12. a. Vaccination and viral infection demonstrate active immunity.
(Objective 3)

13. b. An anaphylactic response is a type of life-threatening allergic response. Basophils and mast cells are white
blood cells that are involved in the immune response.
(Objective 2)

14. b. IgA immunoglobulins are antibodies found in blood, secretions such as tears, and the respiratory system. IgG
antibodies are the most common antibodies involved in the immune response. Production of IgM antibodies
precedes IgG production in acute infections.
(Objective 2)

15. a. Angioedema may be found in local or systemic allergic reactions. All of the other signs or symptoms, if present
during an allergic reaction, would be most often associated with a systemic (anaphylactic) reaction.
(Objective 5)

16. a. Because no systemic signs or symptoms exist, intramuscular diphenhydramine is indicated. Epinephrine 1:1000
should never be given IV to treat anaphylaxis. Oxygen is not indicated because the patient has no signs of
hypoxia.
(Objective 8)

17. d. Chemotactic substances cause the attraction of phagocytic cells toward or away from the antigen, leukotactic
substances attract leukocytes to the pathogenic agent, and opsonins bind phagocytes to the invading
microorganism.
(Objective 9)

18. d. Diphenhydramine is used to treat anaphylaxis after epinephrine is given. Peanuts are an increasingly common
trigger for anaphylaxis.
(Objective 7)

19. a. Each of the other problems could cause death, but upper airway obstruction is associated with the most deaths
from anaphylaxis.
(Objective 9)

20. d. Erythema and urticaria (hives) are the most frequent skin signs associated with anaphylaxis. Rhinorrhea (runny
nose) may be seen but is not a skin sign.
(Objective 9)

21. b
(Objective 6)

22. e
(Objective 9)

23. b. The immune system recognizes body tissues as foreign and attacks them.
(Objective 10)

24. a. In lupus, the body attacks connective tissue. Red blood cells are one type of connective tissue.
(Objective 11)

25. c. Scleroderma is more common in women than men. Raynaud phenomenon (poor circulation in fingers) is a
common early sign.
(Objective 11)

414

26. d. Immunosuppressant drugs to prevent rejection impair the body's ability to prevent cancer.
(Objective 15)

27. a. Anaphylaxis is a type I hypersensitivity reaction.
(Objective 5)

WRAP IT UP

1. a. IgE antibodies are the primary mediators in anaphylaxis. Additional chemicals that are triggered include eosinophil chemotactic factor of anaphylaxis, heparin, kinins, prostaglandins, and thromboxanes.
(Objective 9)

2. Antibiotic (penicillin), aspirin, nonsteroidal antiinflammatory agent (ibuprofen), vaccine, possible insect sting, peanuts (peanut butter crackers), shellfish (fried shrimp), egg white (deviled eggs), strawberries, mangoes, sesame seeds (salad), and milk
(Objective 7)

3. b, c, e, h, j, k, x, y, z, aa, bb, cc
(Objective 9)

4. a. The patient is hypoxic and in shock. Oxygen administration is indicated for both conditions.
b. Epinephrine antagonizes the effects of histamine and exerts beta-2 effects, which dilate bronchioles; beta-1 effects, which improve myocardial contractility; and alpha effects, which provide vasoconstriction to counteract the effects of anaphylaxis.
c. Normal saline bolus is given as an adjunct to epinephrine in the treatment of the shock associated with anaphylaxis.
d. Diphenhydramine is an antihistamine that can help to reverse some of the symptoms (especially cutaneous) of anaphylaxis.
e. Steroids such as methylprednisolone and dexamethasone suppress acute inflammatory responses that accompany anaphylaxis; they also potentiate smooth muscle relaxation by beta-adrenergic agonists (epinephrine, albuterol) and may alter airway hyperreactivity.
f. Albuterol can aid the management of some of the bronchospasm that is unresolved by epinephrine. However, if signs and symptoms of upper airway edema, severe bronchospasm, or shock persist, an additional dose of epinephrine would be indicated in addition to albuterol.
(Objective 9)

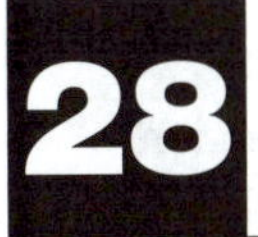 Infectious and Communicable Diseases

Infectious and Communicable Diseases

READING ASSIGNMENT

Chapter 28, pages 843-885, in *Mosby's Paramedic Textbook,* ed. 4.

OBJECTIVES

Upon completion of this chapter, the paramedic student will be able to do the following:

1. Identify general public health principles related to infectious diseases.
2. Describe the chain of elements necessary for an infectious disease to occur.
3. Explain how internal and external barriers affect susceptibility to infection.
4. Differentiate the four stages of infectious disease: the latent period, the incubation period, the communicability period, and the disease period.
5. Describe the mode of transmission, pathophysiology, prehospital considerations, and personal protective measures to be taken for the human immunodeficiency virus (HIV), hepatitis, tuberculosis, meningococcal meningitis, and pneumonia.
6. Describe the mode of transmission, pathophysiology, signs and symptoms, and prehospital considerations for patients who have rabies or tetanus.
7. List the signs, symptoms, and possible secondary complications of selected childhood viral diseases.
8. List the signs, symptoms, and possible secondary complications of influenza, severe acute respiratory syndrome, and mononucleosis.
9. Describe the mode of transmission, pathophysiology, prehospital considerations, and personal protective measures for sexually transmitted diseases.
10. Identify the signs and symptoms and prehospital considerations for scabies and lice.
11. Outline the reporting process for exposure to infectious or communicable diseases.
12. Discuss the paramedic's role in preventing disease transmission.

SUMMARY

- National concerns regarding communicable disease and infection control have resulted in public law, standards, guidelines, and recommendations to protect health care providers and emergency responders against infectious diseases. Paramedics must be familiar with these guidelines. They also must take personal protective measures against exposure to these pathogens.
- The chain of elements needed to transmit an infectious disease includes the pathogenic agent, a reservoir, a portal of exit from the reservoir, an environment conducive to transmission of the pathogenic agent, a portal of entry into the new host, and susceptibility of the new host to the infectious disease.
- The human body is protected from infectious disease by external and internal barriers. These serve as lines of defense against infection. External barriers include the skin, gastrointestinal system, upper respiratory tract, and genitourinary tract. Internal barriers include the inflammatory response and the immune response.
- The progression of infectious disease from exposure to the onset of symptoms follows four stages. These are the latent period, the incubation period, the communicability period, and the disease period.
- The human immunodeficiency virus (HIV) is directly transmitted person to person. This occurs through anal or vaginal intercourse, across the placenta, by contact with infected blood or body fluids on mucous membranes or open wounds, through blood transfusion or tissue transplant, or by the use of contaminated needles or syringes. The virus affects the CD4 T cells. Secondary complications are usually related to opportunistic infections that arise as the immune system deteriorates. Progression of the disease can be divided into category A (acute retroviral infection, seroconversion, and asymptomatic infection), category B (early symptomatic HIV), and category C (late symptomatic HIV and advanced HIV). Paramedics should observe strict compliance with universal precautions for protection against HIV. Patient care should include helping these patients feel that they can obtain acceptance and compassion from health care workers.

417

- **Hepatitis** is a viral disease. It produces pathologic changes in the liver. The three main classes of hepatitis virus are hepatitis A, B, and C. Infection with hepatitis may cause mild symptoms, liver failure, or death.
- **Tuberculosis** is a chronic pulmonary disease. It is acquired through inhalation of tubercle bacilli. The infection is passed mainly when infected people cough or sneeze the bacteria into the air or by contact with sputum that contains virulent TB bacilli. The infection is characterized by stages of early infection (frequently asymptomatic), latency, and a potential for recurrent postprimary disease.
- **Meningococcal meningitis** refers to inflammation of the membranes that surround the spinal cord and brain. It can be caused by bacteria, viruses, and other microorganisms.
- **Bacterial endocarditis** is an inflammation of the endocardium and one or more heart valves. The disease can be rapidly fatal if left untreated.
- **Pneumonia** is an acute inflammatory process of the respiratory bronchioles and alveoli. Bacteria, viruses, and fungi can cause this disease.
- **Tetanus** is a serious, sometimes fatal, disease of the central nervous system (CNS). It is caused by infection of a wound with spores of the bacterium *Clostridium tetani*. The most common symptom is trismus (difficulty opening the mouth).
- **Rabies** is an acute viral infection of the CNS. Humans are highly susceptible to the rabies virus after exposure to saliva from the bite or scratch of an infected animal.
- **Hantaviruses** are carried by rodents. They are transmitted through inhalation of material contaminated with rodent urine and feces. Many forms of this disease occur in specific geographical areas.
- **Rubella** is a mild, febrile, and highly communicable viral disease. It is characterized by a diffuse, punctate, macular rash. The Centers for Disease Control and Prevention recommends that all health care providers receive immunization if they are not immune as a result of previous rubella infection.
- **Rubeola** is an acute, highly communicable viral disease caused by the measles virus. It is characterized by fever, conjunctivitis, cough, bronchitis, and a blotchy red rash.
- **Mumps** is an acute, communicable systemic viral disease. It is characterized by localized unilateral or bilateral edema of one or more of the salivary glands. Occasionally, other glands are also involved.
- **Chickenpox** is highly communicable. It is characterized by a sudden onset of low-grade fever, mild malaise, and a maculopapular skin eruption that lasts for a few hours. This is followed by a vesicular eruption that lasts for 3 to 4 days, leaving a granular scab. The virus may reactivate during periods of stress or immunosuppression. At that time, it may produce an illness known as shingles.
- **Pertussis** is an infectious disease that leads to inflammation of the entire respiratory tract. It causes an insidious cough. The cough becomes paroxysmal in 1 to 2 weeks and lasts for 1 to 2 months.
- **Influenza** is mainly a respiratory infection. It is spread by influenza viruses A, B, and C.
- **Mononucleosis** is caused either by the Epstein-Barr virus or cytomegalovirus. Both of these are members of the herpesvirus family.
- **Syphilis** is a systemic disease. It is characterized by a primary lesion; a secondary eruption involving skin and mucous membranes; long latency periods; and eventually by seriously disabling lesions of the skin, bone, viscera, CNS, and cardiovascular system.
- **Gonorrhea** is caused by the sexually transmitted bacterium *Neisseria gonorrhoeae*. Gonorrhea can be treated with antibiotics. However, some strains brought into the United States from other countries do not respond to the usual antibiotic therapy.
- **Chlamydia** is a major cause of sexually transmitted nonspecific urethritis or genital infection. Signs and symptoms are similar to those of gonorrhea.
- **Herpes simplex virus** is transmitted by skin-to-skin contact with an infected area of the body. The primary infection produces a vesicular lesion (blister). This lesion heals spontaneously. After the primary infection, the virus travels to a sensory nerve ganglion. It remains there in a latent stage until reactivated.
- **Lice** are small, wingless insects that are ectoparasites of birds and mammals. During biting and feeding, lice secrete a substance that causes small red macules and pruritus.
- **The human scabies** mite is a parasite. It completes its life cycle in and on the epidermis of its host. Scabies bites are usually concentrated around the hands and feet, especially in the webs of the fingers and toes.
- Reporting a possible communicable disease exposure permits immediate medical follow-up. It also enables the designated officer to make changes that might prevent exposures in the future. Moreover, it helps employees to obtain the proper evaluation and testing.
- Part of the paramedic's professional duty with regard to infectious disease transmission is to know when not to go to work. Paramedics also have a duty to use the proper body substance isolation (universal precautions) at all times.

418

Match the infectious diseases listed in column II with their descriptions in column I. Use each disease only once.

Column I

1. ___c___ Infection that produces influenza-like symptoms, dark-colored urine, and light-colored stools

2. ___g___ Macular rash that can cause severe birth defects if a susceptible mother is exposed in pregnancy

3. ___i___ Bacterial pulmonary infection spread by airborne droplets

4. ___e___ Viral infection that impairs the ability of the body to fight other infectious disease

5. ___h___ Sexually transmitted disease characterized in the early stage by a painless chancre

6. ___f___ Inflammation of lining of the central nervous system that may produce headache, stiff neck, seizures, and coma

7. ___b___ Bacterial infection that produces mucopurulent discharge but rarely causes septicemia

8. ___j___ Generalized illness accompanied by vesicular lesions, fever, and malaise

Column II

a. Chlamydia
b. Gonorrhea
c. Hepatitis
d. Herpes simplex
e. Human immunodeficiency virus
f. Meningitis
g. Rubella
h. Syphilis
i. Tuberculosis
j. Varicella

9. List the six components of the chain of elements that must be present for an infectious disease to occur.

   a. ___________________________   d. ___________________________

   b. ___________________________   e. ___________________________

   c. ___________________________   f. ___________________________

10. Describe two situations that interfere with the body's external barriers to infection, thereby increasing the risk of infection.

   a. ____

   b. ____

11. Name two factors that can affect the ability of the internal barriers of the body to fight infectious disease.

   a. ____

   b. ____

12. For each of the following patient care scenarios, describe the personal protective measures you should take.

   a. A 23-year-old woman is about to deliver her fourth child. The baby's head is crowning, and you are preparing for delivery.

   ____

   b. A 50-year-old man is complaining of severe substernal chest pain. You are preparing to initiate an intravenous line to administer medications.

   ____

419

c. You are preparing to administer epinephrine intramuscularly to a 25-year-old patient with dyspnea because of anaphylaxis.

____

d. A 17-year-old girl ingested a large amount of alcohol and barbiturates, vomited, and rapidly lost consciousness. You elect to intubate her trachea.

____

e. A 55-year-old man attempted suicide by holding a shotgun under his chin and firing. He is combative and thrashes about as you try to control the large amount of bleeding and secure his airway.

____

f. A butcher sustained a laceration to her hand at work. The wound is oozing a small amount of blood.

____

Questions 13 to 16 refer to the following case study:

While caring for a 40-year-old man who has nausea, vomiting, right upper quadrant abdominal pain, and jaundice, you puncture your finger with a needle contaminated with the patient's blood. The hospital notifies you the next day that he tested positive for hepatitis.

13. What type or types of hepatitis can produce the symptoms experienced by this patient?

____

14. What are the most effective measures you can take to prevent yourself from becoming infected with hepatitis at work?

____

15. Describe the modes of transmission for hepatitis B.

____

16. Can you do anything after you are exposed so that you will not get hepatitis?

____

17. What signs and symptoms may be evident on the prehospital examination of a patient in each of the following stages of infection from the human immunodeficiency virus?

a. Acute retroviral infection:

____

b. Asymptomatic infection:

____

c. Early symptomatic infection:

____

d. Late symptomatic infection:

____

18. A patient with human immunodeficiency virus sustained a sprained ankle at a volleyball game. No other injuries are evident.

    a. What personal protective measures should you take while caring for this patient?

____

    b. How should the ambulance be cleaned before transport of the next patient?

____

19. What is the best way for emergency care workers to monitor whether they have been exposed to a patient with tuberculosis?

____

20. A 23-year-old man has a severe headache and a temperature of 102°F (38.9°C) and complained earlier of a stiff neck. Now he is limp and arouses only to a loud voice. You suspect meningitis.

    a. What personal protective measures should you use on this call? (You plan to initiate an intravenous line and apply oxygen by mask.)

____

    b. If the emergency department contacts you later to inform you that the patient has meningococcal meningitis, should you report an exposure?

____

    c. What is the likelihood that you will be given prophylaxis if you have used appropriate body substance isolation from the beginning of this call?

____

21. List three chronic signs or symptoms that may develop if syphilis is untreated for a number of years.

    a. ____

    b. ____

    c. ____

22. What personal protective measures should be taken when examining the mouth of a child with an outbreak of herpes simplex on the lips?

23. For each of the following ailments, list the signs and symptoms and site of infestation:

    a. Pubic lice:

____

 Chapter **28** **Infectious and Communicable Diseases**

b. Head lice:

____

c. Scabies:

____

Questions 24 to 26 refer to the following case study:

You transport a child who has a temperature of 101°F (38.3°C) and a generalized skin rash that began the previous day. Some lesions are flat and red, some are raised blisters, and others have scabbed. On arrival to the emergency department, the pediatrician confirms that the child has chickenpox.

24. Is this disease communicable at this stage?

____

25. If you have never had chickenpox, how long would you expect to wait before symptoms appear?

____

26. Are you contagious during this entire time?

____

Questions 27 to 35 refer to the following case study:

During your care of a patient at the scene of a motor vehicle crash, you had blood splash into your eyes while your partner was intubating the patient and you were holding inline immobilization of the cervical spine. You had gloves on at the time.

27. Has a significant exposure to blood or body fluids occurred?

____

28. When should you report this exposure?

____

29. Besides evaluation for postexposure prophylaxis, what other emergency care will you need in this situation?

____

The patient refuses to give permission to test for human immunodeficiency virus.

30. Can the emergency department ignore the patient's refusal and run a test for human immunodeficiency virus in this situation? Why?

____

31. What other questions should you ask the patient?

____

32. What are your options for postexposure prophylaxis if the patient refuses testing?

____

____

422

33. After counseling and examination by the emergency department staff, you are offered a course of medicine for postexposure prophylaxis. How will you decide whether to take the medicine?

34. Why do you think some paramedics might need psychological counseling after this incident?

35. How could this exposure have been prevented?

STUDENT SELF-ASSESSMENT

36. Which agency is responsible for establishing the guidelines for body substance isolation and universal (standard) precautions?
   a. Centers for Disease Control and Prevention
   b. Department of Health
   c. Department of Transportation
   d. Occupational Safety and Health Administration

37. How can you interrupt the portal of entry in the chain of elements of an infectious disease?
   a. Take antibiotics to kill a bacterium.
   b. Clean a blood spill with an appropriate agent.
   c. Receive immunizations at appropriate intervals.
   d. Use gloves as defined in the body substance isolation guidelines.

38. Which of the following is an internal barrier to infection?
   a. Flora
   b. Leukocytes
   c. Nasal hairs
   d. Prostatic fluid

39. The internal defense that provides antibodies to destroy invading organisms is produced by which of the following?
   a. Cell-mediated immunity
   b. Complement
   c. Humoral immunity
   d. Killer cells

40. The infectious disease phase that begins when the agent invades the body and ends when the disease process begins is which period?
   a. Communicability
   b. Disease
   c. Incubation
   d. Latent

41. Death caused by hepatitis is most likely to occur from which strain of the virus?
   a. Hepatitis A
   b. Hepatitis B
   c. Hepatitis C
   d. Non-A, non-B hepatitis

42. Which is true regarding hepatitis?
   a. Antibiotics will cure it.
   b. It is spread when a patient coughs.
   c. A skin test can detect it.
   d. Vaccination reduces risk of acquiring it.

43. Which sign or symptom can help to distinguish pneumonia from other respiratory illness?
   a. Fatigue and loss of appetite
   b. Headache and muscle aches
   c. Shaking chills and chest pain
   d. Yellow mucus from productive cough

   Chapter **28** **Infectious and Communicable Diseases**

44. Which of the following is a classic sign or symptom of tetanus?
   a. Flaccid paralysis
   b. Seizures
   c. Trismus
   d. Urticaria

45. What is the reaction causing muscle spasms that prevents a patient with rabies from drinking called?
   a. Hydropenia
   b. Hydrophobia
   c. Polydipsia
   d. Polyuria

46. What is the primary mode of transmission for rubella, mumps, and varicella?
   a. Blood-to-blood contact
   b. Fecal contamination
   c. Lesion contact
   d. Respiratory droplets

47. Which is a complication of varicella?
   a. Candida
   b. Croup
   c. Pericarditis
   d. Reye syndrome

48. Which treatment measure usually is given to patients with chickenpox, influenza, or herpes simplex?
   a. Antibiotic therapy
   b. Aspirin for pain and fever
   c. Comfort measures
   d. Intravenous therapy

49. Which childhood disease is characterized by a violent cough that can persist for 1 to 2 months?
   a. Influenza
   b. Mumps
   c. Pertussis
   d. Pneumonia

50. What secondary complication of influenza often is associated with severe illness or death?
   a. Aspiration
   b. Dehydration
   c. Meningitis
   d. Pneumonia

51. Which sign or symptom associated with mononucleosis could produce a life-threatening condition if the patient is not maintained at rest?
   a. Fever
   b. Lymphadenopathy
   c. Oral rash
   d. Splenomegaly

52. A patient has a headache, malaise, fever, lymphadenopathy, and a symmetrical rash that involves the palms and soles. He states that an ulcerated sore on his penis healed spontaneously 3 weeks earlier. Which infectious disease do you suspect?
   a. Chlamydia
   b. Gonorrhea
   c. Herpes
   d. Syphilis

53. Which body system harbors the dormant herpesvirus?
   a. Cardiovascular system
   b. Gastrointestinal system
   c. Integumentary system
   d. Nervous system

54. Which of the following is the most effective measure that you can take to prevent the spread of severe acute respiratory syndrome?
   a. Antibiotic treatment if exposure is suspected
   b. Hand washing and respiratory protection
   c. Immunization with a pneumonia vaccine
   d. Treatment with bronchodilator drugs

WRAP IT UP

A thin 40-year-old who bystanders say lives in the adjacent park complains of "difficulty breathing." He is coughing vigorously, and you smell whiskey as you approach him. His vital signs are BP 142/88 mm Hg, P 104, R28, and SaO$_2$ 92%, so you apply a nasal cannula. He is cooperative but has slurred speech. He tells you that he cannot catch his breath, so you listen and hear diffuse, coarse crackles in his lungs. You note some purple skin lesions around his bare feet, which he says are numb. His mouth is coated with white plaque. His arms and feet are scarred with old track marks. Although initially reluctant to tell you his history, when you move him to the ambulance, he says he has AIDS. He admits he has not been compliant with his medications and has not been to see a doctor for about 6 months. When you ask about this cough and dyspnea, the patient says that it has been going on for about 3 months and that he has lost weight, has night sweats, and now is coughing up blood. You and your partner don N-95 masks, replace the patient's nasal cannula with an oxygen face mask, and open the window in the back of the ambulance. As you move the patient to the emergency department (ED) stretcher, he has a coughing spasm and expectorates a large amount of bloody sputum, which sprays into your face and eyes. You immediately wash with soap and water and have the ED staff irrigate your eyes. After contacting your supervisor, the appropriate exposure reporting papers are completed, and after the patient's HIV and tuberculosis risk factors and health status have been determined, the ED physician sits down to explain your options. You are told the benefits and risks of tuberculosis and HIV transmission by this exposure and the side effects associated with the prophylactic drugs. You decide to take the prophylactic drugs, and you subsequently miss the next 2 days of work sick from them. Your pregnant wife is upset and fearful that she may become HIV positive. In 6 months and 1 a year, the HIV screening test results come back negative, and at last you stop waking in the night, fearful that you will contract this life-threatening illness.

1. What additional personal protective measure(s) could have decreased your risk for this exposure?

____

2. Identify (a) each of the elements in the chain of transmission of infectious disease that are present on this call and (b) actions that were taken to reduce the risk of transmission at some links in the chain.

Link	How is it present on this call?	Actions taken to reduce the risk of transmission
Pathogenic agent(s)		
Reservoir		
Portal of exit		
Transmission		
Host susceptibility		

3. Place a check mark beside the complications of human immunodeficiency virus or acquired immunodeficiency syndrome that are seen in this patient.
   a. _______ *Candida* spp.
   b. _______ Dementia
   c. _______ Kaposi sarcoma
   d. _______ Pulmonary tuberculosis
   e. _______ *Pneumocystis carinii* pneumonia
   f. _______ Sensory neuropathy
   g. _______ Wasting syndrome

4. What risk factors does this patient have for tuberculosis?

____

____

5. Which is true regarding follow-up after infectious disease exposure?
   a. If proper immunizations have been obtained, medical follow-up is not needed.
   b. Prophylaxis should not be taken without information regarding risks and benefits.
   c. Reporting should be deferred until the end of the paramedic's shift.
   d. The final decision regarding prophylaxis is the choice of the treating physician.

CHAPTER 28 ANSWERS

REVIEW QUESTIONS

1. c
   (Objective 5)

2. g
   (Objective 7)

3. i
(Objective 5)

4. e
(Objective 5)

5. h
(Objective 9)

6. f
(Objective 5)

7. b
(Objective 9)

8. j
(Objective 9)

9. A pathologic agent, a reservoir, a portal of exit from the reservoir, an environment conducive to transmission of the pathogenic agent, portal of entry, and susceptibility of the new host to the infectious disease
(Objective 2)

10. Burns, lacerations, abrasions, intravenous therapy, and urinary catheter
(Objective 3)

11. Human immunodeficiency virus, chemotherapy, and prolonged steroid therapy
(Objective 3)

12. a. Gloves, gown, mask, and eyewear
   b. Gloves
   c. Nothing is necessary according to the Centers for Disease Control and Prevention; however, if bleeding is likely and because the prehospital setting is high risk, gloves are indicated.
   d. Gloves, mask, and eyewear
   e. Gloves, gown, mask, and eyewear
   f. Gloves
   (Objective 1)

13. Hepatitis A, B, or C
(Objective 5)

14. Take hepatitis B virus vaccination and use strict universal (body substance isolation) precautions as warranted by each situation.
(Objectives 1 and 5)

15. Direct introduction of infected blood by needle or transfusion, introduction of serum or plasma through skin cuts, absorption of infected serum or plasma through mucosal surfaces, absorption of saliva or semen through mucosal surfaces, and transfer of infective serum or plasma via inanimate surfaces
(Objective 5)

16. Yes. If the patient is found to have hepatitis A, you may be given an immune globulin injection. If he has hepatitis B and if you are not immune to the hepatitis B virus, a hepatitis B virus vaccine will be given to protect against future exposures, and hepatitis B immune globulin will be given to provide temporary passive immunity to the hepatitis B virus. No immunization or immune globulin exists that is effective to prevent hepatitis C.
(Objective 5)

17. a. Fever, swollen lymph nodes, and sore throat; b. enlarged lymph nodes; c. bacterial pneumonia, oral lesions, shingles, and pulmonary tuberculosis; d. diarrhea, tumors, dementia, neurologic symptoms, and opportunistic infections
(Objective 5)

426

18. a. You should take the same precautions you would take with any patient with this type of injury. If no open
     wounds are present, no body substance isolation is indicated.
   b. Clean the ambulance as you would after any patient.
   (Objectives 1 and 5)

19. Periodic skin test with purified protein derivative (of tuberculin) and chest radiography study if the purified
   protein derivative (of tuberculin) test result is positive or other history exists indicating the need
   (Objective 5)

20. a. Gloves and mask (respiratory spread); wear eye shield if risk of splash or spray exists (e.g., if the patient
     vomits or needs to be intubated)
   b. An exposure should be reported if you did not have appropriate personal protective equipment on or if you
     had contact with blood or body fluids.
   c. The need for prophylaxis will be determined by your occupational health provider but is not likely indicated
     if all body substance isolation precautions were used for the entire call.
   (Objective 5)

21. Paresis, wide gait, ataxia, psychosis, and signs of myocardial insufficiency
   (Objective 9)

22. Gloves (mask and protective eyewear if any risk of splash or spray of body fluids exists)
   (Objective 1)

23. a. Pubic lice look like crabs or gray-blue spots, and nits appear on the abdomen, thighs, eyelashes, eyebrows, and axillary hair.
   b. Head lice have an elongated body with narrow head and three pair of legs, and nits look like dandruff that
     cannot be brushed off.
   c. Scabies produce bites concentrated around webs of hands and feet; a child's face and scalp, a female's nipples,
     and a male's penis; and vesicles and papules that become easily infected because of scratching.
   (Objective 10)

24. Yes. Chickenpox is contagious for 1 to 2 days before the onset of the rash until all of the lesions are crusted and dry.
   (Objective 7)

25. 13 to 17 days
   (Objective 7)

26. Varicella can be transmitted 1 to 2 days before eruption of the rash until the lesions have all scabbed over.
   (Objective 5)

27. Yes. Blood that came in contact with your mucous membranes is a significant exposure.
   (Objective 5)

28. Immediately report the exposure as soon as you arrive at the hospital with the patient. If you did not transport the
   patient to the hospital, you should go there immediately (or follow your local protocol).
   (Objective 5)

29. You should irrigate your eyes immediately after the eye splash exposure.
   (Objective 5)

30. No. The emergency department cannot ignore the patient's request. The patient has the legal right to refuse a test
   for human immunodeficiency virus.
   (Objective 5)

31. Ask if the patient has human immunodeficiency virus and assess for risk factors that would indicate the potential
   for such infection (intravenous drug use, unsafe sex practices).
   (Objective 5)

427

Chapter **28** **Infectious and Communicable Diseases**

32. The emergency department or occupational medicine staff still may offer you prophylactic drug treatment based on the nature of the exposure and the patient's risk factors (antiviral and possibly protease inhibitor drugs).
(Objective 5)

33. The benefits to you (risk of human immunodeficiency virus infection) versus complications of the prophylaxis therapy based on your personal health status will need to be weighed before you decide whether to take the medicine.
(Objective 5)

34. For 1 year, you will undergo periodic evaluation to determine whether you have converted to HIV-positive status. Until that time, you should alter your sexual practices and discontinue breastfeeding if you are lactating. This can be a difficult time for paramedics and their significant others, wondering if the next test result will be positive. Counseling may provide an opportunity to verbalize those feelings in a healthful manner.
(Objective 5)

35. Use of eye shield and face mask likely would have prevented this exposure.
(Objectives 5 and 12)

36. a. The Centers for Disease Control and Prevention establishes guidelines that often are adopted by the Occupational Safety and Health Administration and are incorporated by agencies such as the Department of Health and Department of Transportation into other documents (e.g., National Standard Paramedic Curriculum).
(Objective 1)

37. d. All of the answers reflect something that could break a link in the chain of transmission. Antibiotics can kill the pathogenic agent, cleaning agents with appropriate disinfectants destroy the environment conducive to transmission, and immunizations decrease host susceptibility.
(Objective 2)

38. b. All other answers are external barriers to infection.
(Objective 3)

39. c. Antibodies can fix complement. Killer cells are part of cell-mediated immunity.
(Objective 3)

40. c. The communicability period begins when the latent period ends and continues as long as the agent is present and can spread to others. The latent period begins with invasion of the body and ends when the agent can be shed or communicated. The disease period follows the incubation period and has variable lengths.
(Objective 4)

41. b. Short- and long-term mortality rates are higher from hepatitis B.
(Objective 2)

42. d. It is a virus spread by sexual transmission or blood. Antibiotics are used to treat bacteria. Vaccination greatly reduces risk but is not effective in all recipients.
(Objective 2)

43. c. The patient with pneumonia also may have all of the other signs and symptoms.
(Objective 5)

44. c. Trismus (lockjaw) often occurs and makes opening the mouth difficult. The patient often has muscle tetany and spasms but not urticaria or seizures.
(Objective 6)

45. b. Hydropenia is a lack of water in tissues; polydipsia is increased thirst; and polyuria is increased urination.
(Objective 6)

46. d
(Objective 7)

47. d. Bacterial infection, sterility, and meningitis are also complications.
(Objective 7)

48. c. Antibiotic therapy would be indicated only if a secondary bacterial infection develops. Aspirin is contraindicated for children and patients with chickenpox. Intravenous therapy would be needed only if an acute complication of these viral illnesses develops.
(Objectives 7, 8, and 9)

49. c. Influenza and pneumonia can produce cough; however, they do not persist as long as pertussis.
(Objective 7)

50. d. Pneumonia is an especially dangerous secondary complication for patients who are elderly or have preexisting lung or heart disease.
(Objective 8)

51. d. The enlarged spleen increases the chance of injury if the patient sustains a blow to the abdomen.
(Objective 8)

52. d. Syphilis is associated with systemic and chronic signs and symptoms.
(Objective 9)

53. d. The virus migrates along the sensory nerve pathways and remains in a latent stage on the ganglion.
(Objective 9)

54. b. There is no vaccine to prevent severe acute respiratory syndrome, nor is the disease treatable with antibiotics. Bronchodilators may be used to manage signs and symptoms of severe acute respiratory syndrome but do not prevent its spread.
(Objective 8)

WRAP IT UP

1. Protective eyewear could have prevented this exposure.
(Objective 5)

2.

Link	How is it present on this call?	Actions taken to reduce the risk of transmission
Pathogenic agent(s)	Human immunodeficiency virus, tuberculosis (bacteria)	Face washed with soap and water, eyes irrigated
Reservoir	Patient in poor heath	Mask on patient
Portal of exit	Cough with bloody sputum	Mask on patient
Transmission	Cough with bloody sputum	Mask on patient, N-95 mask, gloves, gloves on paramedics, window open in ambulance
Host susceptibility		Human immunodeficiency virus, tuberculosis prophylaxis drugs

(Objective 2)

3. a. (White, coated tongue), b (slurred speech, confusion), c (skin discoloration on feet), d (cough, hemoptysis, night sweats), f (numbness in feet), g (thin, wasted appearance)
(Objective 5)

4. Alcohol use, intravenous drug user (or former user), positive for human immunodeficiency virus, homeless
(Objective 5)

5. b. Follow-up should be initiated as soon as possible after the exposure for maximum effectiveness. The paramedic should make the decision after being given adequate information about the risks and benefits of treatment.
(Objective 11)

429

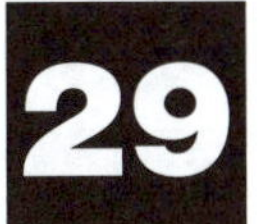 **Abdominal and Gastrointestinal Disorders**

READING ASSIGNMENT

Chapter 29, pages 886-905 in *Mosby's Paramedic Textbook*, ed. 4.

OBJECTIVES

Upon completion of this chapter, the paramedic student will be able to do the following:

1. Label a diagram of the abdominal organs.
2. Describe the function of the abdominal organs.
3. Outline prehospital assessment of a patient who is complaining of abdominal pain.
4. Distinguish between pain characteristics in abdominal pain.
5. Describe general prehospital management techniques for a patient who is complaining of abdominal pain.
6. Describe signs and symptoms, complications, and prehospital management for the following abdominal and gastrointestinal disorders: gastrointestinal bleeding, acute and chronic gastroenteritis, ulcerative colitis, diverticulosis, appendicitis, peptic ulcer disease, bowel obstruction, Crohn disease, pancreatitis, esophagogastric varices, hemorrhoids, cholecystitis, acute hepatitis, and hereditary hemochromatosis.

SUMMARY

- The major organs associated with the gastrointestinal (GI) system include the esophagus, stomach, small and large intestines, liver, gallbladder, and pancreas.
- After the scene survey and primary assessment of a patient with abdominal obtain a thorough history. The physical examination may help to determine whether the pain is visceral, somatic, or referred.
- The type and location of pain may help to narrow the differential diagnosis.
- Important signs and symptoms associated with abdominal pain include nausea, vomiting and anorexia, diarrhea, constipation, stool color, and fever.
- The most common treatment for abdominal pain occurs at the hospital. The paramedic should provide supportive treatment, manage life threats, and transport the patient to an appropriate facility.
- GI bleeding can be slow and chronic or rapid and life threatening. Causes of GI bleeding include esophagogastric varices, Mallory-Weiss syndrome, cancer, medication use, and other systemic disease.
- Gastroenteritis is inflammation of the stomach and intestines secondary to infectious agents, chemicals, or other conditions.
- Gastritis is acute or chronic inflammation of the gastric mucosa. Gastritis commonly results from hyperacidity, alcohol or other drug ingestion, bile reflux, and *Helicobacter pylori* infection.
- Ulcerative colitis is an inflammatory condition of the large intestine. Colitis is characterized by severe diarrhea and ulceration of the mucosa of the intestine (ulcerative colitis).
- Diverticulosis may result in bright red rectal bleeding if perforation occurs.
- Diverticulitis results when a diverticulum becomes obstructed with fecal matter.
- Appendicitis occurs when the passageway between the appendix and cecum is obstructed by fecal material or by inflammation caused by infection.
- Peptic ulcer disease occurs when open wounds or sores develop in the stomach or duodenum.
- Bowel obstruction is an occlusion of the intestinal lumen. It results in blockage of the normal flow of intestinal contents.
- Crohn disease is a chronic, inflammatory bowel disease. The disease is of unknown origin.
- Inflammation of the pancreas is called pancreatitis. It causes severe abdominal pain.
- Esophagogastric varices result from obstruction of blood flow to the liver as a result of liver disease. Rupture of the varices can cause hemorrhage and death.
- Hemorrhoids are distended veins in the rectoanal area.
- Cholecystitis is inflammation of the gallbladder. It most often is associated with the presence of gallstones.
- Hepatitis is characterized by the sudden onset of malaise, weakness, anorexia, intermittent nausea and vomiting, and dull right upper quadrant pain. This is usually followed within 1 week by the onset of jaundice, dark urine, or both.
- Hereditary hemochromatosis is a condition in which the body absorbs and stores too much iron. This can causes severe damage when it collects in the liver, heart, and pancreas.

Match the gastrointestinal disorder in column II with its description in column I. Use each disorder only once.

Column I

1. _________ Occlusion of the intestinal lumen

2. _________ Increased pain after ethyl alcohol ingestion; fever and signs of sepsis and shock also possible

3. _________ Protrusion of viscus from normal position opening in groin or abdominal wall

4. _________ Pain that is most intense at McBurney point

5. _________ Most common cause of massive rectal bleeding in older adults

6. _________ Open erosion wound in digestive system that may bleed

7. _________ Characterized by blood dripping into the toilet after a normal bowel movement

8. _________ Left lower quadrant abdominal pain resulting from a pouch in the colon wall

9. _________ Painless bleeding resulting from a vascular abnormality in the gastrointestinal tract

10. _________ Bright red hematemesis caused by rupture of vessels distended by portal hypertension

11. _________ Inflammation of the gallbladder

12. _________ Inflammation of the gastric mucosa

Column II

a. Appendicitis
b. Arteriovenous malformation
c. Cholecystitis
d. Diverticulitis through
e. Diverticulosis
f. Esophageal varices
g. Esophagitis
h. Gastritis
i. Hemorrhoids
j. Hernia
k. Intestinal obstruction
l. Pancreatitis
m. Peptic ulcer

13. Label the abdominal organs in Fig. 29-1.

a. _________________   f. _________________
b. _________________   g. _________________
c. _________________   h. _________________
d. _________________   i. _________________
e. _________________

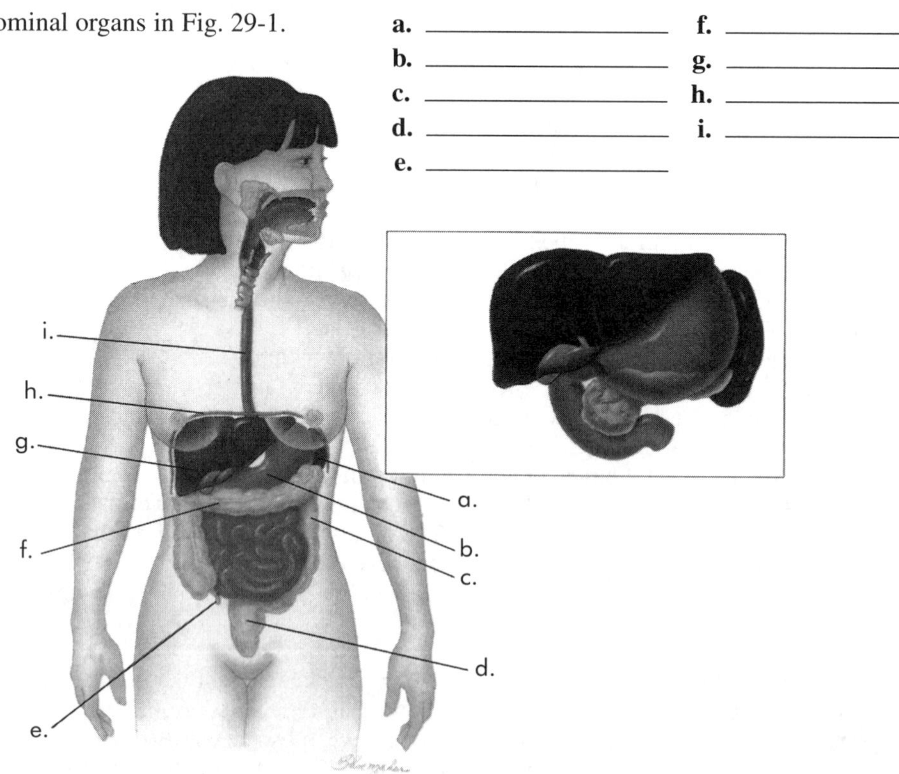

Figure 29-1

14. A 72-year-old man complains of left lower quadrant abdominal pain. State why you would or would not suspect each of the following illnesses as a cause of his pain.

   a. Pancreatitis:

____

   b. Cholecystitis:

____

   c. Diverticulitis:

____

   d. Peptic ulcer:

____

15. A 65-year-old man complains of severe epigastric pain.

   a. List specific questions you must ask this patient to obtain a complete medical history and to determine whether this is a gastrointestinal problem.

____

____

____

   b. What other significant medical problems must you try to rule out by asking these questions?

____

____

16. Name the type of pain described in each of the following statements.

   a. Your patient is supine with his legs flexed and complains of a constant, sharp, stabbing pain.

____

   b. A 40-year-old woman complains of a severe cramping pain at the umbilicus that peaks and then subsides. She is nauseated and has vomited twice.

____

   c. An obese 47-year-old woman complains of right upper quadrant abdominal pain that travels to her right shoulder blade.

____

17. A 17-year-old boy states that he had severe right lower quadrant pain that diminished several hours ago and is now generalized.

  a. What signs and symptoms would indicate that this patient has an acute abdominal condition and may be developing peritonitis?

  ____

  b. Describe the prehospital treatment for this patient.

  ____

  ____

  ____

18. Which of the following abdominal organs is located in the retroperitoneal space?
  a. Liver
  b. Pancreas
  c. Spleen
  d. Stomach

19. A 78-year-old man states that he has been unable to have a bowel movement for 1 week and has been vomiting profusely. What do you suspect?
  a. Appendicitis
  b. Bowel obstruction
  c. Diverticulosis
  d. Peptic ulcer

20. At 1900, a 40-year-old woman complains of intermittent severe right upper quadrant abdominal pain. She is vomiting and has a low-grade fever. What do you suspect?
  a. Colitis
  b. Cholecystitis
  c. Esophagitis
  d. Hepatitis

21. Which of the following is most likely to cause a life-threatening hemorrhage?
  a. Arteriovenous malformations
  b. Diverticulitis
  c. Esophagogastric varices
  d. Hemorrhoids

22. The cause of acute abdominal pain is most accurately assessed in the prehospital setting by which of the following?
  a. Abdominal examination
  b. Patient history
  c. Secondary survey
  d. Vital sign assessment

23. Which of the following is most suggestive of a hemorrhagic gastrointestinal problem?
  a. Anorexia
  b. Fever
  c. Melena
  d. Tachycardia

Questions 24 and 25 refer to the following case study:

A pale, elderly man has had severe vomiting and diarrhea for 3 days. His only history is high blood pressure controlled by an ACE inhibitor and a diuretic. He has severe lower abdominal cramping and is in a fetal position. His wife has a similar illness, but it is not as severe. His blood pressure is 92/50 mm Hg; P, 128 beats/min; and R, 20 breaths/min.

24. What is a likely cause of the man's pain?
  a. Appendicitis
  b. Cholecystitis
  c. Diverticulosis
  d. Gastroenteritis

25. Which is a priority in your care of this patient at this time?
    a. Administer pain medicine to relieve his pain.
    b. Give him some medicine to relieve his nausea.
    c. Position him to allow for maximum comfort.
    d. Start an IV and administer fluids to treat shock.

26. Which of the following conditions may cause jaundice?
    a. Colitis
    b. Gastritis
    c. Hepatitis
    d. Peptic ulcer disease

Questions 27 and 28 pertain to the following case study:

A 57-year-old man with alcoholism complains of nausea and vomiting. He has abdominal pain that starts in the area of the umbilicus and goes to both shoulders. He is hot to the touch. Vital signs are BP, 94/58 mm Hg; P, 132 beats/min; and R, 28 breaths/min.

27. Which intervention is indicated first for this man?
    a. Morphine (4 mg IV push)
    b. Normal saline (200 mL bolus)
    c. Oxygen (15 L/min by mask)
    d. Promethazine (Phenergan), 25 mg IV

28. What abdominal illness is a probable diagnosis for this man?
    a. Crohn disease
    b. Esophageal varices
    c. Pancreatitis
    d. Ulcerative colitis

29. When liver function is impaired, what should you anticipate?
    a. Decreased white blood cell production
    b. Dark green colored stools
    c. Increased risk of bleeding
    d. Scaphoid shaped abdomen

30. What treatment measure is indicated for patients with ulcerative colitis, Crohn disease, and pancreatitis?
    a. Normal saline to maintain blood pressure
    b. Narcotic pain medication intravenous
    c. Administer sodium bicarbonate
    d. Monitor electrocardiogram

WRAP IT UP

At 0300, the horn sounds and the speaker blares, "4017, respond to an EMS call, abdominal pains, Haven Golden Rest Home, 222 Main, cross street Elm." Your patient is an 80-year-old man who has a history of dementia. His medication sheet lists a number of antihypertensives, aspirin, some antiarthritic drugs, and some laxatives and stool softeners. The nurse states that the patient had a shaking chill, vomited twice, seems agitated, and has been moaning and holding his lower abdomen. She thinks his last bowel movement was 4 days ago, and a note in his record states that it was very dark in color. His skin is very warm, moist, and pale, and he is very restless. Vital signs are BP, 100/70 mm Hg; P, 116 beats/min; R, 20 breaths/min; Sao$_2$, 93% on room air; and T (axilla), 100.4°F (38°C). His skin is dry and tents slightly, and his mucous membranes are dry. The rest of his physical examination is unremarkable except that his abdomen is tender to palpation and he is guarding it. Because of his dementia, it is difficult to communicate well enough with him to have him localize the pain. You administer oxygen by nasal cannula at 6 L/min; you then start an IV of normal saline and infuse a bolus of 100 mL, reassessing his breath sounds and vital signs after it has been infused. Medical direction asks you to hold off on pain medicine administration until he can be assessed more thoroughly.

You transport the patient and later find out that free air was present in his abdomen secondary to a ruptured diverticulum. In consultation with his family, after his status deteriorated, the decision was made not to operate.

1. Which abdominal organs could cause pain in the following regions if they are injured, inflamed, or diseased?

   a. Left upper quadrant:

   ____

   b. Right upper quadrant:

   ____

   c. Left lower quadrant:

   ____

   d. Right lower quadrant:

   ____

2. Which of the following describes the correct procedure for an abdominal examination?
   a. Percuss carefully so that painful stimulus can be evaluated.
   b. Auscultate after palpation so you can focus on tender areas.
   c. Begin palpation in an area of no reported pain and move to the painful area last.
   d. Inspection can often reveal the source of the abdominal pain.

3. Put a ✓ beside any illnesses that could be responsible for this patient's signs and symptoms.
   a. ________ Appendicitis   e. ________ Diverticulosis
   b. ________ Bacterial infection   f. ________ Hepatitis B
   c. ________ Cholecystitis   g. ________ Intestinal obstruction
   d. ________ Crohn disease   h. ________ Pancreatitis

4. What additional interventions could have been provided for this patient?

   ____

CHAPTER 29 ANSWERS

REVIEW QUESTIONS

1. k

2. l

3. j

4. a

5. e

6. m

7. i

8. d

9. b

10. f

11. c

12. h
(Questions 1-12, Objective 6)

13. a. Spleen; b. stomach; c. descending colon; d. rectum; e. appendix; f. transverse colon; g. liver; h. diaphragm;
i. esophagus
(Objective 1)

14. a. No. The pain of pancreatitis is located in the epigastric region or right or left upper quadrant. b. No. The
pain of cholecystitis is located in the epigastric region or right upper quadrant. It is more common in women
younger than age 50 years. c. Yes. Diverticulitis is one possibility. It is common in older adults, and the pain is
often in the left lower quadrant. d. No. Pain from a peptic ulcer would typically be in the epigastric area.
(Objective 6)

15. a. Does anything make the pain better or worse? What does the pain feel like (sharp, stabbing, cramping, dull)?
Can you show me where the pain is? Does the pain go anywhere else? On a scale of 0 to 10, with 0 being no
pain and 10 being the worst pain you have ever had, rate the pain. When did the pain begin? Associated signs
and symptoms do you have or have you had any nausea, vomiting, diarrhea, constipation, unusual-colored
stools, chills, fever, or shortness of breath? Medical history and medications.

b. Myocardial infarction and abdominal aneurysm
(Objective 3)

16. a. Somatic; b. visceral; c. referred
(Objective 4)

17. a. Fever, chills, tachycardia, tachypnea, position (lying on side with knees flexed and pulled in toward the chest),
reluctance to move, skin pallor, absent bowel sounds, generalized involuntary guarding, and rigidity of the
abdomen
(Objective 3, 5)

b. Oxygen by non-rebreather mask; IV by 16-gauge catheter with normal saline or lactated Ringer solution (rate
at least 100 mL/hour, determined by patient's vital signs)
(Objective 4)

STUDENT SELF-ASSESSMENT

18. b. All of the other organs are in the abdominal cavity.
(Objective 2)

19. b. Appendicitis would be unusual at this age and typically would not cause the symptoms listed. Diverticulosis
and peptic ulcer would not typically produce the symptoms described.
(Objective 6)

20. b. Her age, the time of day, and the description of the pain are characteristics of cholecystitis
(Objective 6)

21. c. All of the disorders listed cause bleeding, but rupture of the esophagogastric varices usually produces
rapid, life-threatening bleeding. Bleeding from AV malformations may be minor or severe. Bleeding from
diverticulitis may be serious but is not typically an acute life-threatening emergency at onset. Hemorrhoidal
bleeding is usually not severe.
(Objective 6)

22. b. The patient's age and gender and the description of the medical history often disclose more about the cause of the abdominal illness than a physical examination. The severity of the patient's present condition is determined by the physical examination.
(Objective 3)

23. c. Melena (black or maroon stool) indicates the presence of bleeding. Tachycardia can be caused by bleeding, fever, pain, or other fluid loss.
(Objective 3)

24. d. The signs and symptoms, as well as the fact that the man's wife had the same illness, point to this as a probable cause.
(Objective 6)

25. d. The most pressing problem is the shock from fluid loss. IV fluid replacement is needed as soon as possible.
(Objective 6)

26. c
(Objective 6)

27. c. A normal saline bolus is given next as soon as an IV line has been established.
(Objective 6)

28. c. Esophageal varices present with life-threatening bleeding. Crohn disease and ulcerative colitis would be unusual in someone of this age without a history of this.
(Objective 6)

29. c. The liver has an important role in blood clotting. The stools are often light (clay colored). The abdomen is likely to be distended from ascites.
(Objective 2)

30. a. Fluid volume loss is common in the acute phase of all of these illnesses. Pain medication is indicated if the patient has acute abdominal pain.
(Objective 6)

WRAP IT UP

1. Left upper quadrant: Liver, bowel, gallbladder
Right upper quadrant: Stomach, bowel, pancreas, spleen
Left lower quadrant: Bowel
Right lower quadrant: Bowel, appendix
(Objective 1)

2. c. Palpate from an area of no pain (if possible) to the area of greatest pain to facilitate the best exam. The exam should be performed in the following order: inspection, auscultation, palpation, and percussion.
(Objective 5)

3. a, b, c, e, f, g, h
(Objective 6)

4. If the patient's vomiting had persisted, medical direction might have ordered an antiemetic. It's also possible that some pain medicine could have been ordered (a small dose) to relieve his obvious discomfort. This would have had to be done in consultation with medical direction because of the patient's complex history.
(Objective 6)

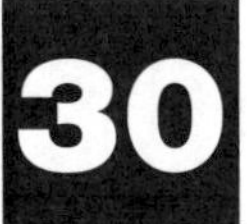 **Genitourinary and Renal Disorders**

READING ASSIGNMENT

Chapter 30, pages 906-927, in *Mosby's Paramedic Textbook*, ed. 4.

OBJECTIVES

Upon completion of this chapter, the paramedic student will be able to do the following:

1. Label a diagram of the urinary system.
2. Distinguish between acute and chronic renal failure.
3. Outline the pathophysiology of renal failure.
4. Identify the signs and symptoms of renal failure.
5. Describe the process of hemodialysis and peritoneal dialysis.
6. Describe signs and symptoms and care of emergent conditions associated with dialysis
7. Describe pathophysiology, signs and symptoms, assessment, and prehospital management of the patient with urinary retention, urinary tract infection, pyelonephritis, urinary calculus, epididymitis, Fourniere gangrene, phimosis, paraphimosis, priapism, benign prostatic hypertrophy, testicular masses, and testicular torsion.
8. Outline the physical examination for patients with genitourinary disorders.
9. Discuss general prehospital management for patients with genitourinary disorders.

SUMMARY

- The urinary system removes waste products from the blood. It helps to maintain a constant body fluid volume and composition as well.
- The nephron is the functional unit of the kidney. It filters blood, removes waste products, and produces urine.
- Renal failure may result in uremia, hyperkalemia, acidosis, hypertension, and volume overload with congestive heart failure.
- Acute renal failure (ARF) occurs when the kidneys are unable to excrete the daily load of toxins in the urine. Its onset may be within hours.
- Prerenal ARF results from poor perfusion of the kidneys. Intrarenal ARF is caused by conditions that damage the tissues of the kidney. Postrenal ARF is caused by obstruction of urine flow from both kidneys.
- Dialysis is a technique used to normalize blood chemistry. Dialysis is used in patients who have acute or chronic renal failure. Dialysis also is used to remove blood toxins. The two dialysis techniques are hemodialysis and peritoneal dialysis. Dialysis emergencies may include problems with vascular access, hemorrhage, hypotension, chest pain, severe hyperkalemia, disequilibrium syndrome, air embolism, and cardiac arrest.
- Urinary retention is the inability to urinate.
- Urinary tract infections can involve the upper or lower urinary tract.
- Pyelonephritis is inflammation of the kidney parenchyma. It can lead to chronic renal problems.
- Urinary calculi are stones that originate in the kidney.
- Epididymitis is inflammation of the epididymis. The epididymis is the tube that carries sperm from the testicle to the seminal vesicles.
- Fournier gangrene is a bacterial infection of the genitals that can lead to death of skin tissue and systemic sepsis.
- Phimosis is tightness of the foreskin of the penis. Paraphimosis occurs when an uncircumcised male is unable to retract the foreskin over the head of the penis.
- Priapism is a painful, sustained erection.
- Benign prostatic hypertrophy is enlargement of the prostate gland. It may be associated with urinary difficulty and urinary tract infections.
- Testicular masses may be benign or cancerous.
- Testicular torsion is a true emergency. In this condition a testicle twists on its spermatic cord. This disrupts the blood supply to the testicle.
- The physical examination for a patient with a urinary tract problem is similar to that performed for abdominal pain. Patients with genitourinary pain should be managed as any other patient with acute pain.

Match the genitourinary problem in column II with the description in column I. Use each disorder only once.

Column I

1. _________ Can cause vascular infarction and loss of function

2. _________ Inflammation of part of the male reproductive system

3. _________ Systemic disease linked with diabetes and hypertension

4. _________ Infectious process that causes dysuria and hematuria

5. _________ Causes include enlarged prostate and CNS dysfunction

6. _________ Caused by an excess of insoluble salts in the urine

7. _________ Upper urinary infection treated with IV antibiotics

Column II

a. Acute renal failure
b. Chronic renal failure
c. Epididymitis
d. Pyelonephritis
e. Testicular torsion
f. Urinary calculus
g. Urinary retention
h. Urinary tract infection

8. Label the parts of the urinary system shown in Fig. 30-1.

a. ____

b. ____

c. ____

d. ____

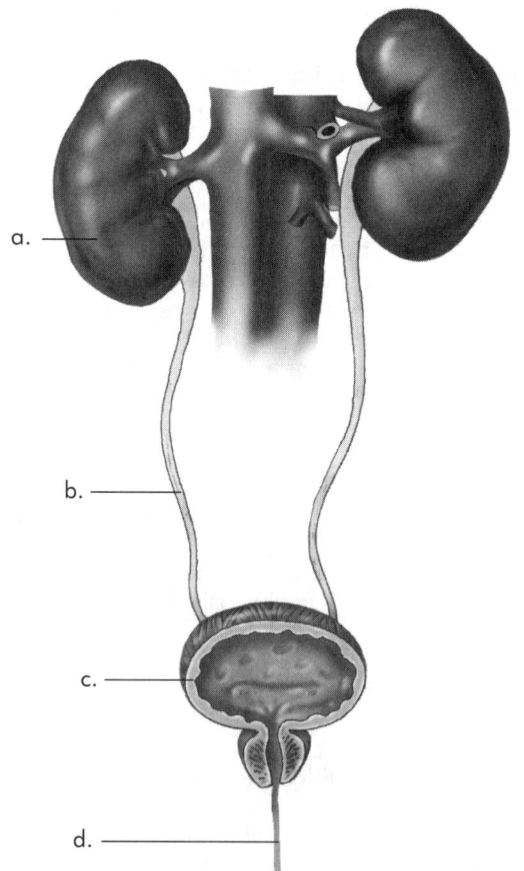

Figure 30-1

Chapter **30** **Genitourinary and Renal Disorders**

9. Identify the genitourinary disorder suspected and the prehospital care needed in each of the following situations.

   a. A 35-year-old afebrile man complains of a sudden onset of severe flank pain that radiates into his testicle.

     Condition:

     Care:

   b. Your 21-year-old patient complains of painful swelling in the scrotal sac that is unrelieved by elevation. He is in acute distress and has vomited twice.

     Condition:

     Care:

   c. A 35-year-old woman with a recent history of recurrent urinary infections complains of fever, chills, and severe flank pain.

     Condition:

     Care:

   d. A 27-year-old woman complains of burning on urination and of feeling as if she must urinate every 20 minutes.

     Condition:

     Care:

10. How can you minimize psychological discomfort for a patient with a urology problem when performing the physical examination?

11. Identify three causes of each of the following disorders.

a. Acute renal failure:

____

b. Chronic renal failure:

____

12. You are called to a dialysis center for a person in shock.

a. What types of patient problems should you anticipate en route to this call?

____

b. If the patient is hypotensive and needs fluid resuscitation, describe how you will initiate fluid therapy and indicate the volume you will infuse.

____

13. Complete the information in the following table regarding dialysis emergencies.

Disorder	Cause	Effect on Patient	Interventions
Hemorrhage			
Hypotension			
Chest pain			
Hyperkalemia			
Disequilibrium syndrome			
Air embolism			

14. You are dispatched to a private residence for a patient in full cardiac arrest. You find a 55-year-old man in asystole. The family reports that he lost consciousness about 5 minutes before your arrival. The patient's history includes renal failure. He missed hemodialysis this week and was feeling bad before cardiac arrest.

a. You begin CPR. List the first three drugs you should administer to this patient, including the dose and route.

____

b. How will the drug therapy help to correct some of the problems that may have caused the patient's cardiac arrest?

____

c. What problem may occur if this combination of drugs is administered improperly?

____

A 31-year-old man calls 9-1-1 complaining of severe flank pain and bloody urine. He said it began suddenly and is sharp and rates it as 10 of 10. He is pale and diaphoretic. Vital signs are BP 136/76, P 118 beats/min, and R 20 breaths/min. He has vomited twice.

15. a. What is the most likely cause of this patient's pain?

b. Where might his pain radiate?

c. Describe your IV therapy for this patient.

d. List two narcotic pain relievers that you may administer to relieve his pain.

e. List one parenteral non-narcotic analgesic you may administer to this patient.

____

f. List two antiemetic drugs that you may administer to relieve his pain.

____

STUDENT SELF-ASSESSMENT

16. Which genitourinary emergency requires treatment within 4 hours to prevent irreversible damage?
   a. Epididymitis
   b. Pyelonephritis
   c. Testicular torsion
   d. Urinary calculus

17. Which of the following is a prerenal cause of acute renal failure?
   a. Kidney infection
   b. Prostatic enlargement
   c. Shock
   d. Ureteral strictures

18. How is prehospital care affected if the patient has a dialysis fistula or shunt?
   a. Blood pressure should be checked in the arm opposite the shunt.
   b. The arm in which the shunt is placed should be elevated.
   c. Vascular access should be initiated in the fistula or shunt.
   d. No special consideration is required.

19. You are caring for a patient with a temperature of 102.5°F (39.2°C) who is on continuous peritoneal dialysis. What is a common cause of fever in patients undergoing this treatment?
   a. Dehydration
   b. Infected fistula
   c. Peritonitis
   d. Pneumonia

20. You are called to the home of an unconscious person in chronic renal failure. The ECG tracing is shown in Fig. 30-2. Which electrolyte imbalance do you suspect?
   a. Hyperkalemia
   b. Hypokalemia
   c. Hypercalcemia
   d. Hypocalcemia

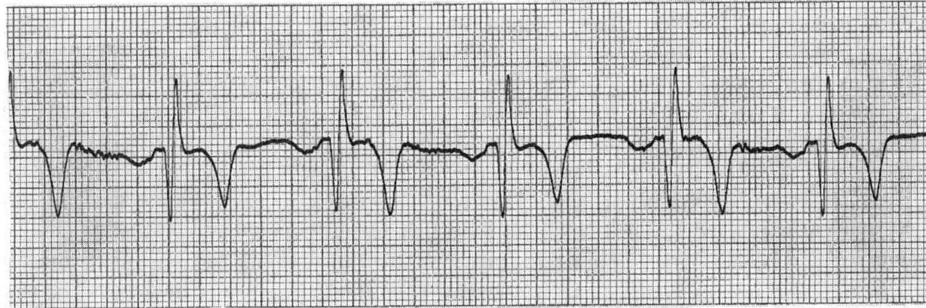

Figure 30-2

21. What drug may be ordered by medical direction to correct the underlying electrolyte imbalance in question 20?
   a. Atropine sulfate (1 mg IV)
   b. Sodium bicarbonate (1 mEq/kg IV)
   c. Magnesium sulfate (1 to 2 g IV)
   d. Verapamil (2.5 mg IV)

22. What physiologic problem makes patients in renal failure more susceptible to hypoxia?
   a. Anemia
   b. Glucose intolerance
   c. Pericarditis
   d. Uremia

23. Which patient may develop acute renal failure related to prerenal disease?
   a. Polycystic kidney disease
   b. Hypovolemic burn shock
   c. Obstruction from urinary calculus
   d. Pyelonephritis

24. What physical finding should you expect when you assess a patient who has untreated chronic renal failure?
   a. Bilateral crackles in the lungs
   b. Jaundice of the skin
   c. Right upper quadrant abdominal pain
   d. Clubbing of the fingers

25. Which is a characteristic dialysate fluid for peritoneal and hemodialysis must have compared with blood so water is removed from the vascular space?
   a. High in potassium
   b. Hypertonic
   c. 0.45% normal saline
   d. Low temperature

26. What is a life-threatening risk of Fournier gangrene?
   a. Loss of genital tissue
   b. Chronic renal failure
   c. Sepsis
   d. Pulmonary emboli

27. What is a risk of benign prostatic hypertrophy if it is untreated?
   a. Cancer will spread
   b. Chronic renal failure
   c. Epididymitis
   d. Urinary calculi

28. Which of the following testicular masses is potentially lethal?
   a. Hydrocele
   b. Spermatocele
   c. Testicular cancer
   d. Varicocele

WRAP IT UP

At 1400, you are dispatched to a dialysis center for a patient who has chest pain. On arrival, you find a 59-year-old man who is anxious, pale, and diaphoretic. He missed dialysis for 1 week because of a severe snowstorm in the area. He came in today fatigued and twitching. About 10 minutes into his dialysis session, he had several episodes of hypotension and then began complaining of chest pain and dyspnea. He has a history of type 1 diabetes, hypertension, and renal failure. He is pale and sweaty and complains of midsternal chest pain. His oxygen saturation is 94% on room air. You administer oxygen at 4 L/min, which quickly improves his Sao$_2$ to 98%. The nurse is keeping pressure on the dialysis fistula site in his left arm, so you go to the right arm to assess vital signs. Your findings are BP, 198/106 mm Hg; P, 110 beats/min; R, 20 breaths/min; and blood glucose, 170 mg/dL. The patient has generalized edema, and you can hear bibasilar crackles in his lungs. You start an IV in the right forearm, administer one spray (0.4 mg) of nitroglycerin, apply the ECG monitor, and then move him by stretcher into the ambulance. You note tall, tented T waves on his ECG. While you are attaching the electrodes to perform a 12-lead ECG, his eyes roll back, and his body goes limp, and you note a very wide, slow ventricular complex on the monitor. You immediately determine that he is not breathing; you assess a carotid pulse but find none, so you begin CPR. Your partner immediately radios for additional help and then takes over CPR. You administer epinephrine IV and set up for intubation.

   You consider possible causes of cardiac arrest in this patient and administer calcium chloride. You flush the line before and after pushing another epinephrine. Then you give sodium bicarbonate. As you are giving the bicarbonate, the patient's rhythm changes to asystole. The ED staff works for another 10 minutes to resuscitate the patient but are unsuccessful, and the man is pronounced dead.

444

1. What risk factors does the patient have for chronic renal failure?

____

____

2. Put a ✓ beside any of the following signs or symptoms of chronic renal failure that you observed in this patient.

a. _______ Anorexia	**h.** _______ Hallucinations	**o.** _______ Pasty, yellow, slow
b. _______ Anemia	**i.** _______ Mental dullness	**p.** _______ Pulmonary edema
c. _______ Anxiety	**j.** _______ Muscle twitching	**q.** _______ Seizures
d. _______ Delirium	**k.** _______ Nausea	**r.** _______ Uremic frost
e. _______ Electrolyte disturbances	**l.** _______ Pericarditis	**s.** _______ Vomiting
f. _______ Fatigue	**m.** _______ Peripheral edema	
g. _______ Glucose intolerance	**n.** _______ Progressive obtundation	

3. Which is true regarding the dialysis fistula?
   a. Blood pressures can be obtained in that arm without harm to the fistula.
   b. Patency should be verified by using Doppler to auscultate pulsation.
   c. Drug administration by this route is contraindicated.
   d. Venous access by this site should be avoided in almost all cases.

4. Explain some possible causes for the following conditions this patient had.

   a. Hypotension:

   ____

   ____

   b. Chest pain:

   ____

   ____

   c. Cardiac arrest:

   ____

   ____

5. Discuss your rationale for the following interventions used in this patient.

   a. Nitroglycerin:

   ____

   ____

   b. Calcium chloride:

   ____

   ____

c. Sodium bicarbonate:

CHAPTER 30 ANSWERS

REVIEW QUESTIONS

1. e
(Objective 2)

2. c
(Objective 2)

3. b
(Objective 5)

4. h

5. g

6. f

7. d
(Questions 4–7, Objective 7)

8. a. Kidney
b. Ureter
c. Bladder
d. Urethra
(Objective 1)

9. a. Urinary calculus: initiate intravenous line; consult with medical direction regarding administration of analgesics such as ketorolac or morphine. b. Testicular torsion: initiate intravenous line; apply ice pack to scrotum and transport rapidly. c. Pyelonephritis: initiate intravenous line; transport. d. Urinary tract infection: transport.
(Objective 7)

10. Protect the patient's privacy with drapes. Have a paramedic who is the same gender as the patient perform the examination if possible. Have a chaperone present during a physical exam of the genitalia (if indicated). Explain all actions to the patient and proceed in a calm, caring manner.
(Objective 8)

11. a. Trauma, shock, infection, urinary obstruction, and multisystem diseases; b. hypertension, diabetes, congenital condition, and pyelonephritis
(Objective 2)

12. a. Too much fluid taken off in dialysis or bleeding at the fistula caused by a pseudoaneurysm (any cause of bleeding is serious because the patient has decreased platelets and is heparinized during dialysis); sepsis; acute myocardial infarction. b. Initiate large-bore intravenous line in the arm without the arteriovenous fistula; infuse a small volume initially (200–300 mL) and reevaluate the patient for signs of fluid overload (crackles, engorged neck veins, pulmonary edema).
(Objective 6)

13.

Disorder	Cause	Effect on Patient	Interventions
Hemorrhage	Decrease in platelet function; anticoagulant use; anemia; bleeding from fistula or graft	Signs and symptoms of shock; dyspnea, angina	Control external bleeding; treat for shock; rapid transport
Hypotension	Hemodialysis because of decreased volume; changes in electrolyte concentration; vascular instability	Decreased blood pressure; signs and symptoms of shock	Small fluid challenge (200–300 mL); monitor for signs and symptoms of congestive hear failure
Chest pain	Hypotension and hypoxia during dialysis	Chest pain, headache, dizziness	Oxygen, fluid replacement, antianginal drugs
Hyperkalemia	Poor diet regulation; missed dialysis	Weakness; may have no symptoms, tall, tented T wave; prolonged PRI (K^+ >6–6.5 mmol/L); depressed S segments and loss of P waves (K^+ >7 mmol/L); wide QRS	Suspect if renal patient in arrest; medical direction may order $CaCl$ and $NaHCO_3$ during cardiac arrest
Disequilibrium syndrome	Increased osmolality of the ECF compared with ICF in the brain or with the CSF	HA, nausea, fatigue; confusion, seizures, coma	Transport; treat seizures with diazepam or lorazepam
Air embolism	Negative pressure in dialysis tubing; malfunction in dialysis machine	Dyspnea, cyanosis, hypotension, respiratory distress	Oxygen rapid transport; position patient on left side with head down

CSF, cerebrospinal fluid; *ECF*, extracellular fluid; *HA*, Headache; *ICF*, extracellular fluid; *PRI*, PR interval.

(Objective 6)

14. a. Epinephrine (1 mg IV) (may substitute vasopressin 40 units for the first or second dose of epinephrine), calcium chloride (10%) 5 to 10 mL (500–1000 mg); sodium bicarbonate (1 mEq/kg IV)
(Objective 6)
b. Epinephrine can increase peripheral vascular resistance and is a sympathomimetic. Calcium chloride stabilizes the myocardial cell membrane. Sodium bicarbonate should be given because it helps move potassium into the cell and helps correct metabolic acidosis.
(Objective 6)
c. Bicarbonate may inactivate epinephrine and precipitate with calcium chloride; therefore, IV tubing should be flushed between drugs.
(Objective 6)

15. a. Urinary calculus (nephrolithiasis)
b. Kidney stone pain often radiates to the testicle, groin, or upper leg on the affected side.
c. Infuse normal saline per protocol. Usually at least 200 to 250 mL/hr if not contraindicated.
d. Fentanyl (Sublimaze); morphine; hydromorphone (Dilaudid)
e. Ketoradol (Toradol)
f. Ondansetron (Zofran); metoclopramide (Reglan)
(Objective 7)

16. c. Because a twisted testicle causes blockage of the blood supply to the testis, intervention within 4 to 6 hours is essential.
(Objective 7)

17. c. Kidney infection is a renal cause, and prostatic enlargement and ureteral strictures are postrenal causes.
(Objective 3)

18. a. Do not assess blood pressure or start an IV on the side where the fistula or shunt is placed. Vascular access should not routinely be obtained through the shunt. In rare cases, because of an cardiac arrest situation, medical direction may authorize vascular access through the shunt.
(Objective 6)

19. c. Infection at the site of catheter insertion is common and may lead to peritonitis.
(Objective 6)

20. a. Peaked, tented T waves are associated with hyperkalemia, a common electrolyte imbalance.
(Objective 6)

21. b. Sodium bicarbonate may temporarily cause movement of potassium out of the vascular space and may relieve the cardiac effects until definitive care (dialysis) can be given.
(Objective 6)

22. a. Anemia secondary to lack of a substance needed for red blood cell production reduces the oxygen-carrying capacity of the blood.
(Objective 3)

23. b. Polycystic kidney disease and pyelonephritis are intrarenal causes and obstruction from urinary calculus is postrenal.
(Objective 3)

24. a. Chronic renal failure can lead to congestive heart failure
(Objective 2)

25. b. Fluid will flow across the membrane toward the hypertonic fluid, so excess fluid is removed from the blood. The goal is to lower potassium so the potassium in the dialysate would need to be lower than in the blood for diffusion to occur. 0.45% normal saline is hypotonic, so fluid would flow from the dialysate into the blood if that were used.
(Objective 5)

26. c. If the bacteria infects the blood, sepsis can develop. Tissue necrosis and loss are possible but not life threatening.
(Objective 7)

27. b. If urinary retention occurs, renal failure can develop over time. Benign prostatic hypertrophy is not cancerous.
(Objective 7)

28. c. If untreated, testicular cancer can be lethal.
(Objective 7)

448

1. Hypertension, diabetes
(Objective 3)

2. c, e, f, j, k, m
(Objective 6)

3. d. If the fistula is damaged during the attempt to access it, the patient's emergency dialysis will be delayed. After venous access has been established, drugs can be given by this route. Patency can be verified by palpation of a bruit over the fistula. Blood pressure assessment and vascular access should not be performed in the arm with the fistula to avoid damaging the fistula.
(Objective 6)

4. a. During dialysis, hypotension can be caused by a rapid reduction in vascular volume, fast changes in electrolytes, or vascular instability.
  b. Hypotension and mild hypoxia, in addition to the patient's high-risk factors, can result in chest pain during dialysis.
  c. Cardiac arrest could be a result of myocardial irritability related to occlusion of blood vessels or of acidosis and electrolyte imbalance related to the patient's week without dialysis.
(Objective 6)

5. a. Nitroglycerin was given to dilate his coronary blood vessels, improving blood flow to the heart, and to decrease preload and afterload, thereby reducing the work the heart must do.
  b. Calcium chloride stabilizes the myocardial cell membrane when hyperkalemia is present.
  c. Sodium bicarbonate was given because of the possibility that acidosis or hyperkalemia (or both) related to the renal failure caused the cardiac arrest.
(Objective 6)

31 Gynecology

READING ASSIGNMENT

Chapter 31, pages 928-941, in *Mosby's Paramedic Textbook,* ed. 4.

OBJECTIVES

Upon completion of this chapter, the paramedic student will be able to do the following:

1. Describe the physiologic processes of menstruation and ovulation.
2. Describe the pathophysiology of the following nontraumatic causes of abdominal pain in females: pelvic inflammatory disease, Bartholin abscess, vaginitis, ruptured ovarian cyst, ovarian torsion, cystitis, dysmenorrhea, mittelschmerz, endometriosis, ectopic pregnancy, vaginal bleeding, uterine prolapse, and vaginal foreign body.
3. Outline the prehospital assessment and management of women with abdominal pain or bleeding.
4. Outline specific assessment and management for patients who have been sexually assaulted.
5. Describe specific prehospital measures to preserve evidence in sexual assault cases.

SUMMARY

- Menstruation is the normal, periodic discharge of blood, mucus, and cellular debris from the uterine mucosa. Ovulation is the release of a secondary oocyte from the ovary.
- Pelvic inflammatory disease results from infection of the cervix, uterus, fallopian tubes, and ovaries and their supporting structures.
- A Bartholin abscess is a buildup of pus in one of the Bartholin's glands.
- Vaginitis is inflammation and infection of the vulva and vagina.
- Ruptured ovarian cyst occurs when a thin-walled, fluid-filled sac located on the ovary ruptures. This can cause internal hemorrhage.
- Ovarian torsion is twisting of the ovary caused by another condition or disease.
- Cystitis is inflammation of the inner lining of the bladder. It usually is caused by a bacterial infection.
- Dysmenorrhea is characterized by painful menses. It may be associated with headache, faintness, dizziness, nausea, diarrhea, backache, and leg pain.
- Mittelschmerz is German for "middle pain." This pain may occur from the rupture of the graafian follicle and bleeding from the ovary during the menstrual cycle.
- Endometritis is inflammation of the uterine lining. Endometriosis is characterized by endometrial tissue growing outside of the uterus.
- An ectopic pregnancy is one that develops outside the uterus. Rupture of an ectopic pregnancy can cause life-threatening hemorrhage.
- Vaginal bleeding is the loss of blood from the uterus, cervix, or vagina.
- Uterine prolapse occurs when the uterus descends into the vagina.
- Vaginal foreign bodies can cause vaginal discharge, pain, and urinary discomfort.
- History of the patient with a gynecologic emergency should include pregnancy history, history of cesearean births, last menstrual period, possibility of pregnancy, history of previous gynecologic problems, blood loss, vaginal discharge, contraceptives used, history of trauma to the reproductive system, and degree of emotional distress.
- The goal of prehospital care of lower abdominal pain in women is to obtain a history (including a gynecologic history); provide airway, ventilatory, and circulatory support as needed; and provide transport for physician evaluation.
- Sexual assault is a crime of violence. It can have serious physical and psychological effects.
- Paramedics should be aware of the need to preserve evidence from a sexual assault crime scene.

Match the gynecologic problems in column II with their description in column I. Use each term only once.

Column I

1. _________ Abdominal pain at ovulation

2. _________ Beginning of menses

3. _________ Intraabdominal growth of the uterine lining

4. _________ Infection of the female pelvic organs

5. _________ Menstrual cramps

6. _________ Fluid sac that ruptures

Column II

a. Dysmenorrhea
b. Endometriosis
c. Endometritis
d. Menarche
e. Mittelschmerz
f. Pelvic inflammatory disease
g. Ruptured ovarian cyst

7. The normal menstrual cycle is about **(a)** _________________ days. The average menstrual flow is

(b) _________________ to _________________ mL and usually lasts from **(c)** _________________

to _________________ days. During the menstrual cycle, some of the primary follicles become

(d) _________________. These enlarge and form a lump on the surface of the ovary and when mature are

known as the **(e)** _________________ or _________________ The release of the oocyte from the follicle

is called **(f)** _________________ After ovulation, the follicle turns into a glandular structure called the

(g) _________________, the cells of which secrete large amounts of **(h)** _________________ and some

(i) _________________ If pregnancy occurs, the fertilized oocyte **(j)** (_________________) begins

releasing a hormone-like substance called **(k)** _________________ that keeps the corpus from degenerating.

8. Other than pain, list three signs or symptoms that a woman may experience during menses.

   a. ____

   b. ____

   c. ____

Questions 9 to 12 refer to the following case study:

A 19-year-old woman is complaining of severe pelvic pain. Her pain began yesterday, and she says it is unbearable now. She has no allergies, takes no medicines, and has no significant medical history.

9. What specific questions related to her obstetric history should you ask her?

   a. ____

   b. ____

   c. ____

   d. ____

   e. ____

   f. ____

   g. ____

   h. ____

   i. ____

   j. ____

She says she has never been pregnant, that she presently has her menstrual period, and that it is of normal color and amount. She denies vaginal discharge or the possibility of pregnancy because she uses birth control pills. She states that she has not had intercourse in 4 months. She denies other symptoms of pregnancy and any history of gynecologic problems.

10. What should you specifically assess on the physical examination?

____

____

Her lower abdomen is diffusely tender. Vital signs are within normal limits, and her skin is warm and dry.

11. What are some potential causes of her pain?

____

____

12. What prehospital interventions will you provide for this patient?

____

____

13. What measures can be taken in the prehospital environment to minimize the fear and stress experienced by a victim of sexual abuse?

____

14. Describe five guidelines for evidence preservation on a sexual abuse call.

a. ____

b. ____

c. ____

d. ____

e. ____

STUDENT SELF-ASSESSMENT

15. How often does a typical woman have menstrual flow?
  a. Every 14 days   **c.** Every 28 days
  b. Every 21 days   **d.** Every 35 days

16. Which hormone initiates the ovarian cycle leading to ovulation?
  a. Estrogen   **c.** Luteinizing hormone
  b. Follicle-stimulating hormone   **d.** Progesterone

17. What is the most common cause of pelvic inflammatory disease?
  a. Gonorrhea
  b. Herpes virus
  c. Human immunodeficiency virus
  d. Syphilis

Chapter **31** **Gynecology**

18. Which of the following factors increases the incidence of dysmenorrhea?
   a. Increased age
   b. Frequent exercise
   c. Childbirth
   d. Infection

19. A ruptured ovarian cyst may mimic all of the following except which disorder?
   a. Appendicitis
   b. Cholecystitis
   c. Ectopic pregnancy
   d. Salpingitis

20. Which of the following is a normal sign or symptom of cystitis?
   a. Blood in the urine
   b. Flank pain
   c. Inability to urinate
   d. Painless urination

21. Which of the following is true regarding endometriosis?
   a. It is an inflammation of the uterine lining.
   b. It is common in young women.
   c. It has no effect on fertility.
   d. Its pain may increase during menstruation.

22. Which of the following gynecological problems may cause severe internal hemorrhage?
   a. Dysmenorrhea
   b. Mittelschmerz
   c. Salpingitis
   d. Ruptured ovarian cyst

23. Which of the following is a traumatic cause of vaginal bleeding?
   a. Abortion attempts
   b. Disorders of the placenta
   c. Onset of labor
   d. Pelvic inflammatory disease

24. What is your top priority when caring for a victim of sexual abuse?
   a. Allow only a paramedic of the same gender to care for the patient.
   b. Provide a safe and secure environment for the patient.
   c. Preserve evidence exactly as outlined by protocol.
   d. Perform a complete history and thorough examination.

25. How should you preserve evidence on a sexual abuse call with a stable patient who has minor scratches?
   a. Ask the patient to shower.
   b. Thoroughly clean wounds.
   c. Leave the patient's clothing on.
   d. Search the scene for evidence.

26. What is the most important action to resolve the life threat from an ectopic pregnancy?
   a. Administer high-concentration oxygen.
   b. Infuse normal saline to maintain blood pressure.
   c. Comfort her on the loss of the pregnancy.
   d. Rapid transport to the closest appropriate hospital.

27. Which of the following distinguishes a Bartolin abscess from pelvic inflammatory disese?
   a. Bacterial infection
   b. Fever
   c. Pain on ambulation
   d. Unilateral vaginal swelling

28. A 23-year-old woman complains of severe right lower quadrant abdominal pain that began during her aerobics class. If her signs and symptoms are related to ovarian torsion, what additional findings might be present?
   a. Foul vaginal odor is detected.
   b. Pain radiates to her back.
   c. Profuse vaginal bleeding is present.
   d. Swelling of both labia is noted.

29. Which patient is most likely to experience uterine prolapse?
   a. 22-Year-old woman with pelvic inflammatory disease
   b. 31-Year-old pregnant woman with right lower quadrant pain
   c. 40-Year-old nullipara with profuse vaginal bleeding
   d. 63-Year-old woman who has four children

454

30. During your care of a seriously injured woman who was sexually assaulted and beaten, you remove several items of bloody clothing. What should you do with it?
   a. Give the clothes to the patient's family.
   b. Ask the patient what she would like done with them.
   c. Bag each item separately in paper bags.
   d. Place the items in a plastic biohazard bag.

WRAP IT UP

"Unit 12, respond to one-two-five-six Weston, cross-street Thames, abdominal pain." You and your partner look hungrily at the dinner you have just set on the table, and you quickly move to the ambulance. Your patient is a 26-year-old woman whose abdominal pain began 2 hours ago. She is pale, and her skin is cool. She is anxious and appears to be in significant pain, especially guarding her left lower quadrant when you palpate her abdomen. Her vital signs are BP 90/50 mm Hg, P 128, R 20, and SaO_2 95%. She has been pregnant four times but has miscarried each within the first 8 weeks. Her last normal menstrual period was 8 weeks ago, so she is concerned that her pain may be related to the pregnancy. She started spotting yesterday but has not soaked a pad yet. You quickly apply oxygen by mask, elevate her legs, and tell your partner to start en route. During transport, you start one IV of normal saline with blood tubing and another with macrodrip tubing using lactated Ringer solution. When you reassess her vital signs, her blood pressure is 74/50 mm Hg, P 134, and R 28, so you open the IVs to administer a fluid challenge. You call the receiving hospital so that they can prepare to resuscitate this patient. On arrival, uncrossmatched blood is given to her, and within 20 minutes, they are rushing her to surgery to treat her ectopic pregnancy.

1. Place a check mark beside the gynecologic condition that you might suspect if this patient's pregnancy status were not known.
   a. _______ Cystitis   **d.** _______ Mittelschmerz
   b. _______ Dysmenorrhea   **e.** _______ Pelvic inflammatory disease
   c. _______ Endometriosis   **f.** _______ Ruptured ovarian cyst

2. Which is true of ectopic pregnancy?
   a. It usually occurs in the fallopian tube.
   b. It is a fluid-filled sac on the ovaries.
   c. Uterine inflammation occurs because of placental tissue retention.
   d. There is ectopic growth and functioning of uterine tissue.

3. Why was it critical to evaluate the possibility of pregnancy in this patient?

____

____

4. Explain your rationale for the following interventions.
   a. Elevation of her legs:

____

____

   b. Intravenous fluid bolus:

____

____

   c. Oxygen therapy:

____

____

455

Chapter **31** Gynecology

GYNECOLOGY

1. e

2. d

3. b

4. f

5. a

6. g
(Questions 1–6, Objective 2)

7. a. 28; b. 25, 60; c. 4, 6; d. secondary follicles; e. vesicular, graafian follicles; f. ovulation; g. corpus luteum; h. progesterone; i. estrogen; j. zygote; k. chorionic gonadotropin
(Objective 1)

8. Headache, faintness, dizziness, nausea, diarrhea, backache, leg pain, chills, nausea, and vomiting
(Objective 2)

9. a. Have you ever been pregnant? If yes, how many pregnancies, and how many have you carried to term?
   b. Have you ever had a cesarean delivery?
   c. When was your last menstrual period? How long did it last? Was it normal? Do you have a regular menstrual cycle? Have you had any bleeding between your periods?
   d. Could you be pregnant now? Is your period late, or did you miss one? Do you have any breast tenderness, increased need to urinate, or morning sickness? Have you had any unprotected sexual activity?
   e. Do you have a history of any gynecologic (female) problems such as bleeding, infections, pain during intercourse, miscarriage, abortion, or ectopic pregnancy?
   f. Are you having any bleeding now? If you are, what color is it, how many pads have you soaked, and how long have you been bleeding?
   g. Do you have any vaginal discharge? What color and how much is there? Does it smell bad?
   h. What kind of birth control do you use? Have you ever forgotten to use it?
   i. Have you had any injury to your genital area?
   j. How are you feeling now?
   Objective 3)

10. Evaluate vital signs and check for signs of blood loss (skin signs, orthostatic vital signs). Palpate the abdomen to assess for masses, tenderness, guarding, distention, and rebound tenderness.
(Objective 3)

11. Pelvic inflammatory disease, ruptured ovarian cyst, dysmenorrhea, endometritis, endometriosis, and appendicitis are potential causes. Ectopic pregnancy and miscarriage should not be discounted completely because sometimes patients do not give a completely accurate sexual history.
(Objective 3)

12. Consider oxygen administration; however, because no signs of shock exist, this may not be necessary. Consider initiating intravenous therapy. Transport in a position of comfort.
(Objective 3)

13. Move to a private, safe location; allow paramedic who is the same sex as the patient to provide care if possible; minimize questions and physical examination as appropriate; and listen and provide comfort.
(Objective 4)

456

14. Handle clothes as little as possible, do not clean wounds, use paper bags for clothing and bag each item separately, ask the victim not to change clothing, and try not to disturb the crime scene.
(Objective 5)

15. c. Menstrual flow varies according to each individual.
(Objective 1)

16. c. Follicle-stimulating hormone stimulates development of the follicle. Estrogen causes a surge in the production of luteinizing hormone, which initiates the ovarian cycle.
(Objective 1)

17. a. Chlamydia organisms and *Chlamydia trachomatis* also often are associated with pelvic inflammatory disease.
(Objective 2)

18. d. All of the other factors often decrease the severity of this condition.
(Objective 2)

19. b. The pain of cholecystitis is usually in the right upper quadrant of the abdomen. All other conditions cause lower abdominal pain.
(Objective 2)

20. a. Urination is usually painful and frequent in cystitis. Flank pain may indicate that the infection has moved to the kidneys.
(Objective 2)

21. d. Endometriosis is an ectopic placement of uterine lining and causes inflammation of the endometrium. It is common in women in their late 30s and is associated with infertility.
(Objective 2)

22. d
(Objective 3)

23. a. All other answers are nontraumatic causes of vaginal bleeding.
(Objective 3)

24. b. Having a paramedic of the same sex as the patient perform care is desirable but may not always be possible. You should attempt to preserve evidence, but this is not always possible if a life-threatening condition exists that requires rapid intervention. Perform only the necessary history and physical examination.
(Objective 4)

25. c. Bag items separately if possible. The patient should not shower, wash, or have wounds cleansed until evidence can be gathered.
(Objective 5)

26. d. Surgery is the definitive care the patient needs to save her life. Each of the other intervenetions should be performed while transporting the patient.
(Objective 2)

27. d. All of the other responses are common to both illnesses.
(Objective 2)

28. b. Other signs may include fever, nausea, vomiting, and signs of shock.
(Objective 2)

29. d. Uterine prolapse is more common in women with multiple deliveries and in postmenopausal women.
(Objective 2)

30. c. The bags should be sealed and remain with you until you hand them to the appropriate law enforcement
officer. Document your actions related to the clothing carefully because it is evidence and part of the
crime scene.
(Objective 5)

WRAP IT UP

1. f. She gave no urinary signs or symptoms, so cystitis would not be a consideration. Pelvic inflammatory disease
is possible, but there is no report of vaginal discharge. The pain of dysmenorrhea and mittelschmerz is not
usually so severe and are not associated with shock.
(Objective 2)

2. a. It can occur less often in the ovary, abdominal cavity, or cervix.
(Objective 2)

3. If the pregnancy status is known, the differential diagnosis can be narrowed.
(Objective 2)

4. a. Elevating her legs may improve her shock temporarily.
b. An intravenous fluid bolus will increase the preload and temporarily increase the blood pressure.
c. Because this patient is in shock, oxygenation is critical, especially because she has internal bleeding.
(Objective 2)

32 Hematology

Chapter 32, pages 942-960, in *Mosby's Paramedic Textbook,* ed. 4.

OBJECTIVES

Upon completion of this chapter, the paramedic student will be able to:

1. Describe the physiology of blood and its components.
2. Discuss pathophysiology and signs and symptoms of specific hematologic disorders.
3. Outline general assessment and management of patients with hematologic disorders.

SUMMARY

- Blood is composed of cells and formed elements surrounded by plasma. About 95% of the volume of formed elements consists of red blood cells (RBCs; erythrocytes). The remaining 5% consists of white blood cells (WBCs; leukocytes) and cell fragments (platelets).
- Anemia is a condition in which the amount of hemoglobin or erythrocytes in the blood is below normal. Two common forms of anemia are iron-deficiency anemia and hemolytic anemia. All forms of anemia share signs and symptoms. These signs and symptoms include fatigue and headaches; sometimes a sore mouth or tongue; brittle nails; and in severe cases, breathlessness, and chest pain. Diagnosis is made by history and from blood tests and bone marrow biopsy.
- Leukemia refers to any of several types of cancer in which an abnormal proliferation of WBCs usually occurs in the bone marrow. The proliferation of leukemic cells crowds and impairs the normal production of RBCs, WBCs, and platelets. Leukemia is classified as acute or chronic. The proliferation of leukemic cells makes the patient highly susceptible to serious infections, anemia, and bleeding episodes. The diagnosis is confirmed by bone marrow biopsy.
- Lymphoma refers to a group of diseases that range from slowly growing chronic disorders to rapidly evolving acute conditions. Hodgkin disease is one type; all others are called non-Hodgkin lymphomas.
- Polycythemia is characterized by an unusually large number of RBCs in the blood as a result of their increased production by the bone marrow. Polycythemia may be a natural response to hypoxia. (This is known as secondary polycythemia.) Polycythemia also may occur for unknown reasons. (This is known as primary polycythemia.)
- Disseminated intravascular coagulopathy (DIC) is a complication of severe injury, trauma, or disease. It disrupts the balance among procoagulants, thrombin formation, inhibitors, and lysis. Signs and symptoms of DIC include dyspnea, bleeding, and those associated with hypotension and hypoperfusion. The treatment is aimed at reversing the underlying illness or injury that triggered the event.
- Hemophilia A is caused by a deficiency of a blood protein called factor VIII. Hemophilia B is caused by a deficiency of factor IX. Bleeding from hemophilia can occur spontaneously, after even minor injury, and during some medical procedures.
- Thrombocytopenia is a low platelet count. It can occur when the body does not produce enough platelets, if too many platelets are destroyed, or if the spleen holds onto too many platelets. Bleeding is the chief complication of thrombocytopenia.
- Sickle cell disease is a debilitating and unpredictable recessive genetic illness. It affects persons of African descent. Less often, it affects persons of Mediterranean origin. Sickle cell anemia produces an abnormal type of hemoglobin. This is called hemoglobin S. This abnormal type has an inferior oxygen-carrying capacity. Complications of sickle cell disease include episodes of severe pain, fatigue, pallor, jaundice, stroke, delayed growth, hematuria, priapism, and splenomegaly.
- Multiple myeloma is a malignant neoplasm of the bone marrow. The tumor destroys bone tissue (especially flat bones). This causes pain, fractures, hypercalcemia, and skeletal deformities.
- In many cases of hematologic disorders, the prehospital treatment is supportive. Treatment includes ensuring adequate airway, ventilatory, and circulatory support.

Match the hematology terms in Column II with the description in Column I. Use each term only once.

Column I

1. _________ Include eosinophils, basophils, and neutrophils

2. _________ Destroy red blood cells

3. _________ Destroy invading organisms and include monophils

4. _________ Waste product after destruction of hemoglobin

5. _________ Activate chemicals that trigger inflammation

6. _________ Contains albumin, globulins, and fibrinogen

7. _________ Composed of water and hemoglobin

Column II

a. Basophils
b. Bilirubin
c. Erythrocytes
d. Macrophages
e. Phagocytes
f. Plasma of hemoglobin
g. Platelets
h. White blood cell inflammation

8. Complete the information in the following table.

Condition	Cause	Signs and Symptoms
Anemia		
Leukemia		
Lymphomata		
Polycythemia		
Disseminated intravascular coagulation		
Hemophilia		
Sickle cell disease		
Multiple myeloma		

9. You respond to a private residence and find a 21-year-old black woman who is complaining of pain in her abdomen, hands, and feet. She said she had the flu and vomited three times yesterday. She tells you that she has sickle cell disease.

    a. What type of sickle cell crisis may present in this manner?

    b. What event may have triggered a crisis in this patient?

    c. What specific organ should you try to palpate on your physical examination of this patient?

    d. Outline the prehospital care of this patient.

10. Which is true regarding red bone marrow?
   a. Only white blood cells are formed here.
   b. It is formed in the liver.
   c. It is composed mainly of connective tissue and fat.
   d. It is found in the vertebrae, pelvis, sternum, and ribs.

11. Which of the following is a normal value for hemoglobin?
   a. 10 g/100 mL   **c.** 35%
   b. 15 g/100 mL   **d.** 50%

12. Which type of anemia may be cured by splenectomy?
   a. Aplastic   **c.** Iron deficiency
   b. Hemolytic   **d.** Sickle cell

13. Which is true of acute myeloblastic leukemia?
   a. It affects mostly young children.
   b. Reed-Sternberg cells are present.
   c. Generalized itching may be present.
   d. It is difficult to cure.

14. Which hematologic disorder is diagnosed using bone marrow biopsy?
   a. Disseminated intravascular coagulation
   b. Leukemia
   c. Hodgkin disease
   d. Sickle cell anemia

15. Which of the following is a target organ in Hodgkin lymphoma?
   a. Kidney   **c.** Spleen
   b. Liver   **d.** Testes

16. What can trigger secondary polycythemia?
   a. Blood loss   **c.** Hypoxia
   b. Hypothermia   **d.** Infection

17. Which of the following occurs when disseminated intravascular coagulation is present?
   a. Coagulation inhibition levels are increased.
   b. Fibrin is deposited in small vessels in multiple organs.
   c. Platelets and fibrinogen V, VIII, and XIII increase.
   d. Thrombin is destroyed.

18. What is needed to stop the bleeding that occurs during hemophilia?
   a. Factor VIII   **c.** Oxygen administration
   b. Intravenous fluids   **d.** Topical thrombin

19. Although all sickle cell disease emergencies can cause death, which one represents an immediate life-threatening situation?
   a. Aplastic crisis   **c.** Splenic sequestration
   b. Hemolytic crisis   **d.** Vasoocclusive crisis

20. In which hematologic disorder of the bone marrow does the tumor destroy bone tissue?
   a. Hodgkin disease   **c.** Lymphoma
   b. Leukemia   **d.** Multiple myeloma

21. Prehospital care for a conscious patient with a hematologic problem should always include which of the following?
   a. Analgesics
   b. Antidysrhythmics
   c. Blood transfusion
   d. Emotional support

22. Which of the following signs or symptoms likely reflects complications related to thrombocytopenia?
   a. Blood glucose is 60 mg/dL.
   b. End-tidal CO_2 is 50 mmHg.
   c. Glasgow Coma Scale score is 13.
   d. Temperature is 102°F (38.9°C).

WRAP IT UP

A 45-year-old white man who is the soccer coach at a local high school complains of difficulty breathing. He experienced shortness of breath and sweating during a practice drill with his team, and a player called 911. You note a pale man in moderate distress. He is alert and oriented and says he was fine until he started running. His initial SaO_2 is 89%, and his breath sounds are clear and equal bilaterally. You mention to him that he appears to have an unusual number of bruises on various areas of his body ranging from old yellow or gray ones to purplish red newer ones. He appears nervous when you ask about his medical history and denies any significant illness, injury, or medications. His vital signs are BP 108/66 mm Hg, P 124, and R 24. You administer oxygen by non-rebreather mask and move him by stretcher into the ambulance. In the privacy of the ambulance, he confides to you that he has been ill and just this week saw his doctor because he has been feeling tired all the time; has generalized bone pain, night sweats, and swollen "glands" in his neck; and has lost 25 lb in the last 8 weeks. This afternoon, his doctor called and said that his blood tests were grossly abnormal and he wanted to hospitalize him to run more tests to rule out leukemia. The coach confesses that he could not believe it and decided to go ahead with practice because he did not know what to tell the kids. His oxygen saturation is now 98%, and you initiate an IV and transport him, completing your physical exam en route. He subsequently is diagnosed with acute myeloblastic leukemia, and 6 months later, you read of his death in the obituaries.

1. Which of the following blood cells increase or decrease in leukemia?
   a. Red blood cells   Increase/decrease
   b. White blood cells   Increase/decrease
   c. Platelets   Increase/decrease

2. What explains the following signs and symptoms that this patient experienced?
   a. Fatigue
   b. Swollen lymph nodes
   c. Difficulty breathing
   d. Bruising

3. What additional findings might you encounter when you assess the abdomen?

4. Place a check mark beside other hematologic conditions you might have suspected based on his history and presenting condition if the patient had not confessed his presumed diagnosis.
   a. _______ Anemia
   b. _______ Hemophilia
   c. _______ Hodgkin disease
   d. _______ Lymphoma
   e. _______ Multiple myeloma
   f. _______ Polycythemia
   g. _______ Sickle cell disease

CHAPTER 32 ANSWERS

REVIEW QUESTIONS

1. h

2. d

3. e

462

4. b

5. a

6. f

7. c

(Questions 1–7, Objective 1)

8.

Condition	Cause	Signs and Symptoms
Anemia	Iron deficiency; decreased production and survival of red blood cells	Fatigue headaches, sore mouth or tongue, brittle nails, breathlessness, or chest pain
Leukemia	Abnormal chromosomes; disorganized proliferation of white blood cells in bone marrow	Bleeding, bone pain, frequent bruising, sternal tenderness, fatigue, headache, weight loss, height sweets; enlarged lymph nodes, liver, spleen; anemia, infections
Lymphomata	Proliferation of cells in lymph tissues (may be genetic link)	Swollen lymph nodes in neck, armpits, groin; fatigue, chills, and night sweats; severe itching, cough, weight loss, dyspnea, chest discomfort
Polycythemia	Unusually large number of red blood cells	Headache, dizziness, blurred vision, generalized itching; hypertension, splenomegaly, platelet disorders, red hands and feet, purple complexion, stroke and development of leukemias
Disseminated intravascular coagulation	Complication of severe injury, trauma, disease imbalance of clotting mechanisms	Dyspnea, bleeding, hypotension, hypoperfusion
Hemophilia	Inherited bleeding disorder; deficiency of factor VIII or less often factor IX	Spontaneous bleeding (joints, deep muscles, urinary tract, and intracranial sites most common) after injury or during medical procedures
Sickle cell disease	Genetic illness; red blood cells are distorted into sickle shape that is easily destroyed and can clog blood vessels	Episodes of severe pain, fatigue, pallor jaundice, stroke; delayed growth, development, and sexual maturation; hematuria, priapism, splenomegaly
Multiple myeloma	Malignant neoplasm of bone marrow	Pain, fractures, hypercalcemia, skeletal deformities, kidney failure, anemia, weight loss, rib fractures, recurrent infections

(Objective 2)

9. a. Possibly a vasoocclusive sickle cell crisis
   b. Dehydration or stress from her illness the day before may have triggered her crisis.
   c. The spleen may enlarge during a sickle cell crisis, so it should be evaluated.
   d. You should administer oxygen by non-rebreather mask at 12 to 15 L/min. You should initiate an intravenous line and administer a fluid bolus under medical direction. Although analgesia will be a high priority for this patient, medical direction may not order it until the abdomen can be examined to ensure that an urgent surgical condition does not exist.

(Objective 2)

10. d. All types of blood cells are formed here. Yellow marrow is composed of connective tissue and fat.
(Objective 1)

11. b. Normal hemoglobin ranges from 13.5 to 18 g/100 mL. Normal hematocrit ranges from 38% to 54%.
(Objective 1)

12. b. Treatment for aplastic anemia may include blood transfusion, folic acid, and bone marrow transplantation. Iron-deficiency anemia is treated with supplemental iron and folic acid.
(Objective 2)

13. d. Acute myeloblastic anemia affects middle-aged adults. Reed-Sternberg cells are characteristic of Hodgkin lymphoma. Itching is not a classic symptom.
(Objective 2)

14. b. Disseminated intravascular coagulation is diagnosed based on clinical history and laboratory values that include clotting studies, platelet count, and fibrin degradation products. Sickle cell anemia is confirmed by laboratory testing.
(Objective 2)

15. c. Hodgkin lymphoma primarily affects lymphoid tissues.
(Objective 2)

16. c. The body produces more red cells in an attempt to improve oxygenation in conditions such as high altitude and chronic lung disease.
(Objective 2)

17. b. Coagulation inhibition levels are decreased. Platelets and coagulation factors are consumed, and thrombin is formed.
(Objective 2)

18. a. Factor VIII is needed to reestablish a normal clotting cascade and stop bleeding.
(Objective 2)

19. c. Splenic sequestration occurs in childhood and is caused by blood trapped in the spleen. Aplastic crisis occurs when the bone marrow temporarily stops making red blood cells. In hemolytic crisis, red blood cell breakdown exceeds production. Vasoocclusive sickle cell crisis occurs when the sickle-shaped cells block blood flow to organs and tissues.
(Objective 2)

20. d. Hodgkin disease is a type of lymphoma and affects the lymph tissue. Leukemia is similar to multiple myeloma, but in multiple myeloma, the primary target is bone.
(Objective 2)

21. d. Acute or chronic hematologic disorders produce tremendous emotional stress on patients and families. You should be empathetic and provide calm support during care and transport. Analgesics and antidysrhythmics occasionally may be indicated. Prehospital blood transfusion usually is done only during interfacility transfers.
(Objective 2)

22. c. Bleeding in the brain can occur when the platelet count is low. (Objective 2)

WRAP IT UP

1. a. Decrease; b. increase; c. decrease
(Objective 2)

2. a. A decrease in red blood cells causes a decrease in oxygen delivery to the cells that could affect adenosine triphosphate (energy) production.
b. Lymph nodes help to rid the body of excess or damaged white blood cells, which are characteristic of leukemia.

464

c. The patient's decrease in red blood cells did not permit his body to transport enough oxygen to meet the increased demand during exertion at practice.

d. Platelets are essential to control bleeding in the body and are greatly decreased in leukemia.

(Objectives 1 and 2)

3. The liver and spleen likely will be greatly enlarged.

(Objective 3)

4. a. Because of his pallor and dyspnea c and

d. Although he is somewhat young, other signs and symptoms would not exclude Hodgkin and other lymphomata.

e. His age and bone pain are consistent with multiple myeloma.

His history does not include hemophilia, which is present at birth; polycythemia is a problem of excess red blood cells and typically would produce red-purple skin, not pallor as in this patient (and this patient does not seem to have risk factors for polycythemia); this patient is white, so sickle cell anemia would be unlikely, and he has no known history of sickle cell disease that would be diagnosed early in life.

(Objective 2)

33 Nontraumatic Musculoskeletal Disorders

READING ASSIGNMENT

Chapter 33, pages 961-980, in *Mosby's Paramedic Textbook,* ed. 4.

OBJECTIVES

Upon completion of this chapter, the paramedic student will be able to do the following:

1. Outline musculoskeletal structure and function.
2. Describe how to perform a detailed assessment of the extremities and spine.
3. Specify questions in the patient history that help identify musculoskeletal problems.
4. Describe assessment and management of specific nontraumatic musculoskeletal disorders based on an understanding of the pathophysiology.

SUMMARY

- Although more common in advanced age, nontraumatic musculoskeletal disorders affect patients of all ages.
- The musculoskeletal system is composed of bones, muscles, tendons, ligaments, and articulating surfaces. Three types of joints are fibrous, cartilaginous, and synovial. Muscles are responsible for movement, posture, and heat production.
- The extremities and spine should be examined to determine structure and function. Specific assessments include range of motion, vascular evaluation, and a motor and sensory examination.
- Prehospital management of nontraumatic musculoskeletal disorders includes routine care and pain management.
- Important historical data to gather on a patient with this type of disorder should relate to the onset of signs and symptoms, nature and location of pain, presence of weakness or other alteration in motor function, and presence of sensory abnormalities.
- Osteomyelitis is a bone infection. It may result from an open fracture, wound infection, or systemic infection. Signs and symptoms include pain, signs of inflammation, fever, pus, and other functional alterations.
- Bone tumors are benign or malignant abnormal cell growth within a bone. Multiple myeloma is the most common type of primary bone cancer. This disorder is characterized by pain and fractures.
- Acute or chronic low back pain is common. It may be caused by trauma, arthritis, infections or congenital abnormalities.
- Intervertebral discs can herniated and compress adjacent nerves, causing severe pain and weakness.
- Cauda equina syndrome is caused by compression of the nerve roots at the distal end of the spine. If the compression is not relieved promptly, permanent paralysis and incontinence can occur.
- A strain is an injury to a muscle or tendon. A sprain is stretching or tearing of a ligament. Both conditions cause pain.
- Arthritis is an inflammatory condition of a joint characterized by pain and swelling. Osteoarthritis is a chronic degenerative joint disease that has a gradual onset. Rheumatoid arthritis is an autoimmune disease that affects synovial joints. It causes severe pain, disability, and deformity. Ankylosing spondylitis is a form of arthritis that primarily affects the spine. It requires modifications in prehospital care. Septic arthritis is infection of a joint. Gout is a type of arthritis caused by deposits of uric acid in the joint space.
- Myalgia is pain in one or more muscles. It can be caused by an autoimmune disorder, overuse, or infection.
- Inflammatory myopathies are a group of diseases characterized by muscle inflammation and weakness. They can be caused by autoimmune disease, injury, infection, or drugs.
- Chronic fatigue syndrome is characterized by severe fatigue not improved by rest.
- Fibromyalgia causes fatigue and "tender points" on the neck, shoulders, back, hips, arms, and legs.
- Bursitis is inflammation of one or more bursae. It is often caused by overuse.
- Muscle strains are slight tears in the muscle caused by overuse or by injury.
- Tendonitis is inflammation of a tendon.
- Carpal tunnel syndrome is a type of neuropathy caused by entrapment of the median nerve after repetitive movement. It causes pain, numbness, and weakness.
- Ulnar nerve entrapment occurs when the ulnar nerve (funny bone) is compressed.

- Fasciitis is inflammation of the connective tissue that lies under the skin. Necrotizing fasciitis (flesh-eating bacteria) is a rare infection that begins in the fascia and can become systemic.
- Gangrene is a complication of tissue necrosis. It occurs when tissue decays.
- Paronychia is a skin infection around the nails.
- Flexor tenosynovitis is often caused by infection. It can lead to dysfunction, necrosis, and systemic infection.

REVIEW QUESTIONS

Match the musculoskeletal condition in column II with the description in column I. Use each disorder only once.

Column I

1. _________ Inflammed connective tissue below the skin

2. _________ Muscle aches associated with influenza

3. _________ Causes numbness and pain of the elbow and fingers

4. _________ Median nerve compression causes pain and numbness

5. _________ Accumulation of pus around the nail bed

6. _________ Inflammation of sacs containing synovial fluid

7. _________ Fatigue with pain of the back and extremities

Column II

a. Bursitis
b. Carpal tunnel syndrome
c. Fasciitis
d. Fibromyalgia
e. Flexor tenosynovitis
f. Myalgia
g. Paronychia
h. Ulnar nerve entrapment

8. Fill in the blanks to name key structure and functions of the musculoskeletal system.

   a. The axial skeletal is composed of the _________________, _________________, _______________ and

   _________________.

   b. Fibrous joints have _____________________ movement. Cartilaginous joints connect bones by

   _____________________ or _________________. Synovial joints contain _______________fluid that permit

   great movement. One example of a synovial joint is the _________________ joint.

   c. Skeletal muscles attach to bones by _________________. Bones are connected to cartilage or other bones by

   _________________.

9. A 70-year-old man complains of severe pain in the right shoulder. He denies traumatic injury. Describe your assessment of her extremity.

   ____

   ____

10. A 40-year-old woman is complaining of fatigue, weakness, and generalized pain. What should you ask in her history to narrow your differential diagnosis?

    ____

    ____

11. What causes pain in fasciitis, bursitis, and arthritis?

    ____

    ____

Questions 12 to 15 relate to the following case.

A 50-year-old man had spine surgery three weeks ago. He has pain in his back and is unable to ambulate without intense pain. His vital signs are BP 128/76, P 116, R 20, T 101.6°F (38.7°C). His surgical incision is reddened and the area around it is tender. There is yellow-green discharge on the dressing.

12. What complication of surgery do you suspect? _______________________________

13. What infectious agent should you suspect? _______________________________

14. Why will his recovery be prolonged if he has this complication?

____

15. Outline your care of this patient.

____

____

16. Which structure causes movement when it contracts?
    a. Bone   **c.** Muscle
    b. Ligament   **d.** Tendon

17. When examining your patient, you note a hunchback appearance. What term would you use to document this?
    a. Kyphosis   **c.** Osteoporosis
    b. Lordosis   **d.** Scoliosis

18. What finding would you expect if there was arterial insufficiency in an extremity?
    a. Clubbing   **c.** Pallor
    b. Bruising   **d.** Rash

19. Which is characteristic of osteosarcoma?
    a. Found in older adults
    b. Tumors occur around the knee
    c. Pain is not affected by movement
    d. Resolves without treatment

20. What causes leg pain in a patient who says they have sciatica from a "slipped disc?"
    a. Compression of spinal nerve roots
    b. Damage to the central spinal cord
    c. Interruption of arterial blood supply
    d. Pressure on peripheral nerves

21. A 65-year-old man is being treated for spinal abscesses 6 months after a knee replacement when he loses sensation in his legs and becomes incontinent. What emergency condition is suspected?
    a. Cauda equina
    b. Guillain-Barré syndrome
    c. Muscular dystrophy
    d. Sepsis

22. What causes arthritic pain?
    a. Damage to peripheral nerves
    b. Ligamentous strain
    c. Joint inflammation
    d. Infected tendons

23. Which is true of ankylosing spondylitis?
  a. Lordosis is a common finding.
  b. It is less painful than osteoarthritis.
  c. Movement of the spine can cause spinal cord damage.
  d. It is usually seen in adults older than the age of 70 years.

24. What distinguishes septic arthritis from osteoarthritis and rheumatoid arthritis?
  a. Infection   **c.** Pain
  b. Inflammation   **d.** Warm joints

25. You document that the patient is experiencing myalgia. What type of pain does this refer to?
  a. Bone   **c.** Nerve
  b. Muscle   **d.** Spine

26. Which is true of chronic fatigue syndrome?
  a. Its signs and symptoms vary greatly from fibromyalgia.
  b. Many patients with its signs have an underlying medical illness.
  c. Antibiotics and antiinflammatory drugs can relieve the symptoms.
  d. Bedrest usually improves the patient's signs and symptoms.

27. What is the primary cause of bursitis?
  a. Overuse of the joint
  b. Infection of the bursa
  c. Lack of synovial fluid
  d. Uric acid deficit destroys bursa

28. What causes necrotizing fasciitis?
  a. Decreased arterial blood supply
  b. Excess exercise of an extremity
  c. Subcutaneous bacterial infection
  d. Torn muscles, ligaments, or tendons

29. You are transporting a patient from a rural hospital to a specialty center for treatment of a gangrenous foot. What is a treatment priority during patient transfer?
  a. Improve oxygenation.
  b. Restore circulatory volume.
  c. Lower body temperature.
  d. Relieve pain.

WRAP IT UP

A 64-year-old man complains of severe lower back pain and a decreased ability to walk. He feels weak and "not himself." He reports no trauma today. On examination, you do not identify any swelling or deformity of his back. He has severe pain on movement and complains of pain and numbness that radiate down his right leg. He cannot raise his legs but feels better when his knees are flexed. His home medications include lansoprazole (Prevacid), simvistatin (Zocor), candesartan (Atacand), and hydrochlorothiazide (HCTZ). His vital signs are BP 158/96 mm Hg, P 102/min, R 20, and T 98.6°F (37°C).

1. What additional questions should you ask this patient to obtain a more complete history?

____

____

____

2. Predict his past medical history based on the medications he is taking.

____

470

3. What additional physical examination should you perform?

____

4. What differential diagnoses are you considering?

____

5. Describe your treatment plan for this patient.

____

____

6. Could any of your treatment plans for this patient be influenced by his home medicines?

____

CHAPTER 33 ANSWERS

REVIEW QUESTIONS

1. c

2. f

3. h

4. b

5. g

6. a

7. d
(Questions 1–7, Objective 4)

8. a. Skull, hyoid, bone, vertebral column, and thoracic cage
  b. little or no; little or no; hyaline or fibrocartilage; synovial; elbow, knee, shoulder, hip and others
  c. tendons; ligaments
  (Objective 1)

9. Inspect the extremity and compare it with the other arm in terms of length, position, and muscle tone. Look for any redness, swelling, or other abnormality of the skin that lies over the affected area. Palpate the shoulder and note any areas of pain. Assess pulse, movement, and sensation distal to the affected shoulder. Assess the patient's range of motion in her shoulder and compare the movement in the affected arm with that of the other arm. (Objective 2)

10. Ask when her signs and symptoms began and whether they vary by time of day or based on activity. Determine the location and nature of her pain. Ask if the pain is affected by movement or other factors. Note the quality and severity of the pain. See if she has any other signs or symptoms such as difficulty breathing; nausea, vomiting, or diarrhea; fever; or other unusual symptoms. Explore her past medical history and whether she has gone through menopause. Determine whether she takes medicine or supplements on a daily basis and if she has any allergies. (Objective 3)

471

11. All of these conditions involve inflammation. Chemicals released in the inflammatory process cause pain. In addition, swelling associated with inflammation can compress tissue and result in pain.
(Objective 4)

12. Osteomyelitis

13. *Staphylococcus aureus*

14. Infection of the bone requires prolonged IV antibiotic treatment.

15. Establish an intravenous (IV) line. Infuse IV fluid at a rate according to protocol. Administer pain medication such as morphine, fentanyl, or hydromorphone titrated to relieve the patient's pain. Position the patient so he is most comfortable on the stretcher. Transport nonemergency to the appropriate health care facility as long as he remains stable.
(Questions 12–15, Objective 4)

STUDENT SELF-ASSESSMENT

16. c. Muscles pull on the other structures when they contract to create movement.
(Objective 1)

17. a. Lordosis is accentuated curve of the lower back (swayback), osteoporosis is demineralization of bones, and scoliosis is lateral curvature of the spine.
(Objective 2)

18. c. Arterial insufficiency decreases blood flow.
(Objective 2)

19. b. Most cases occur in teens. When there is pain, it is typically worsened on movement.
(Objective 4)

20. a. The spinal nerves are compressed when the disc is damaged producing pain along the nerve route.
(Objective 4)

21. a. This patient requires emergent treatment to prevent permanent disability.
(Objective 4)

22. c. The inflammation and swelling cause pain.
(Objective 4)

23. c. Vertebrae become fused, so maneuvers such as normal spinal immobilization techniques can cause spinal damage in this patient.
(Objective 4)

24. a. All of the other responses may be found in all types of arthritis.
(Objective 4)

25. b. "Myo" refers to muscle.
(Objective 4)

26. b. Almost 40% of patients' symptoms are explained by another illness.
(Objective 4)

27. a. Bursitis is one of a number of overuse syndromes.
(Objective 4)

28. c. It often involves a drug resistant bacteria.
(Objective 4)

29. d. Tissue death from gangrene is very painful.
(Objective 4)

WRAP IT UP

1. Ask the patient if he has any other signs or symptoms, what the nature and quality of his pain is, and what the time of onset was. Find out if anything improves his pain or worsens it. Ask him about any old or recent injury to his back or any other significant medical history.
(Objective 2)

2. Ulcers (lansoprazole [Prevacid]), high cholesterol (simvastatin [Zocor]), and hypertension (candesartan [Atacand] hydrochlorothiazide [HCTZ])
(Objective 2)

3. Inspect and palpate the spinal column and lower extremities. Note any pain, deformity, or redness. Note distal pulse, movement, and sensation.
(Objective 3)

4. This patient could have arthritis, muscle strain or sprain, or a disc problem in the spine. Other possibilities include fibromyalgia, chronic fatigue syndrome, or bone cancer.
(Objective 4)

5. Administer medication for pain such as fentanyl (Sublimaze), morphine, or hydromorphone (Dilaudid).
(Objective 4)

6. The non-narcotic pain reliever ketorolac tromethamine (Toradol) is contraindicated in patients with active peptic ulcer disease.
(Objective 4)

34 Toxicology

READING ASSIGNMENT

Chapter 34, pages 981-1024, in *Mosby's Paramedic Textbook,* ed. 4.

OBJECTIVES

Upon completion of this chapter, the paramedic student will be able to do the following:

1. Define poisoning.
2. Describe general principles for assessment and management of the patient who has ingested poison.
3. Describe the causative agents and pathophysiology of selected ingested poisons and management of patients who have taken them.
4. Describe how physical and chemical properties influence the effects of inhaled toxins.
5. Distinguish among the three categories of inhaled toxins: simple asphyxiants, chemical asphyxiants and systemic poisons, and irritants or corrosives.
6. Describe general principles of managing the patient who has inhaled poison.
7. Describe the signs, symptoms, and management of patients who have inhaled cyanide, ammonia, or hydrocarbon.
8. Describe the signs, symptoms, and management of patients injected with poison by insects, reptiles, and hazardous aquatic creatures.
9. Describe the signs, symptoms, and management of patients with organophosphate or carbamate poisoning.
10. Outline the general principles of managing patients with drug overdose.
11. Describe the effects, signs and symptoms, and specific management for selected therapeutic and illegal drug overdoses.
12. Describe the short- and long-term physiologic effects of ethanol ingestion.
13. Describe the signs, symptoms, and management of alcohol-related emergencies.
14. Identify general management principles for the most common toxic syndromes based on knowledge of the characteristic physical findings associated with each syndrome.

SUMMARY

- A poison is any substance that produces harmful physiologic or psychological effects.
- The toxic effects of ingested poisons may be immediate or delayed. This depends on the substance that is ingested. The main goal is to identify effects on the three vital organ systems most likely to produce immediate morbidity and mortality. These are the respiratory system, the cardiovascular system, and the central nervous system (CNS). The goal of managing serious poisonings by ingestion is to prevent the toxic substance from reaching the small intestine. This limits its absorption.
- Strong acids and alkalis may cause burns to the mouth, pharynx, esophagus, and sometimes the upper respiratory and gastrointestinal (GI) tracts. Prehospital care is usually limited to airway and ventilatory support, intravenous (IV) fluid replacement, and rapid transport to the appropriate medical facility.
- The most important physical characteristic in the potential toxicity of ingested hydrocarbons is its viscosity. The lower the viscosity, the higher the risk of aspiration and associated complications. Hydrocarbon ingestion may involve the patient's respiratory, GI, and neurologic systems. The clinical features may be immediate or delayed in onset.
- Methanol is a poisonous alcohol. It is found in a number of products. Methanol itself is no more toxic than ethanol. Yet its metabolites (formaldehyde and formic acid) are very toxic. Ingestion can affect the CNS, the GI tract, and the eyes. It also can cause the development of metabolic acidosis.
- Ethylene glycol toxicity is caused by the buildup of toxic metabolites, especially glycolic and oxalic acids after metabolism. This occurs mainly in the liver and kidneys. This toxicity may affect the CNS and cardiopulmonary and renal systems. It may result in hypocalcemia as well.
- The majority of isopropanol (isopropyl alcohol) is metabolized to acetone after ingestion. Isopropanol poisoning affects several body systems, including the central nervous, GI, and renal systems.

- Infants and children are high-risk groups for accidental iron, lead, and mercury poisoning. This is because of their immature immune systems or increased absorption as a function of age. Ingested iron is corrosive to GI tract mucosa. It may produce lethal GI hemorrhage, bloody vomitus, painless bloody diarrhea, and dark stools.
- *Food poisoning* is a term used for any illness of sudden onset (usually associated with stomach pain, vomiting, and diarrhea) suspected of being caused by food eaten within the previous 48 hours. Food poisoning can be classified as infectious; this results from a bacterium or virus. It also can be classified as noninfectious; this results from toxins and pollutants.
- The toxic effects of major poisonous plant ingestions are predictable. They are categorized by the chemical and physical properties of the plant. Most responses are consistent with the type of major toxic chemical component in the plant.
- The concentration of a chemical in the air helps to predict the severity of an inhalation injury. The duration of exposure helps to determine this as well. Solubility also influences the extent of an inhalation injury. Highly reactive chemicals cause more severe and rapid injury than less reactive chemicals. Properties that determine chemical reactivity are chemical pH, direct-acting potential of chemicals, indirect-acting potential of chemicals, and allergic potential of chemicals.
- Cyanide is any of a number of highly toxic substances that contain the cyanogen chemical group. Regardless of the route of entry, cyanide is a rapidly acting poison. It combines and reacts with ferric ions of the respiratory enzyme cytochrome oxidase. This inhibits cellular oxygenation. This can produce a rapid progression from dyspnea to paralysis, unconsciousness, and death.
- Ammonia is a toxic irritant. It causes local pulmonary complications after inhalation. In severe cases, bronchospasm and pulmonary edema may develop.
- Hydrocarbon inhalation may cause aspiration pneumonitis. It also has the potential for systemic effects such as CNS depression and liver, kidney, or bone marrow toxicity.
- Simple asphyxiants cause toxicity by lowering the ambient oxygen concentration. Chemical asphyxiants possess intrinsic systemic toxicity. This toxicity occurs after absorption into the circulation. Irritants and corrosives cause cellular destruction and inflammation as they come into contact with moisture in the respiratory tract.
- The general principles of managing inhaled poisons are the same as for any other hazardous materials incident.
- Hymenoptera and Arachnida cause the highest incidence of need for emergency care. Arthropod venoms are complex and diverse in their chemistry and pharmacology. They may produce major toxic reactions in sensitized persons. Such reactions include anaphylaxis and upper airway obstruction.
- The two main families of venomous snakes indigenous to the United States are pit vipers and coral snakes. Pit viper venom can produce various toxic effects on blood and other tissues. These effects include hemolysis, intravascular coagulation, convulsions, and acute renal failure. The venom of coral snakes is mainly neurotoxic. Signs and symptoms range from slurred speech, dilated pupils, and dysphagia to flaccid paralysis and death.
- The marine animals most likely to be involved in human poisonings in U.S. coastal waters are coelenterates, echinoderms, and stingrays. Coelenterate envenomation ranges in severity from irritant dermatitis to excruciating pain, respiratory depression, and life-threatening cardiovascular collapse. Echinoderm toxins may cause immediate intense pain, swelling, redness, aching in the affected extremity, and nausea. Delayed effects may include respiratory distress; paresthesia of the lips and face; and in severe cases, respiratory paralysis and complete atonia. Locally, stingray venom produces a painful traumatic injury. It may cause bleeding and necrosis. Systemic manifestations range from weakness and nausea to seizures, paralysis, hypotension, and death.
- Organophosphates and carbamates inhibit the effects of acetylcholinesterase. A mnemonic aid that may help the paramedic to recognize this type of poisoning is SLUDGE, which stands for salivation, lacrimation, urination, defecation, GI upset, and emesis. The most specific findings, however, are miosis, rapidly changing pupils, and muscle fasciculation.
- General principles for managing drug abuse and overdose include scene safety; ensuring adequate airway, breathing, and circulation; history; substance identification; focused physical examination; initiation of an IV; administration of an antidote if needed; prevention of further absorption; and rapid transport.
- Narcotics are CNS depressants. They can cause life-threatening respiratory depression. In severe intoxication, hypotension, profound shock, and pulmonary edema may be present. Naloxone is a pure narcotic antagonist effective for virtually all narcotic and narcotic-like substances.
- Sedative–hypnotic agents include benzodiazepines and barbiturates. Signs and symptoms of sedative–hypnotic overdose are chiefly related to the CNS and cardiovascular symptoms. Flumazenil (Romazicon) is a benzodiazepine antagonist. It is useful in reversing the effects of these agents if they were given in a clinical setting.

476

- Commonly used stimulant drugs are those of the amphetamine family. Adverse effects include tachycardia, increased blood pressure, tachypnea, agitation, dilated pupils, tremors, and disorganized behavior. With sudden withdrawal, the patient becomes depressed, suicidal, incoherent, or near coma.
- Phencyclidine (PCP) is a dissociative analgesic with sympathomimetic and CNS stimulant and depressant effects. In low doses, PCP intoxication produces an unpredictable state that can resemble drunkenness (and rage). High-dose intoxication may cause coma. This may last from several hours to days. Respiratory depression, hypertension, and tachycardia may be present. PCP psychosis is a psychiatric emergency. It may mimic schizophrenia.
- Hallucinogens are substances that cause distortions of perceptions. Depending on the agent, overdose may range from visual hallucinations and anticholinergic syndromes to more serious complications, including psychosis, flashbacks, and respiratory and CNS depression.
- Tricyclic antidepressant toxicity is thought to result from central and peripheral, atropine-like anticholinergic effects, and direct depressant effects on myocardial function. A prolonged QRS complex, a Glasgow Coma Scale score score less than 8, or both should alert the paramedic to a major TCA toxicity.
- Lithium is a mood-stabilizing drug. Toxic ingestion can include CNS effects that can range from blurred vision and confusion to seizure and coma.
- Cardiac drugs are a common cause of poisoning deaths in children and adults. The drugs responsible for the majority of these fatalities are digitalis, beta-blockers, and calcium channel blockers.
- Monoamine oxidase inhibitors block or diminish the activity of the monoamines (norepinephrine, dopamine, serotonin). Toxic effects include CNS depression and various neuromuscular and cardiovascular system manifestations.
- Nonsteroidal antiinflammatory drugs work by blocking the production of prostaglandins. The effects of overdose of ibuprofen are usually reversible, are seldom life threatening, and include mild GI and CNS effects. Salicylate poisoning may cause CNS stimulation, GI irritation, glucose metabolism, fluid and electrolyte imbalance, and coagulation defects.
- Acetaminophen overdose may cause life-threatening liver damage. This results from formation of a hepatotoxic intermediate metabolite if it is not managed within 16 to 24 hours of ingestion.
- Some drugs are abused for sexual purposes or for sexual gratification. These are commonly classified by users as "uppers," "downers," and those that have more than one primary effect ("all-arounders"). Problems associated with their use vary widely.
- Alcohol dependence is a disorder characterized by chronic, excessive consumption of alcohol that results in injury to health or inadequate social function and the development of withdrawal symptoms when the patient stops drinking suddenly. Alcohol causes multiple systemic effects. These include neurologic disorders, nutritional deficiencies, fluid and electrolyte imbalances, GI disorders, cardiac and skeletal muscle myopathy, and immune suppression. Several conditions caused by consumption or abstinence from alcohol that may require emergency care are acute alcohol intoxication, alcohol withdrawal syndromes, and disulfiram-ethanol reaction.
- The most common toxic syndromes are cholinergic, anticholinergic, hallucinogenic, opioid, and sympathomimetic. Using these classifications allows paramedics to group similar toxic agents together. It allows them to more easily remember how to assess and treat poisoned patients.

REVIEW QUESTIONS

Match the illnesses in column II with the toxic syndromes in column I. You may use the signs and symptoms more than once.

Column I

1. _c g_______ Anticholinergic syndrome

2. _a b f h_______ Cholinergic syndrome

3. _b e a_______ Opiate/sedative/ethanol syndrome

4. _b d g_______ Sympathomimetic syndrome

Column II

a. Bradycardia
b. Cardiac dysrhythmias
c. Dry mouth
d. Hypertension
e. Respiratory depression
f. Salivation
g. Tachycardia
h. Urination

Match the poisons in column II with their descriptions in column I. Use each poison only once.

Column I

5. _____ Metabolizes to formic acid and causes toxic visual effects

6. _____ Ingestion of odorless, sweet liquid in antifreeze causes central nervous system depression

7. _____ Inhalation, ingestion, and absorption prevents oxygen from reaching cells

8. _____ Inhalation produces lacrimation, dyspnea, and inflammation of the airway

9. _____ Vomiting should not be induced for phenol and others in this group

10. _____ These chemicals include lye and cause immediate damage to the mucosa

11. _____ The long duration of action requires treatment with atropine and pralidoxime

Column II

a. Acid
b. Alkali
c. Ammonia
d. Carbamate
e. Cyanide
f. Ethylene glycol
g. Hydrocarbon
h. Isopropanol
i. Methanol
j. Organophosphate

12. A young child's family states that he ingested some liquid from a bottle in the garage. He arouses only to painful stimulation. After a rapid assessment of the patient, you contact the regional poison control center.

  a. What information should you be prepared to give the center?

  b. What general care measures should you take when caring for this patient if the source of the poisoning is unknown?

13. You insert a 36- to 40-Fr orogastric tube into a patient.

  a. What position should the patient be in?

  b. What precaution should be taken for an unconscious patient?

  c. How should irrigation be performed?

14. Complete the information missing in the following table.

Ingested Poison	Charcoal (Yes/No)	Other Interventions
a. Bleach		
b. Ammonia		
c. Gasoline		
d. Methanol		
e. Ethylene glycol		
f. Isopropanol		
g. Cyanide		

15. A 65-year-old woman complains of food poisoning after eating at a local seafood restaurant 2 hours earlier.

    a. What is the typical time onset for signs of food poisoning?

    b. What treatment should be provided for a patient with food poisoning?

Questions 16 to 18 refer to the following case study:

A 21-year-old man became extremely ill from eating some wild mushrooms. The patient is awake and complains of nausea, vomiting, and diarrhea. He has pinpoint pupils. Vital signs are BP 90/50 mm Hg, P 48, and R 24. His electrocardiogram rhythm shows a sinus bradycardia with occasional ventricular escape beats.

16. What type of toxic syndrome does this patient appear to be exhibiting?

17. How can you find out more about the specific poison involved in this case?

18. What treatment measures may be indicated for this patient in consultation with medical direction?

19. Complete the information missing in the following table.

Toxic Chemical	Class of Toxin	Signs and Symptoms	Treatment
Copper welding fumes			
Hydrogen sulfide			
Methane gas			
Chlorine gas			

20. A worker in a chemical plant is exposed to ammonia gas and is dyspneic, choking, and wheezing. What treatment should be provided for this patient?

____

____

Questions 21 to 24 refer to the following case study:

A farmer calls you to his ranch after spraying pesticide on a windy day. He is complaining of severe diarrhea and says he cannot stop urinating. Tears are running down his face, and he is coughing up large amounts of phlegm. His electrocardiogram is shown in Fig. 34-1.

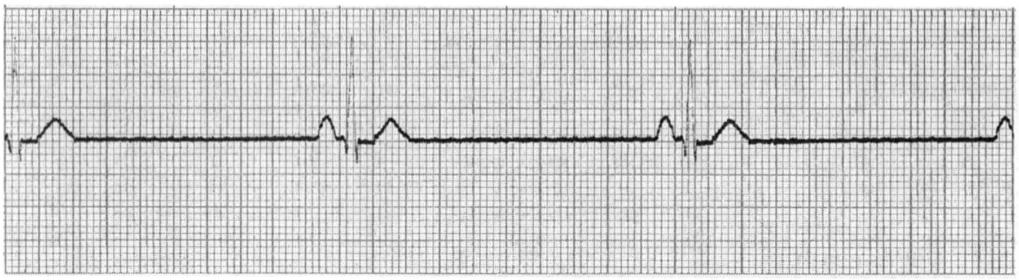

Figure 34-1

21. What poisoning do you suspect?

____

22. What other signs or symptoms might be present?

____

23. What is your interpretation of the electrocardiogram?

____

24. List specific interventions to be used in his care.

____

____

____

25. Interpret the following historical information presented to you at the scene of a potential drug overdose.

   a. "He mainlined some China white."

____

   b. "She was space-basing angel dust and candy."

____

   c. "They were freebasing a rock."

____

d. "He was skin-popping some M."

____

e. "She snorted some PCP before she went crazy."

____

Match the drugs in column II with the appropriate overdose description in column I. Use each drug only once.

Column I

26. _______ Central nervous system stimulant properties can produce violent, unpredictable behavior.

27. _______ It causes visual disturbances, dry mouth, seizures, and tachycardia with a wide QRS complex.

28. _______ It causes tachypnea, central nervous system depression, gastrointestinal irritation, and tinnitus.

29. _______ Mild, influenza-like symptoms are followed by latent liver failure.

30. _______ This stimulant can cause dysrhythmias, myocardial infarction, and hyperthermia.

Column II

a. Acetaminophen
b. Cocaine
c. Heroin
d. Iron
e. Methamphetamine
f. Salicylate
g. Tricyclic antidepressant

Questions 31 and 32 refer to the following case study:

A 32-year-old woman overdosed on sleeping pills 30 minutes ago. She is awake but drowsy.

31. What information regarding the poisoning is critical to the care of this patient?

____

____

32. What dose of activated charcoal should be given?

____

33. Complete the information missing in the following table.

Ingested Poison	Charcoal (Yes/No)	Other Interventions
a. Aspirin		
b. Acetaminophen		
c. Iron		

34. Give two examples of drugs commonly abused in each of the following categories.

a. Narcotics: _______________________________

b. Central nervous system depressants: _______________________________

c. Central nervous system stimulants: _______________________________

d. Hallucinogens: _______________________________

Questions 35 to 37 refer to the following case study:

Your patient injected heroin intravenously and arouses only to pain. He has pinpoint pupils and slow, snoring respirations.

35. What is the primary life threat that must be managed immediately in this patient?

36. How will you manage this life threat until you can administer drugs?

37. List the appropriate drug and dose used to improve this patient's condition.

38. If this man is a chronic heroin abuser and the drug listed previously is administered, what signs and symptoms of narcotic withdrawal will you anticipate?

Questions 39 to 41 refer to the following case study:

A 17-year-old teenager has taken about 50 tablets of chlordiazepoxide and is comatose, with slow, irregular respirations.

39. What is the pupil response likely to be in this patient?

40. Why would administration of flumazenil (Romazicon) to antagonize the effects of this ingestion be risky for this patient?

41. Local college students call you to a party, where participants have been freebasing cocaine. One of the participants has lost consciousness. What life-threatening effects of this drug may have caused loss of consciousness in this patient?

Questions 42 to 44 refer to the following case study:

A popular group is playing at a local club. Security calls you to the parking lot to care for a patient who has reportedly taken bath salts.

42. What should be your primary concern when caring for this patient?

43. Describe the appropriate initial approach to this patient, who is alert and quiet.

44. List signs and symptoms that may be displayed by this patient.

An 18-year-old woman took about 20 tablets of amitriptyline about 1 hour before your arrival at her home. She is drowsy and confused, has a dry mouth, and complains of blurred vision. Her electrocardiogram is shown in Fig. 34-2.

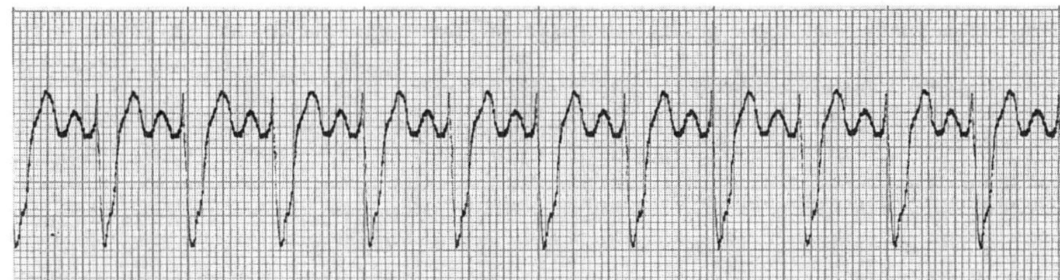

Figure 34-2

45. Should you perform gastric lavage on this patient? Why or why not?

____

____

46. What is your interpretation of the electrocardiogram?

____

47. What drug and appropriate dose may be given to prevent deterioration of this patient's cardiac status?

____

48. What additional signs and symptoms do you anticipate as this patient's condition deteriorates?

____

Questions 49 and 50 refer to the following case study:

Your unit is on the scene of a two-car accident. A 47-year-old male patient appears to be intoxicated. His friend says that he is an alcoholic. The patient states that he drank three beers in the past 5 hours.

49. Should you accept this history of the number of drinks as reliable?

____

50. If the patient is an alcoholic, what chronic physiologic changes in the following areas will make it more difficult to assess his condition and more likely for severe injury to occur?

    a. Neurologic changes:

    ____

    b. Nutritional problems:

    ____

    c. Fluid and electrolyte imbalances:

    ____

483

d. Coagulation disorders:

____

51. Describe the management of a comatose patient suspected to be severely intoxicated by alcohol.

____

____

____

52. Describe the management of a patient experiencing alcohol withdrawal accompanied by severe seizures.

____

____

____

53. List signs and symptoms of delirium tremens.

____

____

54. You are at the first aid station for a church picnic. A 16-year-old boy comes to the station complaining of a bee sting. No signs of anaphylaxis are present.

a. List general care measures for this person.

____

b. Describe the method for removing the stinger.

____

55. List two diseases produced by ticks and possible signs and symptoms for each.

a. ____

b. ____

56. Describe the proper technique for removing a tick.

____

57. A hysterical 20-year-old man states that he has just been bitten by a copperhead snake while camping.

a. List signs and symptoms that would be present if a moderate envenomation had occurred.

____

b. Describe the appropriate prehospital management of this patient.

____

____

58. For each of the following marine animal classifications, list one example and outline general management principles for envenomation:

a. Coelenterates:

____

b. Echinoderms:

____

c. Stingrays:

____

59. Any substance that produces harmful physiologic or psychological effects is known as a(n):
    a. Overdose   **c.** Toxin
    b. Poison   **d.** Venom

60. Which toxic syndrome would present for the patient who has ingested cocaine?
    a. Anticholinergic syndrome
    b. Cholinergic syndrome
    c. Opiate/sedative/ethanol syndrome
    d. Sympathomimetic syndrome

61. What is the primary goal when assessing a poisoned patient?
    a. Begin decontamination of the poison as quickly as possible with activated charcoal.
    b. Determine the exact nature of the poison so that appropriate treatment can be given.
    c. Obtain a history to determine the exact time that the poisoning occurred.
    d. Identify the effects on the respiratory, cardiovascular, and central nervous systems.

62. Charcoal is effective in treating specific overdoses because it does which of the following?
    a. Reverses the effects of the ingested drug
    b. Binds to the drug and prevents absorption
    c. Causes severe nausea and vomiting
    d. Makes the drug speed through the intestine

63. What is the basis for the signs and symptoms of cyanide toxicity?
    a. Cellular hypoxia
    b. Increased metabolism
    c. CO_2 accumulation
    d. Metabolic alkalosis

64. What should be your primary concern when caring for a patient who has ingested hydrocarbon?
    a. Aspiration   **c.** Dysrhythmias
    b. Central nervous system effects   **d.** Hypotension

65. Medical direction may advise administration of sodium bicarbonate in all of the following except which poisoning and overdose situation?
   a. Ethylene glycol
   b. Methanol
   c. Isopropanol
   d. Tricyclic antidepressant

66. Which of the following is true regarding poison plant ingestions?
   a. Dialysis is an effective treatment for most plant poisons.
   b. Ingestion of poisonous plants is common in the United States.
   c. Most signs and symptoms are delayed several days.
   d. Specific treatment should not begin until the plant is identified.

67. Symptoms commonly associated with poisonous mushroom ingestion are likely to include which of the following?
   a. Bradycardia
   b. Dry mouth
   c. Hypertension
   d. Hyperthermia

68. Which hydrocarbon property is associated with the greatest risk?
   a. Low adhesion of molecules along a surface
   b. Low surface tension
   c. High viscosity
   d. High volatility

69. Toxic hydrocarbon inhalation most often is associated with which of the following?
   a. Childhood ingestions
   b. Industrial exposures
   c. Mixing chemicals
   d. Recreational huffing

70. Which of the following overdose or poisoning typically will lead to bradycardia?
   a. Carbamates
   b. Cocaine
   c. Isopropanol
   d. Methanol

71. What should your first priority be when evaluating a patient contaminated with organophosphates?
   a. Administer atropine.
   b. Establish intravenous therapy.
   c. Put on protective gear.
   d. Suction excess secretions.

72. Atropine is supplied in a 10-mL syringe that contains 1 mg of the drug. You wish to administer 2 mg to a patient who has organophosphate poisoning. How many milliliters will you give?
   a. 1 mL
   b. 2 mL
   c. 10 mL
   d. 20 mL

73. Naloxone antagonizes the effects of all of the following except which drug?
   a. Diazepam
   b. Meperidine
   c. Morphine
   d. Vicodin

74. What should your highest priority be when caring for a patient at a methamphetamine lab?
   a. Administration of diazepam to control tremors
   b. Decontamination of the patient
   c. Maintaining scene safety
   d. Talking down the paranoid patient

75. The patient who ingests oil of wintergreen most likely will have which of the following?
   a. Bradycardia, hyperglycemia, and nystagmus
   b. Seizures, hyperglycemia, and ventricular tachycardia
   c. Hypoglycemia, tachypnea, and tinnitus
   d. Hematemesis, metabolic alkalosis, and coma

76. What are the typical findings in patients within the first 24 hours of an overdose of acetaminophen?
   a. Dysrhythmias
   b. Hypoglycemia
   c. No symptoms
   d. Right upper quadrant abdominal pain

486

77. When ingestion of multivitamins is suspected in a child, it is critical to determine whether the preparation contains what?
   a. Ascorbic acid
   b. Folic acid
   c. Iron
   d. Thiamine

78. Which of the following drugs most likely will produce tachycardia if a patient overdoses?
   a. Digoxin (Lanoxin)
   b. Propranolol (Inderal)
   c. Sertraline (Zoloft)
   d. Verapamil (Calan)

79. An alert 4-year-old child ingested about 10 of his grandmother's blood pressure tablets 20 minutes ago. He is awake and alert. What drug should be administered in this situation?
   a. Activated charcoal
   b. Atropine
   c. Calcium chloride
   d. Dopamine

80. Intravenous therapy in the a person with alcoholism with depleted thiamine stores may lead to which of the following?
   a. Disulfiram-ethanol reaction
   b. Guillain-Barré syndrome
   c. Mallory-Weiss tears
   d. Wernicke-Korsakoff syndrome

81. Which of the following is true regarding delirium tremens?
   a. It affects almost all alcoholics going through alcohol withdrawal.
   b. It is associated with a high mortality rate if untreated.
   c. It is characterized by bradycardia, hypotension, and hypothermia.
   d. It usually occurs 12 to 24 hours after cessation of alcohol ingestion.

82. Alcohol withdrawal seizures should be treated with which of the following?
   a. Dextrose 50%
   b. Diazepam
   c. Magnesium sulfate
   d. Thiamine

83. An 18-year-old man who attempts to extract honey from a beehive on a dare sustains 20 to 30 stings. He has a headache, fever, and involuntary muscle spasms and reports a syncopal episode. What type of reaction do you suspect?
   a. Anaphylactic
   b. Delayed
   c. Local
   d. Toxic

84. A 52-year-old man states that he was bitten by a spider at a woodpile. He now is complaining of back, chest, and abdominal pain and has a severe headache. What type of spider envenomation would produce these symptoms?
   a. Black widow
   b. Brown recluse
   c. Tarantula
   d. Wolf

85. A hiker states that he was bitten by a red and yellow snake and is now complaining of slurred speech and dysphagia. His pupils are dilated. You suspect envenomation by what kind of snake?
   a. Copperhead
   b. Cottonmouth moccasin
   c. Coral
   d. Massasauga

86. Which treatment is indicated for a patient who has sustained a venomous coral snake bite to the ankle?
   a. Apply ice to the wound.
   b. Start an intravenous line in the affected extremity.
   c. Elevate the extremity above the heart.
   d. Wrap the affected extremity with an elastic bandage.

87. For which overdose is isoproterenol indicated to treat symptomatic bradycardia?
   a. Digoxin
   b. Nortriptyline
   c. Propranolol
   d. Verapamil

Chapter **34** Toxicology

A 42-year-old man was found "asleep" in the park. Rangers were unable to wake him. He is unresponsive to pain and has snoring respirations at about 2 per minute. His pupils are pinpoint. He has track marks on his arms.

88. What type of overdose would be a likely cause of his decreased level of consciousness?
    a. Cocaine   **c.** Methamphetamine
    b. Heroin   **d.** Bath salts

89. Which intervention will be your first priority in his care?
    a. Assist ventilations with bag-mask device.
    b. Check his blood glucose level.
    c. Deliver a fluid bolus of 200 mL of normal saline.
    d. Give (Narcan) naloxone intravenously.

WRAP IT UP

You are dispatched to a home for a "possible overdose." Your 22-year-old male patient is in the bathtub. He moans and flexes slightly in response to painful stimulus. Emesis is sprayed around the toilet, and a pile of pill bottles is in the sink. The pill bottles are prescribed to several persons and you find Tylenol, aspirin, Vicodin, Glucophage, vitamins with iron, amitryptiline, Ativan, Ritalin, metoprolol, and empty bottles of rubbing alcohol and vodka. You assess him and find his vital signs are BP 100/70 mm Hg, P 104, R 6, and SaO_2 65%. You assist his respirations with a bag-valve mask, and he gags when you try to place an oral airway, so you insert a nasopharyngeal airway. You find his skin to be pale and dry, and his pupils are 2 mm. An IV is started, and his blood glucose reading is 25 mg/dL. You administer naloxone (Narcan) followed by $D_{50}W$. An electrocardiogram tracing shows sinus tachycardia with occasional premature ventricular contractions. His level of consciousness improves slightly, and he is somewhat combative on arrival to the emergency department.

1. Which of the substance(s) that he ingested can cause the following?

    a. Hypoglycemia: ____

    b. Acidosis: ____

    c. Tachycardia: ____

    d. Respiratory depression: ____

    e. Decreased level of consciousness: ____

    f. Pupil constriction: ____

    g. Bradycardia: ____

    h. Cardiac dysrhythmias: ____

    i. Seizures: ____

2. Place a check mark beside the drugs or classifications of drugs that this patient may have taken.
    a. ________ Acetaminophen   **g.** ________ Isopropanol
    b. ________ Benzodiazepine   **h.** ________ Mineral
    c. ________ Beta-blocker   **i.** ________ Opioid or narcotic
    d. ________ Ethanol alcohol   **j.** ________ Organophosphate
    e. ________ Hypoglycemic   **k.** ________ Stimulant
    f. ________ Salicylate   **l.** ________ Tricyclic antidepressant

3. For each of the following drugs this patient has taken, describe the action that is most likely to cause death.

    a. Acetaminophen: ____

    b. Metoprolol: ____

    c. Vodka: ____

    d. Metformin (Glucophage): ____

488

    e. Aspirin: ____

    f. Iron: ____

    g. Hydrocodone/acetaminophen (Vicodin): ______________________________

    h. Tricyclic antidepressant: ____

4. Explain your rationale for the interventions that you performed.

    a. Bag-valve-mask:____

    b. Naloxone: ____

    c. $D_{50}W$: ____

5. Would other antidotes or therapeutic interventions be indicated for this patient if these drugs were taken individually?

____

6. Which of the following is true regarding the care of the overdosed patient?
    a. The most important goal for prehospital treatment is gastric emptying.
    b. Gathering of information from the scene is critical in toxicology emergencies.
    c. Administration of antidotes, when indicated, takes priority over all interventions.
    d. Syrup of ipecac should be given to all overdose patients if not contraindicated.

7. Which of the drugs he ingested, when taken individually, could cause the following toxidromes?

    a. Cholinergic: ____

    b. Anticholinergic: ____

    c. Hallucinogen: ____

    d. Opioid: ____

    e. Sympathomimetic: ____

CHAPTER 34 ANSWERS

REVIEW QUESTIONS

1. c, g

2. a, b, f, h

3. b, e, g

4. b, d, g
(Questions 1–4, Objective 2)

5. i
(Objective 4)

6. f
(Objective 4)

7. e
(Objectives 4 and 6)

8. c
(Objective 8)

9. g
(Objective 4)

10. b
(Objective 4)

11. j
(Objective 9)

12. a. You should be prepared to tell the poison control center the specific agent ingested, amount of agent ingested, time ingested, age, patient weight, medical condition, and treatment rendered before arrival of emergency medical services personnel.
(Objective 3)
  b. Ensure adequate airway, ventilation, and circulation. Obtain a history (especially specific to substance ingested) and perform a physical examination. Assess for hypoglycemia. Consult with medical direction for further treatment guidelines. Monitor vital signs and electrocardiogram. Transport rapidly for definitive treatment.
(Objective 3)

13. a. Position the patient in the left lateral Trendelenburg (swimmer's) position.
  b. Perform rapid-sequence endotracheal intubation before orogastric tube intubation if the patient has a decreased level of consciousness with an absent gag reflex.
  c. After assessment for proper tube placement, normal saline (preferably warmed) should be infused into the orogastric tube in 200- to 300-mL boluses, and the tube should be allowed to drain after each bolus. Continue this process until the gastric drainage returns clear.
(Objective 3)

14. Indicated in alert patient if ingestion < 1 hour prior.

Ingested Poison	Charcoal (Yes/No)	Other Interventions
a. Bleach	No	Dilution with milk or water (200–300 mL for an adult or 15 mL/kg for a child)
b. Ammonia	No	Dilution with milk or water
c. Gasoline	No	Initiation of intravenous line, monitoring of airway, and electrocardiogram
d. Methanol	Controversial	Lavage, indicated in alert patient if in gestion < 1 hour prior; sodium bicarbonate intravenously (30–60 mL), and 80-proof ethanol by mouth
e. Ethylene glycol		Lavage, indicated in alert patient if ingestion < 1 hour prior; sodium bicarbonate intravenously (30–60 mL), 80-proof ethanol by mouth, and (rarely) furosemide, thiamine, and calcium
f. Isopropanol	Yes	Lavage indicated in alert patient if ingestion <1 hour prior
g. Cyanide	No	Hydroxocobalamin or amyl nitrite pearls, 3% sodium nitrite, and 25% sodium thiosulfate

(Objective 4)

15. a. Time varies: chemical, 1 to 2 hours; bacterial toxins, 1 to 12 hours; viral or bacterial, 12 to 48 hours.
    b. Take universal precautions, maintain airway and breathing, and initiate intravenous therapy with crystalloid
       solution to treat dehydration and fluid and electrolyte imbalance.
    (Objective 4)

16. Cholinergic syndrome
    (Objective 2)

17. Ask the patient if he still has a sample of the mushroom and what time he took it. If he does not have a sample,
    have him describe the mushroom. Contact poison control and medical direction (per protocol) for help with
    identification and treatment information. Prehospital treatment likely will be guided by signs and symptoms rather
    than specific identification information.
    (Objective 2)

18. Maintain airway and prepare to suction secretions if needed, administer high-concentration oxygen, monitor
    electrocardiogram and vital signs frequently, initiate an intravenous line and infuse fluids as ordered by medical
    direction, and prepare to administer atropine sulfate as ordered by medical direction.
    (Objective 4)

19. Rescuers should wear appropriate personal protective equipment.

Toxic Chemical	Class of Toxin	Sign and Symptoms	Treatment
Copper welding	Metal fumes	Chills, fever, myalgias; headache, cough, leukocytosis	Remove patient from fumes source, treat symptoms
Hydrogen sulfide	Chemical asphyxiant	Sudden collapse, rotten egg smell, rapid fatigue	Remove patient from source, oxygenate
Chlorine gas	Irritant	Lacrimation, sore throat, stridor, tracheobronchitis, pulmonary edema	Remove patient from source, give humidified oxygen and bronchodilators, manage airway

(Objective 6)

20. Ensure personal protection; open the airway; administer high-flow oxygen; initiate an intravenous line to keep the
    vein open; and if pulmonary edema develops, consider administration of diuretics and bronchodilators.
    (Objective 8)

21. Carbamate or organophosphate
    (Objective 9)

22. Pupil constriction, muscle fasciculation, headache, weakness, dizziness, hypotension, bronchoconstriction, anxiety,
    seizures, and convulsions
    (Objective 9)

23. Sinus bradycardia
    (Objective 9)

24. Wear protective gear; decontaminate as appropriate; suction oral secretions as necessary; prepare to intubate if patient's
    condition deteriorates; initiate intravenous therapy with crystalloid to keep the vein open; administer atropine 2 to 4 mg
    intravenously every 5 to 15 minutes as necessary to induce relative tachycardia, flushing, and decreased secretions;
    monitor for dysrhythmias; administer pralidoxime; and administer diazepam as necessary for seizures.
    (Objective 9)

25. a. He took fentanyl or heroin intravenously.
    b. She was smoking PCP and crack (cocaine).
    c. They were smoking purified crack cocaine.
    d. He injected morphine subcutaneously.
    e. She ingested PCP nasally.
    (Objective 10)

491

26. e

27. g

28. f

29. a

30. b
(Questions 26 to 30, Objective 11)

31. What was taken? Where is the container? How much was in it, and how much is left (may need to estimate based on date prescription issued, amount prescribed daily, and amount left in bottle)? When was the drug taken? Has the patient vomited or taken anything to induce vomiting since the drug was taken? Has any antidote been given to the patient? Ask the patient the following: Why did you do this? Were you trying to hurt or kill yourself?
(Objective 10)

32. 30 to 100 g of activated charcoal
(Objective 10)

33.

Ingested Poison	Charcoal (Yes/No)	Other Interventions
a. Aspirin	Yes	$D_{50}W$ if patient is hypoglycemic
b. Acetaminophen	Usually not (varies by medical direction)	Acetylcysteine (Mucomyst; varies by medical direction)
c. Iron	No	Monitor airway, initiate intravenous line

34. a. Heroin, morphine, OxyContin, Vicodin, and methadone; b. barbiturates (secobarbital, phenobarbital) and benzodiazepines (diazepam, chlordiazepoxide); c. amphetamines and cocaine; d. lysergic acid diethylamide (LSD), phencyclidine (PCP), and salvia
(Objective 10)

35. Respiratory depression (partial airway obstruction and decreased minute volume)
(Objective 11)

36. Assist ventilation with a bag-mask.
(Objective 11)

37. Naloxone (Narcan) 0.4 to 2.0 mg intravenously or 0.4 to 0.8 mg IM or SC (intranasal route is sometimes used). Use smaller doses if known addiction. (Administer enough to ensure adequate airway reflexes and ventilation.)
(Objective 11)

38. Gooseflesh (piloerection), tachycardia, diaphoresis, irritability, insomnia, abdominal cramps, tremors, nausea, vomiting, cold sweats and chills, fever, and diarrhea
(Objective 11)

39. Bilaterally dilated and slow to react to light
(Objective 11)

40. Flumazenil (Romazicon) has serious side effects if the patient is benzodiazepine dependent or if the patient has taken certain other medicines (e.g., TCA).
(Objective 11)

41. Cardiac dysrhythmias, seizures, or cerebrovascular accident (after intracranial hemorrhage)
(Objective 11)

492

42. Personal safety
(Objective 11)

43. Quiet, calm approach. Interview the patient while minimizing external sensory stimuli (for example, bright lights, noise).
(Objective 11)

44. Euphoria, disorientation, seizures, hypertensive crisis, dysrhythmias, catatonia, unresponsiveness, and bizarre and violent behavior. These patients are extremely difficult to manage and dangerous if found in or provoked into violent behavior.
(Objective 11)

45. She is drowsy, and her level of consciousness could deteriorate further. Intubate using rapid-sequence intubation (if authorized) before gastric lavage to prevent aspiration.
(Objective 11)

46. Sinus tachycardia with delayed ventricular conduction (wide QRS complex)
(Objective 11)

47. Sodium bicarbonate 1 to 2 mEq/kg intravenously and normal saline bolus of 500–1000 mL. Medical direction may also order magnesium sulfate.
(Objective 11)

48. Delirium, depressed respirations, hypertension or hypotension, hyperthermia or hypothermia, seizures, coma, and dysrhythmias
(Objective 11)

49. No. People with alcoholism frequently underestimate the number of drinks they have had.
(Objective 13)

50. a. Short-term memory deficit, problems with coordination, and difficulty with concentration can mimic signs and symptoms of head injury.
    b. Nutritional deficiencies can cause muscle cramps, paresthesias, seizures, tremor or ataxia, and poor wound healing.
    c. Chronic dehydration may be difficult to distinguish from a new onset of fluid loss. Patient will decompensate faster if acute fluid loss occurs resulting from trauma.
    d. Clotting factors are suppressed by chronic alcohol abuse, resulting in increased risk of bleeding, especially subdural hematoma, with minor trauma.
(Objective 12)

51. Protect airway (high risk of aspiration); ventilate as necessary; initiate intravenous therapy; draw blood samples per protocol; determine blood glucose levels and if low, administer thiamine 100 mg intravenously and $D_{50}W$ 25 g intravenously; if opiate overdose is suspected or unknown, administer naloxone 2 mg intravenously; and monitor airway, breathing, vital signs, and electrocardiogram.
(Objective 13)

52. Manage as in answer 51 and protect from injury; administer diazepam 2.5 to 5.0 mg or lorazepam 1 to 2 mg intravenously if additional seizures occur; examine for signs or symptoms of traumatic injury.
(Objective 13)

53. Hyperactive motor, speech, and autonomic activity; confusion; disorientation; delusion; hallucinations; tremor; agitation; insomnia; tachycardia; fever; hypertension; dilated pupils; profuse diaphoresis; and in severe cases, cardiovascular collapse
(Objective 13)

54. a. Assess for anaphylaxis, apply ice packs, and immobilize and elevate affected extremity.
    b. Scrape or brush off. Do not squeeze because doing so will inject additional venom.
(Objective 14)

55. a. Lyme disease. Early signs are fever, lethargy, muscle pain, and general malaise; late signs are cardiac abnormalities, cranial nerve palsies, and arthritis.

b. Tick paralysis. Signs include restlessness and paresthesia in the hands and feet progressing to ascending symmetrical flaccid paralysis, which may include respiratory muscles.

(Objective 14)

56. Apply gloves and grasp the tick as close to skin surface as possible (may use tweezers or forceps if available), pull out with steady pressure (avoid squeezing tick), and cleanse the wound and observe for any remnants of the tick.

(Objective 14)

57. a. Fang marks, pain and edema, weakness, diaphoresis, nausea, vomiting, and paresthesias

b. Ensure personal safety from another bite; monitor airway, breathing, and circulation; initiate intravenous therapy in the unaffected extremity; immobilize the affected extremity in a dependent position; and keep the patient at rest.

(Objective 14)

58. a. Jellyfish, fire corals, and sea anemones. Rinse the wound with seawater; apply vinegar, baking soda, isopropanol, ammonia, meat tenderizer (for 5–10 minutes only); remove visible tentacles with forceps; apply shaving cream; gently shave affected area or use knife or spatula to gently scrape remaining tentacles; and rinse again.

b. Sea urchins, starfish, and sea cucumbers. Remove embedded spines with forceps and immerse affected extremity (and unaffected extremity to prevent thermal injury) in hot water during transport.

c. Stingrays. Irrigate wound with saltwater or freshwater; remove venom apparatus if it is visible; and immerse the affected part in hot water.

(Objective 14)

59. b

(Objective 1)

60. d

(Objective 2)

61. d. Life threats that will need immediate management usually are identified by assessing these areas.

(Objective 3)

62. b. Charcoal binds the drug by adsorption. It often is given with a cathartic that speeds the bound drug through the gastrointestinal tract.

(Objective 3)

63. a. Cyanide inhibits use of oxygen in the cell.

(Objective 7)

64. a. Inducing emesis usually is contraindicated for these patients unless the toxicity of the specific hydrocarbon is so great that the risks of absorption in the gastrointestinal tract outweigh the risks of aspiration.

(Objective 4)

65. c. Methanol and ethylene glycol produce metabolic acidosis, so $NaHCO_3$ is indicated. In a tricyclic antidepressant overdose, $NaHCO_3$ will decrease the toxic cardiac side effects. No metabolic acidosis usually is associated with isopropanol ingestion.

(Objective 4)

66. b. The second most common reported category of poisonings is from plants. Dialysis is not effective for most plant poisonings. Most signs and symptoms occur within several hours after ingestion. Treatment should be based on symptoms and not be delayed until the identity of the plant can be determined.

(Objective 4)

67. a. Salivation and hypotension are likely to accompany the bradycardia. Symptoms vary according to the specific variety of mushroom ingested.

(Objective 4)

494

68. d. The lower the viscosity, the higher the risk of aspiration.
(Objective 5)

69. d. Huffing or sniffing substances such as carbon tetrachloride, methylene chloride, or aromatic hydrocarbons such as benzene and toluene is the most common method.
(Objective 8)

70. a. All of the other chemicals are more likely to cause tachycardia.
(Objective 9)

71. c. All other interventions are critical; however, rescuer safety should precede treatment because these poisons are absorbed readily through the skin, by ingestion, or by inhalation.
(Objective 9)

72. d
(Objective 9)

73. a. All of the others are narcotics.
(Objective 11)

74. c. Methamphetamine labs may produce hazards because of booby traps, explosive chemicals, a violent patient, or hazardous material contamination. Scene safety should be the highest priority.
(Objective 11)

75. c. Oil of wintergreen contains a large amount of salicylate and has produced many fatal ingestions.
(Objective 11)

76. c. Unless patients volunteer information regarding an overdose of acetaminophen, they may be asymptomatic or complain of only mild influenza-like symptoms for the first 24 hours after ingestion.
(Objective 11)

77. c. Ingestion of an overdose of iron is often lethal.
(Objective 11)

78. c. All of the other drugs are more likely to produce bradycardia, although digoxin can produce bradycardia or tachycardia.
(Objective 11)

79. a. The immediate goal is to adsorb the drug and prevent its passage into the small intestine where it can be absorbed into the blood. Later, if signs and symptoms develop, they will be treated.
(Objective 11)

80. d. Wernicke-Korsakoff syndrome can lead to irreversible neurologic problems and may be avoided by giving thiamine before administration of $D_{50}W$.
(Objective 12)

81. b. The mortality rate has been reported as high as 15% for delirium tremens. It affects about 5% of hospitalized people with alcoholism undergoing withdrawal and usually occurs 72 to 96 hours after withdrawal of alcohol. Symptoms are associated with autonomic hyperactivity.
(Objective 13)

82. b. Diazepam in doses of 5 mg every 5 minutes up to a total of 30 mg may be needed. Lorazepam 1 to 2 mg intravenously is an alternative.
(Objective 13)

83. d. Anaphylaxis likely would include respiratory distress and urticaria. His reaction was immediate and generalized and involved a large exposure to venom.
(Objective 14)

84. a. The brown recluse spider produces a local reaction, leading to delayed skin necrosis. Envenomation from most other spiders typically causes local versus systemic reactions.
(Objective 14)

85. c. This description matches a coral snake, which is the only neurotoxic snake listed.
(Objective 14)

86. d. Ice or cold packs may increase tissue damage. Establish an IV line in the unaffected extremity.
(Objective 14)

87. c. Isoproterenol may induce or aggravate hypotension and ventricular dysrhythmias and should not be given for drug-induced bradycardia unless massive beta-blocker poisoning has occurred.
(Objective 11)

88. b. The other three are stimulants, and the patient has pinpoint pupils, so an opiate overdose is more likely.
(Objective 11)

89. a. Assist ventilation and then give naloxone.
(Objective 10)

WRAP IT UP

1. a. Hypoglycemia: aspirin, Glucophage, acetaminophen (72–96 hours), ethanol (Vodka)
  b. Acidosis: aspirin, Glucophage
  c. Tachycardia: Ritalin, Elavil
  d. Respiratory depression: Vicodin, Ativan, Elavil, aspirin (late), ethanol alcohol
  e. Decreased level of consciousness: Vicodin, Elavil, Ativan, rubbing alcohol, ethanol (Vodka)
  f. Pupil constriction: Vicodin, Ritalin
  g. Bradycardia: metoprolol
  h. Cardiac dysrhythmias: Elavil, metoprolol, Tylenol (4–14 days)
  i. Seizures: aspirin, Glucophage (hypoglycemia), amitriptyline, metoprolol
  (Objectives 2 and 11)

2. a, b, c, d, e, f, g, h, i, k, l
  (Objective 3)

3. a. Acetaminophen: respiratory depression or cardiac dysrhythmias
  b. Metoprolol: bradycardia, ventricular dysrhythmias
  c. Vodka (ethanol): airway obstruction
  d. Glucophage: hypoglycemic coma
  e. Aspirin: acidosis, convulsions, respiratory arrest, brain death
  f. Iron: gastrointestinal bleeding
  g. Vicodin: respiratory depression
  h. Tricyclic antidepressant: cardiac dysrhythmias, CNS depression
  (Objective 2, 10, and 11)

4. a. Support depressed, slow respirations.
  b. Naloxone is an antidote for narcotic (Vicodin) overdose and its accompanying respiratory depression.
  c. Blood glucose tests revealed hypoglycemia, which occurred as a result of his ingestions.
  (Objectives 10 and 11)

5. Flumazenil (Romazicon) is used to treat benzodiazepine overdose. However, it is only recommended after procedural sedation. It is not used in multiple-drug overdoses because life-threatening side effects can occur in patients who have taken certain other drugs, including tricyclic antidepressants.
  Sodium bicarbonate is indicated in cases of tricyclic antidepressant overdose, and acidosis. Medical control may or may not have ordered it in this polydrug situation.

496

Glucagon can be administered in beta-blocker overdose.
Activated charcoal sometimes is indicated to adsorb drugs that are ingested; however, with the airway not yet secured, this could increase the risk of aspiration.
(Objective 11)

6. b. Gathering information related to the toxic ingestion is a key element in the prehospital care of the poisoned patient. Ipecac should not be used to treat ingestions. Antidotes are available for few poisonings.
(Objective 10)

7. a. None
   b. Elavil
   c. None
   d. Vicodin
   e. Ritalin
(Objective 14)

 # Behavioral and Psychiatric Disorders

READING ASSIGNMENT

Chapter 35, pages 1025-1050, in *Mosby's Paramedic Textbook,* ed. 4.

OBJECTIVES

Upon completion of this chapter, the paramedic student will be able to do the following:

1. Define what constitutes a behavioral emergency.
2. Identify potential causes for behavioral and psychiatric illnesses.
3. List three critical principles that should be considered in the prehospital care of any patient with a behavioral emergency.
4. Outline key elements in the prehospital patient examination during a behavioral emergency.
5. Describe effective techniques for interviewing a patient during a behavioral emergency.
6. Distinguish between key symptoms and management techniques for selected behavioral and psychiatric disorders.
7. Identify factors that must be considered when assessing suicide risk.
8. Formulate appropriate interview questions to determine suicidal intent.
9. Explain prehospital management techniques for the patient who has attempted suicide.
10. Describe assessment of the potentially violent patient.
11. Outline measures that may be used in an attempt to safely diffuse a potentially violent patient situation.
12. List situations when patient restraints can be used.
13. Discuss key principles in patient restraint.
14. Describe safety measures taken when patient violence is anticipated.
15. Explain variations in approach to behavioral emergencies in children.

SUMMARY

- A behavioral emergency is a change in mood or behavior. This change cannot be tolerated by the involved person or others. It calls for immediate attention.
- Physical or biochemical disturbances can result in significant changes in behavior. Psychosocial mental illness is often the result of childhood trauma, parental deprivation, or a dysfunctional family structure.
- Changes in behavior caused by interpersonal or situational stress are often linked to specific incidents, such as environmental violence, death of a loved one, economic or employment problems, or prejudice and discrimination.
- When dealing with behavioral emergencies, the paramedic should contain the crisis. It begins by establishing a rapport with the patient. He or she should provide the proper emergency care as well. Also, the paramedic should transport the patient to an appropriate health care facility.
- During the patient assessment, an attempt should be made to determine the patient's mental state, name and age, significant past medical history, medications (and compliance), and past psychiatric problems, as well as the precipitating situation or problem.
- Effective interviewing techniques include active listening, being supportive and empathetic, limiting interruptions, and respecting the patient's personal space.
- A mental status exam includes assessment of appearance and behavior; speech and language; cognitive abilities; and emotional stability.
- All cognitive disorders result in a disturbance in thinking that may manifest as delirium or dementia.
- Schizophrenia is characterized by recurrent episodes of psychotic behavior. This behavior may include abnormalities of thought process, thought content, perception, and judgment.
- Anxiety disorders may cause a panic attack. Anxiety disorders include phobias, obsessive-compulsive disorders, and posttraumatic syndrome.
- Depression is a mood disorder. A person with depression may have feelings of hopelessness, loss of appetite, decreased libido, and feelings of worthlessness and guilt.
- Bipolar disorder is a manic-depressive illness. In this illness, depressive and manic episodes alternate with one another.
- Suicide threats or attempts indicate the patient has a serious crisis. Certain factors increase the risk of suicide. Patients who express the wish to harm or kill themselves should be transported.

- Somatoform disorders are conditions in which there are physical symptoms for which no physical cause can be found. The cause is thought to be psychological. These include somatization disorder and conversion disorder.
- Factitious disorders are disorders in which symptoms mimic a true illness. However, the symptoms have been invented. They are under the control of the patient.
- Dissociative disorders are a group of psychological illnesses. In these disorders, a particular mental function is separated from the mind as a whole.
- The most common eating disorders considered to be forms of psychiatric illness are anorexia nervosa and bulimia nervosa.
- Impulse control disorders are characterized by the inability to resist an impulse or temptation to do some act that is unlawful, socially unacceptable, or self-harmful.
- Personality disorders are conditions characterized by failing to learn from experience or adapt appropriately to changes. This results in personal distress and impairment of social functioning.
- After ensuring scene safety, the first priority in patient management after a suicide attempt is medical care. If the patient is conscious, developing rapport as soon as possible is crucial.
- Assessment of a potentially violent patient should include past history of violence, posture, vocal activity, and physical activity.
- When trying to defuse a situation involving a potentially violent patient, the paramedic should ensure a safe environment, gather the patient's history, try to gain the patient's cooperation, avoid threats, and explain the paramedic's role in providing care.
- Severely disturbed patients who pose a threat to themselves or others may need to be restrained.
- Reasonable force to restrain a patient should be used as humanely as possible. An adequate number of personnel is needed. This will ensure patient and rescuer safety during restraint. The risk of personal injury and legal liability is always present.
- Personal safety measures while responding to a behavioral emergency should include not allowing the patient to block the exit, keeping large furniture between you and the patient, working as a team, avoiding threatening statements, and using soft objects to absorb the impact of thrown objects.
- When caring for children with behavioral emergencies, the paramedic should attempt to gain their trust, tell them they won't be hurt, keep questions brief, be honest, involve parents (if appropriate), and take threats of violence seriously.

REVIEW QUESTIONS

Match the psychiatric conditions in Column II with their descriptions in Column I. Use each condition only once.

Column I

1. ________ Feelings of worthlessness and guilt

2. ________ Unfounded fear of situation or object

3. ________ Loss of touch with reality in this major mental disorder

4. ________ Loss of sensory or motor function without organic cause

5. ________ Excessive elation, irritability, talkativeness, and delusions

6. ________ Logical, highly developed delusions

Column II

a. Conversion hysteria
b. Depression
c. Mania
d. Neurosis
e. Panic attack
f. Paranoia
g. Phobia
h. Psychosis

7. A 60-year-old man has erratic behavior. He alternates between hysterical bursts of laughter, irritability, sitting quietly, and crying. You find metformin HCL (Glucophage), hydralazine, and thyroxine in the medicine chest and note an ecchymotic area on his left temple. His skin is hot and moist. Based on this patient's history, what are some likely organic causes of his behavior that must be ruled out before assuming that this is a behavioral emergency?

___

___

___

8. a. List three psychosocial causes of mental illness.

____

b. List three sociocultural causes of mental illness.

____

Questions 9 to 11 refer to the following patient case study:

You are called to a private residence to care for a behavioral emergency. Police report that the patient is "OBS." On arrival, you find a 34-year-old woman sitting quietly in a living room chair. She is complaining of depression.

9. What four general management principles should you consider on this and all behavioral calls?

a. ____

b. ____

c. ____

d. ____

10. What should your scene survey include?

____

11. What minimum patient data should be obtained if possible?

____

12. Should a detailed secondary survey be performed on a patient with a behavioral emergency?

____

13. Complete the missing information in the following table.

Illness	Classification	Clinical Presentation	Treatment (Medical or EMS)
Dementia			
Schizophrenia			
Posttraumatic syndrome			
Bipolar disorder			
Somatization disorder			
Bulimia nervosa			

14. A patient with a phobia of heights must be rescued by ladder from a high bridge. What measures can you take to prevent a panic attack?

____

15. A manic patient is being transported to the hospital for psychiatric evaluation. Describe effective patient management techniques in this situation.

____

16. Family members call you to the home of a 25-year-old man who has become increasingly out of touch with reality. He feels that aliens are trying to kidnap him so that they can remove his brain. He tells you that they are trying to control his thoughts. He states, "They're here. Can't you hear them laughing?"

    a. What behavioral illness does this presentation suggest?

    ____

    b. What approach will enable therapeutic communication with this patient?

    ____

17. A 25-year-old woman cut her wrist with a razor blade. She is crying, "Let me go. Why didn't you let me do it?" She has a small laceration with controlled bleeding, minimal blood loss, and stable vital signs.

    a. How can you best assess the patient's suicidal risk?

    ____

    b. What are your goals in caring for this patient during transport?

    ____

Questions 18 to 22 refer to the following case study:

A distraught family calls you to take their son to the hospital for a court-ordered, involuntary psychiatric evaluation. They state that he has been breaking furniture for the past few hours and refuses to take his antipsychotic drugs.

18. What four factors should you assess rapidly to determine the potential for violence in this patient?

    a. ____

    b. ____

    c. ____

    d. ____

    Your patient is pacing, is verbally abusive, and is threatening injury to those who approach. He is not armed.

19. You elect to restrain him. What help should you request?

____

20. When approaching the patient to prepare for restraint, what should you note about the physical environment?

____

21. Assuming that the patient meets the standard for involuntary detention in your state, how should he be restrained (including position and ways to secure extremities and torso)?

____

____

22. After restraints are applied, what should you monitor en route to the hospital?

____

STUDENT SELF-ASSESSMENT

23. What is a change in mood or behavior that cannot be tolerated by the involved person or others and needs immediate attention called?
- **a.** Behavioral emergency
- **b.** Delusion
- **c.** Neurosis
- **d.** Psychosis

24. What is the characteristic of abnormal (maladaptive) behavior?
- **a.** Deviates from the person's normal behavior
- **b.** Does not conform to your idea of normal behavior
- **c.** Interferes with a person's ability to function
- **d.** Violates a societal law

25. Which of the following questions would be most appropriate to begin a conversation with a mentally ill patient?
- **a.** Did you start feeling this way today?
- **b.** Are you feeling bad now?
- **c.** How did this all begin?
- **d.** Are you okay?

26. Which response by the paramedic is most likely to lead to an effective interview in the prehospital setting?
- **a.** Everything will be fine.
- **b.** I know exactly how you feel.
- **c.** Yes, I see those scary bugs too.
- **d.** You look very sad.

27. Which condition is a state of acute mental confusion commonly brought on by a physical illness?
- **a.** Delirium
- **b.** Delusions
- **c.** Dementia
- **d.** Depression

28. A middle-aged woman suddenly loses the ability to speak after catching her husband in an extramarital affair. What behavioral illness may have caused her problem?
- **a.** Conversion hysteria
- b. Depression
- **c.** Panic attack
- **d.** Phobia

29. Which feeling commonly characterize depression?
- **a.** Hopelessness
- **b.** Hunger
- **c.** Increased libido
- **d.** Restlessness

30. You are transporting a man who believes he is Elvis Presley. His wife states that he quit his job, keeps calling her Priscilla, and is preparing to move to Graceland. You suspect that he is suffering from which of the following?
- **a.** Delusions
- **b.** Neurosis
- **c.** Paranoia
- **d.** Phobia

31. A panic attack typically occurs with any of the following except which symptom?
- **a.** Chest pain and vertigo
- **b.** Hyperventilation
- **c.** Suicidal intent
- **d.** Trembling and sweating

32. What is the highest priority on a suicide call?
    a. Ensuring safety of crew members
    b. Managing life threats
    c. Talking the person out of it
    d. Listening empathetically

33. Which of the following statements regarding suicide is true?
    a. Those who talk about killing themselves rarely do it.
    b. Men commit suicide more often than women.
    c. Suicide is an inherited tendency.
    d. When depression lifts, suicide risk disappears.

34. When should a violent patient be released from physical restraints?
    a. Immediately after administration of haloperidol intramuscularly
    b. As soon as the patient assures cooperation
    c. When the police have adequate personnel to control the patient
    d. When a physician at the hospital determines the patient is no longer dangerous

35. You are caring for a violent psychiatric patient. Which of the following drugs is appropriate for chemical restraint?
    a. Etomidate   **c.** Haloperidol
    b. Diphenhydramine   **d.** Fentanyl

36. Which strategy should be used to maintain emergency medical services crew safety when on a behavioral emergency call?
    a. Be firm and tell the patient to behave or you will have to use restraints.
    b. Interview the patient privately while your partner waits outside of the room.
    c. Kneel and put your arm on the patient's shoulder to show you care.
    d. Stay closer to the exit than the patient, with furniture between you and the patient.

37. Which strategy will be helpful when caring for a child who is experiencing a behavioral emergency?
    a. Avoid having the parents present during care.
    b. Do not be concerned about the possibility of violence.
    c. Keep the interview questions brief.
    d. Lie if you need to gain cooperation.

WRAP IT UP

You immediately recognize your patient when you arrive at the call. "Herb" is a 30-year-old homeless man with a history of schizophrenia. He is in and out of treatment facilities, and he is difficult to predict. When he is taking his medications, he is usually reasonable, but when he runs out of his medications, he can be dangerous. The police are with him and have called because he was threatening to kill himself. You introduce yourself, call him by name, and ask how he is feeling. He says, "The voices are telling me to end it all." "What do you mean by end it all?" you ask. "Kill myself you silly, x#@$er," he replies, "What did you think I meant?" His voice tone gets louder as he speaks, and he begins to lean forward menacingly toward you. "I'm here to help you, Herb," you tell him. "Have you thought about how you would do it?" you ask. "Hanging, it's what the voices say I should do," he replies, "that's why I'm headed to the park, lots of good trees for it over there." "Herb, we'd like to take you to the hospital to get you some medicine so you don't hurt yourself," you explain. With that, he suddenly lunges toward you, screaming, "You'll never get me to go back to that place." With police assistance, you subdue him and restrain him supine on your cot, where he continues to struggle forcefully. Then, with the approval of online medical direction, you administer haloperidol intramuscularly. You manage to get a pulse oximeter reading every few minutes and monitor his respirations carefully. Just as you arrive at the hospital, 30 minutes later, you note marked relaxation, and his voice calms. You give report to the ED staff and assist them to secure him to their stretcher after the physician briefly examines him. As you return to the station, you express your frustration about this patient to your partner: it just doesn't seem right that they can't find a treatment to make him well for more than a month or so at a time.

1. What clues led you to believe that the patient's behavior might become violent?

2. Which of the following is true regarding schizophrenia?

   a. It is more common in men than women.

   b. It typically resolves when the patient is in his or her 40s.

   c. Delusions and auditory hallucinations are common.

   d. Suicide rarely is associated with this disease.

3. Explain why asking a patient directly about suicidal intent would or would not be a helpful strategy.

4. Explain your rationale for administering haloperidol.

CHAPTER 35 ANSWERS

REVIEW QUESTIONS

1. b

2. g

3. h

4. a

5. c

6. f
(Questions 1 to 6, Objective 5)

7. Metformin (Glucophage) indicates that he is diabetic; assess for hypoglycemia or hyperglycemia. Thyroxine is prescribed for thyroid disorders, which can cause behavioral alterations. Treatment with hydralazine suggests he has a history of hypertension or heart disease, so he may have had a transient ischemic attack, stroke, or cardiac dysrhythmia. The ecchymotic area on his head could indicate cerebral injury from trauma, causing his behavior. His warm, moist skin could indicate many problems. If he has a fever, an infectious process will have to be ruled out as a cause for his mental status change.
(Objective 2)

8. a. Childhood trauma, parental deprivation, or a dysfunctional family structure
   b. War, riots, rape, assault, death of a loved one, economic and employment problems, or prejudice and discrimination
   (Objective 2)

9. a. Ensure scene safety.
   b. Contain the crisis.
   c. Render appropriate emergency care.
   d. Transport to the appropriate medical facility.
   (Objective 3)

10. Look for evidence of violence, substance abuse, a suicide attempt, and any weapons that may be accessible to the patient.
   (Objective 4)

11. The patient's mental status, name, age, significant medical history, medications, allergies, and the precipitating event for this crisis should be ascertained from the patient, family, or other bystanders.
   (Objective 4)

12. The need to perform a physical assessment should be guided by your initial patient interview. If no possibility to exacerbate a violent situation arises and no life threat exists, the survey can be deferred until you arrive at the hospital. Bulky clothing and bags should be examined for the presence of weapons by law enforcement before transport.
   (Objective 4)

13.

Illness	Classification	Clinical Presentation	Treatment (Medical or EMS)
Dementia	Cognitive disorder	General decline in mental functioning; inability for self-care	Medical interventions
Schizophrenia	Schizophrenia	Recurrent psychotic behavior; abnormal thought processes, delusions, hallucinations, poor judgment	Drug therapy; paramedic should be friendly but neutral do not respond to anger or speak to family in hushed tones; be firm, maintain personal safety.
Posttramatic syndrome	Anxiety disorder	Reaction to severe psychosocial event producing depression, sleep disturbances, nightmares, survivor guilt	Psychotherapy; medication
Bipolar disorder	Mood disorder	Alternating depressive and manic behaviors	Medications; paramedic should be calm and provide firm emotional support; minimize stimulation (no lights or sirens)
Somatization disorder	Somatoform disorder	Chronic physical complaints without any physical problems indentified; associated with anxiety, depression	Psychotherapy
Bulimia nervosa	Eating disorder	Binge eating followed by purging (vomiting or laxatives), depression, self-deprivation	Medication, psychotherapy, hospitalization

(Objective 5)

14. Talk through the steps (rehearse) of the rescue slowly and calmly with the patient.
   (Objective 5)

15. Provide calm, firm, emotional support, and minimize sensory stimuli.
   (Objective 6)

506

16. a. Schizophrenia or paranoia is suggested by this presentation.

b. Be friendly but neutral; modulate your voice so that it does not get louder if the patient does. Do not talk to the family in whispers. Use firmness and tact to guide the patient to the ambulance. Consider asking for police assistance if you suspect a risk of violence.

(Objective 5)

17. a. Ask, "Why did you do that? Were you trying to kill yourself?" Determine whether she had a plan (did she leave a note or call significant others to say good-bye?).

b. Ensure safety (protect the patient from escape or injury), listen in a nonjudgmental way, observe the dressing to ensure bleeding is controlled.

(Objectives 7 to 9)

18. a. Does the patient have a history of violent, aggressive, or hostile behavior?

b. What is the patient's posture? Is he sitting or standing? Does he appear tense or rigid?

c. What does his voice sound like? Is his speech loud, obscene, or erratic?

d. Is he pacing or agitated or displaying aggressive behaviors?

(Objective 10)

19. Ask for police assistance.

(Objective 14)

20. Look for any objects that the patient could use as a weapon.

(Objective 14)

21. A minimum of two rescuers should move swiftly toward the patient and position themselves close to and slightly behind the patient. Each rescuer then should position an inside leg in front of the patient's leg to force the patient into a prone position if needed. The least restrictive restraints needed for a given situation should be used.

(Objective 13)

22. Monitor the patient's level of consciousness, airway, breathing, circulation, vital signs, oxygen saturation (if available), and peripheral pulses while the patient remains in restraints.

(Objective 13)

23. a. Delusional behavior, neurosis, or psychosis may be present during a behavioral emergency.

(Objective 1)

24. c. Many persons break laws without demonstrating abnormal behavior. One person (the paramedic) does not establish norms for society. A person may deviate from usual, normal behavior and not meet the standard for abnormal behavior.

(Objective 1)

25. c. All of the other questions elicit a yes or no answer and yield limited information.

(Objective 5)

26. d. You may acknowledge and label a patient's feelings, but do not patronize or give false reassurances. Correct cognitive misconceptions or distortions in a nonconfrontational manner.

(Objective 4)

27. a. Common signs and symptoms include inattention, memory impairment, disorientation, clouding of consciousness, and vivid visual hallucinations.

(Objective 5)

28. a. In conversion hysteria, painful emotions are converted unconsciously into physical symptoms.

(Objective 5)

29. a. The depressed patient has low self-worth, a loss of appetite, and decreased libido and is tense and irritable.

(Objective 5)

507

30. a. Neurosis is a faulty or inefficient way of coping. Paranoia is an abnormal way of thinking, characterized by delusions of persecution or grandeur usually centered on a theme. A phobia occurs when a person transfers feelings of anxiety onto a situation or object in the form of an irrational, intense fear. (Objective 5)

31. c (Objective 5)

32. a. A small percentage of suicidal patients also will be homicidal. All of the other options are important, but crew safety is your primary responsibility. (Objective 9)

33. b. Women attempt suicide more often, but men succeed at a higher rate. All talk or threats of suicide should be taken seriously. When depression lifts, the person finally may have the energy to follow through on a suicide plan. (Objective 7)

34. d. Releasing a patient from restraints en route can place the crew in great danger. (Objective 13)

35. c. Etomidate is a short-acting agent used for procedural sedation. Diphenhydramine is used to treat allergic reactions. Fentanyl is a narcotic analgesic. (Objective 11)

36. d. Be sure you can exit quickly if the situation deteriorates. Do not threaten the patient. Do not allow the patient to be alone or to be alone with an emergency medical services crew member on the scene. Remain a safe distance from the patient until your assessment reveals no danger. (Objective 14)

37. c. Usually the parents can be helpful in the interview and help to relieve anxiety in children (if the situation worsens when they are present, immediately remove them). Children can become violent and injure themselves or others. Do not lie to children. (Objective 15)

WRAP IT UP

1. His voice was getting louder, his posture became more threatening, and he started to use profane language. (Objective 10)

2. c. The disease occurs as often in women as in men. Schizophrenia is a chronic, lifelong disease that is associated with about a 10% risk of suicide. (Objective 6)

3. It is important to determine suicide risk by asking patients direct questions about their intent, method, and timing of when they intend to commit suicide. This often is not associated with an escalation of the patient's violent behavior. (Objectives 5, 7, and 8)

4. Haloperidol is an antipsychotic drug that can help control violent, aggressive behavior. (Objective 11)

PART EIGHT

Chapter 36   Pathophysiology and Management of Shock

Pathophysiology and Management of Shock

READING ASSIGNMENT

Chapter 36, pages 1051-1074, in *Mosby's Paramedic Textbook*, ed. 4.

OBJECTIVES

Upon completion of this chapter, the paramedic student will be able to do the following:

1. Define *shock*.
2. Outline the factors necessary to achieve adequate tissue oxygenation.
3. Describe how the diameter of resistance vessels influences preload.
4. Calculate mean arterial blood pressure when given a blood pressure.
5. Outline the changes in the microcirculation during the progression of shock.
6. List the causes of hypovolemic, cardiogenic, neurogenic, anaphylactic, and septic shock.
7. Describe pathophysiology as a basis for signs and symptoms associated with the progression through the stages of shock.
8. Describe key assessment findings to distinguish the etiology of the shock state.
9. Outline the prehospital management of the patient in shock based on knowledge of the pathophysiology associated with each type of shock.
10. Discuss how to integrate the assessment and management of a patient in shock.
11. Describe principles of fluid administration in shock.

SUMMARY

- Shock is inadequate tissue perfusion. It is not a single event but rather the culmination of a complex group of physiological abnormalities.
- Perfusion is the adequate oxygenation of tissue cells. The heart, lungs, and blood vessels (and blood volume) must all be working effectively to achieve normal perfusion.
- The blood vessels form the body's container. This container must be able to shrink and grow and must be filled with an adequate volume to achieve normal tissue perfusion.
- Uncorrected shock progresses through a series of stages. These are vasoconstriction, capillary and venous opening, disseminated intravascular coagulation, and multiple organ failure.
- Shock can be categorized using many methods. Hypovolemic shock occurs when excess blood or body fluid is lost.
- Cardiogenic shock results from pump failure related to a heart muscle, valve, or rhythm problem.
- Neurogenic shock occurs when there is vasomotor paralysis high on the spinal cord.
- Anaphylactic shock is a type of severe allergic reaction that causes impaired vasomotor tone, fluid volume loss, airway obstruction, and bronchospasm.
- Septic shock occurs as a result of a systemic infection. Chemical toxins released from the infectious agent cause a cascade of events that impair cardiac output.
- The three stages of shock are compensated, uncompensated, and irreversible shock.
- Treatment of a patient in shock aims to ensure a patent airway, provide adequate oxygenation, and restore perfusion. The means to achieve each of those objectives varies according to the type of shock and condition of the patient.
- Fluid resuscitation in shock varies according to the cause. If the patient has uncorrected internal hemorrhage, isotonic crystalloid solution should be infused to maintain a systolic blood pressure of 90 mm Hg.
- Treatment of cardiogenic shock is aimed at normalizing heart rate and improving pumping action of the heart.
- During neurogenic shock, fluids should be administered cautiously with frequent monitoring of lung sounds.
- Anaphylactic shock is treated with epinephrine, diphenhydramine, and fluid bolus.
- Treatment for patients with septic shock includes fluid resuscitation and possibly administration of vasopressors.

Match the type of shock in column II with the description in column I. Use each answer only once.

Column I

1. _B_ Decreased stroke volume related to decreased contractility

2. _G_ Increased vascular resistance caused by endotoxins

3. _E_ Related to loss of sympathetic stimulation

4. _A_ Systemic response to antigenic exposure

5. _D_ Decreased preload related to reduced total volume

6. _F_ Restricted blood flow prevents blood return to the heart

Column II

a. Anaphylactic
b. Cardiogenic
c. Distributive
d. Hypovolemic
e. Neurogenic
f. Obstructive
g. Septic

7. A 20-year-old butcher sustained a stab wound to the femoral artery. There is a large amount of blood loss from an inguinal wound that is spurting bright red blood. The patient is anxious and confused. Vital signs are as follows: blood pressure, 86/70 mm Hg; pulse, 136 beats/min; respirations, 28 breaths/min; and lungs, clear. The patient's lips and nail beds are pale and cyanotic, and capillary refill is greater than 2 seconds. List the three physiologic components necessary for normal cellular oxygenation.

a. _effective pump_

b. _oxygenation via lungs_

c. _intact vasculature_

8. Complete the following sentences: The pressure that blood exerts against the vessel walls is known as **(a)** _hydrostatic_ pressure. Pressure that results from contraction of the ventricles is **(b)** _systolic_ pressure, and the residual pressure between contractions is **(c)** _diastolic_ pressure. The pulse felt in an artery resulting from the difference in **(b)** and **(c)** pressure is known as **(d)** _pulse_ pressure. Pressure in the vessels is greatest at the **(e)** _____ and least at the **(f)** _____. Mean arterial pressure is the **(g)** _average_ pressure in the vascular system that perfuses the tissues. To calculate mean arterial pressure, add the **(h)** _sys_ pressure to one-third of the **(i)** _pulse_ pressure.

9. Calculate the pulse pressure and mean arterial pressure for each blood pressure in the table.

Blood Pressure (mm Hg)	Pulse Pressure	Mean Arterial Pressure
70/50		
90/54		
120/80		
150/96		
210/140		

10. State the effect that each of the following patient situations has on the size of the patient's vascular container and on preload.

   a. A patient with a cervical spine injury from a motor vehicle collision has the following vital signs: blood pressure, 80/60 mm Hg; pulse, 60 beats/min; and respirations, 28 breaths/min. His skin is cool and pale above the level of the injury and warm and dry below it.

   b. A 55-year-old woman with heavy vaginal bleeding has been dizzy. Vital signs are as follows: blood pressure, 106/92 mm Hg; pulse, 116 beats/min; and respirations, 20 breaths/min.

11. For each of the following intravenous fluids, indicate whether the solution is isotonic, hypotonic, or hypertonic. Indicate whether there will be immediate net movement of fluid into or out of the intravascular space if this fluid is given or whether no movement is observed.

Intravenous Fluid	Isotonic, Hypotonic, or Hypertonic	Fluid Movement
$D_{50}W$		
Lactated Ringer solution		
Normal saline		
0.45% normal saline		
D_5W		

12. A 65-year-old patient complains of severe abdominal pain that radiates to the back. A large pulsatile mass is evident in the abdomen. Vital signs are as follows: blood pressure, 80/70 mm Hg; pulse, 128 beats/min; and respirations, 28 breaths/min. Predict the pathophysiologic changes and associated signs and symptoms that will occur during the stages of shock for this patient.

   a. Stage 1: Vasoconstriction

   b. Stage 2: Capillary and venule opening

   c. Stage 3: Disseminated intravascular coagulation

   d. Stage 4: Multiple organ failure

13. For each of the following situations, list the type of shock and briefly describe interventions necessary for patient management.

    a. A 72-year-old man's wife states that he had chest pain all day yesterday and earlier today. He has no pain when you arrive, but he is confused, pale, and diaphoretic. No bleeding is evident. Lung sounds reveal crackles in the bases. Vital signs are as follows: blood pressure, 86/76 mm Hg; pulse, 128 beats/min and irregular; and respirations, 28 breaths/min.

    Classification: ____

    Interventions: ____

    ____

    ____

    b. A 17-year-old teenager was unrestrained in a motor vehicle collision. He has no sensation below the nipple line and is confused. He has a large laceration on the parietal area and complains of neck pain. No other injuries are evident. His skin is pale and cool above the nipple line and warm and dry below. Vital signs are as follows: blood pressure, 84 mm Hg by palpation; pulse, 56 beats/min; and respirations, 28 breaths/min and very shallow.

    Classification: ____

    Interventions: ____

    ____

    ____

    c. A 26-year-old woman who says her last menstrual period was 8 weeks ago complains of severe right lower quadrant abdominal pain. She is pale, cool, and diaphoretic. Vital signs are as follows: blood pressure, 106/78 mm Hg; pulse, 120 beats/min; and respirations, 20 breaths/min while supine; blood pressure, 88/76 mm Hg; pulse, 136 beats/min; and respirations, 28 breaths/min while standing.

    Classification: ____

    Interventions: ____

    ____

    ____

    d. A 42-year-old woman experiences acute shortness of breath, urticaria, nausea, and dizziness after ingesting a penicillin tablet prescribed by her dentist. Vital signs are as follows: blood pressure, 80 mm Hg by palpation; pulse, 140 beats/min; and respirations, 40 breaths/min and labored.

    Classification: ____

    Interventions: ____

    ____

    ____

    e. A 72-year-old resident of a nursing home has a fever and is restless and agitated. The urine in the indwelling catheter collection bag is milky and green. Vital signs are as follows: blood pressure, 94/60 mm Hg; pulse, 132 beats/min; and respirations, 30 breaths/min.

    Classification: ____

    Interventions: ____

    ____

    ____

f. A 55-year-old office worker complained of a pounding sensation in his chest and fell from his chair, striking his head on the desk. You note a 5-cm laceration on the frontal area that is freely oozing dark red blood (about 20 mL on the floor). The patient is unconscious, and vital signs are as follows: blood pressure, 60 mm Hg by palpation; pulse, 180 beats/min; and respirations, 28 breaths/min.

Classification: ____

Interventions: ____

____

____

14. For each of the following situations, identify whether the patient is in compensated or uncompensated shock and explain why.

a. A 48-year-old man has sustained second- and third-degree burns to 70% of his body. He is pale, cool, and diaphoretic. His nail beds are cyanotic, and his vital signs are as follows: blood pressure, 84/76 mm Hg; pulse, 136 beats/min; and respirations, 32 breaths/min.

____

____

b. A 22-year-old passenger in a high-speed motor vehicle crash was restrained with a lap belt. She complains of severe abdominal pain. Her skin is cool and pale. Vital signs are as follows: blood pressure, 110/86 mm Hg; pulse, 128 beats/min; and respirations, 28 breaths/min.

____

____

15. Describe the characteristics of irreversible shock.

____

16. List three conditions, situations, or characteristics that decrease a patient's ability to compensate in shock.

____

17. For each of the following scenarios, select the appropriate intervention(s) from the following list. Briefly justify your answer.

Pneumatic antishock garment   Drug therapy (specify)   Other: (specify)
Rapid fluid replacement   Blood transfusions

a. A 72-year-old man had a myocardial infarction with pulmonary edema and vital signs as follows: blood pressure, 86/60 mm Hg; pulse, 124 beats/min; and respirations, 28 breaths/min.

____

____

b. A 2-year-old child was struck by an automobile, and you suspect that he has numerous pelvic and abdominal injuries. Vital signs are as follows: blood pressure, unobtainable; pulse, 170 beats/min carotid and weak; and respirations, 40 breaths/min and shallow.

____

____

     Chapter **36** **Pathophysiology and Management of Shock**

c. A 44-year-old man had sudden onset of dizziness followed by syncope and vital signs as follows: blood pressure, 86/68 mm Hg; pulse, 44 beats/min; and respirations, 20 breaths/min.

d. An 18-year-old teenager stung by a bee at a park has generalized redness and hives and is acutely short of breath. Vital signs are as follows: blood pressure, 70 mm Hg by palpation; pulse, 132 beats/min; and respirations, 36 breaths/min.

e. A 53-year-old woman with heavy vaginal bleeding for 1 week became lethargic and confused. Vital signs are as follows: blood pressure, 66 mm Hg by palpation; pulse, 136 beats/min; and respirations, 32 breaths/min.

f. A 19-year-old teenager sustained a gunshot wound to the chest. Vital signs are as follows: blood pressure, 106/88 mm Hg; pulse, 128 beats/min; and respirations, 24 breaths/min. The estimated time of arrival to the hospital is 40 minutes.

STUDENT SELF-ASSESSMENT

18. Your patient is passing bright red blood through the rectum. What is this called?
  a. Coffee-ground emesis   **c.** Hematochezia
  b. Epistaxis   **d.** Melena

19. Which of the following is the best definition of shock?
  a. Systolic blood pressure less than 90 mm Hg
  b. Greater than 25% loss of circulating blood
  c. Inadequate perfusion of the capillaries
  d. Blood flow deficit to the myocardium

20. Which of the following is true so tissue can be oxygenated normally?
  a. Glucose must be available for cellular oxygenation.
  b. Precapillary and postcapillary sphincters must be open for adequate flow.
  c. Red blood cells must be able to load and unload oxygen.
  d. The pH should be at least 6.5 for adequate perfusion to occur.

21. Which of the following blood characteristics is the greatest determinant of afterload (peripheral vascular resistance)?
  a. Vessel diameter   **c.** Viscosity
  b. Vessel length   **d.** Volume

22. A decrease in peripheral vascular resistance causes the container size of the body to __increase__ and the blood pressure to ________________________.
  a. decrease, decrease   **c.** increase, increase
  b. decrease, increase   **d.** increase, decrease

516

23. Which blood vessels act as collecting channels and storage (capacitance) vessels?
   a. Arterioles
   b. Arteries
   c. Capillaries
   d. Venules and veins

24. A patient who was shot in the chest and abdomen is pale and has no palpable radial pulse. Vital signs are blood pressure, 78 by palpation, pulse 72, R 20. His home medicines include nadolol (Corgard), atorvastatin (Lipitor), and chlorothiazide (Diuril). What medicine explains his inadequate ability to compensate for shock normally?
   a. ACE inhibitors reduce blood pressure.
   b. Beta-blockers slow heart rate.
   c. Calcium channel blockers decreased contractility.
   d. Statin drugs lower red blood cell production.

25. In what phase of shock does the microcirculation develop the leaky capillary syndrome?
   a. Capillary and venule opening
   b. Disseminated intravascular coagulation
   c. Multiple organ failure
   d. Vasoconstriction

26. What happens to fluid in stage 2 of the progression of shock?
   a. It is pulled into the intravascular space because of vasoconstriction.
   b. It leaks out of the intravascular space because of vasoconstriction.
   c. It is pulled into the intravascular space because of increased hydrostatic pressure.
   d. It leaks out of the intravascular space because of decreased hydrostatic pressure.

27. What occurs when there is dilation of the precapillary sphincter while the postcapillary sphincter remains constricted during lactic acidosis?
   a. No net movement of fluid between the fluid compartments
   b. Loss of vascular fluid into the interstitial spaces
   c. Movement of fluid from the interstitial spaces to the intravascular spaces
   d. Fluid shunting around the capillaries through the arterioles

28. What is shock caused by heart (pump) failure known as?
   a. Anaphylactic shock
   b. Cardiogenic shock
   c. Hypovolemic shock
   d. Neurogenic shock

29. Which of the following shock states causes compensatory systemic vasoconstriction?
   a. Anaphylactic
   b. Cardiogenic
   c. Neurogenic
   d. Septic

30. Your patient was stabbed in the abdomen 20 minutes ago. Vital signs are as follows: blood pressure, 80/50 mm Hg; pulse, 136 beats/min; and respirations, 26 breaths/min. He is anxious and pale. He is probably in which stage of shock?
   a. Compensated
   b. Irreversible
   c. Transitional
   d. Uncompensated

31. Increases in peripheral vascular resistance can be measured indirectly by noting which of the following?
   a. Diastolic blood pressure
   b. Jugular distention
   c. Pulse rate
   d. Systolic blood pressure

32. For which of the following conditions is the pneumatic antishock garment considered helpful?
   a. Cardiogenic shock
   b. Pelvic fractures
   c. Penetrating chest injuries
   d. Pulmonary edema

33. Which of the following fluids is a colloid solution?
   a. Dextran
   b. 0.45% sodium chloride
   c. Lactated Ringer solution
   d. Normal saline

Chapter **36** **Pathophysiology and Management of Shock**

34. Which of the following blood products has the greatest oxygen-carrying capacity per volume?
    a. Fibrinogen   **c.** Plasma
    b. Packed red blood cells   **d.** Whole blood

35. You arrive at the emergency department with a patient who has been vomiting bright red blood and is exhibiting signs and symptoms of shock. Which fluid is most beneficial to him at this time?
    a. Blood plasma   **c.** Packed red blood cells
    b. Dextran   **d.** Plasmanate

36. Your patient fell 30 feet from scaffolding and is anxious, confused, and in obvious shock. Which of the following is your priority of care, in the proper order?
    a. Rapid transport, oxygen, intravenous therapy
    b. Oxygen, intravenous therapy, rapid transport
    c. Intravenous therapy, rapid transport, oxygen
    d. Oxygen, rapid transport, intravenous therapy

37. What explains why the blood pressure of a patient with a spinal cord injury with neurogenic shock drops?
    a. Decreased venous return
    b. Blood volume is lower
    c. Tachycardia lowers preload
    d. Contractility decreases

38. How would you manage the patient in hypovolemic shock from a gastrointestinal bleed on the scene?
    a. Hang a dopamine drip.
    b. Apply direct pressure.
    c. Infuse 0.45% normal saline.
    d. Administer oxygen.

39. When should fluid therapy in cardiogenic shock be slowed to the keep-open rate ?
    a. If lung crackles (rales) increase
    b. If jugular vein distention decreases
    c. If heart rate decreases
    d. If peripheral edema increases

40. Which treatment for severe anaphylactic shock bronchodilates and vasoconstricts?
    a. Albuterol   **c.** Epinephrine
    b. Diphenhydramine   **d.** Methylprednisolone

41. You suspect that your patient has a ruptured ectopic pregnancy. She is in profound shock. Which intravenous catheter will allow the fastest infusion of fluids?
    a. 14 gauge, 1½ inch   **c.** 18 gauge, 1½ inch
    b. 14 gauge, 3 inch   **d.** 18 gauge, 3 inch

42. A 200-mL fluid challenge is to be infused over 20 minutes. The drop factor is 10 drops/mL. How fast will you run it?
    a. 1 drop/min   **c.** 100 drops/min
    b. 33 drops/min   **d.** 400 drops/min

43. Which of the following is a goal for prehospital care of the patient with severe internal hemorrhage and shock?
    a. Determine the patient's blood type.
    b. Begin hypothermia treatment.
    c. Establish vascular access on the scene.
    d. Rapid transport to the appropriate hospital.

You are dispatched to a construction site for a fall. A 35-year-old worker fell about 30 feet onto a pile of dirt and rock. She is conscious but confused and is bleeding from a large head laceration. You immediately apply direct pressure to the laceration with a 5 × 9 inch dressing as you hold inline immobilization of her head and continue your assessment. Her airway is patent, breathing is rapid, skin is pale and cool, and heart rate is rapid. The bleeding from her head laceration is controlled by direct pressure, so your partner wraps it with a gauze roller bandage as you continue your assessments. Her trachea is midline, neck veins are flat, and breath sounds are clear and equal bilaterally. There is a large reddened area on her lateral chest that extends down across her upper abdomen. There is tenderness to palpation over the left lateral ribs and diffuse tenderness over her abdomen. Both lower legs are swollen, tender, and deformed, with weak pedal pulses noted. She is rolled onto the backboard with spinal precautions and support of her legs and is moved to the ambulance. Vital signs are BP 84/66 mm Hg, P 136, R 28, and SaO_2 not obtainable. Oxygen is delivered by non-rebreather mask at 15 L/min, transport is initiated, and the trauma center is notified that you are en route with an unstable patient who has fallen. En route to the hospital, an IV of normal saline is initiated in the left antecubital space and administered wide open; ECG monitoring is performed, and serial blood pressures obtained by an automatic BP cuff show a slight improvement in mean arterial pressure, although her heart rate does not come down. Her head bandage is reinforced when blood soaks through the first one. The trauma team is awaiting you in the resuscitation room. Immediately, cross-table cervical spine, and chest radiographs are performed. Uncrossmatched blood is transfused, and as the patient's condition rapidly deteriorates, she is rushed to the surgical suite, where her severely injured spleen is removed.

1. Were this patient's signs and symptoms of shock a result of external or internal hemorrhage? Explain your answer.

   ____

2. Which of the following factors needed for adequate tissue perfusion was impaired in this patient?
   a. Adequate oxygen must be available in the lungs.
   b. Oxygen must be able to move freely across the alveolar walls.
   c. Normal hemoglobin levels must exist to carry oxygen.
   d. Tissue cells must close to capillaries so oxygen can offload.

3. Circle the appropriate answer. The pale color of the patient's skin reflected a narrowing/widening of the blood vessels, which would cause a(n) decrease/increase in cardiac preload.

4. Which blood component most urgently needs replacement in this patient?
   a. Erythrocytes
   b. Fibrinogen
   c. Leukocytes
   d. Plasma

5. Your initial assessment of this patient reveals that she is in what stage of shock?
   a. Compensated
   b. Irreversible
   c. Multiple organ dysfunction syndrome
   d. Uncompensated

6. What sites (injuries) were possible causes for her shock?

   ____

7. Pick the compensatory responses in shock that would be responsible for the following signs or symptoms present in this patient.
   a. Sympathetic response   b. Hormonal response   c. Adrenal response

   Sign or Symptom   **Compensatory Mechanism**
   Narrowed pulse pressure: ____

   Pale, cool skin: ____

   Tachycardia: ____

          Chapter **36** **Pathophysiology and Management of Shock**

8. Which of the following represents definitive care for this patient?
   a. Isotonic fluid administration
   b. High-concentration oxygen delivery
   c. Surgical intervention
   d. Uncrossmatched blood transfusion

CHAPTER 36 ANSWERS

REVIEW QUESTIONS

1. b
   (Objective 6)

2. g
   (Objective 6)

3. e
   (Objective 6)

4. a
   (Objective 6)

5. d
   (Objective 6)

6. f
   (Objective 6)

7. a. An adequate amount of oxygen is available to red blood cells. There is a sufficient FIO_2, his airway is patent, and his lungs are clear.
   b. Red blood cells must be circulated to all tissue cells. Based on the history of significant blood loss and the physical findings that indicate decreased cerebral perfusion (anxiety and confusion) and peripheral perfusion (pale, cyanotic lips and nail beds), it is evident that red blood cell transport is inadequate.
   c. Red blood cells must be able to offload oxygen adequately. This seems to be occurring in this situation, although acid–base abnormalities can impair this ability, and insufficient information is available to determine this accurately.
   (Objective 2)

8. a. systemic; b. systolic; c. diastolic; d. pulse; e. heart (or aorta); f. vena cava g. average; h. diastolic; i. pulse
   (Objective 8)

9.

Blood Pressure (mm Hg)	Pulse Pressure (Systolic Blood Pressure – Diastolic Blood Pressure) (mm Hg)	Mean Arterial Pressure Diastolic Blood Pressure + 1/3 Pulse Blood Pressure (mm Hg)
70/50	20	50 + 7 = 57
90/54	44	54 + 15 = 69
120/80	40	80 + 13 = 93
150/96	54	96 + 18 = 114
210/140	70	70 + 47 = 117

(Objective 4)

10. a. Spinal cord injury results in a loss of sympathetic tone and therefore impairs the ability of the blood vessels to constrict below the level of the injury. This increases the container size, decreasing the effective circulating volume and preload.

b. When blood loss occurs, a situation potentially exists in which the container is the same size but the volume has decreased, reducing the preload. Body compensatory mechanisms attempt to decrease the size of the container by vasoconstriction in an effort to match the container to the volume.

(Objective 3)

11.

Intravenous Fluid	Isotonic, Hypotonic, or Hypertonic	Fluid Movement
$D_{50}W$	Hypertonic	Into intravascular space
Lactated Ringer solution	Isotonic	No net movement
Normal saline	Isotonic	No net movement
0.45% normal saline	Hypotonic	Out of intravascular space
D_5W	Isotonic initially but rapidly hypotonic because of glucose metabolism	Out of intravascular space

(Objective 11)

12. a. Oxygen to cells in vasoconstricted areas decreases. Anaerobic metabolism occurs. Leaky capillary syndrome evolves. Pale, sweaty skin; a rapid, thready pulse; elevation in blood glucose; and dilation of coronary, cerebral, and skeletal muscle arterioles occur.

b. Precapillary sphincters open. Blood pools, and vascular space is expanded greatly, resulting in an increased container size. Decreased preload and congestion of the viscera occur. Increased anaerobic metabolism results in increased respiratory rate. Rouleaux formation inhibits perfusion in visceral capillaries and impedes flow. Hypercoagulability develops.

c. Blood coagulates in microcirculation, clogging capillaries and causing congestion, and fibrinolytic mechanisms then are overstimulated, causing pulmonary edema and hemorrhage. Cell membrane function is lost, and anaerobic metabolism increases. Water and sodium leak into cells, and potassium leaks out. Cells swell and die. Oxygen absorption and carbon dioxide elimination are impaired in the lungs, and acute respiratory distress syndrome may result.

d. After 1 to 2 hours, a dramatic decrease in blood pressure occurs. Cellular metabolism stops. Organ failure occurs and may include liver, kidney, and heart failure; gastrointestinal bleeding; pancreatitis; and pulmonary thrombosis.

(Objective 5)

13. a. Cardiogenic shock: Administer high-flow oxygen, continue assessment, initiate intravenous normal saline to keep the vein open, consider a fluid challenge of 100 to 200 mL of lactated Ringer solution or normal saline, monitor lung sounds and patient response carefully, and consider vasopressor drug therapy.

b. Neurogenic shock: Apply cervical spine immobilization, assess the need to assist ventilations, administer high-flow oxygen, initiate intravenous lactated Ringer solution or normal saline (avoiding excessive amounts), monitor lung sounds frequently, apply and inflate pneumatic antishock garments if local protocol advises, continue assessment, and consider vasopressor drug therapy.

c. Hypovolemic shock: Administer high-flow oxygen, place the patient in modified the Trendelenburg position, transport rapidly, initiate two large-bore (14- or 16-gauge) intravenous lines with lactated Ringer solution or normal saline and infuse rapidly.

d. Anaphylactic shock: Ensure a patent airway, administer high-flow oxygen (administer subcutaneous epinephrine), initiate intravenous lactated Ringer solution or normal saline with a 14- or 16-gauge catheter, and consider administration of diphenhydramine (Benadryl).

e. Septic shock: Administer high-flow oxygen, determine whether the patient has preexisting obstructive pulmonary disease, initiate intravenous therapy with a 14- or 16-gauge catheter, and obtain an accurate patient history.

f. Cardiogenic shock: Assess for a patent airway, administer high-flow oxygen, initiate a 16- or 18-gauge intravenous line with normal saline to keep the vein open, institute electrocardiographic monitoring, initiate maneuvers to decrease heart rate based on the electrocardiographic tracing and patient symptoms (drugs, cardioversion), and apply dressing to the head wound.
(Objectives 6, 8 and 9)

14. a. Uncompensated shock: The compensatory mechanisms can no longer sustain a normal systolic blood pressure. The pulse pressure is narrowed. Blood oxygenation is decreased as evidenced by cyanosis.
  b. Compensated shock: Systolic blood pressure is adequate, but other signs of shock are evident (cool, pale skin and increased pulse and respiratory rate).
(Objective 7)

15. Irreversible shock may occur suddenly or 1 to 3 weeks after the event. Clinical signs include bradycardia; pale, cold, clammy skin; and cardiac arrest.
(Objective 7)

16. Preexisting disease, medication, older or young age
(Objective 7)

17. a. Drug therapy: Neither pneumatic antishock garments nor rapid fluid infusion is considered because this patient is already in heart failure. Therapy should be directed at improving the function of the heart with drugs such as dopamine.
  b. Pediatric pneumatic antishock garments (if indicated by local medical direction), rapid fluid replacement, and blood transfusion. The patient has a mechanism of injury for significant blood loss and is exhibiting signs of uncompensated shock. Pneumatic antishock garments may decrease the container size and maximize blood flow to the vital organs. Rapid fluid infusion may restore circulating volume. Blood transfusion may be necessary on arrival to the emergency department to enhance oxygen-carrying capability and restore the vascular volume. Advanced airway with positive-pressure ventilation. Rapid transport is essential.
  c. Drug therapy: The heart rate is slow and is likely the reason why this person is exhibiting signs of shock. None of the other interventions increases heart rate. Medication will depend on ECG rhythm and may include atropine, dopamine, or an epinephrine drip. Transcutaneous pacing may also be indicated.
  d. Drug therapy and rapid fluid replacement: The primary cause of the shock state in this patient is probably histamine release. Drug therapy is the only intervention that can arrest and reverse these symptoms. Rapid fluid replacement also may help restore circulating volume until drug therapy is effective. Drugs may include epinephrine, diphenhydramine, and methylprednisolone.
  e. But rapid fluid replacement should only be infused if the blood pressure drops below 90 mm Hg. At the emergency department, the blood transfusion helps restore oxygen-carrying capacity and circulating volume.
  f. Rapid fluid replacement is not indicated; however, at least two IVs should be established. At this time, the patient is maintaining a normal blood pressure. The pulse and respiratory rate are elevated somewhat, so assessment should be frequent. Rapid fluid replacement may be necessary if the patient's blood pressure drops below 90 mm Hg. The wound should be sealed on three sides with an occlusive dressing.
(Objective 10)

18. c. Coffee-ground emesis indicates gastrointestinal bleeding. Epistaxis is bleeding from the nose. Melena is dark, black, tarry stools.
(Objective 8)

19. c. A systolic blood pressure less than 90 mm Hg may be normal in certain individuals. Loss of blood volume may lead to shock but does not define it. Shock leads to decreased myocardial blood flow.
(Objective 1)

20. c. The Fick principle states that adequate oxygen must be available to red blood cells (RBCs0 through the alveolar cells of the lungs. So hemoglobin can be oxygenated, RBCs0 must be circulated to the tissue cells, and RBCs0 must be able to load oxygen at the lungs and unload oxygen at the peripheral cells.
(Objective 2)

21. a. Vessel length and viscosity are relatively constant. Blood volume may influence pressure but not resistance.
(Objective 2)

522

22. d. As peripheral vascular resistance decreases, vessel capacitance increases, and the container size increases. This makes the existing blood volume insufficient to maintain an adequate preload.
(Objective 3)

23. d
(Objective 3)

24. b. Beta-blockers such as nadolol (Corgard) slow the heart rate and prevent compensation. Atorvastatin (Lipitor) is a statin drug to lower cholesterol, and chlorothiazide (Diuril) is a thiazide diuretic.
(Objective 10)

25. d. Leaky capillary syndrome develops after lactate and hydrogen ions build up in the capillaries and their linings lose their ability to retain large molecular structures within their walls.
(Objective 5)

26. b. This fluid loss is caused by the increased hydrostatic pressure created in this situation.
(Objective 5)

27. b. The precapillary sphincter opens, and the postcapillary sphincter remains closed, increasing the pressure inside the capillary and forcing fluid out through the already compromised capillary walls.
(Objective 5)

28. b. Anaphylactic shock is caused by the release of chemicals after an antigen–antibody reaction. Hypovolemic shock results from a loss of body fluid (water, plasma, blood). Neurogenic shock is a loss of vasomotor tone.
(Objective 7)

29. b. Loss of vasomotor tone is a contributing factor to shock in each of the other types of shock.
(Objective 7)

30. d. The compensatory mechanisms of vasoconstriction, increased heart rate, and increased contractility are no longer sufficient to maintain adequate blood pressure.
(Objective 7)

31. a. As peripheral vascular resistance increases, diastolic blood pressure also increases.
(Objective 8)

32. b. Use of pneumatic antishock garments generally is not recommended for any of the other situations.
(Objective 9)

33. a. All of the others are crystalloid solutions.
(Objective 11)

34. b. Whole blood and packed red blood cells have red blood cells and therefore the greatest ability to carry oxygen. Packed cells do not contain plasma and therefore have a greater concentration of red blood cells per unit volume. Only a small amount of oxygen is carried dissolved in plasma.
(Objective 11)

35. c. This is the only fluid that contains red blood cells.
(Objective 11)

36. d. Priorities of care always follow the ABCs; therefore, oxygen should be first, and intravenous therapy should be initiated en route unless a transportation delay exists; in this case, definitive care may be expedited.
(Objective 10)

37. a. Sympathetic stimulation is blocked below the level of injury. This causes vasodilation that reduces preload and prevents tachycardia to compensate.
(Objective 6)

38. d. Vasoactive drugs are not indicated for use in a patient with hypovolemic shock until adequate fluid volume has been replaced at the hospital. 0.45% normal saline is a hypotonic fluid and will diffuse into the interstitial space quickly, so it is not indicated to treat a patient with hypovolemic shock. (Objective 10)

39. a. Increased lung congestion indicates that the failing heart cannot deal with the existing fluid volume. Jugular venous distension should increase with fluid overload. Peripheral edema has a slow onset and is not an acute sign evident in the prehospital phase of care. A moderate decrease in heart rate indicates patient improvement. (Objective 11)

40. c. Epinephrine is the only treatment that rapidly improves all of the life-threatening effects of anaphylaxis. Other adjunct therapy may be used after epinephrine has been given. (Objective 9)

41. a. The shortest catheter with the widest diameter should be selected. (Objective 11)

42. c. Drops/minute $= \dfrac{200 \times 10}{20} = 100$

(Objective 11)

43. d. IVs should be established en route to the hospital. (Objective 11)

WRAP IT UP

1. This patient had internal bleeding and external bleeding. The internal bleeding was most likely responsible for her shock. (Objective 1)

2. c. Most of the oxygen in the body is carried on hemoglobin. This patient's blood loss has caused a decrease in hemoglobin. (Objective 2)

3. The blood vessels narrow in an attempt to increase the preload. (Objective 4)

4. a. The red blood cells contain hemoglobin, which carries oxygen and is critical for normal tissue oxygenation. (Objective 5)

5. d. Because the blood pressure has decreased, the patient is no longer compensating adequately for the shock. (Objective 6)

6. Bleeding from head, concealed intraabdominal bleeding, or long bone fractures of lower legs (Objective 7)

7. Narrow pulse pressure: a, b, c
Pale, cool, skin: a, b, c
Tachycardia: a, b, c
(Objective 8)

8. c. If the patient had uncontrolled bleeding from the spleen, the only definitive intervention is surgical. Prehospital care includes oxygenation, monitoring, fluid replacement, and transport to the closest appropriate hospital (trauma center preferred). (Objective 10)

<table><tr><td>**37**</td><td># Trauma Overview and Mechanism of Injury</td></tr></table>

READING ASSIGNMENT

Chapter 37, pages 1075-1099, in *Mosby's Paramedic Textbook,* ed. 4.

OBJECTIVES

Upon completion of this chapter, the paramedic student will be able to do the following:

1. Describe the incidence and scope of traumatic injuries and deaths.
2. Identify the role of each component of the trauma system.
3. Predict injury patterns based on knowledge of the laws of physics related to forces involved in trauma.
4. Describe injury patterns that should be suspected when injury occurs related to a specific type of blunt trauma.
5. Describe the role of restraints in injury prevention and injury patterns.
6. Discuss how organ motion can contribute to injury in each body region depending on the forces applied.
7. Identify selected injury patterns associated with motorcycle and all-terrain vehicle collisions.
8. Describe injury patterns associated with pedestrian collisions.
9. Identify injury patterns associated with sports injuries, blast injuries, and vertical falls.
10. Describe factors that influence tissue damage related to penetrating injury.

SUMMARY

- Trauma is the leading cause of death among persons 1 to 44 years of age and is the fifth leading cause of death among all Americans.
- Trauma care is divided into three phases: preincident, incident, and postincident.
- Components of the trauma system include injury prevention, prehospital care, emergency department care, interfacility transportation (if needed), definitive care, trauma critical care, rehabilitation, data collection, and trauma registry.
- Transport decisions for trauma patients should be made based on structured triage guidelines.
- Injuries are caused by a transfer of energy from some external source to the human body. The extent of injury is determined by the type of energy applied, how quickly it is applied, and the part of the body to which the energy is applied.
- Four laws of physics describe energy and forces that produce injury. They are Newton's first law of motion, the conservation of energy law, Newton's second law of motion, and the formula for kinetic energy.
- Kinematics is the process of predicting injuries based on mechanism of injury, forces involved, anatomy, and energy.
- Blunt trauma is an injury produced by the wounding forces of compression and change of speed, which can disrupt tissues.
- Four restraining systems are available in the United States. These are lap belts, diagonal shoulder straps, child safety seats, and air bags. All of these significantly reduce injuries. However, if they are used inappropriately, these protective devices also can produce injuries.
- Organ injuries can result from sudden movement caused by deceleration and compression forces. The recognition of these injuries requires a high degree of suspicion. Paramedics must use the principles of kinematics.
- Small motorized vehicles such as motorcycles, all-terrain vehicles, snowmobiles, motorboats, water bikes, and farm machinery are considered to be more dangerous than other motor vehicles. They are more dangerous because they offer little protection to the rider. They offer minimal protection from the transfer of energy associated with collisions.
- All auto–pedestrian collisions can produce serious injuries. They require a high degree of suspicion for multiple-system trauma.
- Sports provide a variety of health benefits. However, they also can produce severe injury. Sports injuries are related to acceleration/deceleration, compression, twisting, hyperextension, and hyperflexion mechanisms of injury.
- Blast injury is damage to a patient exposed to a pressure field that is produced by an explosion of volatile substances. Blasts release large amounts of energy in the form of pressure and heat. Blast injuries are classified as primary, secondary, tertiary, and miscellaneous.

527

- Falls from greater than three times the height of a person (15–20 feet) are associated with an increased incidence of severe injuries. In predicting injuries associated with falls, the paramedic should evaluate three things: the distance fallen, the body position of the patient on impact, and the type of landing surface struck.
- All penetrating objects, regardless of velocity, cause tissue disruption. The character of the penetrating object, its speed of penetration, and the type of body tissue it passes through or into determine whether crushing or stretching forces will cause injury.

REVIEW QUESTIONS

Match the appropriate energy law listed in column II with its description in column I.

Column I

1. __b__ Force is equal to mass times acceleration or deceleration.

2. __e__ Equal to 1/2 mass × Velocity^2

3. __a__ An object at rest or in motion remains in that state unless force is applied.

4. __c__ Energy can neither be created nor destroyed; it can only change form.

Column II

a. Newton's first law of motion
b. Newton's second law of motion
c. Conservation of energy law
d. Joule's law
e. Kinetic energy law

5. Identify three causes of death for each of the periods of the trimodal distribution of traumatic death; for each period, identify prehospital interventions that may increase patient survival.

   a. Immediate:

   ____

   b. Early:

   ____

   c. Late:

   ____

6. A 17-year-old girl falls asleep at the wheel, rides the median for 50 feet, and then strikes a concrete bridge abutment head on.

   a. Identify the three collisions that occur in this situation.

   ____

   ____

   ____

   b. Assuming that this driver took the down-and-under pathway during the collision, what injuries should you anticipate?

   ____

7. Aside from speed and size, what factor affects the injury pattern found in a lateral impact collision?

   ____

8. In which of the following rear-end collisions will damage be greater, assuming that mass and other factors are equal? Why?

   a. A vehicle traveling 50 mph is struck by a vehicle traveling 70 mph.

   b. A vehicle traveling 5 mph is struck by a vehicle traveling 40 mph.

   ____

   ____

9. For each of the body regions, list the injury or injuries that may occur during sudden, rapid deceleration.

   a. Head and neck injuries:

   ____

   b. Thoracic injuries:

   ____

   c. Abdominal injuries:

   ____

10. You are called to the scene of a high-speed frontal crash caused by a crossover accident. The driver of one of the vehicles complains of severe dyspnea and has a large circular bruise on her chest. You note greatly decreased lung sounds on the right side of the chest and suspect a pneumothorax.

   a. What traumatic mechanism can cause a pneumothorax in this example?

   ____

   b. The driver of the other vehicle has severe abdominal pain and is exhibiting signs of hypovolemic shock. Which abdominal organs or structures can be injured from sudden compression of the abdomen?

   ____

11. Identify the type of motorcycle collision most frequently associated with the pattern of injuries listed.

   a. A seasoned biker has a severely angulated fracture of the right forearm and extensive abrasions to the right side of the body.

   ____

   b. A 47-year-old executive has bilateral fractured femurs and facial injuries.

   ____

   c. A traffic officer has a severe crush injury to the left lower leg.

   ____

12. Identify the injuries to be anticipated in the following situations:

a. A motorist swerves across the highway and is struck by an oncoming vehicle.

____

b. As a young child hurries to avoid being late to school, he is struck by a full-size automobile.

____

____

____

13. When evaluating a sports injury, what principles of kinematics must be considered to determine probable areas of injury?

____

14. A suitcase filled with plastic explosives detonates in a locker at a busy urban airport. Describe the type of injuries the paramedic should anticipate in each of the following categories:

a. Primary blast injuries:

____

b. Secondary blast injuries:

____

c. Tertiary blast injuries:

____

d. Miscellaneous blast injuries:

____

15. You are called to a home to care for a person who has fallen.

a. List three things you must determine to predict injuries associated with this fall.

____

b. What age of patient is most likely to fall?

____

c. If the person who fell is an adult, how is she likely to land?

____

16. Briefly describe the way each of the following ballistic properties influences injury patterns in penetrating trauma.

    a. Character of the penetrating object:

____

    b. Speed of penetration:

____

    c. Distance from patient that a bullet is fired:

____

STUDENT SELF-ASSESSMENT

17. Why is prevention of traumatic injury such a high priority?
    a. Mortality is greater for all ages than heart disease.
    b. It is the top killer of people 1 to 44 years of age.
    c. It involves significant property damage as well.
    d. It is difficult to treat after it occurs.

18. What actions can a paramedic take to intervene at the incident phase of trauma?
    a. Educate the community.
    b. Decrease scene time.
    c. Promote safety legislation.
    d. Wear personal restraint systems.

19. Which of the following is a component of a trauma system?
    a. Emergency medical services education
    b. Fire suppression
    c. Pain management
    d. Rehabilitation

20. What factor influences trauma triage guidelines?
    a. Mechanism of injury
    b. Type of climate
    c. Patient gender
    d. Patient's pain score

21. What is the process of predicting injury patterns that may result from specific force and motion of energy known as?
    a. Force of energy applied
    b. Index of suspicion
    c. Kinematics
    d. Mechanism of injury

22. Injury resulting from blunt trauma most often is caused by which of the following forces?
    a. Compression
    b. Deceleration
    c. Distraction
    d. Torsion

23. Your patient was restrained when her car was struck on the right side on her door at a high rate of speed. What injuries do you predict?
    a. Aortic injury
    b. Liver injury
    c. Pancreatic injury
    d. Splenic injury

24. Which injuries are more likely if the lap belt is applied improperly?
    a. Duodenal injuries
    b. Maxillofacial injuries
    c. Pelvic fractures
    d. Sternal fractures

25. Which of the following is true regarding ejection from a vehicle?
    a. It will not happen if the person is restrained.
    b. It usually happens before impact.
    c. Spinal injuries are common.
    d. There is little risk of death.

531

26. Steering wheel and dash air bags are designed to reduce injuries in which of the following collisions?
   a. Frontal collisions
   b. Lateral collisions
   c. Rollover collisions
   d. Rear-end collisions

27. Which of the following are predictable injuries from all-terrain vehicle crashes?
   a. Abdominal injuries
   b. Kidney injuries
   c. Thoracic injuries
   d. Upper extremity injuries

28. Which of the following is more likely to occur when a child is struck by a car compared with an adult?
   a. The child may strike the hood of the vehicle.
   b. The child may be dragged under the vehicle.
   c. The child may land on the ground.
   d. The child may strike the bumper of the vehicle.

29. A roofer falls from the top of a two-story residence. What type of injuries do you anticipate?
   a. Minor injuries to the feet and spine
   b. Severe injuries to the feet and spine
   c. Minor injuries to the head and neck
   d. Major injuries to the head and neck

30. A 2-year-old child falls from a second-story window. What area of the body is most likely to be injured?
   a. Head and neck
   b. Arm
   c. Leg
   d. Pelvis

31. Which of the following is a high-energy weapon with the potential to cause the greatest injury to tissues?
   a. M-16
   b. .357 magnum
   c. 12-gauge shotgun
   d. Knife

32. Which organ is likely to experience the most severe injury from tissue crushing caused by cavitation after a gunshot wound?
   a. Bowel
   b. Liver
   c. Lung
   d. Muscle

WRAP IT UP

You are dispatched to the interstate highway for a chain reaction collision involving multiple vehicles on a foggy September morning. You and your supervisor arrive on the scene simultaneously, and she sends you to begin triage. As you move from vehicle to vehicle, you note the following. The first two cars appear to have struck each other head on—there is major damage. In vehicle #1, there are two front seat passengers, both restrained with air bags that now are deflated. They are conscious, but the passenger has abdominal and low back pain and lifts his shirt to show you the abrasion over his abdomen. In vehicle #2, the passengers were not restrained. The driver was thrown up and over the steering wheel and into the now starred windshield. He is dyspneic, pale, and anxious. His passenger was ejected and lies motionless at the side of the road; there is no breathing even after you open his airway, so you move on. Vehicle #3, a small sedan, struck vehicle #2 on the right rear fender in a glancing blow and then swerved into the ditch and rolled several times. The front seat passenger, who is belted with her lap and shoulder belt, and her child, appropriately secured in a child seat in the middle rear seat, are crying, are alert, and have normal skin color. As vehicle #3 swerved, it struck a sport utility vehicle (vehicle #4) that spun and came to rest sideways in the highway. The SUV was then struck laterally on the driver door by a delivery truck (vehicle #5). There were no side air bags, and the restrained SUV driver has chest pain and severe arm and hip pain. The truck driver was restrained and is ambulatory with no complaints. A motorcyclist (vehicle #6), seeing an imminent collision with vehicle #5, laid his bike down and slid on his side 30 feet before striking the rear dual wheels of the truck. The protective coating on his helmet has been worn away on the lateral side, as has his jacket, and he is conscious, alert, and complaining of severe pain from his deep skin abrasions. A police officer, struck by a car as he set up traffic cones, is unconscious on the ground. You report to command the number of patients and triage categories so that appropriate transport decisions can be made; the closest level I or II trauma center is 75 miles away.

1. Which phase of trauma care will you be involved with on this scene?
   a. Preincident
   b. Incident
   c. Postincident
   d. Preventive

2. Place a check mark beside the components of a sophisticated trauma system that could (or did) benefit any of the patients on this call.
   a. _________ Injury prevention
   b. _________ Prehospital care
   c. _________ Emergency department care
   d. _________ Interfacility transportation if needed
   e. _________ Definitive care
   f. _________ Trauma critical care
   g. _________ Rehabilitation
   h. _________ Data collection and trauma registry

3. List injuries that you would anticipate based on the mechanism of injury for each of the following patients.

   Patient   **Injuries Predicted**

   a. Passenger vehicle #1:

   ____

   b. Driver vehicle #2:

   ____

   c. Passenger car #2:

   ____

   d. Passenger vehicle #3:

   ____

   e. Driver vehicle #4 (SUV):

   ____

   f. Rider vehicle #6 (motorcycle):

   ____

   g. Police officer:

   ____

CHAPTER 37 ANSWERS

REVIEW QUESTIONS

1. b
(Objective 3)

2. e
(Objective 3)

3. a
(Objective 3)

4. c
(Objective 3)

5. a. Lacerations of the brain, brainstem, upper spinal cord, heart, aorta, and other large vessels; injury prevention
programs
b. Subdural or epidural hematoma, hemopneumothorax, ruptured spleen, lacerated liver, pelvic fracture, and
numerous injuries associated with significant blood loss; decreasing time from injury to definitive care, which
must be brief
c. Sepsis, infection, and multiple organ failure; early recognition and treatment of life-threatening injury in the
field with adequate fluid resuscitation and aseptic technique
(Objective 1)

6. a. The vehicle strikes the abutment, the passenger strikes the inside of the vehicle, and the internal organs pull
forward rapidly and strike the bony structures inside the body.
b. Dislocated knees, patellar fractures, fractured femurs, posterior fracture or dislocation of the acetabulum,
vascular injury, and hemorrhage
(Objective 1)

7. Whether the car struck remains stationary (injuries likely on the side of the impact) or moves away from the point
of impact (injuries likely on the side opposite the impact)
(Objective 4)

8. b. The velocity that produces damage is determined by calculating the difference between the speed of the two
vehicles. In example a it is $70 - 50 = 20$, and in example b, it is $40 - 5 = 35$.
(Objective 3)

9. a. Intracerebral hemorrhage and cervical fracture; b. ruptured aorta; c. kidney, liver, and spleen lacerations
(Objective 4)

10. a. Pneumothorax could be caused by displaced rib fractures that puncture a lung or by a paper bag injury, in which
impact occurs after the patient has inhaled against a closed glottis.
b. Lacerated spleen, liver, or kidney; rupture of the bladder, diaphragm, gallbladder, duodenum, colon, stomach,
and small bowel
(Objective 4)

11. a. Laying down the bike; b. head-on (up and over the handle bars); c. angular
(Objective 7)

12. a. Fractures of the lower legs, femur, pelvis, thorax, and spine; injuries to the intraabdominal or intrathoracic
contents; and head and spinal injuries
b. Fractures of the femur and pelvis; abdominopelvic and thoracic trauma; and head and neck injuries
(Objective 8)

13. Energy forces involved, body part to which energy is transferred, speed of acceleration and deceleration, forces involved (compression, twisting, hyperextension, hyperflexion), protective gear
(Objective 9)

14. a. Hearing loss, pulmonary hemorrhage, cerebral air embolism, thermal injuries, abdominal hemorrhage, and bowel perforation
    b. Lacerations, contusions, fractures, and impaled objects
    c. Fractures and abdominopelvic, thoracic, head, and spine injuries
    d. Radiation exposure and dust inhalation
    (Objective 9)

15. a. The paramedic should evaluate the distance fallen, the body position of the patient on impact, and the type of landing surface.
    b. Children and the elderly are more likely to fall.
    c. An adult is more likely to land on her feet.
    (Objective 9)

16. a. Length and width of knives determine the depth and extent of the injury. With bullets, missile damage increases if the bullet is designed to rotate, flatten, or fragment during or after impact.
    b. Kinetic injury increases with increased speed, and tissue damage increases with increased energy applied.
    c. As the range increases, the damage decreases because of decreased velocity. Close-range injuries produce more damage because of the direct injury of gases from combustion and the explosion of powder.
    (Objective 10)

17. b. Trauma is the fifth leading cause of death overall.
    (Objective 1)

18. d. Community education and legislation are preincident interventions, and decreasing scene time is a postinjury intervention.
    (Objective 1)

19. d. The other components are injury prevention, prehospital care, emergency department care, interfacility transportation, definitive care, trauma critical care, data collection, and trauma registry.
    (Objective 2)

20. a. Other factors include patient condition, injury severity indices, and available patient care resources.
    (Objective 2)

21. c. Kinematics is based on mechanism of injury and force of energy applied. Index of suspicion for certain types of injuries is related to kinematics, the age of the patient, and preexisting illness.
    (Objective 3)

22. a. Direct compression or pressure on a structure is the most common type of force applied in blunt trauma.
    (Objective 4)

23. b. Because she was struck on the right side, injury to the liver is more likely than injury to the spleen.
    (Objective 4)

24. a. All of the other injuries can occur in high-speed crashes in which the lap belt is applied properly.
    (Objective 5)

25. c. A small number of restrained persons are ejected. Risk of death is six times greater than the risk for those who are not ejected. Ejection typically happens after impact.
    (Objective 5)

26. a. The air bag inflates and then rapidly deflates after the first frontal collision.
    (Objective 5)

27. d. Head and neck injuries also are common.
(Objective 7)

28. b. This may compound other injuries and cause traumatic amputation.
(Objective 8)

29. b. Falls from more than three times the height of the individual are likely to produce serious injury. Adults who
fall from a height greater than 15 feet usually land on their feet.
(Objective 9)

30. a. Children tend to fall head first because their heads are proportionately larger.
(Objective 9)

31. a.
(Objective 10)

32. b. Nonelastic organs do not stretch.
(Objective 10)

WRAP IT UP

1. b.
(Objective 1)

2. a. Injury prevention (seat belt education, passive restraint [air bags] systems; prehospital care (triage, treatment,
transport); emergency department care (examination, diagnostics, interventions); interfacility transport, if
needed (to higher-level trauma centers); definitive care (surgery for intraabdominal injuries); trauma critical
care (early postresuscitation care); rehabilitation (physical, head injury); data collection and trauma registry (to
monitor trauma quality, track demographics)
(Objective 2)

3. a. If the lap belt was improperly worn too high, injury to T12, L1, and L2 could occur. If compressed, injury to the
liver, spleen, duodenum, or pancreas could be present.
(Objectives 3, 4, and 5)

b. Rib fractures, ruptured diaphragm, hemopneumothorax, pulmonary contusion, cardiac contusion, myocardial
rupture, or aortic rupture are possible if the thorax absorbed impact. If the abdomen absorbed impact, tears to
the liver, spleen, or blood vessels are possible. Head and neck injuries are also common.
(Objectives 3 and 4)

c. Spinal fracture, death
(Objectives 3 and 4)

d. Rollover: difficult to categorize injuries; none may be present if proper restraints were used.
(Objectives 3 and 4)

e. Lateral impact: fractured ribs, pulmonary contusion, ruptured liver or spleen, fractured clavicle, fractured pelvis,
and head and neck injury
(Objectives 3 and 4)

f. Motorcyclist laying down the bike: abrasions, fractures to the affected side
(Objective 7)

g. Pedestrian struck: lower extremity fractures; femur, pelvis, spine fractures; head injuries, internal hemorrhage
(Objective 8)

 **Bleeding and Soft Tissue Trauma**

READING ASSIGNMENT

Chapter 38, pages 1100-1121, in *Mosby's Paramedic Textbook,* ed. 4.

OBJECTIVES

Upon completion of this chapter, the paramedic student will be able to do the following:

1. Describe the normal structure and function of the skin.
2. Describe the pathophysiologic responses to soft tissue injury.
3. Discuss pathophysiology as a basis for key signs and symptoms and describe the mechanism of injury and signs and symptoms of specific soft tissue injuries.
4. Outline management principles for prehospital care of soft tissue injuries.
5. Describe, in the correct sequence, patient management techniques for control of hemorrhage.
6. Identify the characteristics of general categories of dressings and bandages.
7. Describe prehospital management of specific soft tissue injuries not requiring closure.
8. Discuss factors that increase the potential for wound infection.
9. Describe the prehospital management of selected soft tissue injuries.

SUMMARY

- Hemorrhage can be internal or external.
- The skin and its accessory organs are the main cosmetic structures of the body. These structures perform many functions that are critical to survival. The skin is composed of two distinct layers of tissue, the outer layer (epidermis) and the inner layer (dermis).
- Surface trauma can disrupt the normal distribution of body fluids and electrolytes. Surface trauma also can interfere with the maintenance of body temperature. The two physiologic responses to surface trauma are vascular and inflammatory reactions. These can lead to healing, scar formation, or both. Many factors can affect or alter wound healing.
- Soft tissue injuries are classified as closed or open. Classification is determined by the absence or presence of a break in the continuity of the epidermis. Closed wounds include contusions, hematoma, and crush injury. Open wounds are classified as abrasions, lacerations, punctures, avulsions, amputations, and bites.
- Assessment of life-threatening injuries and resuscitation precedes evaluation and intervention of non–life-threatening soft tissue injuries. General wound assessment should include a history of the event that caused the wound and a careful examination of the injury.
- Methods of hemorrhage control include direct pressure, immobilization by splinting, pneumatic pressure devices, and the use of tourniquets.
- The general categories of dressings used in trauma care are sterile, nonsterile, occlusive, nonocclusive, adherent, and nonadherent. The general categories of bandages are absorbent, nonabsorbent, adherent, and nonadherent.
- Depending on the nature and location of the patient's injury, cleansing, dressings, bandages, and immobilization may be indicated to care for a wound properly.
- The goals of wound care are to prevent infection and protect from infection. Factors that influence the likelihood of infection include unclean wounds and wound mechanisms and a patient's poor state of health.
- Special considerations for specific wounds include penetrating chest or abdominal injury, avulsion, amputation, and crush syndrome.

Match the type of dressing listed in column II with its description in column I. Use each answer only once.

Column I

1. _________ Air does not pass through this dressing.

2. _________ Bacteria have been eliminated from this dressing.

3. _________ This dressing can be used when infection is not a concern.

4. _________ This dressing sticks to the wound surface.

5. _________ This dressing allows air to pass through to the wound.

6. _________ This dressing does not stick to the wound.

Column II

a. Adherent dressing
b. Nonadherent
c. Nonocclusive dressing
d. Nonsterile dressing
e. Occlusive dressing
f. Sterile dressing

7. List at least six structures or tissues located in the dermis.

a. ____

b. ____

c. ____

d. ____

e. ____

f. ____

8. Identify at least three functions of the integumentary system.

a. ____

b. ____

c. ____

9. List the three crucial steps in the clotting mechanism.

a. ____

b. ____

c. ____

10. Why are redness, swelling, warmth, and pain found at the site of an inflammatory response?

____

____

Chapter **38** **Bleeding and Soft Tissue Trauma**

11. List six types of drugs that can impair normal wound healing.

    a. ____

    b. ____

    c. ____

    d. ____

    e. ____

    f. ____

12. List six types of wounds that are likely to require closure.

    a. ____

    b. ____

    c. ____

    d. ____

    e. ____

    f. ____

13. For each of the following scenarios, list the soft tissue injury described and key prehospital interventions to manage the trauma.

    a. A 45-year-old woman is being transported for care after her husband repeatedly struck her head and face with his fist. You note numerous swollen, ecchymotic areas on her face and head.

       Injury: ____

       Interventions:

       ____

       ____

    b. Rescuers have just removed a victim who was trapped in a concrete structure for 2 days. The patient's lower torso had been pinned under a concrete piling. During the rescue phase, the patient was alert but somewhat confused. Vital signs were within normal limits. Shortly after extrication, the patient's physiologic status begins to deteriorate.

       Injury: ____

       Interventions:

       ____

       ____

539

c. A wallpaper hanger has sustained a deep linear wound after cutting himself with an Exacto knife. The wound is oozing dark red blood, and fatty tissue is visible at the edges of the injury.

Injury: ____

Interventions:

____

____

d. A motorcyclist wearing only her swimsuit had to lay down the bike to avoid a collision. The patient states that the bike slid about 100 feet along the asphalt road. She has huge scrape-type injuries on her entire left side. She denies pain or tenderness anywhere else.

Injury: ____

Interventions:

____

____

e. Neighbors direct you to a yard where a young child was attacked by a large dog. No one is sure of the dog's present location. The child is screaming, and his left arm has many puncture wounds and lacerations.

Injury: ____

Interventions:

____

____

f. A hunter was impaled with an arrow. The arrow has penetrated the right upper quadrant of the abdomen. She is pale and cool.

Injury: ____

Interventions:

____

____

g. A mechanic reports an injury to her right hand while working with a high-pressure grease gun. You note a small puncture wound with a drop of grease on it at the distal end of the left thumb.

Injury: ____

Interventions:

____

____

h. A butcher slices off the distal tip of his index finger.

Injury: ____

Interventions:

____

____

i. A factory employee catches his hair in some large machinery and avulses a large portion of the posterior aspect of his scalp.

Injury: ____

Interventions:

____

____

j. A weekend handyman severs his right index finger with a skill saw. He drives himself to a nearby firehouse but does not have the digit with him.

Injury: ____

Interventions:

____

____

Questions 14 and 15 pertain to the following case study:

Your patient was treated and released from the emergency department with a diagnosis of tibial fracture after a fall. He has a plaster splint that was applied there and is complaining of pain so severe, "I just can't take it anymore."

14. What further assessments should you perform on this patient's leg to look for compartment syndrome?

____

15. If he has compartment syndrome, what could a delay in treatment cause?

____

Questions 16 and 17 pertain to the following case study:

You are called to the scene of a construction site, where a 57-year-old workman has lacerated his left hand.

16. What questions should you ask to obtain the wound history on this patient?

____

____

541

17. Outline the physical examination of the wound and hand.

____

____

18. A 17-year-old sustained a partial amputation of his left lower arm after tangling it in a corn picker. There is extensive soft tissue damage and deformity of the extremity, which is squirting bright red blood. Your estimated time of arrival to the nearest hospital is 30 minutes. Describe in the proper sequence four measures you can use to control the bleeding in this patient and briefly describe the proper technique for using each skill.

a. ____

b. ____

c. ____

d. ____

For questions 19 to 23, circle (a) or (b) to indicate the wound that is at _greater risk_ for infection. Explain why you chose your answer in (c).

19. a. A farmer lacerates his hand on a combine.

b. A chef cuts his hand on a butcher knife.

c. ____

20. a. A 25-year-old athlete is stabbed.

b. A 79-year-old nursing home resident is stabbed.

c. ____

21. a. A patient cut his abdomen.

b. A patient's laceration is on his hand.

c. ____

22. a. Your patient reports to the emergency department for sutures 18 hours after the injury.

b. The patient drives to the emergency department 2 hours after injury.

c. ____

23. a. His finger was split open after he jammed it in a door.

b. He sliced his finger on a piece of metal on the door.

c. ____

24. What is the avascular layer of the skin?
    a. Dermis   **c.** Sebaceous
    b. Epidermis   **d.** Subcutaneous tissue

25. Which of the following occurs at the site of injury during the first phase of normal hemostasis?
    a. Thrombocytopenia   **c.** Fibrin break-down
    b. Increased blood flow   **d.** Decreased blood vessel diameter

26. Which medication can interfere with hemostasis?
    a. Acetaminophen   **c.** Decongestants
    b. Aspirin   **d.** Insulin

27. Which of the following medical conditions is associated with delayed healing?
    a. Alcoholism   **c.** Cardiac dysrhythmias
    b. Asthma   **d.** Stroke

28. Which of the following wound forces is least likely to be associated with a high risk for infection?
    a. Foreign bodies   **c.** Injection injuries
    b. Human and animal bites   **d.** Paring knife wounds

29. Which of the following is considered a closed injury?
    a. Avulsion   **c.** Hematoma
    b. Bite   **d.** Puncture

30. High-pressure injection injuries can be limb threatening. Why is the severity of this wound difficult to assess in the prehospital environment?
    a. The light is too poor to evaluate the wound adequately.
    b. The location of the wound is difficult to visualize.
    c. The equipment needed for assessment is not available.
    d. The wound is small with minimal external signs.

31. What is the appropriate prehospital care for avulsed body tissue?
    a. Place it directly on ice.
    b. Seal it in a plastic bag.
    c. Soak it in a cup of lactated Ringer solution.
    d. Débride it of all dirt.

32. Which type of soft tissue injury may result in abscesses, lymphangitis, cellulitis, osteomyelitis, tenosynovitis, tuberculosis, hepatitis B, and tetanus?
    a. Amputation   **c.** Bites
    b. Avulsion   **d.** Crush injury

33. Which of the following is an early finding in crush injury?
    a. Paralysis   **c.** Paresthesia
    b. Paresis   **d.** Pulselessness

34. Where is compartment syndrome most likely to be found?
    a. Abdomen   **c.** Head
    b. Upper arm   **d.** Thorax

35. What causes life-threatening symptoms in patients with crush syndrome after being released from entrapment?
    a. Circulatory overload when blood rushes back to the central circulation
    b. Hypokalemia, hypouricemia, hypercalcemia, and hypophosphatemia
    c. Myoglobin is released and filtered through the liver, causing liver failure.
    d. Toxic substances from anaerobic metabolism are released into the blood.

543

36. Blast pressure forces are likely to rupture which organ?
  a. Bladder   **c.** Lungs
  b. Heart   **d.** Pancreas

37. Which wound is least likely to require physician evaluation if tetanus immunization is up to date?
  a. A needle fragment imbedded in the wound
  b. Weakness in the finger distal to the laceration
  c. Laceration extending over the border of the lip
  d. A painful abrasion on the leg that is oozing slightly

38. Who is a candidate for tetanus toxoid?
  a. A 40-year-old man who has a large contusion on his head
  b. A pregnant woman with a laceration of the leg
  c. A 2-week-old infant whose finger was amputated
  d. A 70-year-old patient with diabetes who received third-degree burns

WRAP IT UP

You are dispatched to a ranger's cabin deep in a rugged national park for "traumatic injuries." A 20-year-old climber was injured when he fell about 12 feet, sliding down a steep rock face 1 day ago. While headed back to the cabin, he was bitten by a wild dog and then cut his forearm in a desperate attempt to enter the cabin when there was no response to his initial knocks at the door. He has numerous swollen, painful blunt injuries because of small collections of blood under the skin; several puncture wounds to the left forearm from the bite around which the skin is now tender, red, warm, and swollen; several areas on his hands, arms, and legs where the skin was scraped off and is oozing clear liquid; and a deep wound on the right forearm from the glass injury that is bleeding freely and in which fatty tissue is visible. You easily control the bleeding and complete your assessment, finding no additional injuries. His vital signs are BP 126/72 mm Hg, P 98, R 16, and SaO$_2$ 98%. You transport him to the local hospital, where he is treated and released 8 hours later.

1. Which of the skin layers were injured?

____

2. What signs and symptoms of inflammation are present from his wounds?

____

3. Place a check mark beside the soft tissue injuries present in this patient.

  a. ________ Closed wounds   **f.** ________ Laceration

  b. ________ Contusions   **g.** ________ Puncture

  c. ________ Crush injury   **h.** ________ Avulsion

  d. ________ Open wounds   **i.** ________ Amputation

  e. ________ Abrasion   **j.** ________ Bites

4. Describe appropriate steps in management of this patient's bleeding.

____

5. How will you treat his other wounds? ____

6. What risk factors are present in this patient for the development of infection?

____

Chapter **38** **Bleeding and Soft Tissue Trauma**

CHAPTER 38 ANSWERS

<u>**REVIEW QUESTIONS**</u>

1. e
(Objective 6)

2. f
(Objective 6)

3. d
(Objective 6)

4. a
(Objective 6)

5. c
(Objective 6)

6. b
(Objective 6)

7. Connective tissue, elastic fibers, blood vessels, lymphatic vessels, motor and sensory fibers, hair, nails, and glands
(Objective 1)

8. Protection and cushioning against injury, barrier against infection, temperature regulation, and preservation of body fluids
(Objective 1)

9. a. Release of platelet factors at injury site
b. Formation of thrombin
c. Trapping of red blood cells in fibrin to form a clot
(Objective 2)

10. The warmth and redness are caused by vasodilation and enhanced blood supply to the affected area. Swelling is caused by increased capillary permeability, which allows plasma, plasma proteins, and electrolytes to leak into extracellular space. Pain is caused by chemicals and increased pressure resulting from fluid buildup.
(Objective 2)

11. a. Corticosteroids; b. nonsteroidal antiinflammatory drugs; c. penicillin; d. colchicine; e. anticoagulants;
f. antineoplastic agents
(Objective 2)

12. a. Wounds to cosmetic regions; b. gaping wounds; c. wounds over tension areas; d. degloving injuries; e. ring finger injuries; f. skin tearing
(Objective 2)

13. a. Contusion or hematoma: Apply ice or cold packs and compression with manual pressure or compression bandage. Assess for underlying injury.
b. Crush syndrome: Provide airway and ventilation support; administer high-flow oxygen; maintain body temperature; rehydrate with expanding intravenous fluids (1–1.5 L initial bolus); and administer pharmacologic agents such as sodium bicarbonate (to help control hyperkalemia and acidosis), glucose and insulin (to decrease serum potassium), and mannitol (to promote diuresis).
c. Laceration: Control hemorrhage and monitor for signs of hypovolemic shock.
d. Abrasions: Clean gross contaminants from injured surface and lightly cover with a sterile dressing.

545

e. Dog bite: Ensure that the animal is contained, control bleeding, rinse off gross contaminants, splint the extremity, and obtain a medical history from the pet owner.

f. Penetrating or impaled object: Leave the object in place, do not manipulate the object unless it is necessary for patient extrication or transport, control bleeding with direct pressure around the impaling object, stabilize the object with bulky dressings, and immobilize the patient. Treat shock if present.

g. Puncture wound: Evaluate the wound, elevate the affected extremity, immobilize, and transport.

h. Avulsion: Control bleeding, retrieve the avulsed tissue, wrap tissue in gauze that is dry or moistened with lactated Ringer or saline solution (per local protocol), seal in a plastic bag, and place the sealed bag on crushed ice.

i. Degloving: Control bleeding, evaluate for hypovolemia, elevate the head of the stretcher after you rule out mechanism for cervical spine injury.

j. Amputation: Control bleeding, retrieve amputated tissue, and treat as for avulsion.

(Objectives 3 and 9)

14. Assess for pain, paresis, paresthesia, pallor, and pulselessness in the affected extremity. Determine whether there is swelling or tightness of the compartment, tenderness to palpation, weakness in the leg, or pain on passive stretch (early sign).
(Objective 3)

15. A delay in treatment of compartment syndrome can cause nerve death, muscle necrosis, and crush syndrome.
(Objective 3)

16. When did you cut yourself? Was it a dirty place where you got the cut? How did the injury happen? Does anything else hurt? How much blood did you lose? Rate your pain on a scale of 1 to 10 with 1 being no pain and 10 the worst pain you have ever had. Do you take any medicines? Do you have any major illnesses? When was your last tetanus shot?
(Objective 4)

17. Inspect the wound for bleeding, size, depth, presence of foreign bodies, amount of tissue lost, edema, and deformity. Inspect the surrounding area for damage to arteries, nerves, tendons, and muscle. Assess the sensory and motor function of his hand. Evaluate the perfusion of the wound and of the tissues of the hand distal to the wound. Assess capillary refill, distal pulse, tenderness, temperature, edema, and crepitus (if underlying bone injury is suspected).
(Objective 4)

18. a. Apply direct pressure to the wound with a gloved hand or handheld dressing (for 4–6 minutes) and then secure a pressure dressing firmly with an elastic bandage. Reinforce the dressing if bleeding continues.

b. Apply a tourniquet if direct pressure is unsuccessful in controlling bleeding quickly. Notify medical control and select a site 2 inches proximal to the wound over the brachial or femoral artery. Place a tourniquet over the artery and a pad over the artery to be compressed. Wind the tourniquet twice around the extremity and tie it in a half knot over the pad. Place a windlass on the half knot and secure it with a square knot. Tighten the windlass until the hemorrhage stops and secure it. Note the time of application and mark "TK" on the patient's forehead and notify the receiving hospital. Carefully monitor the time the tourniquet is on. A commercial tourniquet may also be used.

c. Immobilize by splinting if movement increases the bleeding and if the bleeding was controlled by pressure. (Immobilization is used as an adjunct to other control devices.) Select the appropriate splint for the body area and apply it to minimize blood flow.

d. Use pneumatic pressure devices. (Devices such as air splints or pneumatic antishock garments serve as adjuncts for pressure control after the bleeding is controlled by other methods.)

(Objective 5)

19. a. This wound is likely much more contaminated than one that occurred in a clean indoor setting.
(Objective 8)

20. b. The risk of infection increases in older patients and in those who have preexisting medical conditions.
(Objective 8)

21. b. Injuries of the hand, foot, lower extremity, scalp, and face have a higher than normal risk of infection.
(Objective 8)

22. a. The risk of infection is greater in wounds that are not cleaned and repaired for longer than 8 to 12 hours after the injury.
(Objective 8)

23. a. Injuries associated with a crushing mechanism are more susceptible to infection than those caused by fine cutting forces.
(Objective 8)

24. b. The dermis provides the vascular supply to the epidermis. The sebaceous glands are in the dermis. The subcutaneous tissue lies under the dermis.
(Objective 1)

25. d. Vasoconstriction occurs to reduce blood flow to the area. Platelets are not destroyed nor is fibrin broken down.
(Objective 2)

26. b. Aspirin decreases platelet activity.
(Objective 2)

27. a. Other conditions associated with impaired healing are advanced age, uremia, diabetes, hypoxia, peripheral vascular disease, malnutrition, advanced cancer, hepatic failure, and cardiovascular disease.
(Objective 2)

28. d. A knife wound would be considered high risk if it were contaminated with organic material or if the patient were immunocompromised or had poor circulation.
(Objective 2)

29. c. All of the others are open wounds.
(Objective 3)

30. d. The wound site may only have minimal bleeding, numbness, and blanching. Surgical intervention is often necessary.
(Objective 3)

31. b. All of the other interventions could cause further damage.
(Objective 9)

32. c. Bites may be a combination of puncture, laceration, avulsion, and crush injuries heavily laden with infectious organisms.
(Objective 3)

33. c. All of the others are late findings.
(Objective 3)

34. b. The most common sites are below the knee and above the elbow.
(Objective 3)

35. d. Blood pools in the injured extremity, causing hypovolemia. Elevated blood potassium, phosphate, and uric acid levels and low blood calcium levels occur. Myoglobin is filtered in the kidneys, resulting in acute renal failure.
(Objective 3)

36. c. Other air-filled structures that may be affected are the eardrum, sinuses, stomach, and intestines.
(Objective 3)

37. d. All of the other injuries have a high potential for impaired wound healing or infection if not treated by a
physician.
(Objective 7)

38. d. Tetanus toxoid should not be given to pregnant patients or children younger than 6 weeks of age. Tetanus is not
indicted for closed injuries such as contusions.
(Objective 7)

WRAP IT UP

1. Epidermis and dermis (puncture wounds may be deeper)
(Objective 1)

2. Pain, warmth, redness, swelling
(Objective 2)

3. Closed wounds, contusions, crush injury is possible (from dog bite), open wounds, abrasions, lacerations,
punctures (bites), bites
(Objective 3)

4. Direct pressure may be all that is necessary to control bleeding. If not, elevation of the extremity and
reinforcement of the bandage may be helpful. For severe and persistent bleeding, if direct pressure does not
immediately control bleeding a tourniquet may be applied for a brief period.
(Objective 5)

5. The wounds should be cleansed with clean running water until no debris is seen. If transport time will be
prolonged, wounds may be covered with nonadherent dressings to prevent further contamination. Antibiotic
ointment can be applied to superficial wounds.
(Objectives 7 and 9)

6. Wounds were sustained in a dirty environment; bite wounds are highly susceptible to infection; no wound care
was provided for a prolonged period of time.
(Objective 8)

 **Burns**

READING ASSIGNMENT

Chapter 39, pages 1122-1145, in *Mosby's Paramedic Textbook,* ed. 4.

OBJECTIVES

Upon completion of this chapter, the paramedic student will be able to do the following:

1. Describe the incidence, patterns, and sources of burn injury.
2. Describe the pathophysiology of local and systemic responses to burn injury.
3. Classify burn injury according to depth, extent, and severity based on established standards.
4. Discuss the pathophysiology of burn shock as a basis for key signs and symptoms.
5. Outline the physical examination of the burned patient.
6. Describe the prehospital management of the patient who has sustained a burn injury.
7. Discuss pathophysiology as a basis for key signs, symptoms, and management of the patient with an inhalation injury.
8. Outline the general assessment and management of the patient who has a chemical injury.
9. Describe specific complications and management techniques for selected chemical injuries.
10. Describe the physiologic effects of electrical injuries as they relate to each body system based on an understanding of key principles of electricity.
11. Outline assessment and management of the patient with electrical injury.
12. Describe the distinguishing features of radiation injury and considerations in the prehospital management of these patients.

SUMMARY

- Each year more than 2 million Americans seek medical attention for burns. Morbidity and mortality rates from burn injury follow significant patterns regarding gender, age, and socioeconomic status. A burn injury is caused by an interaction between thermal, chemical, electrical, or radiation energy and biological matter.
- Tissue damage from burns depends on the degree of the heat and on the duration of exposure to the thermal source. As local events occur at the injury site, other organ systems become involved in a general response to the stress caused by the burn.
- Burns are classified in terms of depth as superficial, partial thickness, and full thickness. The rule of nines provides a rough estimate of burn injury size (extent) and is most accurate for adults and for children older than age 10 years. The Lund and Browder chart is a more accurate method of determining the area of burn injury. Severity of burn injury and burn center referral guidelines are based on standards that take into account the depth, extent, and severity of the burn wound; the source of injury; patient age; presence of concurrent medical or surgical problems; and the body region that is burned.
- Shock after thermal injury results from edema and accumulation of vascular fluid. These tissue changes occur in the area of injury and can produce systemic hypovolemia if the burn area is large.
- Emergency care for a burn patient begins with the initial assessment. The goal is to recognize and treat life-threatening injuries.
- Goals for prehospital management of a severely burned patient include preventing further tissue injury, maintaining the airway, administering oxygen and ventilatory support, providing fluid resuscitation, providing rapid transport to an appropriate medical facility, using aseptic (clean) technique to minimize the patient's exposure to infectious agents, managing pain, and providing psychological and emotional support.
- Prehospital considerations in caring for patients with inhalation injuries include recognition of the dangers inherent in the fire environment, pathophysiology of inhalation injury, and early detection and treatment of impending airway or respiratory problems.
- The severity of chemical injury is related to three things: the chemical agent, the concentration and volume of the chemical, and the duration of contact. Treatment is directed at stopping the burning process by using copious irrigation.

- Three types of injury may occur as a result of contact with electrical current: direct contact burns, arc injuries, and flash burns. After the scene is safe, patient intervention may begin. Internal damage from electrical current may be much more significant than external wounds.
- Persons who are injured by radiation rarely require emergency care. Radioactive particles are classified into three types: alpha, beta, and gamma. The Federal Emergency Management Agency recommends that basic radiation protection for the rescuer and the patient include four factors: minimize time in the radiation field, maintain a safe distance from the source, place shielding between the rescuers and the source, and limit the amount of radioactive material in a specific area.

REVIEW QUESTIONS

Match the chemicals listed in column II with the appropriate description in column I.

Column I

1. _________ Chemical used to clean fabric and metal; can cause hypocalcemia and severe burns

2. _________ Noxious gas that, when in solution, can cause blindness if it contaminates the eye

3. _________ Chemical that causes burns after prolonged exposure and also may result in lead poisoning

4. _________ Chemical that produces heat if exposed to water and should be removed or covered with oil

5. _________ Exposure to this chemical may be painless and result in dysrhythmias and central nervous system depression

Column II

a. Alkali
b. Ammonia
c. Hydrofluoric acid
d. Petroleum
e. Phenol

6. Identify the four major sources of burn injury.

a. ____

b. ____

c. ____

d. ____

7. Label the three zones of burn injury on Fig. 39-1 and briefly describe the characteristics of the tissue in each.

a. ____

____

b. ____

____

c. ____

____

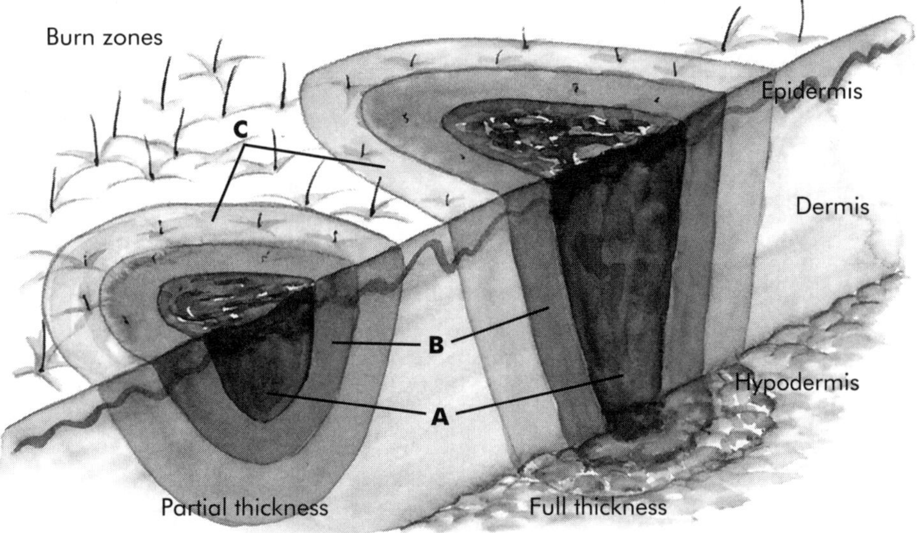

Figure 29-1

8. Explain two mechanisms that cause swelling in the burned tissue.

   a. ____

   b. ____

9. Describe the response in each of the following body systems to a major burn injury:

   a. Cardiovascular:

   ____

   b. Pulmonary:

   ____

   c. Gastrointestinal:

   ____

   d. Musculoskeletal:

   ____

   e. Neuroendocrine:

   ____

   f. Metabolic:

   ____

g. Immune:

____

h. Emotional:

____

10. For each of the following situations, classify the burn according to depth (first, second, or third degree), extent (body surface area), and severity (according to the American Burn Association). Identify patients who meet the American Burn Association criteria for referral to a burn center.

    a. A chef spilled hot grease down the anterior surface of his body. The wound is painful, moist, and red, with many blisters. The burns cover the anterior surface of his chest, abdomen, arms, and left leg.

    Depth: ____

    Extent: ____

    Severity: ____

    Referral: ____

    b. A young motorist opens his radiator cap and sprays hot steam and fluid over the upper half of his torso. The wounds are painful, moist, and red, with some blistering, and they blanch to the touch. The burns cover his face, anterior chest, and abdomen.

    Depth: ____

    Extent: ____

    Severity: ____

    Referral: ____

    c. An 80-year-old woman steps into a tub of extremely hot water. Because of her severe arthritis, she takes a long time to step out. She has circumferential burns around the right lower extremity up to the knee. The burn wound appears white and leathery and has no capillary refill.

    Depth: ____

    Extent: ____

    Severity: ____

    Referral: ____

11. Firefighters carry an approximately 40-year-old, 80-kg man from a residential fire. He is unconscious and has white, leathery burns. The burns cover the entire body surface except the posterior surface of both legs. He has shallow respirations at a rate of 24 breaths/min, and his blood pressure is 106/70 mm Hg. Patchy pieces of his smoldering clothing remain.

    a. Describe your initial assessment of this patient, including depth, extent, and severity of burns.

    ____

b. Describe the prehospital care, including airway and fluid resuscitation, with type of fluid and rate.

____

____

12. Describe the specific interventions to be used when the following third-degree burns are present:

    a. Burns to the face:

____

    b. Extremity burns:

____

    c. Circumferential burns:

____

Questions 13 to 16 pertain to the following case study:

A 13-year-old boy uses gasoline to start a bonfire and ignites his clothing. As he attempts to pull his flaming jacket over his head, it gets stuck while continuing to burn. On your arrival, he is alert after an initial brief loss of consciousness. He has extensive burns on his face, neck, and chest. The burns are white and dry with charred patches. They do not blanch when touched. His nasal hair is singed, and he is coughing up black, sooty sputum.

13. What aspects of the mechanism of injury and history of the event lead you to believe that this patient may have an inhalation injury?

____

14. What physical findings suggest inhalation injury?

____

15. At what point would you consider intubation?

____

16. Do you suspect an inhalation injury above or below the glottis? Explain your answer.

____

17. You are responding to a call for a person who has a chemical burn. En route to the industrial complex, you review the questions you will ask to determine the potential seriousness of the burn.

    a. Provide two examples of these questions.

____

____

b. The patient is covered with a powder known to cause chemical burns to the skin. Describe patient decontamination techniques.

____

____

18. Identify two examples of chemical products that can cause burn injury in each of the following categories:

a. Acids:

____

b. Alkalis:

____

c. Organic compounds:

____

19. The amount of tissue damage caused by an electrical current depends on six factors:
(a) _____________, _____________, _____________, _____________ _____________, and _____________. Amperage is the measure of current **(b)** _____________ per unit time. Voltage is a continuous **(c)** _____________ applied to any electrical circuit causing a flow of electricity. High-voltage electrical injuries result from contact with an electrical source of **(d)** _____________ or greater. Resistance to electricity depends on four factors: **(e)** _____________ _____________, _____________, _____________, and _____________. Resistance to electrical flow in the body is greatest in the **(f)** _____________ tissue. The two types of current commonly used are **(g)** _____________ and _____________. Direct current flows in **(h)** _____________ direction. It is used in **(i)** _____________. Alternating current periodically reverses **(j)** _____________ of flow. This reversal may cause muscle contractions that may **(k)** _____________ the patient to the source. In general, the current pathway in low-voltage current follows the path of **(l)** _____________ _____________, and high-voltage current follows the **(m)** _____________ path. As the duration of contact with the patient increases, tissue damage **(n)** _____________.

20. Name the three burn patterns that can result from electrical current.

a. ____

b. ____

c. ____

21. Briefly describe the potential effects of electrical injury on each of the following body regions.

a. Cutaneous:

____

b. Cardiovascular:

____

c. Neurologic:

____

d. Vascular:

____

e. Muscular:

____

f. Renal:

____

g. Pulmonary:

____

h. Orthopedic:

____

i. Ocular and otic:

____

22. A home owner was trimming trees when he came into contact with overhead electrical wires. When you arrive, he is still in contact with the electrical source.

    a. What must be done before treatment commences?

____

    The patient falls 10 feet from the tree to the ground. The scene is now safe. He is conscious and alert. You note multiple small, round, white burns on his right hand. When his clothing is removed, you discover significant burns and tissue injury to both feet.

    b. Describe your history and physical examination of this patient.

____

____

____

    c. Describe treatment, including fluid resuscitation (rate and type).

____

____

23. Describe the appearance of wounds characteristically associated with lightning burns.

____

24. For each of the following classes of lightning injury, list two physical signs:

a. Minor:

____

b. Moderate:

____

c. Severe:

____

25. Describe the characteristics of the following three types of radiation particles:

a. Alpha:

____

b. Beta:

____

c. Gamma:

____

26. Describe the physical effects that can be expected at the following levels of radiation exposure:

a. Less than 100 rem:

____

b. 100 to 200 rem:

____

c. Greater than 450 rem:

____

Questions 27 to 29 pertain to the following case study:

You arrive at a clinical laboratory, where a significant amount of radioactive material reportedly was released when a worker fell 1 foot from a platform.

27. Describe your approach to the emergency scene.

____

____

556

28. The victim must be accessed. Describe how the crew members designated to perform the rescue can minimize their radiation exposure.

____

____

____

29. Describe any special measures that you should use to care for this patient after you reach him or her.

____

____

STUDENT SELF-ASSESSMENT

30. Which is an example of a thermal mechanism of injury?
- **a.** Arcing
- **b.** Alkali agents
- **c.** Ionizing agents
- **d.** Scalding

31. What risk factor is associated with a high incidence of burn fatality?
- **a.** Female gender
- **b.** Child
- **c.** Industrial setting
- **d.** High-income family

32. What is the most common source of burn injury?
- **a.** Chemical
- **b.** Electrical
- **c.** Radiation
- **d.** Thermal

33. Which of the following is a systemic response to burn injury?
- **a.** Hypoventilation
- **b.** Hyperactive gastrointestinal tract
- **c.** Decreased metabolic rate
- **d.** Depressed inflammatory response

34. A burn characterized by a moist, red appearance with blisters is probably what degree?
- **a.** First
- **b.** Second
- **c.** Third
- **d.** Fourth

35. A 5-year-old patient with third-degree burns of the anterior and posterior surfaces of both legs would be estimated to have a(n) _______ burn.
- **a.** 18%
- **b.** 24%
- **c.** 28%
- **d.** 36%

36. Why does hypovolemia occur in burn injury?
- **a.** Blood loss
- **b.** Condensation of tissue fluid
- **c.** Increased capillary permeability
- **d.** Decrease in fluid intake

37. What should the paramedic do when calculating the extent of burn injury to ensure accurate fluid resuscitation?
- **a.** Calculate the burn size after arriving at the hospital.
- **b.** Estimate size before cooling the burn.
- **c.** Not include first-degree burns.
- **d.** Use the Lund and Browder chart.

38. How should the paramedic cool the burn of a smoldering patient burned on 50% of the body surface area?
   a. Apply ice intermittently in 15-minute cycles.
   b. Leave the patient exposed to air and apply a fan.
   c. Apply room-temperature water and then cover the patient with sheets and blankets.
   d. Continuously apply cool water while en route to the hospital.

39. Using the consensus burn formula, calculate the minimum fluid requirement during the first hour for a 100-kg patient who has 60% third-degree burns covering his body.
   a. 250 mL
   b. 500 mL
   c. 750 mL
   d. 6000 mL

40. Which of the following is a reason to suspect inhalation injury?
   a. Burns involving petroleum products
   b. Documented loss of consciousness
   c. End-tidal CO_2 is 43 mmHg
   d. Burns involving electric energy

41. Which statement is true regarding carbon monoxide poisoning?
   a. Oxygen saturation on the pulse oximeter is 80 or less.
   b. Skin color is cyanotic and often mottled.
   c. Respiratory rate is depressed in the early stages.
   d. Oxygen administration reduces the half-life of carbon monoxide.

42. What is the treatment of choice for most chemical injuries?
   a. Vigorous drying of the chemical
   b. Application of a chemical antidote
   c. Copious irrigation with water
   d. Neutralization with an acid or base

43. What determines the severity of a chemical injury?
   a. Chemical concentration
   b. Viscosity of the chemical
   c. Environmental temperature
   d. Time of injury

44. Calcium gluconate gel and solution are used to treat which of the following chemical injuries?
   a. Ammonia
   b. Hydrofluoric acid
   c. Petroleum
   d. Phenol

45. Electrical burns caused when the heat of the electrical current ignites the patient's clothing are what type of burns?
   a. Alternating
   b. Arc
   c. Direct
   d. Flame

46. Which tissue does electrical current flow through most easily?
   a. Bone
   b. Blood
   c. Muscle
   d. Nerve

47. What causes death most frequently in lightning injury?
   a. Cardiac or respiratory arrest
   b. Central nervous system injury
   c. Coagulation of the blood
   d. Severe burn shock

48. Which type of radiation requires a lead shield to stop penetration?
   a. Alpha
   b. Beta
   c. Gamma
   d. Nonionizing

You are dispatched to a refinery for an explosion. When you arrive, you are directed into a dock area where you find a 37-year-old worker who was touching a forklift when it contacted a high-voltage electrical line, breaking it. He was thrown into some packing material that ignited because of the arcing. It took several minutes for the power to be interrupted so the fire could be extinguished. When you arrive, he is conscious, alert, and complaining of severe pain in his right arm. You immobilize the cervical spine and continue your assessment as your partner applies high-concentration oxygen. You note a brown leathery wound on his left hand and a charred wound on his right foot. He has moist, painful, partially blistered burns on his abdomen and waxy, pale, tan-colored burns on his back from his shoulders to his buttocks. His vital signs are BP 170/100 mm Hg, P 124 irregular, and R 20, and SaO_2 on room air is 95%. You apply a clean sheet over the long spine board, secure him, cover his burns with clean sheets and warm blankets, and move him into the ambulance where you initiate an IV of LR. An ECG monitor is applied, and morphine is administered for his increasing pain. Medical direction advises you to transport him to the burn center. En route, you monitor vital signs and peripheral pulses, which are diminished in the right foot, and continue to administer pain medication. When the urinary catheter is inserted in the ED, you note that it is a dark red wine color. The patient is hospitalized for 3 months, has his right lower leg amputated, and requires numerous skin grafts.

1. What source(s) caused this patient's burns?
   a. Chemical
   b. Electrical
   c. Thermal
   d. Electrical and thermal

2. Why did this patient have no signs of burn shock? _____________________________________

____

3. What was the burn depth? _________________________ Extent? _________________________

   Severity? _________________________

4. Why was it necessary to monitor peripheral pulses? _____________________________________

____

5. Explain the following treatment decisions.

   a. Transport to a burn center ____

   b. Administration of oxygen despite normal SaO_2 _____________________________________

____

   c. Initiating the IV in the left arm

____

   d. Giving morphine intravenously instead of intramuscularly

____

6. What should you specifically assess to determine whether this patient has any indication of inhalation injury?

____

____

7. His electrical wounds were on the hand and on the foot. Explain why you did not find electrical burns in other places.

____

8. Place a check mark beside each of the signs or symptoms this patient had that indicate electrical injury.

a. _______ Hypertension   **f.** _______ Motor/sensory deficits

b. _______ Tachycardia   **g.** _______ Respiratory depression

c. _______ Dysrhythmias   **h.** _______ Peripheral circulation impaired

d. _______ Seizures   **i.** _______ Myoglobinuria

e. _______ Coma

CHAPTER 39 ANSWERS

REVIEW QUESTIONS

1. c
(Objective 8)

2. b
(Objective 8)

3. d
(Objective 8)

4. a
(Objective 8)

5. e
(Objective 8)

6. a. Thermal
b. Electrical
c. Chemical
d. Radiation
(Objective 1)

7. a. Zone of coagulation: nonviable tissue
b. Zone of stasis: seriously injured but potentially viable (cells will die if no supportive measures are taken within 24 hours)
c. Zone of hyperemia: increased blood flow caused by inflammatory response (cells will recover in 7 to 10 days if no shock or infection develops)
(Objective 2)

8. a. Chemical mediators cause increased capillary permeability and a fluid shift from the intravascular space to burned tissues.
b. The sodium pump in cell walls is damaged, and sodium moves into injured cells and increases swelling.
(Objective 2)

9. a. Decreased venous return, decreased cardiac output, increased vascular resistance (except in zone of hyperemia), hemolysis, and rhabdomyolysis that may lead to renal failure

   b. Increased respiratory rate to meet increased metabolic demands

   c. Adynamic ileus, vomiting, and stress ulcer

   d. Decreased range of motion resulting from edema and immobilization; osteoporosis and demineralization later

   e. Increased circulating levels of epinephrine, norepinephrine, and aldosterone

   f. Increased basal metabolic rate

   g. Increased susceptibility to infection and depressed inflammatory response

   h. Pain, isolation, and fear of disfigurement

(Objectives 2 and 4)

10.

Depth	Extent (%)	Severity	Referral
a. Second degree (partial thickness)	36	Major	Yes
b. Second degree (partial thickness)	22.5	Moderate	Yes
c. Third degree (full thickness)	9	Major	Yes (involves feet)

(Objective 3)

11. a. Simultaneously put out the fire and cool the burn with room-temperature, clean water if the skin or clothing is smoldering while performing an initial assessment; monitor vital signs; assess burn depth (third degree), extent (82%), and severity (major); perform a head-to-toe survey; assess lung sounds and distal pulse, movement, sensation, and capillary refill in all extremities.

   b. Cool the burn with clean water for 10 minutes or less; open the airway; intubate as necessary; ventilate with 100% oxygen; prepare to intubate; remove remaining clothing and jewelry; cover the patient to maintain warmth; initiate lactated Ringer solution intravenously at 820 mL/h (2 mL/kg per percent body surface area burned 24 hours [half of daily fluid to be given in first 8 hours]) up to 1640 mL/h (4 mL/kg per percent body surface area burned, over 24 hours) in an unburned extremity; and rapidly transport the patient.

(Objectives 5 and 6)

12. a. Realize that the burns may swell and be associated with airway problems. Raise the head of the stretcher 30 degrees if spinal injury is not suspected. If the ears are burned, do not use a pillow.

   b. Remove jewelry, assess neurovascular status frequently, and elevate the extremities.

   c. Monitor distal pulse, movement, sensation, and respirations and rapidly transport the patient to the nearest appropriate facility.

(Objective 6)

13. His jacket created an enclosed space, and he experienced a loss of consciousness.

(Objective 7)

14. Facial burns, singed nasal hair, and carbonaceous sputum suggest inhalation injury.

(Objective 7)

15. Increased dyspnea, decreased level of consciousness, hoarseness, and stridor indicate the need for intubation.

(Objective 7)

16. Above the glottis is the most likely area of injury. The mechanism of injury does not suggest injury below the glottis.

(Objective 7)

17. a. What type, concentration, and volume of chemical was involved? How did the injury occur? When did the injury occur? Was any first aid given? Does the patient feel any pain?

   b. With appropriate protective clothing, brush most of the powder off and then irrigate profusely (using a shower if available).

(Objective 7)

18. a. Rust removers, bathroom cleaners, and swimming pool acidifiers
   b. Drain cleaners, fertilizers, heavy industrial cleaners, and cement and concrete
   c. Phenols, creosote, and gasoline
   (Objective 8)

19. a. Amperage, voltage, resistance, type of current, current pathway, duration of current flow
   b. Flow (intensity)
   c. Force (tension)
   d. 1000 volts
   e. Resistivity, size of object pathway, length of object pathway, and temperature
   f. Bone
   g. Alternating, direct
   h. One
   i. Industry
   j. Direction
   k. Freeze
   l. Least resistance
   m. Shortest
   n. Increases
   (Objective 10)

20. a. Direct contact
   b. Arc
   c. Flash
   (Objective 10)

21. a. Direct contact can create large areas of coagulation necrosis. The entry wound is often a characteristic bull's eye (dry and leathery), and the exit is ulcerated and explosive.
   b. Dysrhythmias and damage to the myocardium may occur. Cardiac arrest is the most common cause of death after electrical injury. Hypertension caused by increased catecholamine levels is common.
   c. Central nervous system injury may result in coma, seizures, and peripheral nerve injury and may lead to sensory or motor deficits. Brainstem injury may cause respiratory depression or arrest or cerebral edema or hemorrhage, which can lead to death.
   d. Blood vessel necrosis may cause immediate or delayed hemorrhage or thrombosis.
   e. Muscle injury may result in release of myoglobin, which can cause renal failure.
   f. Acute renal failure occurs in 10% of significant electrical injuries.
   g. The patient may have decreased ventilation or respiratory arrest because of central nervous system injury or chest wall dysfunction.
   h. Fractures and dislocations can result from direct electrical injury or from injury caused by a fall or electrocution.
   i. Burns to conjunctiva or cornea and ruptured tympanic membrane are common.
   (Objective 10)

22. a. The electrical source must be removed safely from the patient, preferably by interruption of power by the electric company.
   b. Perform cervical spine immobilization and ABCDEs. Determine the patient's chief complaint, source of electricity, duration of exposure, level of consciousness before and after injury, and medical history. Perform a head-to-toe survey, looking for entry and exit burn wounds and trauma associated with the fall. Assess distal pulse, movement, sensation, and capillary refill in all extremities and document them. Monitor electrocardiographic rhythm.
   c. Immobilize the cervical spine, open the airway, apply 100% oxygen, assess the need to assist ventilations, remove all jewelry, initiate lactated Ringer solution intravenously at 20 to 40 mL/kg, monitor the vital signs and electrocardiogram, and maintain body warmth.
   (Objective 11)

23. Linear, feathery, pinpoint appearance
   (Objective 10)

24. a. The patient is usually conscious and may be confused and amnesic with stable vital signs.
  b. The patient may be combative or comatose, with associated injuries from lightning strike, first- and second-degree burns, tympanic membrane rupture (common), and possible internal injuries.
  c. The patient may have immediate brain damage, seizures, respiratory paralysis, and cardiac arrest.
(Objective 10)

25. a. Alpha particles are positively charged atoms with minimal penetrability; however, they are dangerous when internal exposure occurs.
  b. Beta particles are positively or negatively charged electrons that have more penetrating power than alpha particles and can permeate subcutaneous tissue.
  c. Gamma particles have a much higher penetrating power than alpha or beta rays and require lead shielding to stop penetration. (Protective clothing does not stop these rays.) Exposure may produce local skin burns and extensive internal damage.
(Objective 12)

26. a. Less than 100 rem usually causes no significant acute problems.
  b. A total of 100 to 200 rem can cause symptoms such as nausea and vomiting but is not life threatening.
  c. Exposure of greater than 450 rem has a 50% mortality rate within 30 days.
(Objective 12)

27. The rescuers and emergency vehicle initially should be positioned 200 to 300 feet upwind of the site. No eating, smoking, or drinking should be permitted at the site. The appropriate local authorities and medical control should be notified of the situation.
(Objective 12)

28. Protective clothing should be worn, if available. The victim should be approached quickly by trained rescue teams. Rescue personnel should trade off frequently until the victim is stabilized sufficiently to remove him or her a safe distance from the contaminated area. If possible, the crew members should position themselves behind any protective barrier available.
(Objective 12)

29. If ventilation is required for the radiation-contaminated victim, an airway adjunct should be used. The patient should be moved away from the radiation source as soon as possible, but lifesaving care should not be delayed if the patient cannot be moved immediately. Intravenous lines should be initiated only if absolutely necessary, and good aseptic technique should be used to minimize the risk of introducing contaminants into the patient's body.
(Objective 12)

30. d. Alkali agents cause chemical burns, ionizing agents cause radiation burns, and arcing is caused by electrical energy.
(Objective 1)

31. b. Men die more frequently than women from burns. Three fourths of burn fatalities occur in the home. Deaths are also common in low-income homes.
(Objective 1)

32. d. This source includes flames, scalds, or contact with hot substances.
(Objective 1)

33. d. The patient hyperventilates to adapt to the increased metabolic rate. The gastrointestinal tract slows, and with large burns, adynamic ileus is a frequent complication.
(Objective 2)

34. b. First-degree burns are usually red, dry, and painful without blisters. Third-degree burns are white, yellow, tan, brown, or black; leathery; and often painless.
(Objective 3)

35. c. Each leg is between 13.5% and 14% body surface area.
(Objective 3)

36. c. Evaporation of fluid from the injured area also accounts for significant fluid loss.
(Objective 4)

37. c. The presence of first-degree burns should be noted in the narrative; however, these burns should not be included in the estimate of percent body surface area burned.
(Objective 3)

38. c. The burn should be cooled rapidly and then body temperature should be maintained with sheets and blankets.
(Objective 6)

39. c. $2\,\text{mL} \times 60 \times 100 = 12,000\,\text{mL}$ in the first 24 hours
One half in the first 8 hours $= 6000\,\text{mL}$
$6000\,\text{mL} \div 8 = 750\,\text{mL}$
The formula states that 2 to $4\,\text{mL/kg}$ per percent body surface area burned is given in 24 hours, so the range would be 750 to $1500\,\text{mL}$.
(Objective 6)

40. b. Petroleum products are not associated with inhalation burns unless they occur in an enclosed space. That is a normal end-tidal CO_2.
(Objective 6)

41. d. Oxygen saturation levels may be normal because the hemoglobin still is saturated (with carbon monoxide, not oxygen), and the oximeter may not differentiate between the two. Intravenous fluid therapy is not helpful in these patients.
(Objective 7)

42. c. Drying the chemical or delaying treatment only prolongs contact with the skin and increases the burn injury. Application of a chemical antidote is recommended only for a few chemicals.
(Objective 8)

43. a. The concentration or "dose" has a large influence on injury severity.
(Objective 7)

44. b. Subcutaneous injection of the calcium gluconate gel under the burn eschar is the most effective method.
(Objective 9)

45. d. An arc occurs when electrical energy "jumps" from its source through the air to another conductive medium. Direct burns result when the current passes through a person. Alternating is a description of a type of electrical current.
(Objective 10)

46. d. Bone provides the most resistance to electrical energy.
(Objective 10)

47. a. All of the other pathologic conditions can occur after lightning injury but cause death less frequently than cardiac or respiratory arrest.
(Objective 10)

48. c. Gamma rays have 10,000 times the penetrating power of alpha particles and 100 times the penetrating power of beta particles.
(Objective 12)

564

1. d. Direct contact electrical and flame burns.
   (Objective 1)

2. Burn shock evolves over 8 to 24 hours after injury and often is not seen immediately after injury.
   (Objective 2)

3. Depth: Second- and third-degree (partial and full thickness)
   Extent: ~24% (rule of nines); ~28% (Lund and Browder chart)
   Severity: Major burn (>25%; electrical injury; significant involvement of hands or feet)
   (Objective 3)

4. Damage from direct electrical current is often greatest in the tissues between the entrance and exit wounds. If the swelling occurs in the tissue compartments, severe circulatory compromise to the extremities can occur, causing progressive loss of pulses.
   (Objective 5)

5. a. Care at a burn center is indicated because he has full-thickness burns and electrical injuries.
   b. Anticipate progressive burn shock. Administer oxygen despite an initially normal SaO_2. If carbon monoxide exposure exists, SaO_2 will be normal despite tissue hypoxia.
   c. Electrical burns were present in the right hand and right foot. The current traveled through the right arm to reach the foot, so that arm should be avoided because of the potential for impaired circulation.
   d. As burn shock progresses, blood flow to the muscles declines, resulting in ineffective management of pain.
   (Objective 6)

6. Did the burns occur in an enclosed space? Does the patient have any stridor, facial burns, soot in the nose or mouth, facial burns, singed facial or nasal hair, edema of the lips or oral cavity, coughing, difficulty swallowing, a hoarse voice, or circumferential neck burns?
   (Objective 7)

7. Electrical current usually follows the path of least resistance to ground. Body tissues with the least resistance include the nerves and the blood vessels, not external skin structures.
   (Objective 10)

8. a, b, c, h, i
   (Objective 10)

40 Head, Face, and Neck Trauma

READING ASSIGNMENT

Chapter 40, pages 1146-1175, in *Mosby's Paramedic Textbook,* ed. 4.

OBJECTIVES

Upon completion of this chapter, the paramedic student will be able to do the following:

1. Describe the mechanisms of injury, assessment, and management of maxillofacial injuries.
2. Describe the mechanisms of injury, assessment, and management of ear, eye, and dental injuries.
3. Describe the mechanisms of injury, assessment, and management of anterior neck trauma.
4. Describe the mechanisms of injury, assessment, and management of injuries to the scalp, cranial vault, and cranial nerves.
5. Distinguish between types of traumatic brain injury based on an understanding of pathophysiology and assessment findings.
6. Outline the prehospital management of the patient with cerebral injury.
7. Calculate a Glasgow Coma Scale score, trauma score, Revised Trauma Score, and pediatric trauma score when given appropriate patient information.

SUMMARY

- Major causes of maxillofacial trauma are motor vehicle crashes, home accidents, athletic injuries, animal bites, intentional violent acts, and industrial injuries.
- With the exception of compromised airway and the potential for significant bleeding, damage to the tissues of the maxillofacial area is seldom life threatening. Some facial fractures are associated with basilar skull fracture. Blunt trauma injuries may be classified as fractures to the mandible, midface, zygoma, orbit, and nose.
- Injury to the ears, eyes, or teeth may be minor or may result in permanent sensory function loss and disfigurement. Trauma to the ear may include lacerations and contusions, thermal injuries, chemical injuries, traumatic perforation, and barotitis. Evaluation of the eye should include a thorough history. Assessment also should include measurement of visual acuity, pupillary reaction, and extraocular movements.
- Anterior neck injuries may result in damage to the skeletal structures, vascular structures, nerves, muscles, and glands of the neck. The patient should be assessed for airway compromise, bleeding, and cervical spine injury.
- Injuries to the skull may be classified as soft tissue injuries to the scalp and skull fractures. Skull fractures may be classified as linear fractures, basilar fractures, depressed fractures, and open vault fractures.
- The categories of brain injury include diffuse axonal injury (DAI) and focal injury. DAI may be mild (concussion), moderate, or severe. Focal injuries are specific, grossly observable brain lesions. Included in this category are lesions that result from skull fracture, contusion, edema with associated increased intracranial pressure, ischemia, and hemorrhage.
- The prehospital management of a patient with head injuries is determined by a number of factors. One factor is the mechanism of injury. A second factor is the severity of injury. A third factor is the patient's level of consciousness. Associated injuries affect the priorities of care.
- Several injury rating systems are used to triage, guide patient care, predict patient outcome, identify changes in patient status, and evaluate trauma care. Rating systems commonly used in emergency care include the Glasgow Coma Scale, trauma score/Revised Trauma Score, and pediatric trauma score.

Match the type of skull fracture listed in column II with the appropriate description in column I. Use each answer only once.

Column I

1. ________ Associated with Battle sign and raccoon's eyes

2. ________ Skull fracture with a low complication rate

3. ________ Communication between scalp laceration and brain tissue

4. ________ Fracture when bone is pushed downward; often associated with scalp laceration

Column II

a. Basilar
b. Depressed
c. Linear
d. Open vault

Match the cranial nerve in column II with the abnormal sign or symptom associated with it in column I. Use each cranial nerve only once.

Column I

5. ________ Hearing loss

6. ________ Loss of vision in one eye

7. ________ Weakness of one side of the face

8. ________ Double vision

9. ________ Loss of sense of smell

Column II

a. Olfactory
b. Optic
c. Oculomotor
d. Facial
e. Acoustic
f. Glossopharyngeal

10. An unrestrained 6-year-old child strikes his face on the stick shift of a truck in a head-on collision. On arrival, you find him seated in the cab of the truck, alert, crying, and complaining of pain in his face. Blood is oozing from his mouth.

    a. Describe your focused assessment of his head and face.

    ____

    ____

    b. You note that the child has difficulty closing his mouth. There is a space between his two lower front teeth, as well as a laceration that extends down through the gums. The bleeding continues, and you note excessive oral secretions. Vital signs are stable. Describe how you would transport and manage this child.

    ____

    ____

11. Briefly describe the evaluation of a suspected eye injury on a patient with no life threats.

    ____

    ____

12. For each of the following patients, identify the injury you suspect and list prehospital management techniques:

    a. A 10-year-old boy complains of severe pain in the right eye after he was struck in the face with a handful of sand. The right eye is reddened and tearing.

    ____

b. A 35-year-old person has a partially avulsed right upper eyelid.

____

____

c. A fish hook is embedded in the eye of a 42-year-old woman.

____

____

d. A handball player is struck directly in the eye by the ball. He is having difficulty seeing from the injured eye. You note blood in the anterior chamber of the eye.

____

____

e. During hockey playoffs, a high stick strikes a player in the eye. You note an irregular pupil on the affected side. A jellylike substance extrudes from an apparent laceration to the globe.

____

____

Questions 13 and 14 pertain to the following case study:

You are en route to a domestic disturbance in which a 45-year-old man reportedly has been stabbed in the neck with an ice pick.

13. What signs and symptoms of penetrating neck trauma should you anticipate?

____

On arrival, you note an ashen-colored unconscious patient who is breathing and has a weak pulse. A large pool of blood surrounds him, and a large amount of blood is coming from his neck.

14. How should you manage this patient's neck wound?

____

____

15. Briefly list the signs and symptoms associated with the following brain injuries and state whether the injury is a diffuse axonal injury or focal brain injury:

a. Concussion:

____

b. Contusion:

____

569

c. Subdural hematoma:

____

d. Epidural hematoma:

____

e. Severe diffuse axonal injury:

____

16. A man was struck on the head with a baseball bat. He is alert and oriented with an obvious depression and laceration at the right temporal area. Describe the signs and symptoms you will see if his intracranial pressure progressively rises en route to the hospital.

____

17. A patient sustained an isolated head injury in a motorcycle accident. Initially, he was awake and talking, but over the past 10 minutes, his condition has deteriorated rapidly. He now has a fixed, dilated right pupil; irregular respirations; a blood pressure of 170/100 mm Hg; and a pulse of 64 beats/min. Identify treatment modalities you would provide for this patient.

____

____

18. Calculate the score indicated (Glasgow Coma scale score [GCS], Revised Trauma Score [RTS], pediatric trauma score [PTS]) for each of the following patient examples:

a. Your patient opens her eyes to voice, is confused, and pulls her hand away when you start intravenous therapy. Her vital signs are blood pressure, 90/70 mm Hg; pulse, 120 beats/min; and respirations, 24 breaths/min and unlabored. Capillary refill is 1 second.

GCS______ RTS______

b. Your patient opens his eyes to deep pain, moans some unrecognizable sounds, and withdraws slightly from pain. His vital signs are blood pressure, 70 mm Hg by palpation; pulse, 136 beats/min; and respirations, 30 breaths/min and shallow. His capillary refill is 4 seconds.

GCS______ RTS______

c. Your 10-day-old, 4-kg patient fell to the floor. She is crying vigorously. You note a small abrasion on her head, with a slight amount of swelling but no palpable crepitus. No other injuries are noted. Her blood pressure is 80 mm Hg.

PTS ______

STUDENT SELF-ASSESSMENT

19. Which of the following is a sign of midface fracture?
    a. Diplopia
    b. Lengthening of the face
    c. Mastoid ecchymosis
    d. Numbness of the forehead

20. Your patient has signs and symptoms of midface fractures. Her Glasgow Coma Scale score is 6. Which of the following is an appropriate prehospital intervention?
    a. Elevation of the head of the cot
    b. Nasogastric intubation
    c. Orotracheal intubation
    d. Pressure dressing over the nares

21. What is the name of the bone that, when fractured, often is associated with signs and symptoms similar to orbital fractures?
   a. Frontal
   b. Mandible
   c. Maxilla
   d. Zygoma

22. Your patient has been struck in the eye with a ball. She has diplopia, subconjunctival ecchymosis, enophthalmos, and numbness in the cheek. Which bone fracture is consistent with these findings?
   a. Mandible
   b. Maxilla
   c. Orbit
   d. Zygoma

23. When are displaced nasal fractures most significant?
   a. If they are displaced to one side
   b. When they are associated with bleeding
   c. If the dorsum of the nose is depressed
   d. When they occur in children

24. The upper segment of the patient's pinna was torn off in a motor vehicle collision. Which of the following treatments is appropriate for this patient?
   a. Approximate the edges of the avulsed tissue to the ear and apply a pressure dressing.
   b. Care for the remaining ear only. No chance exists to reimplant avulsed ear tissue.
   c. Scrub the avulsed tissue before wrapping it for transport to prevent infection.
   d. Wrap the avulsed tissue in moist gauze, seal it in a plastic bag, and place the bag on ice.

25. How should you manage ear pain after barotrauma?
   a. Administer nitrous oxide by inhalation.
   b. Ask the patient perform the Valsalva maneuver.
   c. Deliver oxygen to increase the absorption of trapped air.
   d. Place the patient in the lateral recumbent position.

26. How should you transport an avulsed tooth?
   a. In a mild soap solution
   b. In sterile water
   c. In a dry gauze dressing
   d. In fresh whole milk

27. Zone I neck injuries are associated with the highest mortality because they contain which of the following structures?
   a. Brainstem, carotid artery, and nasopharynx
   b. Carotid artery, jugular vein, trachea, larynx, esophagus, and cervical spine
   c. Distal carotid arteries, salivary glands, and pharynx
   d. Subclavian and jugular vessels, lung, esophagus, trachea, cervical spine, and cervical nerve roots

28. Which sign or symptom may indicate compromise of the upper airway associated with a hematoma in the neck?
   a. Cough
   b. Dysphagia
   c. Stridor
   d. Wheezing

29. Why may intubation of the patient with laryngeal or tracheal trauma be difficult?
   a. Absence of spontaneous respirations
   b. Collapse of the trachea and bronchial tubes
   c. The presence of acute hypoxia
   d. Distorted and invisible vocal cords

30. Which injury is associated with focal brain injury?
   a. Concussion
   b. Contusion
   c. Minute petechial bruising of brain tissue in several areas
   d. Mechanical disruption of axons in both cerebral hemispheres

31. Which is the earliest reliable indicator of increasing intracranial pressure?
  a. Deteriorating level of consciousness
  b. Nausea and vomiting
  c. Increased blood pressure and decreased pulse
  d. Unilateral dilated pupil

32. Which breathing patterns may be exhibited by the patient with increased intracranial pressure?
  a. Eupnea
  b. See saw
  c. Hypoventilation
  d. Kussmaul respirations

33. What is a characteristic sign or symptom of subarachnoid hemorrhage?
  a. Dilated pupil on one side that does not react to light
  b. Gradual onset of unilateral weakness of the arms
  c. Intermittent pain and double vision in both eyes
  d. Sudden onset of "the worst headache I've ever had"

34. Which is the most rapid and effective intervention to decrease intracranial pressure in a patient with a severe head injury and a Glasgow Coma Scale score of 6?
  a. Elevation of the head
  b. Administration of mannitol
  c. Adequate ventilation
  d. Massive doses of steroids

35. You wish to give 40 g of mannitol to a patient who has a head injury. You have a 20% solution of the drug. How many milliliters do you give?
  a. 8
  b. 50
  c. 80
  d. 200

36. Which drug may be administered before intubation to prevent a sudden increase in intracranial pressure?
  a. Atropine
  b. Lidocaine
  c. Mannitol
  d. Midazolam

WRAP IT UP

You are working at an amusement park when a call comes over your walkie-talkie for a person who has fallen off a ride. You respond in a golf cart and find a 17-year-old girl who has fallen about 20 feet from a ride onto the concrete. Bystanders found her prone and rolled her onto her back. Your direct a security officer to maintain spinal immobilization. Her only response to painful stimulation is flexion of her arms. She is making no sounds and her eyes remain closed; pupils are midline, 5 mm, and reactive. She has multiple contusions and lacerations to her face, her nose is flattened, and there is thin bloody drainage from it. You insert an oral airway. Because her respirations are shallow and only about 8 breaths/min, you begin to ventilate her with a bag-valve mask resuscitator connected to oxygen as the local ambulance crew arrives. Her radial pulse is 98 beats/min, her skin is pale and cool, and her blood pressure is 80/50 mm Hg. She is logrolled with spinal precautions; her back is examined quickly; and after she is secured to the long spine board and stretcher, she is moved into the ambulance, where the paramedic intubates her trachea. An ECG and noninvasive blood pressure monitor are attached, and an IV of normal saline is initiated. After a bolus of 200 mL is given, her pressure rises to 100/70 mm Hg. Physical exam shows no crepitus or deformity anywhere except her face. Moments before arrival at the ED, her right pupil dilates to 7 mm and becomes nonreactive, BP is 130/50 mm Hg, pulse is 50 beats/min, and she has no motor response to painful stimulus and no spontaneous respirations when bagging is paused. You hyperventilate at 20 per minute. She is diagnosed with a severe diffuse axonal injury and dies during the flight to the regional trauma center.

1. If this patient had a gag reflex, should you have considered nasal instead of oral intubation?
  a. No, there is a possibility of midface fracture and penetration of the cranial vault.
  b. No, there would not have been a need to intubate if the patient had a gag reflex.
  c. Yes, nasal intubation would have been less likely to raise intracranial pressure.
  d. Yes, nasal intubation would have tamponaded the nasal bleeding when in place.

2. Based on the information given, which type of skull fractures would you anticipate?
   a. Basilar
   b. Depressed
   c. Linear
   d. a and b
   e. a and c

3. What type of brain hemorrhage is present in diffuse axonal injury?
   a. Cerebral hematoma
   b. Epidural hematoma
   c. Subarachnoid hemorrhage
   d. Subdural hematoma
   e. None of the above

4. Explain your rationale for providing the following treatment:

   a. Tracheal intubation: ____

   b. Fluid bolus with normal saline: ____

   c. Hyperventilation after the pupil dilated: _________________________________

   ____

5. Calculate the following scores for this patient:

	Glasgow Coma Scale score	**Revised Trauma Score**
Initial	__________________________	__________________________
During transport	__________________	__________________________

6. Place a check mark beside the indicators of increasing intracranial pressure that were present in this patient.

a. _______ Headache		**g.** _______ Widening pulse pressure	
b. _______ Nausea or vomiting		**h.** _______ Fixed, dilated pupil	
c. _______ Altered level of consciousness		**i.** _______ Central neurogenic hyperventilation	
d. _______ Blood pressure rises		**j.** _______ Abnormal posturing	
e. _______ Pulse slows		**k.** _______ Ataxic respirations	
f. _______ Cheyne-Stokes respirations		**l.** _______ Irregular pulse rate	

CHAPTER 40 ANSWERS

REVIEW QUESTIONS

1. a
(Objective 4)

2. c
(Objective 4)

3. d
(Objective 4)

4. b
(Objective 4)

5. e. This nerve is associated with basilar skull fracture.
(Objective 4)

6. b. Injury to the brain affecting the optic nerve may cause blindness in one or both eyes or visual field defects.
(Objective 4)

7. d. Damage involving the facial nerve may cause immediate or delayed facial paralysis and is associated with basilar skull fracture.
(Objective 4)

8. c. Injury affecting the oculomotor nerve can result in double vision because of the inability of the eye to move medially and down and out. Ptosis and pupil dilation or unresponsiveness to light also may occur.
(Objective 4)

9. a. Loss or alteration of sense of smell associated with injury affecting the olfactory nerve is a common finding associated with basilar skull fracture.
(Objective 4)

10. a. Inspect and palpate the head for lacerations, contusions, and deformities. Inspect the face for asymmetry and soft tissue injury. Evaluate the child's vision by holding up fingers and assessing pupil response. Assess for EOMs by asking the child to look up and down and side to side. Look for nasal deformity and for any drainage of blood or cerebrospinal fluid. Inspect the oral cavity for bleeding, soft tissue injury, and missing teeth. Palpate the face for crepitus and question the child about tenderness or numbness. Ask the child to open and close the mouth and move the lower jaw from side to side. Gently palpate for loose teeth.
   b. Immobilize the cervical spine and secure the child to the backboard while frequently suctioning the oral cavity. Tilt the backboard to the side and secure it firmly with straps. Suction the oral cavity frequently and instruct the child to signal when he needs additional suctioning or if he has difficulty breathing. Continually reevaluate for life threats.
(Objective 1)

11. Obtain a history to include the exact mode of injury; previous ocular, medical, and drug history, including cataracts, glaucoma, and presence of hepatitis or human immunodeficiency virus; use of eye medications; use of corrective glasses or contact lenses; presence of ocular prostheses; and symptoms and treatment interventions that may have been attempted before emergency medical services arrival. Observe the patient for signs of external trauma, discoloration, injury to the lid, fluid or jelly extruding from the eye, bleeding, blood in the anterior chamber, and the presence of contact lenses. Measure visual acuity with a handheld acuity chart or any printed material with small, medium, and large point sizes. Record the distance at which the visual material was held. Measure each eye separately and assess vision with and without corrective lenses. Evaluate pupil reaction to ensure that they constrict in concert when light is applied and dilate in response to darkness. Assess extraocular muscles by asking the patient to track an object with the eyes (without head movement) up, down, right, and left.
(Objective 2)

12. a. Injury: foreign body (or corneal abrasion); management: irrigate with normal saline.
   b. Injury: eyelid avulsion; management: assess for underlying injury to the eye; control bleeding with gentle pressure; for transport, cover with a dressing moistened with normal saline and an eye shield.
   c. Injury: embedded foreign body; management: patch the uninjured eye; stabilize the hook and cover with cardboard cup secured with tape.
   d. Injury: traumatic hyphema; management: elevate the head of the ambulance cot or spine board 40 to 45 degrees; instruct the patient to avoid straining.
   e. Injury: ruptured globe; management: cover the affected eye with damp, sterile dressings and an eye shield.
(Objective 2)

13. Bleeding, shock, hematoma, pulse deficit, neurologic deficit, dyspnea, hoarseness, stridor, subcutaneous emphysema, hemoptysis, dysphagia, and hematemesis
(Objective 3)

14. Secure the airway and breathing. Maintain spinal immobilization. Apply firm, direct pressure to the affected vessels and tamponade the vessel by direct pressure with a gloved finger only to the affected vessel(s). If venous injury is suspected, keep the patient supine or in the Trendelenburg position to prevent an air embolism. If air embolism is suspected, turn the immobilized patient on the left side with the head lower than feet to attempt to trap the air embolus in the right ventricle. Apply an occlusive dressing if bleeding is controlled.
(Objective 3)

15. a. Diffuse axonal injury; loss of consciousness (usually <5 minutes), retrograde or antegrade amnesia, vomiting, combativeness, transient visual disturbances, and problems with coordination; should all improve, not deteriorate
   b. Focal injury; seizures, hemiparesis, aphasia, personality changes, and loss of consciousness (lasting hours, days, or longer)
   c. Focal injury; headache, nausea, vomiting, decreasing level of consciousness, coma, abnormal posturing, paralysis, and bulging fontanelles in infants
   d. Focal injury; transient loss of consciousness followed by a lucid interval (6–18 hours) and a subsequent decreasing level of consciousness, headache, and contralateral hemiparesis (opposite the side of the bleeding); 50% unconscious without improvement
   e. Diffuse axonal injury; patients being usually unconscious for prolonged periods; may have posturing and signs of increased intracranial pressure
(Objective 5)

16. Headache, nausea, vomiting, altered level of consciousness, increased systolic blood pressure, widened pulse pressure, decreased pulse rate, abnormally slow respiratory pattern, unilateral dilated pupil, and abnormal posturing
(Objective 5)

17. Intubate tracheally (possibly nasally if signs of basilar skull fracture are not present) using spinal precautions. Hyperventilate the lungs with 100% oxygen at a rate of 20 per minute (maintain etCO$_2$ at 35 mmHg). Consider gastric tube insertion if available. Maintain fluids to keep the vein open unless signs of shock develop. Consider pharmacologic agents, such as mannitol and furosemide, in consultation with medical direction. Notify medical direction and transport the patient to the closest appropriate trauma center.
(Objective 6)

18. a. GCS is 12, and RTS is 11.
   b. GCS is 8, and RTS is 7.
   c. PTS is 7.
(Objective 7)

19. b. A "donkey face" is associated with this injury. Edema, unstable maxilla, epistaxis, numb upper teeth, nasal flattening, and cerebrospinal fluid rhinorrhea are also signs of midface fracture.
(Objective 1)

20. c. Neither an endotracheal tube nor a gastric tube should be placed nasally in the patient with midface fracture because they may pass into the cranial vault. Elevation of the head of the cot would be appropriate only after the cervical spine is cleared by radiographs in the emergency department. Cerebrospinal fluid drainage often accompanies these injuries and should be allowed to drain freely.
(Objective 1)

21. d. The zygoma commonly is called the *cheek bone*.
(Objective 1)

22. c. Orbital fractures often are associated with other fractures, such as Le Fort II and III and zygomatic fractures.
(Objective 1)

23. d. In children, minimal displacement may result in growth changes and ultimate deformity.
(Objective 1)

24. d. A chance to reimplant does exist, so if possible, the ear should be transported as described. However, ear injuries that involve cartilage often heal poorly and are infected easily.
(Objective 2)

25. b. Nitrous oxide is contraindicated and may increase the pain. Other measures that may help include requests that the patient yawn, swallow, and move the lower jaw.
(Objective 2)

26. d. Milk may be used if a commercial tooth solution, such as Hank's solution, is not available.
(Objective 2)

27. d. Zone II injuries (b) occur more often but are associated with lower mortality.
(Objective 3)

28. c. Stridor indicates that the upper airway is compromised significantly.
(Objective 3)

29. d. Attempting intubation actually may increase the damage associated with the injury and, if unsuccessful, cause partial airway obstruction to become complete.
(Objective 3)

30. b. Contusion is bruising of a specific area of the brain. All of the other answers reflect injuries that represent diffuse axonal injury.
(Objective 5)

31. a. This is the earliest sign and is consistent with all patients who have increased intracranial pressure.
(Objective 5)

32. c. The patient in diabetic ketoacidosis demonstrates Kussmaul respirations in an attempt to correct acidosis. Eupnea is normal breathing. See-saw breathing is seen in extreme respiratory distress.
(Objective 5)

33. d. Other common signs and symptoms include dizziness, neck stiffness, unequal pupils, vomiting, seizures, and loss of consciousness.
(Objective 5)

34. c. All other interventions are indicated (depending on medical control) to decrease intracranial pressure; however, ventilation at a rate not to exceed 20 per minute is the fastest method with the least risk to the patient.
(Objective 6)

35. d. $\dfrac{40\text{g} \times 100\,\text{mL}}{20\text{g}} = 200\text{mL}$

or $20\,\text{g}:100\,\text{mL} = 40\,\text{g}:x\ \text{mL}$

$4000 = 20x$

$200\,\text{mL} = x$

36. b. Atropine may be given to children before intubation to counteract the vagal stimulation. Mannitol is an osmotic diuretic given to decrease intracranial pressure but usually is not given for this purpose. Midazolam (Versed) is often given during rapid-sequence induction procedures to sedate the patient.
(Objective 6)

1. a. The nasal bleeding, massive facial trauma, and flattened nose are indicators of midface fractures. Nasal intubation of this patient is associated with the risk of perforation of the cranial vault.
(Objective 1)

2. e. Midface fractures are associated with basilar skull fractures. There is no indication of depression of the skull bones.
(Objective 1)

3. e. Diffuse axonal injury is associated with severe shearing, stretching, or tearing of the nerve fibers of the brain rather than a large collection of blood in an area of the brain.
(Objective 4)

4. a. Intubation will protect the airway of a patient with a severe head injury with altered level of consciousness as evidenced by a Glasgow Coma Scale score of less than 8.
(Objective 6)

   b. Fluid bolus is given to raise the blood pressure. Because the cerebral perfusion pressure (pressure needed to deliver oxygenated blood to the brain tissue) is equal to the mean arterial pressure less the intracranial pressure, if the blood pressure falls too low, the blood delivery to the brain is severely compromised. A fluid bolus may be needed to increase the blood pressure.
(Objective 6)

   c. Hyperventilation guided by capnography is indicated when there is evidence of herniation. This will cause constriction of the blood vessels in the brain and a resulting decrease in the intracranial pressure, which will decrease the risk of brain herniation.
(Objective 6)

5. Initial Glasgow Coma Scale score: 5; initial Revised Trauma Score: 6
Transport Glasgow Coma Scale score: 3; transport Revised Trauma Score: 4
(Objective 7)

6. c, d, e, g, h, j. There is insufficient information given to determine whether the patient had ataxic or Cheyne-Stokes respirations.
(Objective 5)

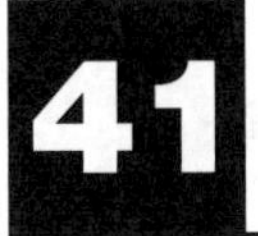# Spine and Nervous System Trauma

READING ASSIGNMENT

Chapter 41, pages 1176-1202, in *Mosby's Paramedic Textbook,* ed. 4.

OBJECTIVES

Upon completion of this chapter, the paramedic student will be able to do the following:

1. Describe the incidence, morbidity, and mortality related to spinal injury.
2. Predict mechanisms of injury that are likely to cause spinal injury.
3. Describe the anatomy and physiology of the spine and spinal cord.
4. Outline the general assessment of a patient with suspected spinal injury.
5. Distinguish between types of spinal injury.
6. Describe prehospital evaluation and assessment of spinal cord injury.
7. Identify prehospital management of the patient with spinal injuries.
8. Distinguish between spinal shock, neurogenic shock, and autonomic hyperreflexia syndrome.
9. Describe selected nontraumatic spinal conditions and the prehospital assessment and treatment of them.

SUMMARY

- Most spinal cord injuries (SCIs) are the result of motor vehicle crashes. Other causes are falls, penetrating injuries from acts of human violence, and sport injuries.
- The spinal column is composed of 33 vertebrae. These are divided into five sections. The sections are seven cervical, 12 thoracic, five lumbar, five sacral (fused), and four coccygeal (fused).
- The paramedic can classify the mechanism of injury (MOI) as positive, negative, or uncertain. This classification is combined with the clinical guidelines for evaluating SCI, which include the following signs and symptoms: pain, tenderness, painful movement, deformity, cuts or bruises over the spinal area, paralysis, paresthesias, and weakness. This system can help to identify cases in which spinal immobilization is appropriate.
- The specific MOIs that frequently cause spinal trauma are axial loading; extremes of flexion, hyperextension, or hyperrotation; excessive lateral bending; and distraction.
- Spinal injuries may be classified as sprains and strains, fractures and dislocations, sacral and coccygeal fractures, and cord injuries. The spinal cord may sustain a primary or a secondary injury. Lesions (transections) of the spinal cord are classified as complete or incomplete.
- With spinal injuries, the first priority is to evaluate and manage any threats to life. The second priority is to preserve spinal cord function. This includes avoiding secondary injury to the spinal cord. These goals are best met by maintaining a high degree of suspicion for the presence of spinal trauma by providing early spinal immobilization, rapidly correcting any volume deficit, and administering oxygen.
- General principles of spinal immobilization include prevention of further injury; treating the spine as a long bone with a joint at either end (the head and pelvis); always using complete spinal immobilization; beginning spinal immobilization in the initial assessment and maintaining it until the spine is immobilized completely on the long spine board; and placing the patient's head in a neutral, inline position unless contraindicated.
- Spinal shock refers to a temporary loss of all types of spinal cord function distal to the injury.
- Neurogenic shock produces a loss of sympathetic tone to the vessels. This causes relative hypotension; warm, dry, and pink skin; and relative bradycardia.
- Autonomic hyperreflexia syndrome results from a massive, uncompensated cardiovascular response that stimulates the sympathetic nervous system. This response in turn causes an increase in blood pressure and other symptoms.

Match the spinal illness or injury in column II with the description in column I. Use each term only once.

Column I

1. _______ Temporary paralysis and sensory loss after spinal injury

2. _______ Nontraumatic structural defect that involves the lamina or vertebral joint

3. _______ Paralysis and decreased pain and temperature sensation below a flexion injury

4. _______ Sprain causing partial dislocation of intervertebral joints

5. _______ Hemitransection of cord with weakness on the injured side

6. _______ Whiplash from a low-speed rear-end collision

7. _______ Sudden, rapid increase in blood pressure, relieved by emptying of the bladder

8. _______ Bradycardia, warm skin, and low blood pressure

9. _______ Abnormal tissue growth in the spine that may cause spasticity

10. _______ Injury characterized by paralysis of the arms with sacral sparing

Column II

a. Anterior cord syndrome
b. Autonomic hyperreflexia syndrome
c. Brown-Séquard syndrome
d. Central cord syndrome
e. Herniated nucleus pulposus
f. Hyperextension strain
g. Neurogenic hypotension
h. Spinal cord tumors
i. Spinal shock
j. Spondylosis
k. Subluxation

11. In each of the following situations, state whether the mechanism of injury is negative, positive, or uncertain related to your assessment of the spine.

    a. A soccer player falls and twists her knee. _______________________________

    b. A patient is ejected during a rollover crash. _______________________________

    c. A hunter falls 25 feet from a deer stand. _______________________________

    d. A young man falls 3 feet off a porch. _______________________________

    e. A patient is the restrained driver in a motor vehicle crash, and the rear hood is buckled.

    ____

    f. A child dives off the high board and strikes the bottom of the pool with his head.

    ____

    g. A woman who was running slips and falls, striking her head on a ceramic tile floor.

    ____

12. List five preexisting conditions that can increase the risk of spine injury or complicate the injury.

    a. ____

    b. ____

    c. ____

    d. ____

    e. ____

13. Spinal sprains and strains usually result from **(a)** _______________ and **(b)** _______________ forces. A hyperflexion sprain occurs when a tear is present in the posterior **(c)** _______________ and _______________, which allows partial **(d)** _______________ of the intervertebral joints. Hyperextension strains are common with low-velocity, rear-end automobile collisions and are known commonly as **(e)** _______________. The most frequently injured spinal regions, in descending order, are **(f)** _______________ to _______________, **(g)** _______________ to _______________, and **(h)** _______________ to _______________. The most common are wedge-shaped **(i)** _______________ fractures. **(j)** _______________ and **(k)** _______________ are extremely unstable injuries caused by a combination of severe hyperflexion and compression forces.

14. A cyclist was thrown from his bike and has severe pain in the back between his scapulae. List signs and symptoms that can indicate a complete spinal cord lesion as a result of this injury.

____

____

Questions 15 to 17 pertain to the following case study:

A 75-year-old woman was involved in a motor vehicle crash with moderate damage, which you classify as an uncertain mechanism for spine injury. She says she is fine and just wants to be "checked out" at the hospital.

15. Which conditions or situations would make her unreliable to perform spinal examination for clinical criteria?

____

____

16. Describe your examination for motor findings suggestive of spine injury.

____

____

17. Describe how to perform the sensory examination to evaluate for spine injury on this patient.

____

18. Identify five situations involving suspected cervical spine injury when the head should *not* be moved to a neutral inline position with manual immobilization.

   a. ____

   b. ____

   c. ____

   d. ____

   e. ____

19. Identify the steps involved in rolling of a supine patient (Fig. 41-1), including positioning of rescuers.

A. ____

B. ____

C. ____

D. ____

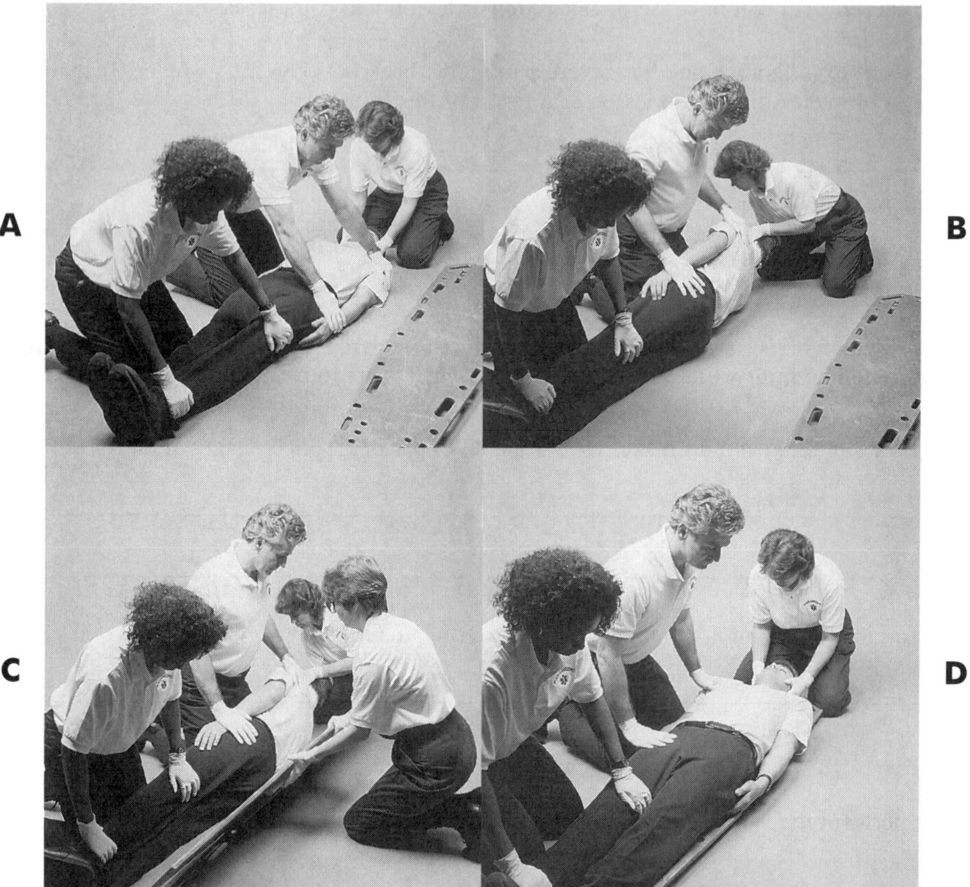

Figure 41-1

20. Identify drugs that may be used for each of the following spinal cord emergencies.

a. Spinal cord injury with paralysis:

____

b. Spinal cord injury with hypotension and bradycardia:

____

21. What causes most spinal injuries?
    a. Falls
    b. Motor vehicle crashes
    c. Sports-related injuries
    d. Penetrating injuries from acts of violence

22. How would a fall from the roof of a single-story residence be classified?
    a. Alternative mechanism of injury
    b. Negative mechanism of injury
    c. Positive mechanism of injury
    d. Uncertain mechanism of injury

23. Which patient would be considered reliable to assess for spinal cord injury?
    a. A patient who witnessed the death of his or her child in crash
    b. A patient with a severely angulated, partially amputated foot
    c. A patient who cannot communicate in a language you understand
    d. A patient who is complaining of knee and hip pain with no deformity

24. Which is the most flexible area of the spine?
    a. Cervical spine   **c.** Sacral spine
    b. Lumbar spine   **d.** Thoracic spine

25. A side-impact motor vehicle collision is most likely to produce spinal injury from extremes in which motion?
    a. Axial loading   **c.** Flexion
    b. Distraction   **d.** Lateral bending

26. Which finding on a patient with uncertain mechanism of injury should cause you to immobilize the spine?
    a. High blood pressure
    b. History of Parkinson's disease
    c. Laceration on the scalp
    d. Pain or tenderness of the neck

27. Hyperflexion sprains can cause partial dislocation of the intervertebral joints. What is this condition known as?
    a. Axial loading   **c.** Subluxation
    b. Herniated disks   **d.** Whiplash

28. What might fractures at the level of S1 and S2 may lead to?
    a. Loss of bowel and bladder function
    b. Neurogenic shock
    c. Paralysis of the legs
    d. Transection of the spinal cord

29. Paralysis and loss of sensation below the umbilicus indicate an injury at the level of which of the following?
    a. C4   **c.** T10
    b. T4   **d.** S1

30. Which sign would you expect to find in a patient with a complete transection of the spinal cord at the eighth cervical level?
    a. Bradycardia   **c.** Profuse sweating
    b. Hypertension   **d.** Polyuria

31. Which of the following signs or symptoms is associated with central cord syndrome?
    a. Intact light touch and position sensation
    b. Greater motor weakness or paralysis in the arms than legs
    c. Loss of pain and temperature sensation on the side of injury
    d. Weakness in the upper and lower extremities on the side opposite the injury

32. Which patient injury is associated with respiratory distress?
   a. Brown-Séquard syndrome
   b. Herniated thoracic disk
   c. Hyperextension strain
   d. Spinal cord transection at C5

33. Why should the paramedic immobilize the spine of patients suspected to have spinal injury ?
   a. To apply traction to pull apart injured bones
   b. To minimize neurogenic shock
   c. To prevent primary injury
   d. To prevent additional cord hypoxia or edema

34. When a patient is immobilized on a long spine board, which body region is secured first?
   a. Arms
   b. Head
   c. Legs
   d. Torso

35. Which cord injury presentation involves flaccid paralysis that resolves within 24 hours?
   a. Autonomic hyperreflexia syndrome
   b. Neurogenic hypotension
   c. Spinal shock
   d. Spondylosis

36. What causes neurogenic shock after spinal cord transection?
   a. Fluid volume loss from capillary leak
   b. Blocked sympathetic stimulation
   c. Vagal activation from cord edema
   d. Interruption of key blood vessels

37. A 32-year-old patient with quadriplegia complains of a severe headache. He is anxious and sweating and seated in his wheelchair. Vital signs are BP 240/150 mmHg, P 40/min, and R 20/min. What intervention has the highest priority?
   a. Assess his urinary catheter for signs of obstruction.
   b. Administer atropine 0.5 mg IV over 30 seconds.
   c. Place him in the left lateral recumbent position.
   d. Place him on a non-rebreather mask with O_2 at 15 lpm.

WRAP IT UP

You are dispatched to a call to "assist the invalid." As per protocol, you respond "on the quiet" with no lights or sirens. The 87-year-old patient's wife tells you that he tripped over a videotape in the living room and fell forward, striking his forehead on the coffee table. As you approach him, he apologizes for calling you to help him up off the floor. He is conscious, alert, and oriented, and you can see a small abrasion on his midforehead. When you ask him if anything hurts, he reaches around to his neck, rubs it vigorously, and says that his neck is sore. You palpate his neck, and he says the cervical spine area is tender, but you feel no crepitus and note no deformity. Your partner begins cervical spine immobilization as you continue your exam. The patient's breathing is normal, and his radial pulse is normal with a regular rate. His skin is warm and dry. His head-to-toe exam is unremarkable except for his persistent complaint of an "electric shock" sensation in his extremities. You explain to the patient your concern that he may have a spine injury, and he consents to transport. After application of the cervical collar, you logroll him and secure him to the long backboard. Vital signs are BP 134/78 mm Hg, P 60, R 20, and SaO$_2$ 96%. You initiate an IV and contact medical direction, who advises no further. The patient's condition remains stable, and you give report to the charge nurse in the ED. Later, the charge nurse calls you to let you know that the patient has an unstable fracture of C2 and C3. A halo vest has been applied, and his condition remains stable.

1. Why is the patient at risk for spinal injuries?
   a. Fall height
   b. His age
   c. Low heart rate
   d. Warm, dry skin

2. Which mechanism of injury occurred in this case?
   a. Negative   **c.** Uncertain
   b. Positive

3. Place a check mark beside the signs or symptoms that made you determine that spinal immobilization was indicated for this patient.
   a. _______ Trauma with use of intoxicating substances
   b. _______ Seizure activity
   c. _______ Complaints of pain in neck or arms
   d. _______ Tender neck on examination
   e. _______ Unconscious after head injury
   f. _______ Significant injury above clavicle
   g. _______ Fall greater than three times the patient's height
   h. _______ Fall and bilateral heel fracture
   i. _______ Injury from high-speed motor vehicle collision
   j. _______ Abnormal sensory exam results

4. Which forces likely injured the spine in this case?
   a. Axial loading
   b. Distraction
   c. Lateral bending
   d. Hyperextension and/or hyperflexion

5. If you had merely assisted the patient to his feet without performing a history or examination on him, what could have happened to his spinal cord?

____

6. List some signs or symptoms that would indicate that this patient had a spinal cord injury.

____

7. Place a check mark beside the signs or symptoms you would anticipate if the spinal cord were injured and the patient was developing neurogenic shock.
   a. _______ Bradycardia   **e.** _______ Hypotension
   b. _______ Cool skin   **f.** _______ Moist skin
   c. _______ Dry skin   **g.** _______ Tachycardia
   d. _______ Hypertension   **h.** _______ Warm skin

CHAPTER 41 ANSWERS

REVIEW QUESTIONS

1. i
   (Objective 9)

2. j
   (Objective 9)

3. a
   (Objective 5)

4. k
   (Objective 5)

5. c
   (Objective 5)

6. f
(Objective 5)

7. b

(Objective 8)

8. g
(Objective 8)

9. h
(Objective 9)

10. d
(Objective 5)

11. a. Negative
b. Positive
c. Positive
d. Uncertain
e. Uncertain
f. Positive
g. Uncertain
(Objective 2)

12. Damage from spinal injury can occur more easily or be complicated by one or more of the following:
a. Increased age
b. Osteoporosis
c. Spondylosis
d. Rheumatoid arthritis
e. Paget disease
f. Congenital spinal cord anomalies (fusion, narrow spinal canal)
g. Down syndrome
(Objective 4)

13. a. Hyperflexion
b. Hyperextension
c. Ligamentous complex and joint capsule
d. Dislocation (subluxation)
e. Whiplash
f. C5 to C7
g. C1 to C2
h. T12 to L2
i. Compression
j. Teardrop fractures
k. Dislocations
(Objective 5)

14. Absence of motor and sensory function below the nipple, relative bradycardia, hypotension, priapism, unstable body temperature, loss of bowel and bladder control, and decreased depth of respiration (loss of innervation of most intercostal muscles)
(Objective 6)

15. To be reliable, she must be calm, cooperative, sober, alert, and oriented. If she exhibits any of the following, she should be considered unreliable: acute stress reaction, brain injury, dementia, intoxication, abnormal mental status, distracting injuries, or problems in communication.
(Objective 4)

16. Motor evaluation: Ask the patient to move her arms and legs. Ask her to flex her elbow, grab and squeeze your fingers, and extend her elbows. Have the patient spread the fingers of both hands and keep them apart while you squeeze the second and fourth fingers. A normal exam produces springlike resistance. Support the patient's lower arm and ask her to hold her wrists or fingers out straight while you press down on her fingers. Moderate resistance should be felt. Place your hands at the sole of each foot and ask the patient to push against your hands. Both sides should feel equal and strong. Then hold the patient's feet (with fingers on her toes) and instruct her to pull them back to her nose. Both sides should feel equal and strong.
(Objectives 4 and 6)

17. Sensory evaluation: Question the patient about pain in the neck or back and any feelings of numbness or tingling in the body. Assess light touch on each hand and each foot (with the patient's eyes closed) and then, if necessary, prick the hands and feet with a sharp object (without breaking the skin).
(Objectives 4 and 6)

18. a. Increasing pain or neurologic deficits during movement
    b. Resistance to movement
    c. Muscle spasm
    d. Airway compromise caused by repositioning
    e. Severe misalignment of head from midline
(Objective 7)

19. a. Rescuer 1 is positioned at the patient's head, providing inline manual stabilization. Rescuers 2 and 3 are positioned at the patient's midthorax and knees.
    b. While maintaining immobilization, the rescuers, in one organized move, slowly logroll the patient onto his or her side, perpendicular to the ground.
    c. Rescuer 4 positions the long spine board by placing the device flat on the ground or at a 30- to 40-degree angle against the patient's back.
    d. In one organized move, the rescuers slowly logroll and center the patient onto the long spine board.
(Objective 7)

20. a. Methylprednisolone 30 mg/kg bolus followed by 5.4 mg/kg/h for 23 hours (controversial)
    Other experimental treatments include naloxone and calcium channel blockers (consult medical direction).
    b. Dopamine
(Objective 7)

21. b. In order of frequency of occurrence, they are motor vehicle crashes, falls, penetrating injuries, and sports injuries.
(Objective 1)

22. c. Most single-story homes are more than three times a person's height, which is classified as positive mechanism of injury.
(Objective 5)

23. d. The patient in (a) may be experiencing a stress reaction. The patient in (b) has a distracting injury. You cannot examine the patient in (c) well enough to rule out spinal injury by clinical criteria because of the language barrier.
(Objective 2)

24. a. The cervical spine allows the head to rotate with an almost 180-degree range of motion, 60 degrees of flexion, and 70 degrees of extension.
(Objective 3)

25. d. Axial loading occurs when the spine is compressed vertically. Distraction results from excessive "pulling" on the spinal cord. Flexion is a bending motion that decreases the angle between two joints, which more often results from anterior/posterior-type motion.
(Objective 2)

26. d. Pain or tenderness of the neck with or without palpation always should indicate immobilization of the spine.
(Objective 4)

27. c. Axial loading is a vertical loading mechanism of injury. A herniated disk occurs when the cartilage surrounding an intervertebral disk ruptures and releases the pulpy elastic substance that cushions the vertebrae above and below, causing pain and damage to nerve roots.[1]
(Objective 5)

28. a. The spinal cord terminates at L2.
(Objective 5)

29. c. C3 and C4 would involve sensory loss at the top of the shoulder, T4 at the nipple, and S1 on the lateral foot.
(Objectives 4 and 6)

30. a. Hypotension, priapism, loss of sweating and shivering, poikilothermy, and loss of bowel and bladder control are also signs.
(Objective 6)

31. b. This weakness usually results from hyperextension or hyperflexion injuries.
(Objective 5)

32. d. Transection of the spinal cord above C3 usually results in respiratory arrest. Lesions that occur at C4 may result in diaphragmatic paralysis. Lesions at C5–C6 spare the diaphragm but result in loss of significant intercostal muscle function.
(Objective 6)

33. d. Traction should not be applied on the spine in the field. Primary injury occurs at the time the initial forces are applied.
(Objective 7)

34. d. Immobilize the torso first to prevent angulation of the cervical spine.
(Objective 7)

35. c. Spinal shock results from a temporary loss of all spinal cord function distal to the injury.
(Objective 8)

36. b. The sympathetic outflow tracts are interrupted. This causes largely unopposed parasympathetic nervous system stimulation.
(Objective 8)

37. a. Autonomic hyperreflexia syndrome is often caused by bladder distention or rectal impaction. Relieving either of those problems will usually cause prompt restoration of normal vital signs. If that is not possible on the scene, the patient needs rapid transport to resolve these problems.
(Objective 8)

WRAP IT UP

1. b. Risk of spinal injury increases with age.
(Objective 1)

2. c. This was a single-level fall.
(Objective 2)

3. c, d, j. Neck pain is the most important predictor of cervical spine injury. The patient also complained of an "electric shock"–like sensation.
(Objective 4)

4. d. The mechanism of injury and abrasion to his forehead lead us to believe that his head was flexed or extended forcefully.
(Objective 2)

5. It could have caused a partial or complete cord injury (causing paralysis) if the unstable cervical spine impinged on the delicate spinal cord.
(Objective 2)

6. The patient was complaining of radicular (electrical shock) pain, a symptom of cord injury. Additional signs or symptoms could include paralysis, paresthesias, weakness, neurologic deficit, priapism, loss of sweating or shivering, poikilothermy, and loss of bowel and bladder control.
(Objective 6)

7. a, c, e, h
(Objective 8)

42 Chest Trauma

Chapter 42, pages 1203-1219, in *Mosby's Paramedic Textbook*, ed. 4.

OBJECTIVES

Upon completion of this chapter, the paramedic student will be able to do the following:

1. Discuss mechanism of injury associated with chest trauma.
2. Describe the mechanism of injury, signs and symptoms, and management of skeletal injuries to the chest.
3. Describe the mechanism of injury, signs and symptoms, and prehospital management of pulmonary trauma.
4. Describe the mechanism of injury, signs and symptoms, and prehospital management of injuries to the heart and great vessels.
5. Outline the mechanism of injury, signs and symptoms, and prehospital care of the patient with esophageal and tracheobronchial injury and diaphragmatic rupture.

SUMMARY

- Chest injuries are caused by blunt or penetrating trauma. Such trauma often results from motor vehicle crashes, falls from heights, blast injuries, blows to the chest, chest compression, gunshot wounds, and stab wounds.
- Fractures of the clavicle, ribs, or sternum, and as well as flail chest, may be caused by blunt or penetrating trauma. Complications of skeletal trauma of the chest may include cardiac, vascular, or pulmonary injuries.
- Closed pneumothorax may be life threatening if (1) it is a tension pneumothorax, (2) it occupies more than 40% of the hemithorax, or (3) it occurs in a patient in shock or a preexisting pulmonary or cardiovascular disease.
- Open pneumothorax may result in severe ventilatory dysfunction, hypoxemia, and death unless it is quickly recognized and corrected.
- Tension pneumothorax is a true emergency. It results in profound hypoventilation. It may result in death if it is not quickly recognized and managed.
- Hemothorax may result in massive blood loss. These patients often have hypovolemia and hypoxemia.
- Pulmonary contusion results when trauma to the lung causes alveolar and capillary damage. Severe hypoxemia may develop. The degree of hypoxemia is directly related to the size of the contused area.
- Traumatic asphyxia results from forces that cause an increase in intrathoracic pressure. When it occurs alone, it is often not lethal. However, brain hemorrhages, seizures, coma, and death have been reported after these injuries.
- The extent of injury from myocardial contusion may vary. The injury may be only a localized bruise. However, it also may be a full-thickness injury to the wall of the heart. The full-thickness injury may result in cardiac rupture, ventricular aneurysm, or a traumatic myocardial infarction.
- Pericardial tamponade occurs if 150 to 200 mL of blood enters the pericardial space suddenly. This results in a decrease in stroke volume and cardiac output. *Myocardial rupture* refers to an acute traumatic perforation of the ventricles or atria. It is nearly always immediately fatal. However, death may be delayed for several weeks after blunt trauma.
- Aortic rupture is a severe injury. There is an 80% to 90% mortality rate in the first hour. The paramedic should consider the possibility of aortic rupture in any trauma patient who has unexplained shock after a rapid deceleration injury.
- Esophageal injuries most frequently often are caused by penetrating trauma (e.g., missile projectile and knife wounds). Tracheobronchial injuries are rare. (They occur in fewer than 3% of victims of blunt or penetrating chest trauma, but the mortality rate is over 30%.) A tension pneumothorax that does not improve after needle decompression or the absence of a continuous flow of air from the needle after decompression should alert the paramedic to the possibility of a tracheobronchial injury.
- Diaphragmatic ruptures may allow abdominal organs to enter the thoracic cavity. There they may cause compression of the lung, resulting in a reduction in ventilation, a decrease in venous return, a decrease in cardiac output, and shock.

Questions 1 to 3 pertain to the following case study:

A 26-year-old woman was a passenger in a car struck laterally on her door. She has a fractured right humerus and multiple fractures of ribs 3 to 8. En route to the trauma center, you note paradoxical movement of her chest.

1. What chest injury do you suspect?

2. Why is the patient likely to become hypoxic after this injury?

3. What patient care measures should you use to improve ventilation?

4. Identify three symptoms common to all types of pneumothorax.

    a.

    b.

    c.

5. A deer hunter is shot accidentally with a 30-30 caliber rifle. The hunter has an open wound inferior to the right nipple, and you cannot find an exit wound.

    a. Why is this patient likely to become hypoxic?

    b. What interventions must be taken immediately to correct the hypoxia?

6. A patient from a motor vehicle crash sustained severe blunt chest trauma. He has diminished breath sounds on the right side of the chest. He is anxious and dyspneic.

    a. What additional signs and symptoms would indicate that he has developed a tension pneumothorax?

    b. Describe how to perform the prehospital intervention for tension pneumothorax.

Chapter **42** **Chest Trauma**

7. What two life-threatening conditions may be caused by hemothorax?

   a. ____

   b. ____

8. A worker was crushed momentarily between a truck and a loading dock. His face and head are a bright, reddish purple, and his jugular veins are greatly distended.

   a. What injury do you suspect?

   ____

   b. What treatment would you provide?

   ____

9. A 28-year-old woman struck her chest on the steering wheel in a frontal vehicle collision. She complains of crushing substernal chest pain and palpitations. Her blood pressure is normal, her pulse is 110 beats/min and irregular, and her lungs are clear.

   a. What injury do you suspect?

   ____

   b. What treatment measures should be instituted for this patient?

   ____

10. A 27-year-old man was splitting wood when a metal splinter flew off the ax and penetrated his chest. He is confused, with a systolic blood pressure of 80 mm Hg, a narrow pulse pressure, muffled heart sounds, and distended neck veins. You notice bulging veins on his forearm when you prepare to start an IV.

    a. What chest injury do you suspect?

    ____

    b. What prehospital care should be rendered?

    ____

11. What signs should be anticipated in a patient with an aortic dissection caused by a rapid deceleration injury?

    ____

STUDENT SELF-ASSESSMENT

12. Which of the following is true regarding chest trauma?
    a. It is associated with a small number of deaths each year.
    b. It only occurs with motor vehicle crashes and penetrating injury.
    c. It only includes soft tissue injuries to the chest.
    d. The use of seat belts decreases the mortality associated with it.

13. Which is true regarding clavicle fractures?
    a. Clavicle fractures are unusual injuries.
    b. They are never serious injuries.
    c. They usually occur when the arm is twisted.
    d. They can be treated with a sling and swath.

14. Which of the following is true regarding rib fractures?
    a. They are more common in children.
    b. The first rib frequently is fractured.
    c. They are associated with pancreatic injury.
    d. Ribs 3 to 8 are most commonly fractured.

15. What is most likely to cause respiratory distress in a patient who has flail chest?
    a. Impaired mechanics of respiration
    b. Open chest wounds
    c. Severe pain that increases with respiration
    d. Underlying pulmonary contusion

16. What other injury should you anticipate if your patient has a sternal fracture?
    a. Airway compromise   c. Myocardial injury
    b. Flail chest   d. Spleen injury

17. Which is the most common cause of pneumothorax?
    a. Excessive pressure on the chest wall
    b. Penetration from a gun or knife
    c. Penetration from a rib fracture
    d. Spontaneous pneumothorax

18. A 22-year-old female involved in an MVC has bruising across the anterior chest with normal chest wall movement. No other injuries are identified. Breath sounds are slightly diminished over the right lung. Vital signs are BP 118/84 mm Hg, P 98, R 24, and SaO_2 94%. Which of the following injuries is most likely?
    a. Closed pneumothorax
    b. Tension pneumothorax
    c. Hemopneumothorax
    d. Pulmonary contusion

19. Your patient has a pneumothorax and may be developing a hemothorax. What signs or symptoms will you anticipate?
    a. Bradypnea   c. Neck vein distension
    b. Hypotension   d. Widened pulse pressure

20. What pathophysiologic change should you anticipate after paper-bag effect injury?
    a. Negative chest pressure on inspiration
    b. Shearing and tearing of alveoli
    c. Excess air in pleural space
    d. Transection of bronchioles

21. What often occurs as a result of pulmonary contusion?
    a. Hypovolemia   c. Pericardial tamponade
    b. Hypoxia   d. Pneumothorax

22. Which sign is associated with pericardial tamponade?
    a. Atrial fibrillation   c. Narrowing pulse pressure
    b. Carotid bruit   d. Tracheal deviation

23. Which assessment is most likely to lead to detection of aortic injury?
   a. Performing a 12-lead electrocardiogram
   b. Analyzing end-tidal CO_2 levels
   c. Palpating both carotid pulses
   d. Assessing blood pressure in both arms

24. Your patient was involved in a high-speed motor vehicle crash. Which of the following signs may signal aortic dissection?
   a. Congestive heart failure
   b. Decreased breath sounds
   c. Hypertension
   d. Jugular venous distension

25. Your patient was in a motorcycle crash and has dyspnea and bowel sounds at the nipple line on the left side of the chest. You suspect which of the following?
   a. Pericardial tamponade
   b. Liver rupture
   c. Diaphragmatic rupture
   d. Kidney injury

WRAP IT UP

You respond to a "vehicle accident" with possible rescue. A single car struck a light standard, knocking it to the ground. The safety officer verifies that the vehicle is not in contact with the pole and that the scene is blocked from oncoming traffic. You open the driver door to access your only patient, an 18-year-old man who was not restrained. He was driving an older car with no air bags. He is conscious and alert with a laceration on his forehead. He is moaning loudly and complaining of pain in his legs. Your partner takes spinal precautions while you quickly assess his condition. He has a weak, rapid radial and carotid pulse with pale, cool skin and rapid respirations. His breath sounds are diminished slightly on the left. He has tenderness and redness over his anterior chest and both lower legs. You apply oxygen and a cervical collar and perform a rapid extrication, moving him quickly to the ambulance. His vital signs are: BP 130/80 mm Hg (right arm) and 166/90 (left arm), P 128, R 24, and SaO_2 on non-rebreather mask is 95%. His breath sounds are difficult to hear, but it seems they are still decreased on the left. The rest of your exam shows bilateral tenderness, deformity, and swelling in the lower legs with weak pedal pulses palpable. You are en route to the trauma center quickly and initiate two IVs and call a report during transport. Repeat vital signs remain unchanged during transport. Your medical officer calls back an hour later and is told that the patient was diagnosed with concussion, left pneumothorax, a fractured second left rib, and bilateral closed fractures of the tibia and fibula and that they are monitoring the patient for an aortic tear because the initial radiographs show some widening in the mediastinum. He is presently stable with a chest tube in the left side of his chest.

1. Circle the classifications of chest trauma with which the patient has been diagnosed or for which he is being evaluated.
   a. Diaphragmatic injury
   b. Heart and great vessel injury
   c. Pulmonary injury
   d. Skeletal injury

2. What signs or symptoms were present that indicated possible bony chest injury?

____

3. i. Place a check mark beside the signs or symptoms of pneumothorax that this patient displayed.

   ii. Place a *t* beside additional signs or symptoms that would have indicated this patient was developing a tension pneumothorax.

   a. _______ Chest pain

   b. _______ Cyanosis

   c. _______ Decreased breath sounds on affected side

   d. _______ Distended neck veins

   e. _______ Dyspnea

   f. _______ Hypotension

   g. _______ Subcutaneous emphysema

   h. _______ Tachycardia

   i. _______ Tachypnea

   j. _______ Tracheal deviation

595

4. How did you treat the pneumothorax in the field?

5. Which of the following is true regarding aortic rupture?
   a. Fracture of the second rib is associated with this injury.
   b. Hypotension will always be seen.
   c. Immediate death rarely is seen with aortic tears.
   d. Quadriplegia can be associated with this injury.

6. What exam findings indicate possible aortic dissection

CHAPTER 42 ANSWERS

REVIEW QUESTIONS

1. Flail chest
(Objective 2)

2. The pulmonary contusion and injured segment of the chest will not expand; therefore, insufficient negative pressure is generated in the chest to draw in a normal amount of air.
(Objective 2)

3. Intubate if the Glasgow Coma Scale score is less than 8 or if the patient has severe hypoxia and assist ventilations with positive pressure (demand valve, bag-valve) with 100% oxygen. Monitor vital signs, electrocardiogram, and oxygen saturation.
(Objective 2)

4. Dyspnea, tachypnea, diminished breath sounds on the affected side, and chest pain on inspiration
(Objective 3)

5. a. During inspiration, some air will enter the wound instead of the trachea, which decreases air entering the lung for ventilation
   b. Seal the wound on three sides with occlusive dressing. Administer high-flow oxygen by non-rebreather mask.
(Objective 3)

6. a. Cyanosis, tracheal deviation, tachycardia, hypotension, and distended neck veins
   b. Insert a 14-gauge catheter in the midclavicular line of the second or third intercostal space on the side of the pneumothorax. Listen for a rush of air, consider a flutter valve, reevaluate the patient, and repeat these steps en route if the needle clots.
(Objective 3)

7. Hypoxia and hypovolemic shock
(Objective 3)

8. a. Traumatic asphyxia
   b. Oxygenate and maintain airway and ventilation and evaluate for associated injuries.
(Objective 3)

9. a. Myocardial contusion
   b. Oxygen administration, electrocardiographic monitoring, and treatment of dysrhythmias per protocol
(Objective 4)

10. a. Pericardial tamponade
   b. Oxygen administration, fluid replacement, rapid transport, consideration of pericardiocentesis (only with authorization and specialized training)
   (Objective 4)

11. Upper extremity or generalized hypertension, systolic murmur, paraplegia (rare), and severe shock
   (Objective 4)

12. d. At least 25% of trauma deaths are associated with chest trauma. Falls, crush injuries, blast injuries, and blows to the chest also can cause significant thoracic trauma.
   (Objective 1)

13. d. The clavicle is one of the most commonly fractured bones. Rarely, clavicle fracture can be complicated by injury to the subclavian vein or artery from bony fragment penetration. The mechanism typically involves a fall on outstretched arms or the shoulder.
   (Objective 2)

14. d. Children have more elastic chests and are less likely to have rib fractures. The first rib is rarely fractured. The pancreas lies protected behind other abdominal organs and is unlikely to be affected by rib fractures.
   (Objective 2)

15. d. The damaged tissue often results in significant hypoxia.
   (Objective 2)

16. c. The heart lies under the sternum and may be compressed if it is injured.
   (Objective 2)

17. c. Excessive pressure on the chest wall can cause pneumothorax (paper-bag effect). Spontaneous pneumothorax occurs when a rupture or tear develops in the lung parenchyma for no apparent reason.
   (Objective 3)

18. a. Tension pneumothorax and hemopneumothorax would be accompanied by signs of shock. Pulmonary contusion is usually seen when flail chest is present.
   (Objective 3)

19. b. Hypotension will develop as a result of hypovolemic shock. Tachypnea, deviation to the affected side (rare), and narrowed pulse pressure also may occur.
   (Objective 3)

20. c. Inertial effect is a stretching and shearing of alveoli and intravascular structures. Negative pressure in the chest on inspiration is normal.
   (Objective 3)

21. b. Profound hypoxia can result from abnormal lung function.
   (Objective 3)

22. c. Tracheal deviation is associated with tension pneumothorax. Carotid bruit is found in carotid stenosis.
   (Objective 4)

23. d. A significant difference in blood pressure in each arm may signal aortic rupture.
   (Objective 4)

24. c. Pulses may be decreased in the lower extremities.
   (Objective 5)

25. c. When the bowel moves into the chest, severe respiratory compromise occurs.
   (Objective 5)

1. b, c, d
   (Objective 1)

2. Pain, redness of the skin over the area, tenderness on palpation
   (Objective 2)

3. i. a, c, e, h, i

   ii. b, d, f, g, j
   (Objective 3)

4. High-concentration oxygen
   (Objective 3)

5. a. Hypertension can be seen initially if vessel tamponade has occurred. There is an 80% to 90% chance of immediate death. Paraplegia is possible.
   (Objective 4)

6. His blood pressure varied between the right and left arms and his pedal pulses were weak despite normal blood pressure.
   (Objective 4)

43 Abdominal Trauma

Chapter 43, pages 1220-1229, in *Mosby's Paramedic Textbook,* ed. 4.

OBJECTIVES

Upon completion of this chapter, the paramedic student will be able to do the following:

1. Identify mechanisms of injury associated with abdominal trauma.
2. Describe mechanisms of injury, signs and symptoms, and complications associated with abdominal solid organ, hollow organ, retroperitoneal organ, and pelvic organ injuries.
3. Outline the significance of injury to intraabdominal vascular structures.
4. Describe the prehospital assessment priorities for the patient suspected of having an abdominal injury.
5. Outline the prehospital care of the patient with abdominal trauma.

SUMMARY

- Blunt trauma to abdominal organs usually results from compression or shearing forces.
- Penetrating injury may result from stab wounds, gunshot wounds, or impaled objects.
- The two solid organs most commonly injured are the liver and the spleen. Both of these organs are primary sources of death from hemorrhage. Injuries to the hollow abdominal organs may result in sepsis, wound infection, and abscess formation.
- Injury to the retroperitoneal organs (kidneys, ureters, pancreas, duodenum) may cause massive hemorrhage.
- Injury to the pelvic organs (bladder, urethra) usually results from motor vehicle crashes that produce pelvic fractures.
- Injuries to abdominal vascular structures may be life threatening because of their potential for massive hemorrhage.
- The most significant sign of severe abdominal trauma is the presence of unexplained shock.
- Emergency care of patients with abdominal trauma usually is limited to two courses of action. One is to stabilize the patient. The other is to rapidly transport the patient to a hospital for surgery to repair the injury.

REVIEW QUESTIONS

1. A 12-year-old boy recovering from mononucleosis was hit on the left side during a football game. He complains of severe left upper quadrant abdominal pain and left shoulder pain. He has signs of shock.

   a. What solid organ has most likely been injured in this situation?

   ____

   b. Why would the boy complain of shoulder pain?

   ____

   c. What care should you provide for him?

   ____

2. Describe complications that may result when hollow organs of the abdomen are injured.

____

____

3. List nine signs or symptoms associated with abdominal trauma.

a. ____

b. ____

c. ____

d. ____

e. ____

f. ____

g. ____

h. ____

i. ____

STUDENT SELF-ASSESSMENT

4. Which of the following is true of abdominal trauma?
  a. Blunt injuries do not occur when personal restraints are used.
  b. Complications of penetrating abdominal trauma appear immediately.
  c. Penetrating injury is associated with higher mortality than blunt trauma.
  d. Shearing forces may produce a tear or rupture of solid organs or blood vessels.

5. Which is the most commonly injured solid organ?
  a. Spleen   **c.** Liver
  b. Kidney   **d.** Pancreas

6. What do patients often experience after injury to the liver?
  a. Bowel obstruction   **c.** Peritoneal irritation
  b. Gastrointestinal bleeding   **d.** Renal failure

7. Which of the following is true about renal trauma?
  a. Bleeding is usually minimal.
  b. Fractures often need surgical repair.
  c. It occurs only as a result of posterior trauma.
  d. Urine output stops.

8. Which of the following mechanisms of blunt trauma is most often associated with pancreatic injury?
  a. Bicycle handlebar impalement
  b. Falls from higher than 20 feet
  c. Punch injuries from abuse
  d. Restrained passenger in head-on crash

9. What sign or symptom is a contraindication to insertion of a urinary catheter?
  a. Blood at the urinary meatus   **c.** Burning during urination
  b. Bruising over the flank   **d.** Microscopic hematuria

600

10. Which is a characteristic of intraabdominal arterial and venous injuries?
   a. Always present with a palpable mass
   b. Have the potential for massive hemorrhage
   c. Involve only the aorta or vena cava
   d. Occur only with penetrating trauma

11. A patient was involved in a high-speed motor vehicle crash. He refuses care. When he stands to leave, he becomes pale and states that he feels nauseated and dizzy. What should you suspect is a possible cause of these signs and symptoms?
   a. Hyperventilation
   b. Preexisting medical problem
   c. Severe abdominal injury
   d. Vagal reaction to pain

12. What is the highest priority for a patient who has severe signs of shock from abdominal injury?
   a. Comprehensive physical examination
   b. Initiation of IV fluid therapy
   c. Rapid transport to the hospital
   d. Oxygen administration

Questions 13 to 15 pertain to the following case study:

A 30-year-old woman was shot in the right upper quadrant of the abdomen. She is pale and restless and has cool, clammy skin. Vital signs are blood pressure, 76/58 mm Hg; pulse, 128 beats/min; and respirations, 28 breaths/min.

13. You would suspect injury to the (1) chest, (2) liver, (3) spleen, or (4) urinary bladder?
   a. (1) and (2)
   b. (1) and (3)
   c. (2) and (4)
   d. (3) and (4)

14. What interventions are indicated for this patient?
   a. Oxygen (4 L/min via nasal cannula) and intravenous lactated Ringer solution to keep the vein open
   b. Oxygen (10 L/min via mask) and intravenous lactated Ringer solution to keep the vein open
   c. Oxygen (4 L/min via nasal cannula) and intravenous lactated Ringer solution via rapid infusion
   d. Oxygen (10 L/min via mask) and intravenous lactated Ringer solution via rapid infusion

15. Your *first* priority on arrival at this call would be
   a. Airway maintenance
   b. Administration of oxygen
   c. Scene safety
   d. Stopping the bleeding

16. What will pain after pancreatic injury be largely related to?
   a. Peritoneal irritation
   b. Stretch receptors
   c. Lack of endorphins
   d. Kehr sign

17. What are signs and symptoms associated with diaphragmatic rupture associated with?
   a. Impaired diffusion
   b. Disruption in ventilation
   c. Airway obstruction
   d. Bronchial constriction

18. What is decreased cellular perfusion in a patient with a liver laceration primarily related to?
   a. Decreased preload
   b. Decreased contractility
   c. Decreased thrombocytes
   d. Decreased vascular resistance

19. Which sign or symptom will you most likely find in a patient who has a serious kidney injury caused by a 20-foot fall sustained 5 minutes before you arrived on the scene?
   a. Cullen sign
   b. Gray-Turner sign
   c. Flank pain
   d. Right shoulder pain

20. What sign or symptom might be expected when you find crepitus on palpation of the iliac crests?
   a. Blood at the urethra
   b. Vomiting blood
   c. Pain over the lower ribs
   d. Bowel sounds in the chest

Dispatch radios you to respond to a call for a "cutting," stating that the scene is not safe and the police are en route. You stage in the area and proceed in when police notify you that the scene has been secured. A 55-year-old obese man was stabbed in the abdomen with a 6-inch kitchen knife by an "unknown" assailant. He is awake and alert but very anxious. He wants to get up and walk around despite his blood-soaked shirt. You note his pale, cool skin; feel a thready, rapid, radial pulse; and then quickly pull off his shirt and pants. One stab wound is visible in the right upper quadrant of his abdomen just below his rib cage. He denies being short of breath when you question him, and you hear clear and equal breath sounds bilaterally, but his abdomen is rigid and tender to palpation. No other wounds are visible on your quick head-to-toe assessment. You administer oxygen and move him to the ambulance, where you assess his vital signs: BP, 78/50 mm Hg; P, 136/min; R, 28/min; Sao_2 is unobtainable. The patient is a critical trauma case, but your rural location is too far from the trauma center, and no helicopter is available. You tell your partner to head for the nearest hospital. Then you continue care; you insert one IV of normal saline, wide open on blood tubing, and another in the other arm of lactated Ringer solution. By the time you establish the second line, you have arrived at the hospital. There the patient is transfused with uncrossmatched blood. Luckily, the surgeon is available in house; she determines that immediate surgery is indicated. The patient is rushed to the operating room, where his lacerated liver is repaired. He is discharged home in 10 days.

1. What other mechanisms can cause injuries to the abdominal organs?

   ____

2. Which of the following is true regarding his injury?
   a. Liver contents spilling into the peritoneal cavity cause no signs or symptoms.
   b. The liver is a solid organ, so the chief concern after injury is bleeding.
   c. The liver is very vascular and can be removed to prevent death from uncontrolled hemorrhage.
   d. Retroperitoneal bleeding can be severe and is hard to control after liver injury.

3. Place a check mark beside the signs or symptoms of peritoneal irritation that this patient displayed.

   a. _______ Distension   d. _______ Pain

   b. _______ Fever   e. _______ Tenderness to palpation

   c. _______ Guarding or rigidity

4. What major artery that supplies the liver could have been injured by this penetrating wound?
   a. Celiac artery   c. Inferior mesenteric artery
   b. Iliac artery   d. Hepatic artery

5. What three critical interventions needed to enhance the chance of survival for patients with abdominal trauma were performed on this patient?

   a. ____

   b. ____

   c. ____

6. How would your care change if his initial vital signs were BP 108/78, P 120, R 24/min, and SaO_2 96%?

   ____

CHAPTER 43 ANSWERS

1. a. Spleen; b. referred pain caused by irritation of the diaphragm by a splenic hematoma or blood in the peritoneum (Kehr sign); c. This child should have a rapid assessment. Oxygen should be administered, and rapid transport to the closest appropriate trauma center should begin immediately. Intravenous therapy using an isotonic solution should be administered at 20 mL/kg during transport. A repeat IV bolus may be indicated based on the reevaluation.
(Objective 2)

2. Sepsis, infection, abscess formation, and peritonitis (resulting from leakage of the contents of hollow organs).
(Objective 2)

3. a. Unexplained shock; b. bruising and discoloration of the abdomen; c. abrasions; d. obvious bleeding; e. pain, abdominal tenderness, or guarding; f. abdominal rigidity, distention; g. evisceration; h. rib fractures; i. pelvic fractures
(Objective 4)

STUDENT SELF-ASSESSMENT

4. d. This injury is caused by stretching of organs and blood vessels.
(Objective 1)

5. c. The other organ most often injured is the spleen.
(Objective 2)

6. c. Shock also occurs often.
(Objective 2)

7. b. Bleeding can be severe and difficult to detect. Injury can result from anterior or posterior trauma. Urine output may contain blood.
(Objective 2)

8. a. Steering wheel trauma and penetrating trauma are also associated with pancreatic injury.
(Objective 2)

9. a. This may indicate urethral injury, which could be complicated by insertion of a catheter.
(Objective 2)

10. b. The patient often presents with signs and symptoms of shock.
(Objective 3)

11. c. With unexplained shock in a trauma patient, abdominal injury should always be at the top of your "rule out" list.
(Objective 4)

12. c. All are important, but definitive care is only available at the hospital. Further examination and treatment may be performed en route to the hospital.
(Objective 5)

13. a. The liver is located in the right upper quadrant. The diaphragm extends low, so the chest cavity is easily penetrated in these types of injuries.
(Objective 1)

14. d. Administration of high-concentration oxygen and fluid resuscitation are indicated.
(Objective 5)

15. c. Scene safety should always be the first priority on every call, especially when a crime has been committed.
   (Objective 5)

16. a. Pancreatic juices will damage and inflame the peritoneum. The Kehr sign is referred pain to the shoulder associated with splenic injury.
   (Objective 2)

17. b. Abdominal contents herniated into the chest and prevent lung expansion.
   (Objective 2)

18. a. Reduced blood volume associated with massive hemorrhage will decrease preload.
   (Objective 2)

19. c. The Gray-Turner and Cullen sign are associated with bleeding related to kidney injury, but they do not occur immediately. Right shoulder pain (Kehr sign) is associated with splenic injury.
   (Objective 2)

20. a. Urethral trauma is associated with pelvic fracture.
   (Objective 2)

WRAP IT UP

1. Blunt: assault, motor vehicle collisions, falls, industrial injuries, pedestrian injuries, blast injuries; penetrating: impaled objects, gunshot wounds
   (Objective 1)

2. b. When bile and blood spill into the peritoneal cavity after liver injury, signs and symptoms of peritoneal irritation occur. The liver is necessary for life; it can be partially removed, but complete removal results in death.
   (Objective 2)

3. c, d, e
   (Objective 2)

4. a. The iliac and inferior mesenteric arteries are lower in the abdomen. The portal vessel is a vein, not an artery.
   (Objective 3)

5. a. Rapid transport for definitive care (surgery)
   b. Oxygenation
   c. Fluid resuscitation
   (Objective 5)

6. Venous access would be obtained with a large-bore catheter, but fluids would be run at a keep-open rate unless his systolic blood pressure dropped below 100 mm Hg.
   (Objective 5)

44 Orthopedic Trauma

READING ASSIGNMENT

Chapter 44, pages 1230-1252, in *Mosby's Paramedic Textbook,* ed. 4.

OBJECTIVES

Upon completion of this chapter, the paramedic student will be able to do the following:

1. Describe the features of each class of musculoskeletal injury.
2. Describe the features of bursitis, tendonitis, and arthritis.
3. Given a specific patient scenario, outline the prehospital assessment of the musculoskeletal system.
4. Outline the general principles of splinting.
5. Describe the significance and prehospital management principles for selected upper extremity injuries.
6. Describe the significance and prehospital management principles for selected lower extremity injuries.
7. Identify prehospital management priorities for open fractures.
8. Describe the principles of realignment of angular fractures and dislocations.

SUMMARY

- Injuries that can result from traumatic force on the musculoskeletal system include fractures, sprains, strains, and joint dislocations. Problems associated with musculoskeletal injuries include hemorrhage, instability, loss of tissue, simple laceration and contamination, interruption of blood supply, and long-term disability.
- Common signs and symptoms of extremity trauma include pain on palpation or movement, swelling or deformity, crepitus, decreased range of motion, false movement, and decreased or absent sensory perception or circulation distal to the injury.
- After the paramedic has assessed for life-threatening conditions, the extremity injury should be examined for pain, pallor, paresthesia, pulses, paralysis, and pressure. In addition, DCAP-BTLS (deformity, contusions, abrasions, penetrations or punctures, burns, tenderness, lacerations, and swelling) should be evaluated for the injured extremity.
- Immobilization by splinting helps alleviate pain; reduces tissue injury, bleeding, and contamination of an open wound; and simplifies and facilitates transport of the patient. Splints can be categorized as rigid, soft or formable, and traction splints.
- Upper extremity injuries can be classified as fractures or dislocations of the shoulder, humerus, elbow, radius and ulna, wrist, hand, and finger. Most upper extremity injuries can be adequately immobilized by application of a sling and swathe.
- Lower extremity injuries include fractures of the pelvis and fractures or dislocations of the hip, femur, knee and patella, tibia and fibula, ankle and foot, and toes.
- Most open fractures are obvious because of associated hemorrhage. However, a small puncture wound may not be initially apparent. In addition, bleeding may be minimal. Therefore, the paramedic must consider any soft tissue wound in the area of a suspected fracture to be evidence of an open fracture. Open fractures are considered a true surgical emergency because of the potential for infection.
- Only *one* attempt at realignment should be made. This should be done *only* if severe neurovascular compromise is present (e.g., extremely weak or absent distal pulses). Moreover, it should be done *only* after consultation with medical direction.

Match the type of fracture in column II with the description in column I. Use each answer only once.

Column I

1. _______ A cancer patient sustains a fracture despite no apparent trauma.

2. _______ A fracture is incomplete, and the bone is bent.

3. _______ Bone is sticking out of a laceration.

4. _______ A runner feels increased pain in the foot and is found to have a fracture.

5. _______ A patient's arm is broken after having been twisted in an auger.

6. _______ The skin over a deformed ankle is intact.

7. _______ The fracture extends through the growth plate.

8. _______ The radiograph reveals a shattered bone.

9. _______ The fracture appears to be at a 45-degree angle across the bone.

Column II

a. Closed
b. Comminuted
c. Epiphyseal
d. Greenstick
e. Oblique
f. Open
g. Pathological
h. Spiral
i. Stress
j. Transverse

Select all the appropriate immobilization devices from column II that would be used to treat the fractures in column I. You may use each term more than once.

Column I

10. _______ Shoulder

11. _______ Humerus

12. _______ Elbow

13. _______ Forearm

14. _______ Wrist

15. _______ Hand

16. _______ Finger

17. _______ Pelvis

18. _______ Hip

19. _______ Femur

20. _______ Knee or patella

21. _______ Tibia or fibula

22. _______ Ankle or foot

23. _______ Toes

Column II

a. Buddy splint
b. Formable splint
c. Long spine board
d. Rigid splint
e. Pneumatic antishock garment
f. Sling
g. Swathe
h. Traction splint

Questions 24 to 26 pertain to the following case study:

A 16-year-old adolescent injured his wrist playing hockey.

24. What is your primary objective when performing the initial assessment on this patient?

____

Chapter **44** **Orthopedic Trauma**

25. What are the six *P*s of assessment for this injury?

P ____

P ____

P ____

P ____

P ____

P ____

26. As you examine this patient, you inspect and palpate the extremity to identify

D ____

C ____

A ____

P ____

B ____

T ____

L ____

S ____

27. Identify at least 11 general principles of splinting.

a. ____

b. ____

c. ____

d. ____

e. ____

f. ____

g. ____

h. ____

i. ____

j. ____

k. ____

Questions 28 and 29 pertain to the following case study:

A 55-year-old patient has a shortened and externally rotated hip with no pedal pulse distal to the injury. You anticipate a 45-minute transport to the nearest medical center.

28. Why is it appropriate to attempt to realign this dislocation?

____

29. Explain the procedure for attempting to realign the hip in this situation.

____

STUDENT SELF-ASSESSMENT

30. Which of the following is true about a sprain?
  a. It means injury to a tendon.
  b. No tissue disruption occurs, but bruising does occur.
  c. Severe hemorrhage can occur.
  d. Joint instability and dislocation may result.

31. A *subluxation* is another name for which of the following?
  a. Complete dislocation
  b. Incomplete dislocation
  c. Open fracture
  d. Strain

32. What sign or symptom indicates a need to reposition a deformed forearm fracture before splinting?
  a. Capillary refill one second
  b. Severe pain after narcotics are given
  c. Cold, blue fingers
  d. Tenting of the skin over the fracture

33. Which preexisting condition increases susceptibility to fracture?
  a. Bursitis
  b. Costochondritis
  c. Arteriosclerosis
  d. Osteoporosis

34. Signs or symptoms of extremity trauma that have a high urgency include which of the following?
  a. Absent distal pulses
  b. Crepitus
  c. Decreased range of motion
  d. Swelling and deformity

35. Your patient has been intubated and has signs of severe shock. His right wrist is swollen and deformed, and crepitus is present. How will you manage this extremity injury during your 7-minute transport time to the hospital?
  a. Elevation and application of ice
  b. Forearm splint
  c. Long spine board
  d. Sling and swathe

36. Boxer's fracture is the most common fracture of which bone(s)?
  a. Carpals
  b. Metacarpal
  c. Phalanges
  d. Radius

37. When a patient has a dislocation of the hip, how would you find the affected leg?
  a. Lengthened and externally rotated
  b. Lengthened and internally rotated
  c. Shortened and externally rotated
  d. Shortened and internally rotated

38. When should you apply a traction splint?
  a. Angulation of the knee
  b. Hip pain with shortened leg
  c. Swollen deformed mid-thigh
  d. Crepitus over the symphysis pubis

608

39. Your patient has severe deformity of the knee and a diminished pulse in the foot on the affected leg. Which artery is likely injured?
   a. Femoral artery
   b. Dorsalis pedis artery
   c. Popliteal artery
   d. Posterior tibial artery

40. A bone is protruding through a wound on the lower leg. When you immobilize the fracture, the bone end slips back into the wound. What action should you take?
   a. Cover the wound with a dry sterile dressing.
   b. Irrigate the wound with sterile normal saline.
   c. Move the leg gently until the bone reappears.
   d. Soak the wound with Betadine solution.

41. Your patient fell and has a grossly deformed shoulder. Which of the following is likely to be associated with complications if you realign it?
   a. Absent radial pulse
   b. Paresthesias
   c. Severe pain
   d. Thoracic spine injury

42. A woman injured her ankle while skating. You splint the ankle, elevate it, and apply ice. What should you administer to treat her pain?
   a. Hydromorphone 4 mg IV
   b. Fentanyl 4 mg IV
   c. Morphine 4 mg IV
   d. Narcotics are not indicated for this injury

WRAP IT UP

You know that you are the closest volunteer responding to a vehicle collision in your township, so you respond in your truck. The ambulance will be about 10 minutes behind you. Your patient is a 45-year-old nurse who you recognize from the emergency department (ED). She apparently dozed off, and her car ran off the road, striking a tree. Major damage was done to the front of her car, and her airbags deployed. She is conscious and crying. She says the only thing she remembers is looking up, seeing the tree, and holding on to the steering wheel. As you speak with her, you unbuckle her belt. Her skin is pink and warm, and her heart rate is increased. She tells you she thinks she has broken her arms and legs. She denies any other pain or difficulty breathing. She has equal breath sounds and no obvious chest or abdominal trauma. Her wrists are both tender and deformed but have good pulses. Her right femur is swollen and very tender; her left lower leg is deformed, and a laceration is slowly oozing blood over the painful area. She has good sensation and movement distal to all of her extremity injuries. You and another volunteer administer oxygen, assess her vital signs (BP, 110/70 mm Hg; P, 124/min; R, 20/min), initiate an IV of normal saline in the left antecubital space, and splint her left lower leg. As the ambulance arrives, she vomits and says she is feeling faint. A repeat set of vital signs shows BP, 106/70 mm Hg; P, 128 beats/min; and R, 20 breaths/min. Even though the patient denies neck pain or tenderness, a collar is applied, and she is rapidly extricated to the long spine board. A traction splint is applied to her right leg, and she is secured to the stretcher and moved to the ambulance. Under the guidance of medical direction, IV morphine is given in 2-mg doses to relieve her pain. Her forearms are splinted and elevated on pillows, and ice is applied to all injured extremities. Continuous monitoring of vital signs and extremity pulses, movement, and sensation shows no change during transport. After a total of 6 mg of morphine, the patient reports that the pain has dulled from a "10" to a "7," so you give an additional 2 mg, knowing that the movement on arrival at the ED will be painful. You apply a sterile 4 ×4 gauze to the wound on her left lower leg. You note fat globules in the oozing dark blood.

   On your next trip to the hospital, you visit the patient. She will miss at least 3 months of work because of her multiple fractures. She thanks you repeatedly for giving her the pain medicine; she says her attitude toward patients who are in pain has been changed forever.

1. List six things you should assess each time you think a patient has fractured an extremity.

____

2. Describe how you would have changed your treatment if you suspected a fracture in her lower right leg as well.

____

  Chapter **44** **Orthopedic Trauma**

3. Which splint (or splints) would be appropriate for each of the patient's injuries on this call?
   a. Sling and swathe
   b. Rigid splint
   c. Formable splint
   d. Traction splint
   e. Pillow splint
   _______ Right and left upper extremity injuries
   _______ Right upper leg injury
   _______ Left lower leg injury

4. What principles should be followed when applying the splints to both arms and the left lower leg?

____

5. Why is the wound over the patient's painful leg deformity significant?
   a. It could greatly increase the risk of blood loss.
   b. It could signify an open fracture, which poses a high risk of infection.
   c. Unless bone can be seen sticking out, it is not significant.
   d. Unless the bleeding is uncontrolled, the wound should not be covered.

6. Explain the rationale for administering oxygen and initiating an IV in this patient.

____

CHAPTER 44 ANSWERS

REVIEW QUESTIONS

1. g

2. d

3. f

4. i

5. h

6. a

7. c

8. b

9. e
   (Questions 1–9, Objective 1)

10. f and g

11. b, d, f, and g

12. b, d, f, and g

13. b, d, and f

14. b, d, and f

15. b and d

610

16. a, b, and d
(Questions 10–16, Objectives 4 and 5)

17. c and e

18. c

19. c and h

20. b and d

21. b and d

22. b

23. a
(Questions 17–23: Objectives 4 and 6)

24. With every patient, you must assess for the presence of life threats in the initial assessment.
(Objective 3)

25. The six *P*s are pain, pallor, paresthesia, pulses, paralysis, and pressure.
(Objective 3)

26. The initials *DCAP-BTLS* refer to deformity, contusions, abrasions, penetrations or punctures, burns, tenderness, lacerations, and swelling.
(Objective 3)

27. The general principles of splinting are splint joints above and below, as well as bone ends; immobilize open and closed fractures in the same manner; cover open fractures to minimize contamination; check pulses, sensation, and motor function before and after splinting; stabilize the extremity with gentle, inline traction to the position of normal alignment; immobilize a long bone extremity in a straight position that can easily be splinted; immobilize dislocations in a position of comfort; ensure good vascular supply; immobilize joints as found; align joint injuries only if no distal pulse is detected; apply cold to reduce swelling and pain; apply compression to reduce swelling; and elevate the extremity if possible.
(Objective 4)

28. No pulse is present distal to the injury; this is an indication to attempt realignment in the prehospital setting.
(Objective 6)

29. Administer an analgesic, benzodiazepine, or both (with appropriate monitoring) if not contraindicated by other injuries. Apply inline traction along the shaft of the femur with the hip and knee flexed at 90 degrees. Apply slow and steady traction to relax the muscle spasm. Listen for a "pop" with accompanying sudden relief of pain and easy manipulation of the leg to full extension. Immobilize the leg in full extension with the patient supine on a long spine board; reevaluate pulses and neurovascular status. If attempt is unsuccessful, place the patient supine and use pillows or blankets to immobilize the leg at a flexion not exceeding 90 degrees.
(Objective 6)

30. d. Sprains represent injuries to ligaments.
(Objective 1)

31. b. A complete dislocation is a *luxation*.
(Objective 1)

32. c. These signs indicate poor blood flow.
(Objective 5)

33. d. During assessment, ask the patient about a history of osteoporosis This weakens the structure of the bones, increasing susceptibility to fracture.
(Objective 3)

34. a. Treatment is needed for all the other signs; however, emergent interventions are needed to preserve the limb when distal pulses are absent.
(Objective 4)

35. c. Because of the life threats present in this patient, it is unlikely you would have to treat this isolated injury except to provide full-body immobilization on a spine board.
(Objective 5)

36. b. The fifth metacarpal is broken in a boxer's fracture.
(Objective 5)

37. d. After a hip fracture, the extremity is usually shortened and externally rotated.
(Objective 6)

38. c. It is not indicated for hip, knee, or pelvic fracture.
(Objective 6)

39. c. Injury to the popliteal artery is associated with knee trauma.
(Objective 6)

40. a. Make sure that this is reported to the receiving medical personnel and documented in the patient care report. Assess distal pulse and sensation.
(Objective 7)

41. d. The movement necessary to realign the arm could cause further injury to the back.
(Objective 5)

42. c. The dose of each of the other drugs is excessive.
(Objective 5)

WRAP IT UP

1. Assess for pain, tenderness, deformity, swelling, crepitus, and any soft tissue wounds in the area of a suspected fracture, as well as distal pulses, sensation, and movement before and after splinting.
(Objective 3)

2. A traction splint would not have been appropriate if the lower leg also had been fractured. The patient could have been splinted on the spine board using blankets or pillows to stabilize the extremity or perhaps long board splints.
(Objective 6)

3. Upper extremity injuries: b or c. Although a sling may be helpful for immobilizing and elevating the splinted isolated upper extremity, in this case, because the patient was supine on the spine board, it wouldn't have been indicated.
(Objective 5)

   Right upper leg injury: d
   (Objective 6)

   Left lower leg injury: b or c
   (Objectives 6)

4. The distal pulse, movement, and sensation should be assessed before and after splinting. The splint should be applied to include the joints above and below the injury and should be secured firmly. The extremity should be elevated if possible and ice applied.
(Objective 4)

5. b. Although significant open fractures pose an increased risk of bleeding, the chief concern is infection of the bone, which is very difficult and time consuming to treat.
(Objective 7)

6. Aside from the potential for chest and abdominal injuries based on the mechanism of injury, there is significant risk of internal bleeding from long bone fractures. This is particularly true for the femur and secondarily for the tibia and fibula.
(Objective 1)

45 Environmental Conditions

Chapter 45, pages 1253-1272, in *Mosby's Paramedic Textbook,* ed. 4.

OBJECTIVES

Upon completion of this chapter, the paramedic student will be able to do the following:

1. Describe the physiology of thermoregulation.
2. Discuss the risk factors, pathophysiology, assessment findings, and management of specific hyperthermic conditions.
3. Discuss the risk factors, pathophysiology, assessment findings, and management of specific hypothermic conditions and frostbite.
4. Discuss the risk factors, pathophysiology, assessment findings, and management of submersion and drowning.
5. Identify the mechanical effects of atmospheric pressure changes on the body based on a knowledge of the basic properties of gases.
6. Discuss the risk factors, pathophysiology, assessment findings, and management of diving emergencies and high-altitude illness.

SUMMARY

- Body temperature is regulated by a thermoregulatory center in the posterior hypothalamus. The body temperature can be increased or decreased in two ways. One of these ways is through the regulation of heat production. (This is known as thermogenesis.) The other way is through the regulation of heat loss. (This is known as thermolysis.).
- Heat illness results from one of two basic causes. First, the normal temperature-regulating functions can be overwhelmed by conditions in the environment. These conditions can include heat stress. More often, though, they involve excessive exercise in moderate to extreme environmental conditions. The other cause is a failure of the body's thermoregulatory mechanism. This may occur in older adults or ill or debilitated individuals.
- Heat cramps are brief, intermittent, and often severe. They are muscular cramps that occur in muscles fatigued by heavy work or exercise.
- Heat exhaustion is characterized by minor aberrations in mental status, dizziness, nausea, headache, and a mild to moderate rise in the core body temperature (CBT) ($\leq$103°F [39°C]).
- Heat stroke occurs when the temperature-regulating functions break down entirely. This failure results in body temperature rises to 105.8°F (41°C) or higher. Temperatures this high damage all tissues and lead to collapse.
- Hypothermia (a CBT <95°F [35°C]) can result from a decrease in heat production, an increase in heat loss, or a combination of these two factors. The progression of clinical signs and symptoms of hypothermia is divided into three classes based on the CBT: mild (CBT 93.2°–96.8°F [34°–6°C]), moderate (CBT 86°–°F [30°–4°C]), and severe (CBT <86°F [30°C]). Severely hypothermic patients have no vital signs, including respiratory effort, pulse, and blood pressure.
- Frostbite is a localized injury. It results from environmentally induced freezing of body tissues. This freezing leads to the damage to blood vessels. Ischemia often produces the most damaging effects of frostbite. In deep frostbite, this can include mummification and sloughing of nonviable skin and deep structures.
- Drowning is a process that results in primary respiratory impairment from submersion or immersion in a liquid medium that prevents the person from breathing air. Regardless of the type of water aspirated, the pathophysiology of drowning is characterized by hypoxia, hypercapnia, and acidosis, which result in cardiac arrest.
- The three laws pertaining to the basic properties of gases that are involved in all pressure-related diving emergencies are Boyle's, Dalton's, and Henry's laws. Increased pressure dissolves gases into blood; oxygen metabolizes, and nitrogen dissolves.
- Barotrauma is tissue damage. It results from compression or expansion of gas spaces when the gas pressure in the body differs from the ambient pressure. The type of barotrauma depends on whether the diver is in descent or ascent. Air embolism is the most serious complication of pulmonary barotrauma. It is a major cause of death and disability among sport divers.
- High-altitude illness results from exposure to reduced atmospheric pressure, which results in hypoxia. Forms of high-altitude illness include acute mountain sickness, high-altitude pulmonary edema, and high-altitude cerebral edema.

615

Match the terms related to environmental conditions in column II with the appropriate description in column I. Use each term only once.

Column I

1. ________ Goose bumps

2. ________ Dissipation of heat in the body by various mechanisms

3. ________ Sudden return of cold blood and wastes to the core

4. ________ Temperature difference between body and environment

5. ________ Gas volume inversely related to its pressure

6. ________ Decompression sickness

7. ________ Heat immersion causing hypotension from vasodilation

8. ________ Total pressure of gases equaling the sum of partial pressure of component gases

9. ________ Regulation of heat production in the body

10. ________ Amount of gas dissolved in fluid volume is proportional to pressure of gas with which it is in equilibrium

Column II

a. Afterdrop phenomenon
b. Boyle's law
c. Cold diuresis
d. Dalton's law
e. Dysbarism
f. Henry's law
g. Piloerection
h. Rewarming shock
i. Thermal gradient
j. Thermogenesis
k. Thermolysis

11. Briefly describe how each of the following contributes to heat production in the body.

   a. Chemical control:

   ____

   b. Musculoskeletal system:

   ____

   c. Endocrine system:

   ____

12. For each of the following situations, select the mechanisms of heat loss that apply (conduction, convection, evaporation, and radiation). You may use each answer more than once.

   a. On a windy autumn evening, you remove the clothing of a trauma patient to assess his injuries more accurately. On arrival to the emergency department, his temperature is 94°F (34.4°C). _____________.

   b. During a multiple patient situation, you extricate a partially clothed patient onto a cold metal backboard. On arrival to the emergency department, her temperature is 96°F (35.6°C). _____________.

   c. On a dry, cool spring evening you transport a wet patient who injured her neck after diving into a swimming pool. On arrival at the emergency department, her temperature is 94.6°F (34.8°C). _____________.

   d. A patient with a 40% body surface area burn is cooled continuously with normal saline en route to the hospital. On arrival to the emergency department, his temperature is 93.5°F (34.2°C). ______.

Chapter **45** **Environmental Conditions**

13. You are on the scene of a multiple-car collision on a hot July day. List four ways your body will compensate to prevent your temperature from rising.

a. ____

b. ____

c. ____

d. ____

14. You are assisting with a search-and-rescue effort after a winter storm. It is cold, wet, and windy. List four ways your body will attempt to maintain a normal temperature.

a. ____

b. ____

c. ____

d. ____

15. For each of the following examples, identify the type of heat illness and briefly describe the appropriate prehospital patient care.

a. You are working at an amusement park on a 95°F (35°C) humid day. A hot, sweaty 45-year-old woman comes to your aid station complaining of severe cramping in her calves. Her vital signs are BP 116/72 mm Hg, P 116, and temperature 98.6°F (37°C).

Illness:

____

Management:

____

b. A 55-year-old man is complaining of dizziness, nausea, and vomiting while participating in a long-distance walk fund-raiser. His vital signs while lying down are BP 104/70 mm Hg and P 108. His vital signs while standing are BP 86/50 mm Hg and P 128, and his temperature is 101°F (38.3°C).

Illness:

____

Management:

____

c. On a 100°F (37.8°C) day, an 80-year-old woman becomes confused and agitated and has a seizure in her apartment, which does not have air conditioning. She is responsive to pain, has jugular venous distension, and has hot, dry skin. Her vital signs are BP 92/70 mm Hg, P 120, R 24, and temperature 106°F (41.1°C).

Illness:

____

Management:

____

16. Why is the increased metabolic rate in mild hypothermia undesirable for a patient who already has an injury or medical illness?

____

____

You are caring for a snowmobiler whose rig broke through the ice 30 minutes ago. He pulled himself out of the water and collapsed before rescuers reached him 20 minutes later. He has been moved to a safe area.

17. Describe general measures of care to begin immediately on this patient.

____

____

18. You determine that he is apneic and pulseless. His electrocardiogram displays the rhythm shown in Fig. 45-1. What actions should be taken?

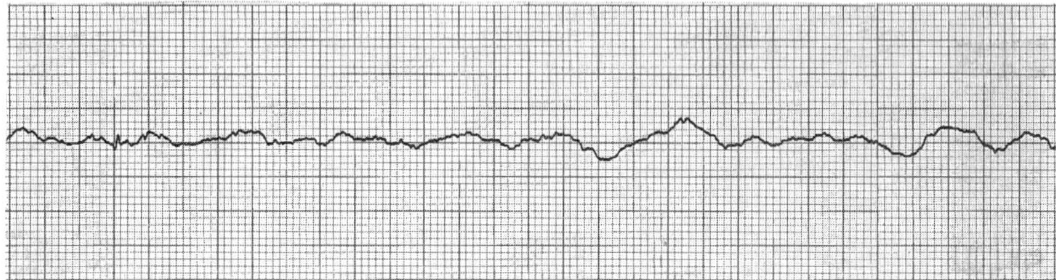

Figure **45-1**

19. When should resuscitation efforts be terminated?

____

20. You are transporting a hiker who became lost on a trail. He is shivering and hungry and has a temperature of 97°F (36.1°C). How would you treat this patient?

____

____

21. A firefighter dives into an ice-covered pond to rescue a child who has fallen through the ice on a windy, cold January evening. On the 10-minute walk back to the fire truck, the firefighter develops slurred speech and ataxia and complains that his heart is pounding. At the ambulance, his temperature is 89.5°F (31.9°C). His electrocardiogram is shown in Fig. 45-2.

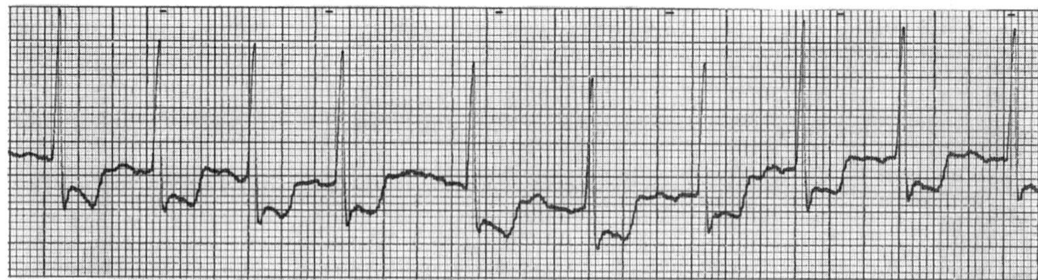

Figure **45-2**

a. What is your interpretation of the electrocardiogram tracing?

____

618

b. Describe your management of this patient.

____

____

____

Questions 22 to 24 refer to the following case study:
During a cross-country ski meet, a participant complains of coldness, numbness, and extreme pain in the fingers of his right hand.

22. Differentiate between the findings you would anticipate for superficial frostbite and deep frostbite.

____

____

23. List four factors that increase susceptibility to frostbite that you should look for in this patient.

a. ____

b. ____

c. ____

d. ____

24. How would you treat frostbite in this patient?

____

____

Questions 25 to 27 refer to the following case study:
A 2-year-old child pulled from a backyard pool is apneic and pulseless.

25. Identify four factors that will influence this patient's clinical outcome.

a. ____

b. ____

c. ____

d. ____

26. What complications do you anticipate if the patient is resuscitated?

____

____

____

619

27. Describe prehospital management of this child.

____

____

28. List five body areas on the patient where pain may occur resulting from SQUEEZE.

    a. _________________________________   **d.** _________________________________

    b. _________________________________   **e.** _________________________________

    c. _________________________________

29. A diver experiences acute distress immediately after rapidly surfacing from a deep dive.

    a. List five signs or symptoms of air embolism.

        a. _________________________________   **d.** _________________________________

        b. _________________________________   **e.** _________________________________

        c. _________________________________

    b. Describe special considerations necessary for care of this patient while you are providing advanced life support and transport.

____

____

30. A tourist at a local resort complains of severe joint pain, fatigue, vertigo, and paraesthesia 12 hours after returning from his first dive.

    a. What diving injury do you suspect?

____

    b. Describe prehospital management of this patient.

____

____

31. You respond to a mountain resort where a participant in a cycling event has become ill.

    a. List the three types of high-altitude illness.

        a. _________________________________

        b. _________________________________

        c. _________________________________

b. What single intervention is most critical to long-term improvement of a patient with high-altitude illness after the ABCs have been managed?

____

32. What is the most important organ that regulates body temperature?
  a. Heart
  b. Lungs
  c. Pituitary gland
  d. Skin

33. You are assessing firefighters in the rehab area of a major fire on a summer day. Your patient is dizzy and nauseated and has orthostatic hypotension. What should you do?
  a. Administer medication for his nausea.
  b. Ask him to rest for 15 minutes before returning to the fire.
  c. Have him drink a fluid-replacement beverage.
  d. Initiate an intravenous line and administer a fluid bolus.

34. What causes shock to develop in the patient with heat stroke?
  a. Fluid loss
  b. Myocardial depression
  c. Peripheral vasodilation
  d. All of the above

35. What is the most critical intervention for heat stroke?
  a. Fluid resuscitation
  b. Medication administration
  c. Rapid cooling in transit
  d. Rapid transport to a hospital

36. When does shivering stop in a hypothermic patient?
  a. The body temperature drops to 90°F (32.2°C).
  b. Glucose or glycogen is depleted.
  c. Excessive amounts of insulin are excreted.
  d. P_{CO_2} increases to more than 50 mm Hg.

37. How will you care for a frostbitten extremity?
  a. Apply a tourniquet.
  b. Elevate the affected extremity.
  c. Rewarm rapidly in hot water.
  d. Refreeze the injured extremity.

38. All drownings are characterized by which of the following?
  a. Hypovolemia, hypoxia, and acidosis
  b. Hypoxia, acidosis, and hypothermia
  c. Hypoxia, acidosis, and hypercapnia
  d. Hypovolemia, acidosis, and hypercapnia

39. Which of the following best describes the term *drowning*?
  a. Death from submersion up to 24 hours after arrival in the emergency department
  b. Death related to submersion that occurs at any time after the incident
  c. Impaired breathing from submersion or immersion in a liquid
  d. Swimming-related distress sufficient to require support in the prehospital setting

40. What is the single most important factor in determining survival after submersion injury?
  a. Age of the patient
  b. Contaminants in the water
  c. Duration of submersion
  d. Water temperature

41. Which law of physics states that the volume of gas is related inversely to its pressure at a constant temperature?
  a. Boyle's law
  b. Dalton's law
  c. Henry's law
  d. Newton's law

621

42. A diver is in respiratory distress after ascent. You palpate subcutaneous emphysema. He probably has which of the following conditions?
  a. Barotrauma of descent
  b. Decompression sickness
  c. Pulmonary air embolus
  d. Pulmonary overpressurization syndrome

43. What is the primary danger of nitrogen narcosis?
  a. Hypoxemia
  b. Impaired judgment
  c. Respiratory acidosis
  d. Shock resulting from hypovolemia

44. What is the critical sign or symptom that indicates deterioration in a patient with acute mountain sickness?
  a. Ataxia
  b. Headache
  c. Irritability
  d. Vomiting

WRAP IT UP

Searchers are trying to find a 50-year-old hunter who is evidently lost in a marshy area and has not been heard from in 18 hours. The weather is cold and windy, with temperatures the night before dropping to 40°F (4°C) and winds of up to 20 mph. An excited transmission on the radio lets you know that he has been found alive. Crews are going to bring him out to your staging area. He arrives in the bed of a pickup truck conscious but confused. Rescuers found him staggering in the swamp. His overalls are soaked, and his boots are full of water. You move him in the warm ambulance and quickly but gently remove his clothes and cover him with warm, dry blankets. Your partner puts a warm pack on his antecubital space to try to expose a vein to start an IV. Warmed, humidified oxygen is administered by mask, and his vital signs are taken. Because of the large number of exposure incidents in your area, you have a hypothermia thermometer and obtain a core temperature of 87°F (30.5°C), BP 100/60 mm Hg, P 56, R 16, and SaO_2 unobtainable; his skin is cool and pale. You initiate an IV of warmed normal saline and obtain a blood glucose, which is 78 mg/dL; electrocardiogram rhythm is sinus bradycardia. As you go en route to the hospital, medical direction asks you to infuse a fluid challenge of 250 mL and reassess the patient. You are sweating because of the heat in the patient compartment and check the heat packs you have placed in his armpits and groin to ensure they are still warm. While you perform your comprehensive exam, you note that his feet have a waxy, white appearance and that he appears to have severe pain when you palpate them. On arrival to the emergency department, his vital signs are BP 110/64 mm Hg, P 58, R 20, and temperature 90°F (32°C).

1. What was the equivalent wind chill factor at the coldest part of the night?

2. Which of the following mechanisms of heat loss played a role in this situation? Circle all that apply.
  a. Conduction
  b. Convection
  c. Evaporation
  d. Radiation

3. Place a ✓ beside the signs or symptoms that demonstrate moderate hypothermia that are found in this patient.

  a. _________ Atrial fibrillation
  b. _________ Ataxia
  c. _________ Bradycardia
  d. _________ Cardiac instability
  e. _________ Confusion
  f. _________ Fixed, dilated pupils
  g. _________ Loss of deep tendon reflexes
  h. _________ Shivering

4. Explain why the following interventions could be harmful in this patient.

  a. Vigorous movement

  ____

  b. IV lactated Ringer solution

  ____

c. Placing the patient in a high Fowler position

---

5. Which is true regarding the assessment findings of his feet?
 a. They are likely just cold and will rewarm last because of the distal circulation.
 b. This is evidence of extensive frostbite, and he will probably need amputations.
 c. Rewarming should not be attempted because of possible tissue damage.
 d. Trench foot is possible, and blisters may begin to form as he rewarms.

CHAPTER 45 ANSWERS

REVIEW QUESTIONS

1. g
(Objective 1)
2. k
(Objective 1)
3. a
(Objective 3)
4. i
(Objective 1)
5. b
(Objective 5)
6. e
(Objective 6)
7. h
(Objective 3)
8. d
(Objective 5)
9. j
(Objective 1)
10. f
(Objective 5)

11. a. Oxidation of energy sources; b. shivering can increase heat production by 400%; c. increased basal metabolic
 rate and vasoconstriction
(Objective 1)

12. a. Conduction, convection, and radiation; b. conduction and radiation; c. conduction, radiation, convection, and
 evaporation; d. conduction, radiation, convection, and evaporation
(Objective 1)

13. Skin vasodilation (becomes warm and flushed), sweating, decreased hormone secretion, and decreased
 muscle tone
(Objective 1)

14. Peripheral vasoconstriction (cool, pale skin), goose bumps, shivering, increased voluntary activity, increased
 hormone secretion, and increased appetite
(Objective 1)

15. a. Heat cramps. Remove the patient from the hot environment, replace sodium and water, and intravenously infuse
 saline solution if the patient's condition is severe.
 b. Heat exhaustion. Remove the patient from the hot environment and intravenously infuse saline solution.
 c. Heat stroke. Secure the airway, assess breathing, ventilate if indicated, administer high-flow oxygen, move
 the patient to a cool environment, remove all clothing, wet the skin with cool fluid, fan the patient, initiate
 intravenous fluid therapy with normal saline, consult with medical direction regarding a fluid challenge, and
 monitor for signs of fluid overload. If seizures recur, administer diazepam, assess for hypoglycemia, and
 administer D50W if indicated.
(Objective 2)

16. Increasing the metabolic rate increases the heart rate and contractility and increases the body's use of oxygen and other nutrients. The patient with preexisting trauma or illness will not tolerate these extra demands, which may compromise organ response to illness or injury.
(Objective 3)

17. Assess and secure the airway, assess breathing, and assist with 100% oxygen (warmed and humidified if available); if indicated, assess circulation and begin cardiopulmonary resuscitation only after verifying that no pulse is present. Move the patient to a warm environment and remove all clothing. Assess the body temperature. Begin warming.
(Objective 3)

18. Cardiopulmonary resuscitation; defibrillation at 360 J; monophasic; biphasic per manufacturer, usually 120 to 200 J intubation; ventilation with warm, humid oxygen; intravenous infusion of warm normal saline; withhold drugs until temperature is above 30°C (86°F); provide active internal rewarming and transport to the hospital.
(Objective 3)

19. Resuscitation may be withheld if there are obvious lethal injuries or if the body is frozen, preventing chest compression or airway management. Resuscitation could stop when the patient's core temperature has reached 94° to 95°F (34° to 35°C) and all resuscitation efforts are still unsuccessful.
(Objective 3)

20. Move the patient to a warm area, remove any wet clothing, and wrap the patient in a warm blanket. If he is awake and alert, administer warm, sugar-sweetened drinks (no alcohol, coffee, or tea). If necessary, apply hot packs wrapped in towels to the neck, armpits, and groin.
(Objective 3)

21. a. Atrial fibrillation
    b. Put the patient at rest and move to a warm environment after ensuring adequate airway, breathing, and circulation. Carefully remove all wet clothing and wrap the patient in a blanket. Administer 100% oxygen (heated and humidified if possible) by non-rebreather mask. Initiate intravenous therapy of normal saline (initial fluid challenge of 250–500 mL may be ordered by medical direction, and use warmed fluids if available). Transport gently, apply warm packs covered in towels to the groin and axilla, and monitor the patient carefully en route.
(Objective 3)

22. In deep frostbite, the underlying tissue is hard and not compressible, but in superficial frostbite, the underlying tissue springs back when palpated.
(Objective 3)

23. No protective clothing; preexisting illness or injury (diabetes or vascular insufficiency); fatigue; tobacco; tight, constrictive clothing; alcohol ingestion; and vasodilatory medications (some antihypertensives)
(Objective 3)

24. Elevate and protect the affected extremity, provide rapid transport to a medical facility, and assess for hypothermia.
(Objective 3)

25. Temperature of water, length of submersion, cleanliness of water, and age of patient
(Objective 4)

26. Acute respiratory failure, dysrhythmias, decreased cardiac output, cerebral edema leading to central nervous system dysfunction, and renal dysfunction (rare)
(Objective 4)

27. Ensure scene safety, initiate cardiopulmonary resuscitation, secure the airway with an endotracheal tube and ventilate with 100% oxygen, assess cardiac rhythm and follow advanced life support protocols to manage appropriately, assess for hypothermia, and transport to an appropriate medical facility.
(Objective 4)

28. Ears, sinuses, lungs and airways, gastrointestinal tract, thorax, and teeth
(Objective 6)

29. a. Focal paralysis or sensory changes, aphasia, confusion, blindness or another visual disturbance, convulsion, loss of consciousness, dizziness, vertigo, abdominal pain, and cardiac arrest

b. If the patient's trachea is intubated, fill the balloon with normal saline instead of air; evaluate for pulmonary over pressurization syndrome (POPS); and transport in the left lateral recumbent position with a 15-degree elevation of the thorax.
   (Objective 6)

30. a. Decompression sickness
    b. Administer high-flow oxygen, initiate intravenous therapy, and rapidly transport for recompression (follow local protocol so that patient can reach hyperbaric chamber as quickly as possible).
    (Objective 6)

31. a. Acute mountain sickness, high-altitude pulmonary edema, and high altitude cerebral edema; b. Descent to a lower altitude
    (Objective 6)

32. d. Vasoconstriction and vasodilation of the blood vessels in the skin are the major ways the body releases or conserves heat.
    (Objective 1)

33. d. Based on his symptoms, you suspect heat exhaustion. Because he is nauseated and has orthostatic hypotension, he needs intravenous rather than oral rehydration. He should be moved to a cool environment and not returned to the fire.
    (Objective 2)

34. d
    (Objective 2)

35. c. Damage to the body continues as long as the temperature remains elevated.
    (Objective 2)

36. b. Shivering should continue until the core temperature reaches 86°F (30°C). A tremendous amount of energy is needed for shivering, so glucose and glycogen must be available to fuel this increased muscle activity.
    (Objective 3)

37. b. Rapid rewarming in warm water is indicated only when sanctioned by medical direction if no chance of refreezing exists. Refreezing is damaging to the tissues.
    (Objective 3)

38. c. The lack of ventilation causes a buildup of carbon dioxide, which coupled with the lack of oxygen intake (hypoxia) leads to acidosis.
    (Objective 4)

39. c. The Utstein definition of drowning is now recommended.
    (Objective 4)

40. c. Although each factor listed influences patient outcome after submersion, the duration of submersion and degree of hypoxia are the critical elements that determine the odds of survival.
    (Objective 4)

41. a. Dalton's law states that the total pressure of a mixture of gases is equal to the sum of the partial pressures of the component gases. Henry's law states that the amount of gas dissolved in a given volume of fluid is proportional to the pressure of the gas with which it is in equilibrium. Newton's law states that a body at rest will remain at rest until acted on by an outside force, and a body in motion will remain in motion until acted on by an outside force.
    (Objective 5)

42. d. As trapped air in the lungs expands on rapid ascent, it ruptures alveoli and allows gas to leak into the subcutaneous tissues.
    (Objective 6)

43. b. The neurodepressant effects of nitrogen narcosis may lead to diving accidents resulting from impaired judgment.
    (Objective 6)

44. a. Ataxia signals progression of the illness, and coma may result within 24 hours of its onset.
    (Objective 6)

625

Chapter **45** **Environmental Conditions**

1. 18°F (-8°C)
   (Objective 1)

2. a, b, d. Conduction causes heat loss from warm skin to cold air or water; convection causes heat loss from the 20 mph wind blowing over; radiation is the heat radiating off his skin.
   (Objective 1)

3. b, c, e. Loss of deep tendon reflexes and dilated pupils are signs of severe hypothermia. Shivering typically has stopped by when the patient has moderate hypothermia.
   (Objective 3)

4. a. The heart become irritable in hypothermia, and vigorous movement can trigger ventricular fibrillation.
   b. The cold liver is unable to metabolize the lactate.
   c. Orthostatic hypotension may result if the patient is moved to a sitting position.
   (Objective 3)

5. d. Prolonged exposure to very cold water can cause trench foot. He will likely develop signs and symptoms similar to frostbite as he rewarms.
   (Objective 3)

46 | Obstetrics

READING ASSIGNMENT

Chapter 46, pages 1273-1306, in *Mosby's Paramedic Textbook,* ed. 4.

OBJECTIVES

Upon completion of this chapter, the paramedic student will be able to do the following:

1. Describe the basic anatomy and physiology of the changes in the female reproductive system.
2. Outline fetal development from ovulation through birth.
3. Explain normal maternal physiologic changes that occur during pregnancy and how they influence prehospital patient care and transportation.
4. Describe appropriate information to be elicited during the obstetric patient's history.
5. Describe specific techniques for assessment of the pregnant patient.
6. Describe the general prehospital care of the pregnant patient.
7. Discuss the special implications of trauma in pregnancy.
8. Outline principles of care for a pregnant patient in cardiac arrest or peri-arrest.
9. Recognize and begin treatment for complications of pregnancy such as hyperemesis gravidarum, Rh sensitization, diabetes mellitus, and infection.
10. Describe the assessment and management of patients with preeclampsia and eclampsia.
11. Explain the pathophysiology, signs and symptoms, and management of vaginal bleeding in pregnancy.
12. Outline the physiologic changes that occur during the stages of labor.
13. Describe the role of the paramedic during normal labor and delivery.
14. Compute an Apgar score.
15. Describe assessment and management of postpartum hemorrhage.
16. Discuss the identification, implications, and prehospital management of complicated deliveries.

SUMMARY

- Cultural differences may influence a woman's response to pregnancy and childbirth. Paramedics should be sensitive to these cultural beliefs.
- Fertilization of an ovum by a sperm forms a zygote that divides as it passes through the fallopian tube to become a morula. The trophoblast cells of the morula implant within 7 days after fertilization and transform into the life support systems of the embryo. The blastocyst cells develop into the embryo.
- The placenta is a disklike organ. It is composed of interlocking fetal and maternal tissues. It is the organ of exchange between the mother and fetus. Blood flows from the fetus to the placenta through two umbilical arteries. These arteries carry deoxygenated blood. Oxygenated blood returns to the fetus through the umbilical vein. The amniotic sac is a fluid-filled bag. It completely surrounds and protects the embryo.
- The developing ovum is known as an embryo during the first 8 weeks of pregnancy. After that time and until birth, it is called a fetus. Gestation (fetal development) usually averages 40 weeks from the time of fertilization to the delivery of the newborn.
- At birth, in normal newborns, the atriovenous shunts present in fetuses close.
- Gravida is the total number of current and past pregnancies. *Para* refers to past pregnancies that resulted in a live birth.
- The pregnant woman undergoes many physiologic changes that affect the genital tract, breasts, gastrointestinal system, cardiovascular system, respiratory system, and metabolism.
- The patient history should include obstetric history; presence of pain; presence, quantity, and character of vaginal bleeding; presence of abnormal vaginal discharge; presence of "bloody show"; current general health and prenatal care; allergies and medicines taken; and maternal urge to bear down.
- The goal in examining an obstetric patient is to rapidly identify acute life-threatening conditions. A part of this involves recognizing imminent delivery. Then the paramedic must take the proper management steps. In addition to the routine physical examination, the paramedic should assess the abdomen, uterine size, and fetal heart sounds.
- If birth is not imminent, the paramedic should limit prehospital care for the healthy patient. It should be limited to basic treatment modalities. It should include transport for physician evaluation as well.

- Causes of fetal death from maternal trauma include death of the mother, separation of the placenta, maternal shock, uterine rupture, and fetal head injury.
- To treat a critically ill pregnant patient, administer high-concentration oxygen. Tilt the patient left lateral. Administer intravenous fluid if there are signs of shock. Aggressively resuscitate the mother in an attempt to save the baby. Cardiac arrest can occur from a number of causes. Rapid transport is indicated.
- Hyperemesis gravidarum presents with severe nausea, vomiting, weight loss, and electrolyte disturbance. Fluid therapy is indicated if there are signs of dehydration.
- Rh sensitization occurs if the mother has Rh negative blood and the baby Rh positive blood. It can cause anemia, jaundice, edema, an enlarged liver or spleen, and hydrops.
- Gestational hypertension is onset of blood pressure greater than 140/90 mm Hg during pregnancy. It can indicate preeclampsia.
- Preeclampsia occurs after 20 weeks' gestation. The criteria for diagnosis include hypertension, protein in the urine, and excessive weight gain with edema. Eclampsia is characterized by the same signs and symptoms with the addition of seizures or coma.
- Gestational diabetes mellitus is diabetes caused by pregnancy.
- Infection during pregnancy can place the mother and fetus at risk. TORCH is an acronym for infections the mother can pass to the fetus that cause fetal death or complication.
- Vaginal bleeding during pregnancy can result from abortion (miscarriage), ectopic pregnancy, abruptio placentae, placenta previa, uterine rupture, or postpartum hemorrhage. Abortion is the termination of pregnancy from any cause before 20 weeks' gestation. Ectopic pregnancy occurs when a fertilized ovum implants anywhere other than the uterus. Abruptio placentae is partial or complete detachment of the placenta at more than 20 weeks' gestation. Placenta previa is placental implantation in the lower uterine segment partially or completely covering the cervical opening. Uterine rupture is a spontaneous or traumatic rupture of the uterine wall.
- The first stage of labor begins with the onset of regular contractions and ends with complete dilation of the cervix. The second stage of labor is measured from full dilation of the cervix to delivery of the infant. The third stage of labor begins with delivery of the infant and ends when the placenta is expelled and the uterus has contracted.
- One of the primary responsibilities of the EMS crew is to prevent an uncontrolled delivery. The other is to protect the infant from cold and stress after birth.
- Criteria for computing the Apgar score include appearance (color), pulse (heart rate), grimace (reflex irritability), activity (muscle tone), and respiratory effort.
- More than 500 mL of blood loss after the delivery of a newborn is called a postpartum hemorrhage. It often results from ineffective or incomplete contraction of the uterus.
- Paramedics should be alert to factors that point to a possible abnormal delivery.
- Cephalopelvic disproportion produces a difficult labor because of the presence of a small pelvis, an oversized uterus, or fetal abnormalities. Most infants are born head first (cephalic or vertex presentation). However, sometimes a presentation is abnormal. In breech presentation, the largest part of the fetus (the head) is delivered last. Shoulder dystocia occurs when the fetal shoulders impact against the maternal symphysis pubis. This blocks shoulder delivery. Shoulder presentation (transverse presentation) results when the long axis of the fetus lies perpendicular to that of the mother. The fetal arm or hand may be the presenting part. Cord presentation occurs when the umbilical cord slips down into the vagina or presents externally.
- A premature infant is born before 37 weeks' gestation.
- A multiple gestation is a pregnancy with more than one fetus. It is accompanied by an increased complication rate.
- A precipitous delivery is a rapid spontaneous delivery with less than 3 hours from the onset of labor to birth. The main danger to the fetus is from cerebral trauma or tearing of the umbilical cord.
- Uterine inversion is a rare complication of childbirth. It is a serious complication. With this condition, the uterus turns "inside out."
- The development of pulmonary embolism during pregnancy, labor, or the postpartum period is a significant cause of maternal death.
- Premature rupture of the membranes is a rupture of the amniotic sac before the onset of labor regardless of gestational age.
- An amniotic fluid embolism may occur when amniotic fluid enters the maternal circulation during labor or delivery or immediately after delivery.

Match the complications of pregnancy in column II with their description in column I. Use each term only once.

Column I

1. _______ Can cause dehydration and electrolyte imbalance

2. _______ Unintentional termination of pregnancy before 20 weeks

3. _______ Cause of sudden maternal death

4. _______ Infections of pregnant woman harmful to the fetus

5. _______ Sydrome associated with liver problems and abnormal clotting

6. _______ Causes large infant weight and difficult delivery

Column II

a. Amniotic fluid embolus
b. Erythroblastosis fetalis
c. Gestational diabetes
d. HELLP
e. Hyperemesis gravidarum
f. Spontaneous abortion
g. TORCH

Match the problems of pregnancy in column II with their description in column I. Use each problem only once.

Column I

7. _______ Painless bleeding in third trimester of pregnancy

8. _______ Hypertension, proteinuria, and visual disturbance in the third trimester

9. _______ Severe abdominal pain, shock, and easily palpable fetal parts

10. _______ Painful third-trimester bleeding

11. _______ Third-trimester seizure after a new onset of hypertension

12. _______ Abdominal pain, scant vaginal bleeding, and shock in the first trimester

Column II

a. Abortion
b. Abruptio placentae
c. Eclampsia
d. Ectopic pregnancy
e. Placenta previa
f. Preeclampsia
g. Uterine rupture

13. In what lunar month do the following fetal development characteristics typically occur?

a. Fetal movement felt by the mother:

____

b. Fetal heart beat:

____

c. Distinct fingers and toes:

____

d. Eyebrows and fingernails:

____

e. Possible viability if born:

____

14. What causes the arteriovenous shunts to close at birth?

____

____

15. What do the following pregnancy terms mean?

    a. A patient is gravida 6 para 5 (G6P5).

    ____

    b. She is a multipara.

    ____

    c. The patient has postpartum bleeding.

    ____

    d. You are called to care for a nullipara who is term.

    ____

16. A woman in her 40th week of pregnancy complains of heartburn, dizziness, and frequency of urination. Her heart rate is 100 beats/min; respirations are 20 breaths/min and deep; and blood pressure is 90/60 mm Hg. (She says her normal is 100/70 mm Hg.) She has slight edema of the ankles and tortuous varicose veins. Explain how the physiologic alterations of pregnancy cause each of the signs or symptoms she is experiencing.

    a. Heartburn:

    ____

    ____

    b. Dizziness:

    ____

    ____

    c. Frequency of urination:

    ____

    ____

    d. Hypotension:

    ____

    ____

    e. Pedal edema and varicose veins:

    ____

    ____

17. Briefly explain why each of the following historical findings would cause concern if delivery is imminent in the field:

   a. No prenatal care:

   b. Diabetic mother:

   c. Vaginal bleeding:

   d. Current heroin intoxication:

   e. Foul-smelling vaginal discharge and maternal fever.

Questions 18 to 20 refer to the following case study:

A 28-year-old woman who is in her third trimester complains of abdominal pain after an automobile accident in which she was the unrestrained driver. She is pale, and her vital signs are blood pressure, 90/60 mm Hg; pulse, 134 beats/min; and respirations, 28 breaths/min. Her abdomen is tender to palpation, and you note some vaginal bleeding.

18. What other subjective information do you need from the mother?

19. How can you determine whether the infant is in distress?

20. Describe prehospital care and transport of this patient.

633

A 30-year-old woman says she is 9 weeks pregnant and complains of severe cramping pain in the lower abdomen and vaginal bleeding. She states that she has saturated six sanitary napkins and passed some "white, stringy stuff" that her husband shows you in the toilet.

21. What condition of pregnancy do you suspect?

22. What actions should you take so that the physician can determine whether she has had a complete abortion?

23. Estimate her blood loss if you believe the history was accurate.

24. Why might this patient be exhibiting a grief reaction?

25. An obstetrician calls you to his office to transport a 28-year-old woman who has an ectopic pregnancy (determined by ultrasonography). She complains of severe abdominal pain and has frank signs of shock.

    a. What other signs or symptoms might she experience?

    b. Describe interventions you will use on your 20-minute trip to the emergency department.

26. What general patient care measures should be taken for any patient who has third trimester bleeding without shock?

Questions 27 to 31 refer to the following case study:

A 40-year-old primipara in the third trimester complains of headache, dizziness, and nausea. Vital signs are blood pressure, 160/100 mm Hg; pulse, 110 beats/min; and respirations, 20 breaths/min. Her hands and feet are considerably swollen, and you note intermittent facial twitching. She says her doctor was worried about protein in her urine.

27. What complication do you suspect?

28. In what position should you transport this patient?

634

29. List two drugs with appropriate doses that may be ordered by medical direction to stop seizure activity in these types of patients.

____

30. Besides medication, what emergency medical services actions can minimize the risk of seizures?

____

31. What risks to the fetus exist with this condition?

____

____

Questions 32 to 36 refer to the following case study:

You are called to a private residence 30 minutes from the nearest hospital to care for a woman in labor.

32. What information in the patient's medical history is important to help gauge how quickly labor will progress?

____

____

33. What specific signs or symptoms during labor would lead you to believe that delivery is imminent?

____

____

34. As the baby's head delivers, what assessment and interventions should you perform?

____

____

35. Describe the procedure to clamp the umbilical cord.

____

____

36. When should the Apgar score be calculated?

____

37. If necessary, when should oxytocin be administered, and what is the proper dose and route?

____

38. Labor fails to progress after a baby in breech position is delivered to the level of the chest. Describe the steps you should take in this situation.

____

____

39. After the head of a baby with shoulder dystocia is delivered, what can you do to deliver the shoulders while minimizing fetal injury?

40. A 35-year-old woman who is G6P5 states that she is ready to deliver her baby at home. Her membranes have ruptured, her contractions are frequent, and she wants to push. When you examine her perineum, you see the umbilical cord protruding from the vagina.

    a. What actions should you take immediately to prevent fetal hypoxia?

    b. Should you attempt to deliver this baby on the scene?

STUDENT SELF-ASSESSMENT

41. Which of the following is a function of the placenta?
    a. Detoxifies wastes
    b. Hormone production
    c. Metabolism of drugs
    d. Food digestion

42. What is the primary role of amniotic fluid?
    a. Excretion
    b. Hydration
    c. Nutrition
    d. Protection

43. Which fetal structure allows blood to bypass the liver and go directly into the inferior vena cava?
    a. Ductus arteriosus
    b. Ductus venosus
    c. Foramen ovale
    d. Umbilical vein

44. What does the umbilical cord carry?
    a. Deoxygenated blood by one umbilical artery and oxygenated blood by one umbilical vein
    b. Deoxygenated blood by two umbilical arteries and oxygenated blood by one umbilical vein
    c. Oxygenated blood by one umbilical artery and deoxygenated blood by one umbilical vein
    d. Oxygenated blood by two umbilical arteries and deoxygenated blood by one umbilical vein

45. Where should the uterus be palpable at week 20 of gestation?
    a. At the lower border of the umbilicus
    b. Between the symphysis pubis and umbilicus
    c. Halfway between the umbilicus and the xiphoid
    d. Just above the symphysis pubis

46. Which of the following is the normal fetal heart rate?
    a. 80 to 120 beats/min
    b. 120 to 160 beats/min
    c. 160 to 200 beats/mine
    d. 200 to 240 beats/min

47. In which position should the hypotensive pregnant patient who is more than 4 months' gestation be transported?
    a. High Fowler
    b. Left lateral recumbent
    c. Prone
    d. Supine

48. Immediately after the delivery of a healthy baby, your patient's eyes roll back, and she becomes pulseless. She has no previous medical history. What is a likely cause of her cardiac arrest?
    a. Abruptio placentae
    b. Amniotic fluid embolism
    c. Aortic dissection
    d. Congestive cardiomyopathy

636

49. When attempting to resuscitate a patient in cardiac arrest who is 8 months pregnant, what special care measures should you use to be most effective?
    a. Decrease ventilation volumes to minimize gastric distension.
    b. Increase the dose of epinephrine to maximize vasoconstriction.
    c. Perform chest compressions lower on the sternum.
    d. Use your hands to displace the uterus to the left.

50. How is eclampsia distinguished from preeclampsia?
    a. Edema
    b. Glucosuria
    c. Hypertension
    d. Seizures

51. What assessment finding indicates a complication from administration of magnesium sulfate?
    a. BP 190/110 mmHg
    b. Blood glucose 200 mg/dL
    c. $etCO_2$ 50 mmHg
    d. Heart rate 140/min

52. What may occur if the paramedic applies excessive traction on the umbilical cord during placental delivery?
    a. Fetal distress
    b. Placenta previa
    c. Uterine inversion
    d. Uterine rupture

53. Which of the following occurs in the second stage of labor?
    a. Cervical dilation
    b. Delivery of the infant
    c. Expulsion of the placenta
    d. Fetal descent into the birth canal

54. When delivering a baby's head, you note that the umbilical cord is wrapped around the baby's neck. What is the first action you should take?
    a. Cut the cord in two places, clamp it, and proceed with delivery.
    b. Elevate the mother's hips and have her pant until you reach the hospital.
    c. Gently unloop the cord around and over the baby's head.
    d. No special action is needed; the cord will free itself as the shoulders deliver.

55. One minute after delivery, a baby has a weak cry, a pink body with blue extremities, and a pulse of 128 beats/min; he actively moves about and sneezes when a catheter is introduced into his nose. What is the Apgar score?
    a. 6
    b. 7
    c. 8
    d. 9

56. A large amount of blood and clots are flowing from the mother's vagina 10 minutes after the placenta is delivered. Which measure is most important to slow the hemorrhage?
    a. Infuse normal saline boluses.
    b. Administer magnesium sulfate.
    c. Pack the vagina with sterile dressings.
    d. Provide vigorous uterine massage.

57. For which of the following is the premature infant at risk?
    a. Gestational diabetes
    b. Hypothermia
    c. Placenta previa
    d. Seizures

58. What is a frequent complication of multiple gestation?
    a. Eclampsia
    b. Placenta previa
    c. Premature delivery
    d. Uterine rupture

59. Which complication of pregnancy is most likely to require delivery by cesarean section?
    a. Breech presentation
    b. Cephalopelvic disproportion
    c. Shoulder dystocia
    d. Vaginal bleeding

60. A 30-year-old woman develops dyspnea and severe chest pain 24 hours after delivery of her third child. She is hypotensive and in acute distress. Based on her history, you suspect which of the following?
    a. Eclampsia
    b. Myocardial infarction
    c. Pneumonia
    d. Pulmonary embolism

61. What is the primary danger to an infant delivered during a precipitous delivery?
    a. Abruptio placentae
    b. Cerebral trauma
    c. Nuchal cord
    d. Placenta previa

62. Which of the following describes chorioamnionitis?
    a. Amniotic fluid embolism
    b. Excessive amniotic fluid
    c. Infection of fetal membranes
    d. Premature rupture of the membranes

637

63. Which intervention is most appropriate if your patient has severe hyperemesis gravidarum?

    a. Ondansetron (Zofran) 4 mg IV

    b. Metoclopramide (Reglan) 25 mg IV

    c. Prochlorperazine (Compazine) 5 mg IV

    d. Promethazine (Phenergan) 25 mg IV

WRAP IT UP

You are dispatched for a "maternity case." Your 30-year-old patient is on the sofa, saying, "I've got to push!" As you prepare to check her perineum, you obtain a quick history: She is due in 8 weeks, her bag of waters ruptured with clear fluid, there is one fetus, and she denies using narcotic drugs. Her perineum is bulging, and there is evidence of mucousy bloody show, so you call for additional personnel. Your partner hears fetal heart tones inferior to the umbilicus at 150 beats/min. The patient has another contraction, moaning loudly, "The baby's coming." The baby's head is now visible at the perineum, so you prepare for imminent delivery and open the OB kit. She says she has two children at home and no miscarriages or other health problems. Your partner moves to the ambulance to open the pediatric resuscitation bag and set up for neonatal resuscitation. You don a face shield, gown, and a clean pair of gloves, and then the patient's next contraction begins—you estimate they are 2 to 3 minutes apart. You encourage her to push, and you see the baby's forehead appear and then retract slightly when the contraction ends. Coaching her breathing, you arrange towels under her buttocks, elevating them slightly, and prepare some clean towels and blankets for the baby. With the next contraction, the baby's head delivers face down. While supporting the baby's head with one hand, you insert a finger in the vagina and sweep around the neck to feel for the presence of the cord; there is none. Then, taking the bulb syringe from your kit, you suction the fluids from the baby's mouth and then nose, clearing the thick, clear mucus. As the next contraction begins, the baby rotates laterally, and you guide the baby downward to deliver the first shoulder and up to free the other; then the baby slips quickly from the birth canal. It's a girl, and she is very slippery and hard to hold on to. You hold her level with her mother's perineum and begin to warm and dry her, vigorously rubbing her back to stimulate the floppy baby to breathe. The umbilical cord is clamped and cut after it stops pulsating, and at 1 minute, you note the baby is still pale and blue. Her heart rate is 100 beats/min; she grimaces and has some flexion, but her muscle tone is generally floppy; and she has slow, irregular respirations. You apply oxygen, position her on her back with her shoulders slightly elevated, and flick her feet to stimulate her. She is becoming pinker and has brisk capillary refill, and at 5 minutes, her heart rate is 140 beats/min, but even though she is breathing, there is no brisk cry or cough, she grimaces, and her body is now completely pink; in fact, it looks very red. You remove the wet towel and cover her (including her head) with warm blankets, apply an oxygen saturation monitor, and continue the blow-by oxygen, continually monitoring her respiratory effort. She is very small, around 5 lb (2.3 kg), you guess. In the meantime, your partner has been caring for the mother, who has delivered the placenta. She has brisk bleeding from the vagina and cramping. He has started an IV and administered oxytocin intramuscularly. Her vital signs are stable, and she is asking about her baby. Your partner massages the mother's fundus, which she finds uncomfortable. You arrive at the hospital in 8 minutes, where the neonatal resuscitation team is awaiting your arrival. They immediately take the baby; evaluate her in the emergency department, where her saturation and heart rate are good; allow the mother to hold the baby for a moment and then take the baby to the neonatal ICU, where they tell the mother they will intubate her because of her premature status. One week later, baby is discharged to home in good health.

1. What stage of labor is the mother in when you arrive?

2. Why is this baby at risk for complications during or after delivery?

3. What was the baby's Apgar score?

    a. At 1 minute:

    b. At 5 minutes:

4. What additional resuscitation measures would you have performed immediately if the baby's color and heart rate did not improve after oxygen administration?
   a. Begin ventilation using a bag-mask device and oxygen.
   b. Give epinephrine 0.01 mg/kg.
   c. Initiate vascular access by cannulation of the umbilicus.
   d. Intubate the trachea and ventilate at a rate of 20 per minute.

5. **a.** What head presentation did you note at delivery?

   b. Is this normal or abnormal?

   ____

6. What action would you have taken if you palpated the cord around his neck?

   ____

7. Why did you hold the baby at the level of the mother's perineum until the umbilical cord was cut?

   ____

8. What should be done with the placenta?

   ____

9. Where should the cord be cut?

   ____

10. Explain your rationale for the following interventions:

    a. Stimulation of the baby:

    ____

    ____

    b. Elevation of the baby's shoulders:

    ____

    c. Massage of the mother's abdomen:

    ____

    d. Administration of oxytocin:

    ____

CHAPTER 46 ANSWERS

REVIEW QUESTIONS

1. e
   (Objective 9)

2. f
   (Objective 9)

3. a
(Objective 9)

4. g
(Objective 9)

5. d
(Objective 10)

6. c
(Objective 9)

7. e
(Objective 9)

8. f
(Objective 10)

9. g
(Objective 11)

10. b
(Objective 11)

11. c
(Objective 10)

12. d
(Objective 11)

13. a. Fifth
b. Fourth
c. Third
d. Sixth
e. Eighth
(Objective 2)

14. The rapid increase in systemic vascular resistance, aortic pressure, and left ventricular and left atrial pressures after placental flow stops and the decrease in pulmonary vascular resistance resulting from expansion of the lungs cause atrioventricular shunts to close within a few hours after birth.
(Objective 2)

15. a. She has had six pregnancies and delivered five children.
b. She has had two or more deliveries.
c. The patient had bleeding after delivery of her baby.
d. You are called to care for a woman who has never delivered and whose pregnancy has reached 40 weeks of gestation.
(Objective 4)

16. a. Decreased tone and motility of the gastrointestinal tract, which leads to slow gastric emptying and relaxation of the pyloric sphincter
b. Decreased Pco_2 caused by increased respiratory rate and tidal volume late in pregnancy
c. Pressure that the gravid uterus places directly on the bladder when the fetal head moves down in the pelvis near term
d. Blood pressure decreases 10 to 15 mm Hg during the second semester and gradually increases to prepregnant levels near term. (The patient should be questioned about her normal blood pressure.)
e. Impaired venous return resulting from the pressure the uterus exerts
(Objective 3)

640

17. a. Problems such as maternal nutrition, growth of fetus, maternal diabetes, and preeclampsia would not have been managed; an increased risk of fetal and maternal problems at birth exists.
   b. Increased birth weight of the baby may make field delivery difficult or impossible if cephalopelvic disproportion is present.
   c. Vaginal bleeding may indicate abruptio placentae, placenta previa, or uterine rupture. All of these conditions cause an increase in fetal mortality rate and pose a risk of maternal shock and death.
   d. Recent maternal narcotic intoxication causes neonatal respiratory depression and increases the risk of complications in the field.
   e. Bacterial infection can cause infant illness or death.
   (Objective 9)

18. When did she last feel fetal movement? What other medical problems does she have? What other medications does she take? Is she having any contractions?
   (Objective 5)

19. Assess fetal heart tones. (A persistent fetal heart rate of greater than 160 beats/min or less than 120 beats/min is an early sign of fetal distress and fetal or maternal hypoxia.) Ask the mother to report fetal movement to you.
   (Objective 5)

20. Administer 100% oxygen by non-rebreather mask (monitoring oxygen saturation with pulse oximeter, if available). Immobilize the patient on a backboard and roll the backboard to the left side. Initiate intravenous lactated Ringer solution or normal saline (two large-bore lines) en route to the nearest appropriate trauma center and frequently reassess vital signs, fetal heart tones, and the amount of vaginal bleeding en route.
   (Objective 7)

21. Spontaneous abortion
   (Objective 9)

22. Retrieve the tissue from the toilet and give it to the emergency department staff so a pathologist can examine it for completeness.
   (Objective 9)

23. 6 sanitary napkins × 20 to 30 mL/pad = 120 to 180 mL of blood lost.
   (Objective 9)

24. Pregnant women are often attached to the fetus and grieve when they know that their baby has died. This fact is especially true if a similar event has happened to the patient in the past.
   (Objective 5)

25. a. Vaginal bleeding, shoulder pain, nausea, vomiting, and syncope
   b. Administer 100% oxygen by non-rebreather mask. Consider use of pneumatic antishock garments (controversial). While en route, initiate two large-bore intravenous lines and infuse boluses of normal saline or lactated Ringer solution. Place the patient in modified Trendelenburg position if signs and symptoms of shock do not improve, and report her condition and diagnosis to the receiving hospital so that operative preparations can be made.
   (Objective 9)

26. Administer 100% oxygen by a non-rebreather mask. Place the patient in the left lateral recumbent position. Initiate precautionary intravenous lactated Ringer solution or normal saline en route to the hospital. Rapidly transport the patient to the closest appropriate medical center and monitor maternal vital signs and fetal heart tones.
   (Objective 6)

27. Preeclampsia
   (Objective 10)

28. Left lateral recumbent
   (Objective 10)

29. Magnesium sulfate 10% (1–4 g slow intravenous infusion) and diazepam (5 mg slow intravenous) or lorazepam (1-4 mg slow IV) over 2 minutes
(Objective 10)

30. Minimized stimulation and gentle patient handling. Avoid lights and sirens if possible.
(Objective 10)

31. Abruptio placentae is a complication, and maternal apnea during a seizure may cause fetal hypoxia.
(Objective 10)

32. How many previous deliveries has she had, and how quickly did they progress? How long has she been in labor, and how close are the contractions?
(Objective 4)

33. Contractions lasting 45 to 60 seconds at 1- to 2-minute intervals; measurement from beginning of one contraction to the beginning of the next; patient who wants to bear down or have a bowel movement; large amount of bloody show; crowning; and mother's feeling that delivery is imminent
(Objective 12)

34. Examine for the presence of a nuchal cord. If this cord is present, gently slip it over the infant's head or, if this is not possible, clamp it in two places and cut between the clamps to release the cord. If the cord is cut, ensure that the rest of the delivery proceeds rapidly because the baby has no source of oxygen. Suction the fluids from the baby's mouth and nose with a bulb syringe. Deliver the shoulders.
(Objective 13)

35. Clamp 6 to 9 inches from the infant in two places. Cut between the clamps with sterile scissors or a scalpel. Examine the cord to ensure that no bleeding exists.
(Objective 13)

36. At 1 minute and 5 minutes of age
(Objective 14)

37. After delivery of the baby, 10 units of oxytocin in 1000 mL of lactated Ringer solution infused at 20 to 30 gtt/min on microdrip tubing
(Objectives 15)

38. If the head does not deliver immediately, place a gloved hand in the vagina with the palm toward the baby's face. Form a V, with the index and middle fingers on either side of the baby's nose, and push the vaginal wall from the face until delivery. If the head does not deliver within 3 minutes, maintain the airway as described and transport the patient to the receiving hospital.
(Objective 16)

39. Position the mother on her left side in the knee-chest position. Guide the baby's head downward to allow the anterior shoulder to slip under the symphysis pubis; avoid excess force. Rotate the fetal shoulder girdle into the wider oblique pelvic diameter and deliver the posterior and then the anterior shoulders.
(Objective 16)

40. a. Elevate the mother's hips, administer oxygen, and ask the mother to pant with contractions to avoid bearing down. With gloved hand, gently push the baby's presenting part back into the vagina and elevate it to relieve pressure on the cord. Maintain this position while rapidly transporting the patient to the receiving hospital.
b. No, this baby will have to be delivered by cesarean section.
(Objective 16)

41. b. The placenta secretes estrogen and progesterone. It excretes rather than detoxifying wastes. It prevents passage of some drugs from the maternal circulation.
(Objective 1)

42. d. Although amniotic fluid originates from fetal urine and secretions from the respiratory tract, skin, and amniotic membranes, its primary function is protection.
(Objective 1)

642

43. b. The ductus arteriosus connects the aorta and pulmonary artery, and the foramen ovale provides a passageway for blood directly from the right to the left atrium. The umbilical cord connects the placenta to the embryo and is its lifeline. (Objective 2)

44. b
(Objective 1)

45. a. At week 12, the uterus is just above the symphysis pubis; at week 16, it is between the symphysis pubis and the umbilicus; and at week 28, it is halfway between the umbilicus and the xiphoid. (Objective 5)

46. b. A persistent rate greater than 160 beats/min or below 120 beats/min is a sign of fetal distress and fetal or maternal hypoxia. (Objective 5)

47. b. This position prevents pressure from being exerted on the inferior vena cava. (Objective 6)

48. b. Maternal mortality from pregnancy-related causes is rare. If the patient had abruptio placentae, a healthy delivery would be unlikely. Aortic dissection and congestive cardiomyopathy may cause maternal death, but amniotic fluid embolism is more likely at the time of delivery. (Objective 8)

49. d. Drug doses and ventilations do not need to be modified. Alternately, the patient may be tilted 30 degrees to the left using a wedge. (Objective 8)

50. d. Edema and hypertension are found in both. (Objective 10)

51. c. Magnesium also can cause clinically significant hypotension. (Objective 10)

52. c. Uterine inversion also may happen, although less frequently, after a contraction, cough, or sneeze. (Objective 13)

53. b. During the prodromal period, the fetus descends into the birth canal. In the first stage, the cervix dilates completely, and in the third stage, the placenta is delivered. (Objective 12)

54. c. Usually the cord can be freed in this manner. If this action fails and the decision is made to cut the cord after your medical direction protocols, delivery must be expedited or the baby will experience severe hypoxia and risk of death. (Objectives 16)

55. c. Weak cry (1); plus pink body and blue extremities (1); plus pulse at 128 beats/min (2), plus active movement (2); plus sneeze (2) = 8 (Objective 14)

56. d. The IV fluid is indicated but will not slow bleeding. Oxytocin is given, not magnesium sulfate. Magnesium sulfate is indicated for eclampsia in pregnancy. Packing is not indicated. (Objective 15)

57. b. Premature infants have a large surface area-to-mass ratio and are susceptible to hypothermia. In addition, a potential for cardiorespiratory dysfunction exists because of immaturity. (Objective 16)

58. c. Other complications include abruptio placentae, postpartum hemorrhage, and abnormal presentation. (Objective 16)

643

59. b. In this condition, the pelvic ring is too small to allow passage of the baby's head.
(Objective 16)

60. d. Pulmonary embolism or, more rarely, amniotic fluid embolism can cause these signs and symptoms.
(Objective 9)

61. b. Tearing of the umbilical cord is also a risk.
(Objective 16)

62. c. This condition often occurs after prolonged premature rupture of the membranes.
(Objective 9)

63. a. Ondansetron and metoclopramide both have Category B recommendations in pregnancy; however, the dose of Reglan listed is incorrect. The other drugs are Category C drugs in pregnancy and would therefore not be as safe.
(Objective 9)

WRAP IT UP

1. Stage II (expulsion stage)
(Objective 12)

2. Baby is premature based on mother's history
(Objective 14)

3. a. 1-minute Apgar: 4
b. 5-minute Apgar: 7
(Objective 14)

4. a. Assisted ventilation may be all that is necessary to open the small airway and stimulate normal breathing in the infant.
(Objectives 16)

5. a. Vertex (cephalic); this is normal
(Objective 12)

6. Gently try to slip the cord over the head.
(Objective 16)

7. Elevation of the baby below the perineum could result in undertransfusion of blood from the cord; lowering the baby below the perineum could result in overtransfusion of cord blood.
(Objective 13)

8. The placenta surface should be inspected to see whether it is intact (retained fragments can cause postpartum hemorrhage), and then it should be placed in a plastic bag and transported with the mother to the hospital.
(Objective 13)

9. Clamp the cord in two places 6 inches from the baby and then cut between the clamps.
(Objective 13)

10. a. Stimulation of the baby is designed to promote effective respiratory effort.
b. Elevation of the baby's shoulders positions the airway in the most effective manner to promote effective ventilation.
c. Massage of the mother's abdomen stimulates uterine contractions that help to slow vaginal bleeding.
d. Administration of oxytocin causes uterine contraction and slows vaginal bleeding.
(Objective 13 and 15)

47 Neonatal Care

READING ASSIGNMENT

Chapter 47, pages 1307-1332, in *Mosby's Paramedic Textbook,* ed. 4.

OBJECTIVES

Upon completion of this chapter, the paramedic student will be able to do the following:

1. Identify risk factors associated with the need for neonatal resuscitation.
2. Describe physiological adaptations at birth.
3. Describe pathophysiology and implications of selected genetic anomalies present in some neonates.
4. Outline the prehospital assessment and management of the neonate.
5. Describe resuscitation of the distressed neonate.
6. Discuss postresuscitative management and transport.
7. Describe signs and symptoms and prehospital management of specific neonatal resuscitation situations.
8. Identify injuries associated with birth.
9. Describe appropriate interventions to manage the emotional needs of the neonate's family.

SUMMARY

- Low birth weight and a variety of antepartum and intrapartum risk factors affect the need for resuscitation.
- Some of the more common congenital anomalies include choanal atresia, tracheobronchial fistula and atresia, Pierre Robin syndrome, cleft lip and cleft palate, congenital heart anomalies, pyloric stenosis, diaphragmatic hernia, omphalocele, and spina bifida.
- At birth, newborns make three major physiological adaptations necessary for survival: (1) emptying fluids from their lungs and beginning ventilation, (2) changing their circulatory pattern, and (3) maintaining body temperature.
- The initial steps of neonatal resuscitation (except for those born through meconium) are to prevent heat loss, clear the airway by positioning and suction if needed, provide tactile stimulation and initiate breathing if necessary, and further evaluate the infant.
- If neonatal resuscitation is needed, the paramedic should reevaluate the initial steps of stabilization (warm, position, clear airway, dry, stimulate, reposition). If there is no change, resuscitation proceeds in 30-second increments with ventilation, chest compressions, and, if needed, administration of epinephrine.
- The three most common complications during the postresuscitation period are endotracheal tube position change (including dislodgment), tube occlusion by mucus or meconium, and pneumothorax. During transport of the neonate, it is important to maintain body temperature, oxygen administration, and ventilatory support.
- Specific situations that may require advanced life support for the neonate include meconium staining, apnea, diaphragmatic hernia, bradycardia, premature infants, respiratory distress and cyanosis, hypovolemia, seizures, fever, hypothermia, hypoglycemia, vomiting and diarrhea, and birth injuries.
- Primary apnea is common immediately after birth and is self-limiting. Secondary apnea is a pause in breathing that exceeds 20 seconds.
- Bradycardia is a heart rate less than 100 beats/min. It is most often caused by hypoxia.
- Premature infants have an increased risk of respiratory suppression, hypothermia, and head and brain injury. In addition to low birth weight, various antepartum and intrapartum risk factors may affect the need for resuscitation.
- Prematurity is the most common cause of respiratory distress in neonates.
- Hypovolemia in infants may result from dehydration, hemorrhage, trauma, or sepsis.
- Seizures in a newborn signal an underlying abnormality.
- A temperature of greater than 100.4°F (38.0°C) is a fever and often signals a viral or bacterial infection.
- Hypothermia is a core body temperature below 95°F (35°C). It increases metabolic demand and can cause metabolic acidosis, pulmonary hypertension, and hypoxemia.
- Blood glucose less than 40 mg/dL indicates hypothermia in the neonate.
- Injuries at birth may include cranial trauma, intracranial hemorrhage or brain injury, spine and spinal cord injury, peripheral nerve injury, spleen or liver injuries, fractures, or soft tissue injury.
- Paramedics should be aware of the normal feelings and reactions of parents, siblings, other family members, and caregivers while providing emergency care to an ill or injured child.

645

Match the structures described in column I with the correct term in column II.

Column I

1. ________ A vertical split in the lip

2. ________ Abnormalities that include a small mandible and defects of the eyes and ears

3. ________ Occlusion that blocks the passage between the nose and pharynx

4. ________ Protrusion of stomach through the diaphragm

Column II

a. Choanal atresia
b. Cleft lip
c. Diaphragmatic hernia
d. Gastroesophageal reflux
e. Pierre Robin syndrome

5. List two risk factors that may indicate the need for neonatal resuscitation in each of the following categories:

a. Antepartum risk factors:

____

b. Intrapartum risk factors:

____

6. What three major adaptations are necessary for the survival of neonates at birth?

a. ____

b. ____

c. ____

7. List three actions that help maintain body warmth of neonates.

a. ____

b. ____

c. ____

8. Arrange the following steps in neonatal resuscitation (assuming you have a blue infant with slightly decreased respirations and a heart rate of 70 beats/min that does not improve at each step) in the correct order in the following table.

Incorrect Order	Correct Order
Administer epinephrine.	
Obtain vascular access.	
Administer oxygen at 5 L/min.	
Ventilate with bag-mask device.	
Perform chest compressions.	
Warm, dry, suction if indicated, and stimulate.	

A 3-kg baby is delivered, and he has been positioned properly. Tactile stimulation has been provided; however, he is still not breathing.

9. At what rate should you ventilate the neonate?

After ventilations are initiated, you detect a pulse of 70 beats/min.

10. Where should you palpate the pulse on a neonate?

11. What steps should you take now?

After you initiate chest compressions, there is no improvement. Your partner has intubated the baby.

12. What size of endotracheal tube would be appropriate for this infant?

13. What are your options to obtain vascular access?

14. What drug and dose should you administer when vascular access has been established?

15. List an intervention for each of the following neonatal postresuscitation complications:

    a. Endotracheal tube dislodgment:

    b. Endotracheal tube occlusion by mucus:

    c. Pneumothorax:

STUDENT SELF-ASSESSMENT

16. When should you anticipate the need for neonatal resuscitation?
    a. Contractions have been occurring for 6 hours.
    b. The physician states that the baby weighs 3600 g (7½ lb).
    c. Rupture of the membranes occurred 12 hours ago.
    d. The baby is at 36 weeks' gestation.

17. What initiates respiration in the newborn?
    a. Chemical and temperature changes
    b. Chest compression
    c. Closure of the patent ductus
    d. Cutting the umbilical cord

18. What is a proper position to maximize the airway of a neonate?
    a. Prone with the neck slightly extended
    b. Supine with the neck slightly flexed
    c. Supine with a towel under the shoulders
    d. Supine with a towel under the head

19. When is neonatal suctioning appropriate after delivery if the amniotic fluid is clear?
    a. Tracheal suction using an endotracheal tube until clear and reevaluate.
    b. Suction if secretions obstruct breathing or if you need to bag-mask ventilate.
    c. Suction all infants immediately after delivery to clear the airway and promote breathing.
    d. Suctioning should not be performed unless the infant is cyanotic or dyspneic.

20. Priorities of care for neonatal resuscitation are as follows:
    a. Prevent heat loss, administer intravenous fluids, and allow the infant to feed at the breast.
    b. Position the neonate, minimize external stimulation, and initiate intravenous fluids.
    c. Prevent heat loss, position the neonate, suction if secretions interfere with breathing, and provide stimulation.
    d. Position the infant, suction to clear the airway, administer intravenous fluids, and provide stimulation.

21. What can deep suctioning of the posterior pharynx of the neonate cause?
    a. Bradycardia
    b. Central nervous system depression
    c. Hypocarbia
    d. Tachypnea

22. After delivery, the infant is warmed, dried, and stimulated. Respirations are 30 breaths/min, and heart rate is 110 beats/min, but the baby's lips and ears are still blue. What should you do?
    a. Administer oxygen at 5 L/min by holding the tubing 1/2 inch from the nose.
    b. Begin bag-mask ventilation with 100% oxygen until the color improves.
    c. Initiate bag-mask ventilation and chest compressions.
    d. No intervention is needed; this is a normal finding in a newborn.

23. Which is an acceptable method of neonatal stimulation?
    a. Shouting loudly close to the baby's ear
    b. Holding the baby by the ankles and slapping the buttocks
    c. Slapping or flicking the soles of the feet or rubbing the back
    d. Vigorously shaking the baby by firmly grasping the shoulders

24. When should the paramedic consider intubation of the neonate?
    a. If the heart rate increases after bag-mask ventilation is performed
    b. If prolonged ventilation is likely to be needed
    c. Immediately after absent respirations are noted
    d. When the gestational age is less than 39 weeks

25. What is the normal heart rate of an infant?
    a. 60 beats/min   c. 120 beats/min
    b. 80 beats/min   d. 160 beats/min

26. Which finding may indicate a postresuscitation complication related to intubation in a neonate?
    a. Decreased resistance to ventilation
    b. Diminished breath sounds
    c. Increase in chest expansion
    d. Return of tachycardia

648

Chapter **47** **Neonatal Care**

27. Apnea in infants may be related to which of the following?
   a. Central nervous system disorders   **c.** Meconium aspiration
   b. Excessive stimulation   **d.** Use of stimulants

28. The most common factor for respiratory distress and cyanosis in a neonate is prematurity. Which of the following factors also can be responsible for this condition?
   a. Cleft lip congenital anomaly
   b. Mucus obstruction of the nasal passages
   c. Premature rupture of membranes
   d. Postterm delivery

29. What is the correct first drug and dose used for the treatment of neonatal bradycardia in the presence of adequate ventilation and oxygenation?
   a. Atropine 0.01 mg/kg IV
   b. Atropine 0.02 mg/kg IV
   c. Epinephrine 0.01 mg/kg (1:1000) IV
   d. Epinephrine 0.01 mg/kg (1:10,000) IV

30. Which is a risk factor associated with cardiac arrest in a newborn?
   a. Amniotic fluid aspiration
   b. Gestational diabetes
   c. Intrauterine asphyxia
   d. Premature cutting of the cord after birth

31. Which is true regarding vomiting in neonates?
   a. An intravenous line should be established if this is observed.
   b. It is unusual and is associated with serious illness.
   c. It is a frequent occurrence and should be of no concern.
   d. Persistent bile-stained vomit may indicate a bowel obstruction.

32. What sign or symptom can be found after phototherapy for hyperbilirubinemia?
   a. Bradycardia   **c.** Seizures
   b. Diarrhea   **d.** Vomiting

33. You are called to evaluate a 4-day-old breastfed infant whose mother states the child has diarrhea. When asked, she says the child is having five or six "loose" yellow stools per day. What is your assessment of this situation?
   a. This number of stools is normal for a breastfed baby.
   b. This indicates a serious situation that requires immediate intravenous therapy.
   c. This indicates bowel obstruction from a congenital defect.
   d. The yellow stools could indicate hepatitis, and the mother should be assessed for risk.

34. A mother states that she has observed repetitive eye deviation and blinking and sucking and swimming movements of the 2-day-old infant's arms. This may indicate which of the following?
   a. Focal clonic seizures   **c.** Subtle seizures
   b. Multifocal seizures   **d.** Tonic seizures

35. What should be assessed in the prehospital setting when evaluating an infant with apparent seizures?
   a. Blood glucose level   **c.** Child's ability to feed normally
   b. Blood pressure   **d.** Glasgow Coma Scale score

36. Which is true of a temperature of 100.4°F (38.0°C) in a neonate?
   a. It is a normal result of immature temperature control and does not require treatment.
   b. It may indicate a life-threatening infection and requires immediate transport.
   c. It often results in the development of febrile seizures that are difficult to control.
   d. Prehospital care should involve ice packs in the groin area to lower temperature.

   Chapter **47**   **Neonatal Care**

37. A 3-kg infant delivered at home yesterday is limp and has irregular respirations. You assess the child, maintain warmth, assist ventilations, and initiate vascular access. The blood glucose drawn when the intravenous line was started is 40 mg/dL. What should you administer?
    a. 3 g of a $D_{10}W$ solution
    b. 3 g of a D50W solution
    c. 6 g of a $D_{10}W$ solution
    d. 6 g of a D50W solution

38. Which of the following birth injuries may damage the brachial plexus?
    a. Clavicle or extremity fracture
    b. Liver or spleen injury
    c. Spine or spinal cord injury
    d. Brain injuries

39. Which of the following statements by the paramedic would be helpful when speaking to the parents of an infant who is being resuscitated in the prehospital setting?
    a. Everything's going to be okay.
    b. Everything possible is being done for your baby.
    c. I can't tell you anything at all about your baby.
    d. I think your baby's going to make it; this is a great crew.

40. The femoral pulses of a newborn a difficult to palpate. What alteration in physiology caused by a congenital problem can cause this finding?
    a. Impaired blood flow through the aorta
    b. Hole between the left and right ventricle
    c. Patent connection between the aorta and pulmonary artery
    d. Obstruction of the mitral valve

41. Which congenital heart defect may cause cyanosis in a newborn?
    a. Atrial septal defect
    b. Coarctation of the aorta
    c. Hypoplastic left heart syndrome
    d. Patent ductus arteriosus

42. What maternal factor is associated with congenital heart defects?
    a. Age younger than 25 years if the mother is a primipara
    b. Infection with German measles during pregnancy
    c. Maternal weight is greater than 1½ times normal BMI
    d. Diagnosis of hypertensive illness during pregnancy

43. A term newborn is cyanotic, dyspneic, and limp. Which congenital defect should be considered?
    a. Atrial septal defect
    b. Mitral valve stenosis
    c. Coarctation of the aorta
    d. Tetralogy of Fallot

44. What causes the signs and symptoms associated with pyloric stenosis?
    a. Inability to swallow
    b. Enhanced gag reflex
    c. Impaired stomach emptying
    d. Excess secretion of gastric juice

45. What risk factor is most strongly associated with birth injury such as head, spine, or extremity trauma?
    a. Sudden, rapid, unexpected delivery
    b. Maternal use of drugs or alcohol
    c. Premature birth
    d. Lack of prenatal care

650

The dispatcher calls, "Respond to a call for maternity." You figure this will be another false alarm. When you arrive, the father meets you at the door yelling, "The baby, the baby!" You find an 18-year-old woman squatting by the bed, pants around her ankles, screaming. You can see thick, chunky, green liquid running down her legs and a baby's head crowning at her perineum. You pull out the OB kit while your partner calls for a pumper assist and hurries to get the pediatric resuscitation bag from your ambulance. As the head delivers, you suction secretions from the mouth and then nose with the bulb syringe, pulling out thick meconium with each aspiration. The chest delivers, and there is no immediate spontaneous respiration, so you insert an endotracheal tube, quickly applying suction to the end. As you pull it out, some residual green meconium is aspirated, and you repeat it twice until there is no aspirate. Your partner holds an oxygen mask close to the baby's face and checks his heart rate after you position him on his side, dry him, and stimulate him; it is 50 beats/min, and he is floppy and does not grimace to suction, so your partner begins ventilation with a bag mask. After 30 seconds, there is no improvement in heart rate, so you have a firefighter perform chest compressions. There is no change in 30 seconds, so you intubate the baby's trachea and verify placement using capnography. You explain quickly to the mother that the baby has not responded to initial treatment, so you are helping his blood circulate with chest compressions and are going to give him some medicines to help stimulate his heart. There is still no improvement, so you initiate a scalp vein IV and administer epinephrine. Reassessment shows a heart rate of 150 beats/min, which quickly slows when you stop ventilation for a moment. You continue ventilation with frequent reevaluation of tube placement and cover him to keep him warm until you arrive at the ED 10 minutes later. After 1 month in NICU, he is released home, and his mother brings him to visit 2 months later.

1. What scene finding made you prepare for neonatal resuscitation?
   a. Age of the mother
   b. Baby crowning on arrival
   c. Presence of meconium on the mother's legs
   d. Resuscitation is needed on most field deliveries

2. What four newborn characteristics, assessed immediately after birth, would suggest that no resuscitation is needed?

   a. ____

   b. ____

   c. ____

   d. ____

3. What physiological change at birth explains the

   a. Presence of secretions in the baby's nose and mouth:

   ____

   b. Need to dry and warm the infant:

   ____

   c. Circulatory changes after the cord is cut:

   ____

4. Place a check mark beside the steps in the neonatal resuscitation pyramid that you performed on this baby.

a. ________ Position, suction, stimulate   **d.** ________ Chest compression

b. ________ Oxygen   **e.** ________ Intubation

c. ________ Bag-mask ventilation   **f.** ________ Medication

5. Why was the baby intubated and secretions suctioned before any other resuscitation measures?
  a. All babies with meconium in the amniotic fluid need intubation.
  b. If the paramedic is skilled at intubation, it should be done first.
  c. It takes longer to insert an umbilical catheter, so it is left until later.
  d. The baby was depressed, and the meconium was thick.

6. Why is it important to give the family some preliminary information about the baby's condition?

CHAPTER 47 ANSWERS

REVIEW QUESTIONS

1. b
(Objective 1)

2. e
(Objective 1)

3. a
(Objective 1)

4. c
(Objective 1)

5. a. Multiple gestation, inadequate prenatal care, mother's age, history of perinatal morbidity or mortality, postterm
gestation, drugs or medication, toxemia, hypertension, and diabetes
  b. Premature labor, meconium-stained amniotic fluid, rupture of membranes more than 24 hours before delivery,
use of narcotics within 4 hours of delivery, abnormal presentation, prolonged labor or precipitous delivery,
prolapsed cord, bleeding
(Objective 1)

6. a. Emptying fluid from the lungs and beginning ventilation
  b. Changing the circulatory pattern
  c. Maintaining body temperature
(Objective 2)

7. a. Dry the infant's head and body thoroughly; remove any wet coverings; cover the head and body of the baby
with warm blankets; turn the heat up high in the ambulance; use chemical warm packs (with blankets between
the pack and the infant). Wrap low-birth-weight infants in plastic food wrap.
(Objective 4)

8.

Incorrect Order	Correct Order
Administer epinephrine.	Warm, dry, clear airway, and stimulate.
Obtain vascular access.	Administer oxygen at 5 L/min.
Administer oxygen at 5 L/min.	Ventilate with bag-mask device.
Ventilate with bag-mask device.	Perform chest compressions.
Perform chest compressions.	Obtain vascular access.
Warm, dry, suction if indicated, and stimulate.	Administer epinephrine.

(Objective 5)

9. Initiate positive pressure breathing with 100% oxygen by bag mask at 40 to 60 breaths/min.
(Objectives 4 and 5)

10. At the brachial artery, at the umbilical cord, or by auscultation
(Objective 4)

11. Continue positive-pressure ventilations for 30 seconds; if heart rate does not begin to improve, start chest compressions 1/2 to 3/4 inch at 120 per minute.
(Objective 5)

12. 2.5 or 3.0
(Objective 5)

13. Initiate a peripheral intravenous line, an intraosseous line, or an umbilical vein cannulation (if specially trained and authorized).
(Objective 4)

14. Epinephrine 0.01 to 0.03 mg/kg (1:10,000)
(Objective 5)

15. a. If breath sounds are audible only on the right, pull back slightly and reevaluate; if the tube is in the correct location, secure it. If breath sounds are absent, remove the tube and reintubate.
(Objective 6)

    b. Suction the tube with a suction catheter and reevaluate.
(Objective 6)

    c. Assess for presence of tension pneumothorax and treat if present. If at a hospital, prepare to assist with chest tube placement.
(Objective 6)

16. d. A premature infant refers to a baby born before 37 weeks' gestation (weight usually 0.6–2.2 kg [11.5–5 lb]). The incidence of complications increases as gestational age (and weight) decreases. A normal birth weight is 7.5 lb; 6 hours is not a lengthy labor. Rupture of membranes more than 24 hours before birth would be a concern.
(Objective 1)

17. a. As the chest recoils during delivery, chemical and temperature changes initiate the first breath. Cutting the umbilical cord initiates changes in fetal circulation.
(Objective 2)

18. c. The torso should be elevated 3/4 to 1 inch so the neck is slighted extended in the sniffing position.
(Objective 4)

19. b. Suctioning unnecessarily can cause bradycardia in a newborn.
(Objective 4)

20. c. Intravenous fluids are rarely necessary in the normal infant if appropriate resuscitation is done.
(Objective 4)

21. a
(Objective 4)

22. a. Continue the oxygen administration until the color improves (keep the baby warm).
(Objective 4)

23. c. The goal is to stimulate the neonate without risk of injury.
(Objective 4)

24. b. Often the infant will initiate adequate spontaneous respirations after a brief period of bagging and will not
require intubation. Increasing heart rate is a positive indicator.
(Objective 5)

25. c. A heart rate greater than 100 beats/min is desirable. Chest compressions should be initiated for a persistent
heart rate less than 80 beats/min that does not respond to ventilation.
(Objective 4)

26. b. Decreased chest wall movement, return of bradycardia, unilateral decrease in chest expansion, altered intensity
to pitch or breath sounds, and increased resistance to hand ventilation are signs that may point to tube
migration, occlusion, or pneumothorax.
(Objective 6)

27. a. Other causes include narcotic or central nervous system depressant use, airway or respiratory muscle weakness,
oxyhemoglobin dissociation curve shift, septicemia, and metabolic disorders.
(Objective 7)

28. b. Infants are obligate nose breathers; suctioning of mucus from the nasal passages will correct this problem.

29. d. Inadequate ventilations and oxygenation are the most common causes of bradycardia and should be reassessed
continually.
(Objective 7)

30. c. Other causes are drugs taken by the mother, congenital diseases or malformations, and intrapartum hypoxemia.
(Objective 7)

31. d. Some vomiting is normal; however, if it is persistent or bile stained or contains dark blood, a serious underlying
illness may exist. Vascular access would not be indicated unless needed to treat dehydration or bradycardia
because of the vagal stimulation this can produce.
(Objective 7)

32. b. Other causes of diarrhea in the neonate are gastroenteritis, lactose intolerance, neonatal abstinence syndrome,
thyrotoxicosis, and cystic fibrosis
(Objective 7)

33. a. The baby should be assessed for clinical signs of dehydration or other signs of illness (e.g., fever, lethargy, and
feeding habits), but typically this stool pattern is normal in this situation.
(Objective 7)

34. c. All types of seizures in this age group are considered pathological.

654

35. a. Hypoglycemia may produce seizure activity. Determining the presence of this condition and correcting it are urgent matters.
(Objective 7)

36. b. Even small temperature elevations in this age group can signal impending sepsis. Febrile seizures are unusual in this age group and would not be expected (especially at this temperature). Ice packs should never be applied to a neonate.
(Objective 7)

37. a
(Objective 7)

38. a. This can cause temporary or permanent functional impairment of the arm.
(Objective 8)

39. b. Honest, frequent updates about the baby's condition should be given during the resuscitation so that family members can prepare themselves for the outcome.
(Objective 8)

40. a. This is called coarctation of the aorta and is caused by a narrowing of the aorta. Septal defects are present when there is an opening between the right and left side of the heart. Patent ductus arteriosus exists in c.
(Objective 3)

41. c. Although the other defects are serious, they do not typically cause cyanosis initially.
(Objective 3)

42. b. Rubella, maternal alcohol or drug ingestion, and maternal history of congenital heart defect are associated with congenital heart defects.
(Objective 3)

43. d. Tetralogy of Fallot includes a large ventricular septal defect, pulmonary stenosis, right ventricular hypertrophy, and an overriding aorta.
(Objective 3)

44. c. The pyloric sphincter is narrowed slowing or preventing gastric emptying.
(Objective 3)

45. a. The other factors may be associated with other problems at birth.
(Objective 8)

WRAP IT UP

1. c. Meconium points to a high-risk delivery, especially if it is thick and dark. Other indicators of birth complications are early delivery, maternal use of drugs, and multiple births.
(Objective 1)

2. a. Full-term baby
   b. No meconium or signs of infected amniotic fluid
   c. The baby is breathing or crying
   d. The baby has good muscle tone

3. a. Fluid is squeezed from the chest into the nose and mouth during delivery and should be suctioned if it is thick and impairs ventilation.
   b. Infants have a large body surface area; immature temperature regulation mechanisms; and are born into a cool, wet environment. Maintaining warmth is a critical aspect of neonatal resuscitation.
   c. Cutting the cord shuts down placental circulation, closing some of the circulatory pathways established in utero.
(Objective 2)

4. a, b, c, d, e, f. On most deliveries, progression past (a) or (b) is never needed.
(Objectives 3 and 4)

5. d. This is the only situation when intubation would be near the first step.
(Objectives 4 and 6)

6. The family should be given brief, accurate information often to give them a realistic idea of the condition of their baby.
(Objective 8)

48 Pediatrics

OBJECTIVES

Upon completion of this chapter, the paramedic student will be able to do the following:

1. Identify the role of the Emergency Medical Services for Children program.
2. Identify age-related illnesses and injuries in pediatric patients.
3. Outline the general principles of assessment and management of the pediatric patient.
4. Identify modifications in patient assessment techniques that assist in the examination of patients at different developmental levels.
5. Describe the pathophysiology, signs and symptoms, and management of selected pediatric respiratory emergencies.
6. Describe the pathophysiology, signs and symptoms, and management of shock in the pediatric patient.
7. Describe the pathophysiology, signs and symptoms, and management of selected pediatric dysrhythmias.
8. Describe the pathophysiology, signs and symptoms, and management of pediatric seizures.
9. Describe the pathophysiology, signs and symptoms, and management of hypoglycemia and hyperglycemia in the pediatric patient.
10. Describe the pathophysiology, signs and symptoms, and management of infectious pediatric emergencies.
11. Identify common causes of poisoning and toxic exposure in the pediatric patient.
12. Describe special considerations for assessment and management of specific injuries in children.
13. Outline the pathophysiology and management of sudden infant death syndrome.
14. Describe the risk factors, key signs and symptoms, and management of injuries or illness resulting from child abuse and neglect.
15. Identify prehospital considerations for the care of infants and children with special needs.

SUMMARY

- Paramedics must continually maintain their knowledge of pediatric emergency care.
- The Emergency Medical Services for Children (EMSC) program was designed to enhance and expand emergency medical services for acutely ill and injured children. The program has defined 12 basic components of an effective EMSC system.
- Children have unique anatomic, physiologic, and psychological characteristics, which change during their development.
- Airway structures are narrower and less stable than those of adults. This increases the risk of upper and lower airway obstruction related to injury or illness.
- Principles of assessment are similar to adults, but pediatric-sized equipment and specific adaptations to the examination should be made.
- Some childhood diseases and disabilities can be predicted by age group.
- Many elements of the initial evaluation can be done by observing the child. The child's parent or guardian also should be involved in the initial evaluation. The three components of the pediatric assessment triangle are appearance, work of breathing, and circulation.
- Paramedics must recognize and distinguish among respiratory distress, respiratory failure, and respiratory arrest.
- Obstruction of the upper or lower airway by a foreign body usually occurs in toddlers or preschoolers. Obstruction may be partial or complete.
- Croup is a common inflammatory respiratory illness. It usually is seen in children between the ages of 6 months and 4 years. Symptoms are caused by inflammation in the subglottic region.
- Epiglottitis is a rapidly progressive, life-threatening bacterial infection. It causes edema and swelling of the epiglottis and supraglottic structures. It often affects children between 3 and 7 years of age.

- Bacterial tracheitis is an infection of the upper airway and subglottic trachea usually seen in infants and toddlers; it often occurs with or after croup.
- Asthma is common in children who are older than 2 years of age. Asthma is characterized by bronchoconstriction that results from autonomic dysfunction or sensitizing agents.
- Bronchiolitis is a viral disease frequently caused by respiratory syncytial virus infection of the lower airway; it usually affects children ages 6 to 18 months of age.
- Pneumonia is an acute infection of the lower airways and lungs involving the alveolar walls and the alveoli.
- Pertussis is a bacterial respiratory infection associated with a long course of illness; a violent cough with a characteristic "whoop"; and a risk of pneumonia and death, especially in infants.
- Bronchopulmonary dysplasia is a chronic lung disease resulting from intervention with oxygen and ventilation as a neonate. It causes alveolar damage and chronic pulmonary dysfunction that can lead to death.
- Several special differences must be remembered when caring for a child in shock. These include circulating blood volume, body surface area and hypothermia, cardiac reserve, and vital signs and assessment. A child in shock may appear normal and stable until all compensatory mechanisms fail. At that point, pediatric shock progresses rapidly, with serious deterioration.
- When dysrhythmias occur in children, they usually result from hypoxia or structural heart disease.
- Goals of postresuscitation stabilization in children include preserving brain function, avoiding secondary injury, identifying causes of illness, managing pain, and transport to an appropriate facility.
- Meningitis is inflammation of the meninges. It can lead to neurologic damage, hearing or vision impairment, and death.
- The most common causes of seizure in adult and pediatric patients are noncompliance with a drug regimen for the treatment of epilepsy in addition to head trauma, intracranial infection, metabolic disturbance, or poisoning. The most common cause of new onset of seizure in children is fever.
- Hypoglycemia and hyperglycemia should be suspected whenever a child has an altered level of consciousness with no explainable cause. Consider diabetes as a possible cause in children even in the absence of a history of diabetes.
- Blood disorders that may affect children include sickle cell disease, leukemia, clotting disorders, and others.
- Gastrointestinal disorders in children can lead to serious illness, including life-threatening dehydration and death.
- Children with infection may have a variety of signs and symptoms. These depend on the source and extent of infection and the length of time since the patient was exposed.
- Most poisoning events in the United States involve children. Signs and symptoms of accidental poisoning vary, depending on the toxic substance and the length of time since the child was exposed.
- Blunt and penetrating trauma is a chief cause of injury and death in children. Head injury is the most common cause of death in pediatric trauma patients. Early recognition and aggressive management can reduce morbidity and mortality caused by traumatic brain injury in children.
- Because of the pliability of the chest wall, severe intrathoracic injury can be present without signs of external injury. The liver, kidneys, and spleen are the most frequently injured abdominal organs. Extremity injuries are more common in children than adults.
- Sudden infant death syndrome is the leading cause of death in American infants younger than 1 year of age. The syndrome is defined as the sudden death of a seemingly healthy infant. The death cannot be explained by history and an autopsy.
- Child abuse and neglect is the maltreatment of children by their parents, guardians, or other caregivers. Forms of maltreatment include infliction of physical injury, sexual exploitation, and infliction of emotional pain and neglect.
- Some infants and children are born with or develop conditions that pose special needs. These children may require special medical equipment to sustain life. Often these children are cared for at home. Many are dependent on specialized medical equipment such as tracheostomy tubes, home artificial ventilators, central venous lines, gastrostomy tubes, and shunts. They may have emergencies associated with airway obstruction, impaired ventilation, infection, or increased intracranial pressure.

Match the drugs in column II with their appropriate initial pediatric dose in column I. Use each drug only once.

Column I

1. _______ 0.1 mL/kg

2. _______ 2 to 20 mcg/kg/min

3. _______ 1 mEq/kg per dose

4. _______ 0.1 mg/kg

5. _______ 1 mg/kg

6. _______ 0.02 mg/kg

7. _______ 5 mg/kg

Column II

a. Adenosine
b. Amiodarone
c. Atropine sulfate
d. Diazepam
e. Dopamine hydrochloride
f. Epinephrine (1:10,000)
g. Lidocaine
h. Sodium bicarbonate

8. In what pediatric age group(s) are you most likely to see the following illness or injuries?

a. Sepsis:

____

b. Febrile seizures:

____

c. Jaundice:

____

d. Ingestions:

____

e.. Falls:

____

f. Child abuse:

____

g. Drowning or near drowning:

____

h. Suicidal gestures:

____

Questions 9 to 12 pertain to the following case study:

A 7-year-old boy is in acute respiratory distress after visiting a friend's home. He gives a history of asthma and allergy to dogs (his friend has three). His home medicines include an Atrovent (ipratropium) inhaler; montelukast sodium (Singulair) tabs, which he takes daily; and pirbuterol (Maxair) by nebulizer as necessary, which he has not used for 1 week. He has circumoral cyanosis, is working very hard to breathe, and has faint inspiratory and expiratory wheezes.

9. What interventions are appropriate for this child? Include two possible beta-agonist drugs you could administer (with appropriate doses and routes).

____

10. What side effects do you anticipate from the administration of these drugs?

____

11. In 15 minutes, you see no clinical improvement, and your estimated arrival time is 20 minutes. What do you do?

____

12. What aspects of the physical examination will change when the patient improves?

____

____

13. List three characteristic signs or symptoms of epiglottitis.

    a. ____

    b. ____

    c. ____

14. A 20-month-old with croup is in mild respiratory distress on a cool October evening.

    a. What intervention should you try before entering the ambulance that may cause rapid improvement in the patient's signs and symptoms?

    ____

    b. When in the ambulance, how will you care for this child?

    ____

    ____

    c. Why is albuterol _not_ indicated for this child?

    ____

    ____

Questions 15 to 19 pertain to the following case study:

A limp, 11-month-old boy is carried into the ambulance base by his mother. She states that he has had a fever with vomiting and diarrhea for 3 days. His eyes are sunken, his tongue is furrowed, and his lips are cracked. Physical examination reveals rapid respirations and cold, mottled extremities. His electrocardiogram is shown in Fig. 48-1.

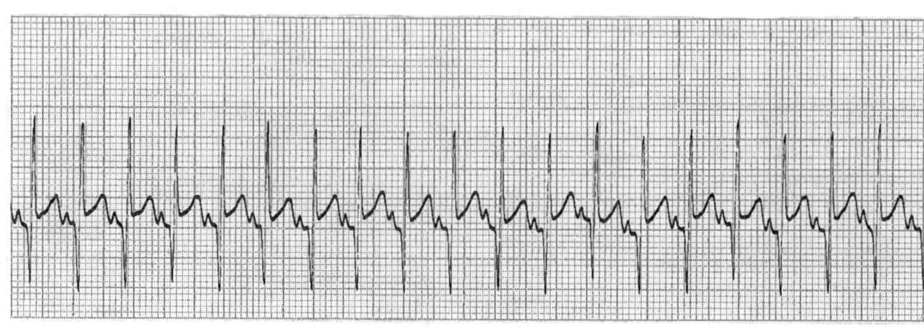

Figure 48-1

15. What condition does this child have?

____

16. Interpret the electrocardiogram.

____

17. Describe management of this child, assuming a 45-minute transport time.

____

____

18. What are the appropriate vital signs for this child?

____

19. What clinical signs of improvement will you watch for in addition to improvement in vital signs?

____

Questions 20 to 23 refer to the following case study:

A 3-year-old, 33-pound (15-kg) child is found unconscious after suffocation with a plastic bag. On arrival, you find a dusky, pale child who is unresponsive and apneic. Occasionally, you can palpate a faint pulse at the carotid artery, but you obtain no blood pressure reading. The electrocardiogram is shown in Fig. 48-2.

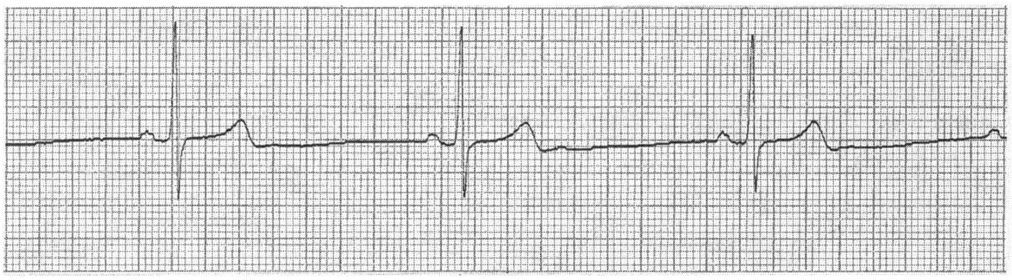

Figure 48-2

20. Interpret the electrocardiogram tracing.

____

21. What actions will you take immediately, up to and including the first drug (with appropriate dose and route)?

____

____

22. If an intravenous line cannot be immediately established, what two actions can be taken?

    a. ____

    b. ____

23. After your initial interventions result in no patient improvement, what is the next drug (and dose and route) indicated?

____

24. A 3-week-old, 5-kg infant with a history of congenital heart defects suddenly loses consciousness and stops breathing. On arrival, you find him pulseless and apneic. Cardiopulmonary resuscitation is initiated by the police emergency medical responders. The electrocardiogram tracing in Fig. 48-3 is noted.

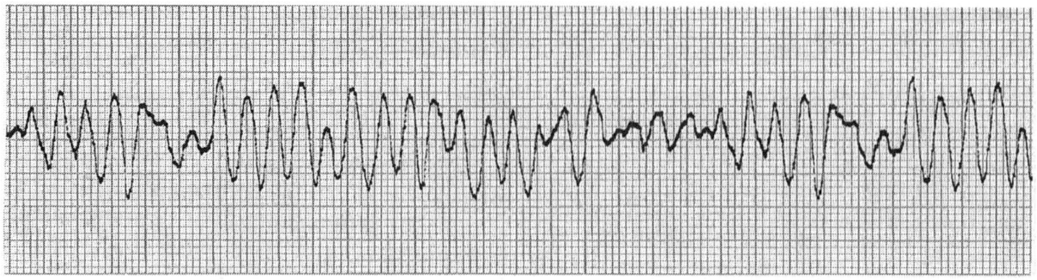

Figure 48-3

    a. Outline your continued care of this patient up to and including the first two drugs (including doses and routes).

____

____

____

    b. If a repeat dose of epinephrine is necessary, what is the correct dose and concentration?

____

Questions 25 to 27 refer to the following case study:

A frightened mother tells you that when she put her 4-year-old, 14-kg child to bed, he complained of a slight earache and had a low-grade temperature. She heard a noise several hours later and found her child having a grand mal seizure, which stopped after approximately 1 minute. The child's temperature is 105.5°F (40.8°C). He appears to be postictal at this time.

25. After you have ensured that the child is stable, what history should you obtain from the mother?

____

____

26. What care should be provided en route to the hospital?

____

____

27. If the child has a seizure during transport, list two anticonvulsant drugs that may be given, including the appropriate doses and routes.

    a. ____

    b. ____

662

28. You are called to an elementary school to care for a 6-year-old girl who is "acting funny." She is responsive only to pain. The nurse says the child has a history of diabetes. You check a finger-stick glucose level and determine that this child's blood sugar is 35 mg/dL.

    a. What drug should you administer (including dose and route)?

    b. What other signs or symptoms may this child have had before becoming this ill?

29. Your 3-year-old patient weighs 17 kg. He was involved in a head-on motor vehicle collision and was restrained only by a lap belt. He says his "tummy hurts." The physical examination reveals an anxious, pale child with a rigid, tender abdomen. Discuss the significance of the following physiologic differences in children and specific ways they will influence your care of this child.

    a. Children have a greater percentage of circulating blood volume than adults.

    b. Children have a large body surface area in proportion to body weight.

    c. Children's hearts function at near-maximal performance in a normal, healthy state.

    d. Volume replacement in children is weight related.

    e. Intravenous access is difficult to establish in children.

30. How do you determine whether an intraosseous needle has been properly placed?

____

Questions 31 to 33 pertain to the following case study:

At 1 AM on a February morning, you are dispatched for a "baby choking." You find a well-nourished 4-month-old baby boy apneic and pulseless in his crib. There is frothy sputum in the nose and mouth, and his diaper is wet and full of stool. The child is cold, and dependent lividity is present. The hysterical mother states that he and his older sister have both had a slight cold but that otherwise he was healthy.

31. What characteristics of sudden infant death syndrome are consistent with this call?

____

32. What other findings should you document in this situation?

____

You comfort the family and make the appropriate notifications and then ride back quietly to the firehouse with your normally talkative partner. You ask if he is OK, and he says, "Of course, I'm fine." Then he immediately rushes to the phone, where you hear him awaken his wife and ask her to check on their 6-month-old daughter.

33. Should you ignore your partner's unusual behavior because he told you he is OK? If not, what action(s) can you take?

____

____

Questions 34 to 36 pertain to the following case study:

A mother says her 8-month-old son fell off his tricycle early in the day but seemed to be feeling fine. Later she could not wake him from his nap. On physical examination, you find a dirty child who has agonal respirations, a slow pulse, and extension posturing. No visible signs of trauma are present on the head, although small bruises are noted on the shoulders.

34. What should your immediate interventions be for this child?

____

____

35. What findings might lead you to suspect child abuse?

____

____

36. After you deliver the child to the appropriate medical center, what are your responsibilities?

____

____

37. What history and physical examination should be performed on a child who is a victim of sexual abuse?

____

____

STUDENT SELF-ASSESSMENT

38. Which is a component of an effective EMSC system?
 a. Access to care **c.** Legislative committees
 b. Immunization programs **d.** Medical direction

39. Which examination strategy can help reduce anxiety in school-age children?
 a. Allow them to take part in decisions about their care.
 b. Reassure them that they are not being punished.
 c. Let them play with equipment.
 d. Use deep breathing and relaxation techniques.

40. Which age group fears bodily injury and mutilation and interprets words literally?
 a. Adolescents **c.** School-age children
 b. Preschoolers **d.** Toddlers

41. A 6-month-old child has respiratory distress. What is the most likely cause of this complaint in this age group?
 a. Asthma **c.** Epiglottitis
 b. Bronchiolitis **d.** Chronic bronchitis

42. A great deal of the child's physical examination can be done by which step?
 a. Assessing the skin temperature and moisture
 b. Auscultating the breath sounds
 c. Observing the child's behavior
 d. Palpating the central and distal pulses

43. Which of the following is a sign of respiratory distress in a child?
 a. Crying **c.** Flushed skin
 b. Elevated temperature **d.** Head bobbing

44. Which of the following is a bacterial infection of the upper airway and subglottic trachea that occurs during or after croup?
 a. Bronchiolitis **c.** Pneumonia
 b. Epiglottitis **d.** Tracheitis

45. Which of the following may be indicated for the management of severe respiratory distress associated with bronchiolitis?
 a. Albuterol, 0.15 mg/kg by inhalation
 b. Atropine, 0.01 mg/kg by inhalation
 c. Epinephrine, 0.1 mg/kg subcutaneously
 d. Terbutaline, 0.2 mg/kg subcutaneously

46. Which of the following is an appropriate intervention for a child in whom epiglottitis is suspected?
 a. Administer albuterol by nebulizer
 b. See if the epiglottis is swollen.
 c. Infuse intravenous normal saline fluids at 20 mL/kg.
 d. Allow the child to assume a comfortable position.

47. Which drug may initially relieve respiratory distress in a child with bronchiolitis?
 a. Albuterol **c.** Epinephrine
 b. Alupent **d.** Diphenhydramine

48. Which finding would be your first indication that an infant needs a fluid bolus?
   a. Decreasing blood pressure and poor skin turgor
   b. Flat fontanelle and warm skin
   c. Loss of appetite and nausea
   d. Very dry mucous membranes and tachycardia

49. A 20-kg child is lethargic and tachycardic and has dry mucous membranes after a 3-day history of "flu." Medical direction asks for a fluid bolus of normal saline. How much will you administer initially?
   a. 20 mL   c. 200 mL
   b. 100 mL   d. 400 mL

50. A 4-year-old child has fatigue, difficulty breathing, and peripheral edema. Crackles are audible in the bases of both lungs. Which illness do you suspect?
   a. Anaphylaxis   c. Cardiomyopathy
   b. Asthma   d. Pneumonia

51. A 5-year-old, 44-lb child is in ventricular fibrillation. Which is the correct initial energy level for defibrillation?
   a. 20 joules   c. 80 joules
   b. 40 joules   d. 88 joules

52. What is the maximum single dose of atropine that should be given to a 6-year-old child?
   a. 0.05 mg   c. 0.1 mg
   b. 0.01 mg   d. 0.5 mg

53. Which drug(s) is/are appropriate for an unresponsive child who became bradycardic after endotracheal suctioning after cardiopulmonary resuscitation has been initiated?
   a. Atropine and epinephrine   c. Atropine only
   b. Epinephrine and atropine   d. Epinephrine only

54. An infant who "wasn't acting right" has a heart rate of 230 beats/min. He is awake but lethargic, and his skin is pale with delayed capillary refill. He has SVT, and vagal maneuvers do not convert the rhythm. Your partner has established vascular access. What is the initial treatment of choice for this child?
   a. Adenosine   c. Synchronized cardioversion
   b. Digoxin   d. Verapamil

55. Which of the following is not likely to cause seizures?
   a. CNS infection   c. Prolonged dehydration
   b. Metabolic abnormalities   d. Serious head trauma

56. After intravenous administration of diazepam, you should monitor closely for which of the following?
   a. Decreased pulse   c. Respiratory depression
   b. Increased blood pressure   d. Vomiting or nausea

57. Your 7-year-old patient is lethargic and has a blood pressure of 70/50 mm Hg and a pulse of 138 beats/min. Respirations are 40 breaths/min, and his breath smells fruity. His mother says he has been losing weight and has had increased urination and thirst for several weeks. What condition should you consider?
   a. Head injury   c. Hyperglycemia
   b. Hydrocarbon ingestion   d. Hyperthermia

58. What life-threatening condition may be found in a child after ingestion of alcohol?
   a. Hypoglycemia   c. Hypokalemia
   b. Hypothermia   d. Hypocalcemia

59. What clinical finding may be present in a child who has ingested a large amount of aspirin?
   a. Bradycardia   c. Hypothermia
   b. Hiccoughs   d. Tachypnea

60. You are caring for a teenager who was "huffing" toluene. What effects could this produce?
   a. Pulmonary edema
   b. Renal failure
   c. Uncontrolled bleeding
   d. Visual disturbances

61. A 14-year-old adolescent is anxious and has tremors and chest pain after smoking crack cocaine. His vital signs are BP, 180/100 mm Hg; P, 130/min; and R, 20/min. Which drug is indicated?
   a. Naloxone
   b. Epinephrine
   c. Lorazepam
   d. Flumazenil

62. A 4-year-old girl took 10 tricyclic antidepressant tablets. Her BP is 60 mm Hg by palpation; P is 130/min; and she is drowsy. Which intervention is indicated to improve her cardiac output?
   a. Lidocaine (1 mg/kg)
   b. Dopamine (5 mcg/kg/min)
   c. Oxygen (2 L/min)
   d. Sodium bicarbonate (1 mEq/kg)

63. For which drug is glucagon given as an antidote?
   a. Beta blockers
   b. Heroin
   c. Cocaine
   d. Tricyclic antidepressants

64. Which mechanism of injury accounts for the largest number of trauma deaths in children?
   a. Drowning
   b. Falls
   c. Fire
   d. Motor vehicle crashes

65. Which is a sign of increasing intracranial pressure unique to an infant?
   a. Bulging fontanelle
   b. Cheyne-Stokes respirations
   c. Hypotension
   d. Tachycardia

66. Why are children more vulnerable to liver and splenic injuries?
   a. Those organs are larger in children younger than the age of 8 years.
   b. Mechanisms of injury in children are more likely to affect these areas.
   c. The abdominal musculature is minimal and does not protect these organs.
   d. These organs are more fragile in children and injure more easily.

67. Which is a risk factor associated with a higher incidence of SIDS?
   a. High maternal or paternal age
   b. Rank of first in the birth order
   c. Premature birth and low birth weight
   d. Higher socioeconomic groups

68. Which injuries should be considered the result of possible abuse?
   a. Any fractures in a child younger than 5 years of age
   b. Injuries localized to one area of the body
   c. Bruises or burns in unusual patterns
   d. Lacerations on the forehead of a toddler

69. A 10-month-old child "didn't wake up from his nap." He is unconscious and has vomited. What other physical findings may indicate abuse?
   a. Dirty diaper
   b. Increased respiratory rate
   c. Other children in the room
   d. Retinal hemorrhage

70. A child who has a tracheostomy is dyspneic. The tube appears to be partly obstructed. What is your first intervention?
   a. Intubate the child orally.
   b. Insert a tracheal dilator to enlarge the hole.
   c. Remove and replace the tracheostomy.
   d. Suction the tracheostomy.

71. A child is experiencing signs and symptoms of hypoxia while on a home ventilator. On arrival, you should immediately perform which of the following?
   a. Begin ventilation with a bag-valve device.
   b. Check the connections on the machine and oxygen.
   c. Contact medical direction to help troubleshoot.
   d. Request that the home health agency repair the ventilator.

72. A frantic mother calls you to check her son's central venous catheter because it is leaking. On arrival, you note that the catheter is cracked and leaking. The child's condition is stable. What action should you take?
   a. Clamp the line.   **c.** Remove the line.
   b. Flush the line.   **d.** Tape around the crack.

73. A child with a gastric feeding tube develops respiratory distress. For what complication should you assess?
   a. Allergic reaction   **c.** Hypoglycemia
   b. Aspiration   **d.** Pulmonary embolism

WRAP IT UP

You are dispatched to a home for an "unresponsive child." As you pull up to the house, a woman runs toward your ambulance with a limp, 3-week-old infant in her arms. "He's had a runny nose and been listless today," she explains. "Then he started shaking all over, and now I can't wake him." "Febrile seizure," you hear your partner mutter under his breath. In the ambulance, oxygen is administered as you begin to assess the baby. He is floppy and limp, but he grimaces, whines weakly, opens his eyes when you rub his sternum, and his arms flex. You note rapid breathing with retractions of the ribs. The skin is pale and cool and shows sluggish capillary refill (about 3 seconds). Vital signs are BP, 70/50 mm Hg; P, 168/min; and R, 40/min. Oxygen saturation is intermittently showing about 95%, and the infant's lungs are clear. A temperature shows 99°F (37°C) axilla, and the diaper is wet when you remove it. Pupils are 3 mm and react to light; skin turgor seems normal; ECG shows a rapid, narrow complex tachycardia; and blood glucose is 98 mg/dL. No other significant findings are noted on the detailed exam. The baby's mother says he was term with no birth complications and no illnesses or injuries that she is aware of. You are able to start a 22 g IV in the AC space TKO and continue to monitor the baby's condition, which is unchanged en route. In the ED, a determination of sepsis is made, and the infant is admitted to the ICU.

1. Put a ✓ beside some possible causes of this baby's condition based on your initial impression.

   a. _________ Abuse   **e.** _________ Jaundice

   b. _________ Croup   **f.** _________ Meningitis

   c. _________ Dehydration   **g.** _________ Sepsis

   d. _________ Febrile seizure

2. Which aspects of the physical examination indicated that the baby was in distress?

   ____

   ____

3. What treatment should have been given to treat the heart rate or rhythm?
   a. Adenosine   **c.** Vagal maneuvers
   b. Diltiazem   **d.** None of the above

4. What was the baby's score on the Glasgow Coma Scale?

   ____

5. What should you monitor most closely as you continue transport?

____

____

6. a. List at least three possible causes of seizure in a baby this age.

____

____

    b. What interventions would you consider if the child has another seizure?

____

____

7. Why should you assess the blood glucose level in this child even though you know that the onset of type 1 diabetes does not usually occur until later in childhood?

____

____

CHAPTER 48 ANSWERS

REVIEW QUESTIONS

1. f

2. e

3. h

4. a

5. g

6. c

7. b
(Questions 1–7, Objective 7)

8. a. Neonate

    b. Infant, toddler, and preschooler

    c. Neonate

    d. Infant and toddler

    e. Infant, toddler, and school-age child

   f. Young infant, infant, toddler, school-age child, and adolescent (sexual abuse)

   g. Preschooler and school-age child

   h. Adolescent
(Objective 2)

9. Humidified oxygen by non-rebreather mask, position of comfort (to maximize respiratory efficiency), albuterol 0.01 to 0.03 mL (0.05 to 0.15 mg)/kg/dose to maximum of 0.5 mL/dose diluted in 2 mL of 0.9% NS, or epinephrine 0.01 mL/kg subcutaneous (1:1000), maximum 0.3 mL
(Objective 5)

10. Tachycardia and anxiousness
(Objective 5)

11. Repeat drugs, initiate IV, and continue to reassess.
(Objective 5)

12. The patient will state improvement, respiratory rate will decrease, oxygen saturation will improve, use of accessory muscles will decrease, wheezing will diminish (inspiratory wheeze and then expiratory wheeze should dissipate), and heart rate may decrease (although possibly not because of the effects of beta-agonists).
(Objective 5)

13. Drooling, stridor, sudden onset of high fever, and dysphagia
(Objective 5)

14. a. Take the patient into the cool night air or into a steam-filled bathroom.
   b. Allow the child to assume a position of comfort and administer high-flow oxygen (humidified) by whatever means is least threatening to the child.
   c. Albuterol dilates lower airway structures. Croup causes upper airway narrowing.
(Objective 5)

15. Moderate to severe dehydration
(Objective 6)

16. Sinus tachycardia
(Objective 6)

17. Open airway, ventilate with 100% oxygen; initiate lactated Ringer solution or normal saline intravenously (intraosseously if intravenous line cannot be established), and infuse an initial fluid bolus of 20 mL/kg; reassess and repeat until perfusion improves.
(Objective 6)

18. BP, 82/44 mm Hg; P, 80 to 140/min; R, 30 to 40/min
(Objective 4)

19. Improved level of consciousness, skin color, and temperature
(Objective 6)

20. Sinus bradycardia, rate 30 beats/min
(Objective 7)

21. Assess the ABCs; secure the airway; administer 100% oxygen using bag-mask device; perform chest compressions; start an intravenous or intraosseous line; assess vital signs; and if bradycardia continues, administer epinephrine 0.1 mL/kg (1:10,000) intravenously or intraosseously.
(Objective 7)

670

22. Infuse the medication intraosseously or administer epinephrine 0.1 mL/kg (1:1000) endotracheally diluted to 3 to 5 mL. NOTE: The endotracheal dose is 10 times greater than the intravenous dose.
(Objective 7)

23. Atropine 0.02 mg/kg intravenously to a maximum single dose of 0.5 mg (child) and 1 mg (adolescent); minimum dose, 0.1 mg
(Objective 7)

24. a. Defibrillate at 2 J/kg; give 5 cycles of CPR; defibrillate 4 J/kg; CPR; start IV; give epinephrine 0.01 mg/kg (1:10,000)IV/IO every 3 to 5 minutes; secure the airway when possible; confirm placement; defibrillate 4 J/kg, CPR; consider amiodarone or magnesium sulfate
b. 0.01 mg/kg (0.1 mL/kg 1:10,000)
(Objective 7)

25. Description of seizure activity, vomiting during seizure, history of epilepsy or another major medical illness, other current medicines, potential for toxic ingestion, recent head injury, and complaints of headache or a stiff neck
(Objective 8)

26. Maintain airway and breathing; monitor vital signs; cool the child with tepid water and fanning; monitor electrocardiogram and oxygen saturation (if available); depending on the patient's vital signs and level of consciousness, initiate lactated Ringer solution intravenously to keep vein open and obtain a blood sample; assess blood sugar and treat if it is below 60 mg/dL.
(Objective 8)

27. a. Diazepam 1 mg every 2 to 5 minutes by slow IV; if intravenous or intraosseous infusion is not possible, administer medication rectally at a higher dose (0.5 mg/kg).
b. Lorazepam 0.05 to 0.15 mg/kg/dose intramuscularly, intravenously, or intraosseously to maximum dose 4 mg (rectal dose, 0.1–0.2 mg/kg)
(Objective 8)

28. a. 50% dextrose 1 to 2 mL/kg/dose or 25% dextrose 2 to 4 mL/kg/dose intravenously
(Objective 9)
b. Presenting symptoms of mild hypoglycemia may be hunger, weakness, tachypnea, and tachycardia. Presenting symptoms of moderate hypoglycemia may be sweating, tremors, irritability, vomiting, mood swings, blurred vision, stomachache, headache, and dizziness.
(Objective 9)

29. a. Because a relatively small loss of blood can be devastating, fluid resuscitation should be anticipated for blood volume losses that would seem small in an adult.
b. This makes children susceptible to hypothermia. Measures should be used on the scene to maintain body warmth.
c. This leaves them little reserve for a stressed situation such as shock. Energy and oxygen requirements should be reduced to a minimum by assisting ventilations and using measures to decrease anxiety and promote body warmth.
d. Volume replacement with lactated Ringer solution or normal saline should be initiated at 20 mL/kg given rapidly and repeated if no response is seen. If a good response is obtained, the fluids should be continued at a weight-related maintenance rate obtained from medical direction.
e. Intravenous access should first be attempted in a peripheral vein in the arms, hands, or feet. If access cannot be easily established and the patient's condition deteriorates, intraosseous infusion should be used.
(Objectives 6, 12)

30. Aspiration of marrow may rarely be obtained. The intravenous fluid will run freely with no evidence of infiltration.
(Objectives 2, 6)

31. Occurrence between midnight and 6 AM, male child younger than 6 months of age, occurrence between October and March, frothy sputum, wet diaper with stool, second child, and recent mild viral illness.
(Objective 13)

32. Document death as required by protocol and observe carefully for any obvious external signs of trauma.
(Objective 13)

33. Encourage your partner to verbalize, perhaps stating, "It's frightening to go on a call like this when you have a baby at home." Listen if he wants to talk; if he does not, check on him again in the morning. Initiate the CISD team following local protocol (if available).
(Objective 13)

34. Protect the cervical spine while opening the airway; hyperventilate with 100% oxygen and consider intubation; verify perfusion with slow pulse; if it is inadequate, initiate cardiopulmonary resuscitation; en route to the hospital, initiate an intravenous or intraosseous line and administer medicines if indicated.
(Objective 12)

35. The story does not match the physical findings or the child's developmental stage. An 8-month-old child is too young to ride a tricycle. A fall from a tricycle is unlikely to produce intracerebral bleeding. The child had no external signs of head trauma but had bruises at the shoulders, it may suggest shaking. The child was dirty (this could be normal).
(Objective 14)

36. Report the suspected abuse to the receiving facility and to other authorities as indicated by local protocol and state law. Carefully document all physical findings and statements made by the mother, using exact quotes if possible. This document is likely to be questioned in court if abuse is suspected.
(Objective 14)

37. Only enough data to address the immediate threats to the health of the sexually abused child should be elicited. The child should be made to feel safe and secure, and the detailed history and physical examination should be performed by child sexual abuse specialists if they are available in your area.
(Objective 14)

STUDENT SELF-ASSESSMENT

38. a. The other 11 components are system approach, education, data collection, quality improvement, injury prevention, prehospital care, emergency care, definitive care, rehabilitation, finance, and ongoing health care from birth to young adulthood.
(Objective 1)

39. b. Have them repeat things back to you in their words to be sure they understand. Give them choices when possible. Anticipate questions about the long-term effect of care, injuries, and so on.
(Objective 4)

40. b. Toddlers fear separation and loss of direction; school-age children fear bodily injury and mutilation but are less likely to interpret words literally.
(Objective 4)

41. b. Asthma is usually not diagnosed until a child is 3 to 5 years of age. Epiglottitis is more common in children 3 to 5 years of age.
(Objective 2)

42. c. Each component is important, but information about level of consciousness, color, respiratory effort, and muscle tone often can be assessed by observing children before touching them.
(Objective 3)

672

43. d. Other signs are use of accessory muscles, nasal flaring, tachypnea, bradypnea, irregular breathing pattern, grunting, and absent or abnormal breath sounds.
(Objective 3)

44. d. It may produce stridor and complete airway obstruction.
(Objective 5)

45. a. The correct dose of epinephrine is 0.01 mL/kg subcutaneously (1:1000), and the correct dose of terbutaline is 0.01 mg/kg of a 1 mg/mL solution subcutaneously.
(Objective 5)

46. d. The child should be permitted to assume a position of comfort, which typically is sitting up with the chin jutted forward to maximize airflow. Examination of the airway can produce obstruction and is contraindicated. Initiation of an intravenous infusion will not improve the child's condition and may cause the child to become agitated and cry, increasing the respiratory distress. Albuterol is not indicated. Epiglottitis is an upper airway problem.
(Objective 5)

47. a. Albuterol can provide temporary symptomatic relief with limited side effects.
(Objective 5)

48. d. Fluid resuscitation should not be delayed until the blood pressure drops, or resuscitating the child may be difficult. The fontanelle likely would be flat and the skin cool.
(Objective 6)

49. d. The recommended fluid bolus is 20 mL/kg.
20 mL/kg × 20 kg = 400 mL
(Objective 6)

50. c. Crackles and edema are characteristics of congestive heart failure associated with cardiomyopathy.
(Objective 6)

51. b. 44 lb = 20 kg; initial defibrillation is 2 joules/kg; 2 joules × 20 kg = 40 joules
(Objective 7)

52. d. Atropine 0.02 mg/kg to a maximum dose of 0.5 mg in a child
(Objective 7)

53. b. Epinephrine is the drug of choice in patients with bradycardia with hemodynamic compromise followed by atropine if the bradycardia was caused by vagal stimulation (e.g., suctioning).
(Objective 7)

54. a. If his condition deteriorates, synchronized cardioversion may be considered.
(Objective 7)

55. c. Unless the dehydration produces severe electrolyte imbalance, it is much more likely to produce shock and death than seizures.
(Objective 8)

56. c. Ventilatory equipment should be available, and the respiratory rate and depth should be closely monitored. Pulse oximetry should be used if available.
(Objective 8)

57. c. Undiagnosed type 1 diabetes can manifest in this manner with severe hyperglycemia and ketoacidosis. This child is critical and needs urgent transport with airway management, oxygenation, and fluid resuscitation. (Objective 9)

58. a. Hypoglycemia can lead to death if left uncorrected. (Objective 11)

59. d. Tachypnea, gastrointestinal irritation, hypoglycemia, cardiac dysrhythmias (ventricular), seizure, coma, coagulation defects, and death can occur from salicylate poisoning. (Objective 11)

60. d. Changes in color perception, hallucinations, and blindness can occur, as well as other central nervous system and gastrointestinal effects. (Objective 11)

61. c. Naloxone is indicated for opioid narcotic overdose. Epinephrine would be indicated only if cardiac arrest ensues. Lorazepam is administered to treat anxiety and seizures. Flumazenil is an antidote to benzodiazepine overdose. (Objective 11)

62. d. Sodium bicarbonate may be given to improve myocardial contractility and cardiac output. Lidocaine would be given to treat ventricular dysrhythmias (if present). Normal saline (10 mL/kg bolus) may be given to improve cardiac output. Oxygen should be given at high flow based on the patient's physical findings. (Objective 11)

63. a. Other prehospital interventions may include oxygen administration, ventilatory support (if indicated), ECG monitoring, treatment for shock, epinephrine infusion, sodium bicarbonate, and calcium chloride (controversial). (Objective 11)

64. d. Motor vehicle crashes are the leading cause of death and serious injury in children. (Objective 12)

65. a. Other findings include hypertension, bradycardia, and Cheyne-Stokes respirations. (Objective 12)

66. c (Objective 12)

67. c. Low maternal or paternal age, low socioeconomic group, and rank of second or third in the birth order are associated with an increased incidence. (Objective 13)

68. c. Fractures in a child younger than 2 years of age should be cause for suspicion. (Objective 14)

69. d. Retinal hemorrhage is a sign of a shaken baby. (Objective 14)

70. d. If suctioning does not improve the situation, removing and replacing the tracheostomy may be necessary. If this is not possible or proves unsuccessful, oral intubation or intubation through the stoma may be necessary. (Objective 15)

71. a. Correcting the hypoxia is the priority. The machine can be checked and fixed after the hypoxia has been corrected.
(Objective 15)

72. a. If the child develops signs of air embolism, position him on the left side with his head lowered and administer high-flow oxygen.
(Objective 15)

73. b. If the tube becomes dislodged, the feeding could be delivered to the lung, causing aspiration.
(Objective 15)

WRAP IT UP

1. a, c, f, g. The baby is too young for croup and for febrile seizures (and the temperature is not high). No evidence of yellow skin or eyes was noted, which would be apparent in jaundice. Dehydration is less likely because skin turgor is normal and the diaper is wet.
(Objective 2)

2. Decreased muscle tone and level of consciousness; labored, rapid breathing; rapid heart rate; skin color
(Objective 3)

3. d. Based on the information available, this baby's rapid heart rate probably is sinus tachycardia. If the rhythm were SVT, the heart rate could be expected to be about 220 beats/min. Treatment should focus on the underlying cause of the tachycardia.
(Objective 7)

4. Opens eyes to pain (2) + Flexion to pain (4) + Whines (3) = 9
(Objective 3)

5. Respiratory status should be monitored closely by observing rate; effort; Sao_2; skin color; heart rate; and, if available, end-tidal CO_2.
(Objective 3)

6. a. Head trauma, intracranial infection, metabolic disturbance, poisoning, epilepsy
b. Secure the airway, manage breathing, and consider administration of lorazepam or diazepam.
(Objective 8)

7. Blood glucose can be altered by other illnesses and should be assessed in any child with an altered level of consciousness.
(Objective 3)

49 Geriatrics

READING ASSIGNMENT

Chapter 49, pages 1388-1414, in *Mosby's Paramedic Textbook,* ed. 4.

OBJECTIVES

Upon completion of this chapter, the paramedic student will be able to do the following:

1. Explain the physiology of the aging process as it relates to major body systems and homeostasis.
2. Describe general principles of assessment specific to older adults.
3. Describe the pathophysiology, assessment, and management of specific illnesses that affect selected body systems in the geriatric patient.
4. Identify specific problems with sensations experienced by some geriatric patients.
5. Discuss effects of drug toxicity and alcoholism in the older adult.
6. Identify factors that contribute to environmental emergencies in the geriatric patient.
7. Discuss prehospital assessment and management of depression and suicide in the older adult.
8. Describe the epidemiology, assessment, and management of trauma in the geriatric patient.
9. Identify characteristics of elder abuse.

SUMMARY

- The aging process proceeds at different rates in different persons. Respiratory function in older adults generally is compromised. This is a result of changes in pulmonary physiology that go along with the aging process. Cardiac function also declines with age. This is a result of normal physiologic changes and the high incidence of coronary artery disease. Renal blood flow falls an average of 50% between 30 and 80 years of age. A gradual decrease in neurons, decreased cerebral blood flow, and changes in the location and amounts of specific neurotransmitters probably contribute to changes in the central nervous system. As the body ages, muscles shrink, muscles and ligaments calcify, and the intervertebral disks become thin. Other physiologic changes that occur with aging include changes in body mass and total body water, a decreased ability to maintain internal homeostasis, a decrease in the function of immunological mechanisms, nutritional disorders, and decreases in hearing and visual acuity.
- Normal changes with aging and existing illnesses may make evaluation of ill or injured geriatric patients a challenge.
- Pneumonia is a leading cause of death in the geriatric age group. It often is fatal in frail adults. Chronic obstructive pulmonary disease (COPD) is a common finding in geriatric patients with a history of smoking. The disease usually is associated with various other diseases that result in reduced expiratory airflow. Pulmonary embolism is a life-threatening cause of dyspnea. Pulmonary embolism is associated with venous stasis, heart failure, COPD, malignancy, and immobilization. All of these are common in older adults.
- A lack of the typical chest pain can cause myocardial infarction to go unrecognized in geriatric patients. Heart failure is more frequent in geriatric patients and has a larger incidence of noncardiac causes. The most common cause of dysrhythmias in geriatric patients is hypertensive heart disease. Abdominal aortic aneurysm affects 2% to 4% of the U.S. population older than 50 years of age. This aneurysm is most prevalent between 60 and 70 years of age. The incidence of hypertension in geriatric patients increases when atherosclerosis is present.
- Risk factors for cerebral vascular disease in older adults include smoking, hypertension, diabetes, atherosclerosis, hyperlipidemia, polycythemia, and heart disease.
- Delirium is an abrupt disorientation of time and place. Delirium is commonly a result of physical illness.
- Dementia is a slow, progressive loss of awareness of time and place. It usually involves an inability to learn new things or remember recent events. This condition often is a result of brain disease. Alzheimer disease is the most common cause of dementia. Alzheimer's disease is a condition in which nerve cells in the cerebral cortex die and the brain substance shrinks.
- Parkinson disease is a brain disorder. It causes muscle tremor, stiffness, and weakness.
- About 20% of older adults have diabetes. Almost 40% have some impaired glucose tolerance. Hyperglycemic hyperosmolar nonketotic coma is a serious complication of elderly patients with type 2 diabetes. It has a mortality rate of 20% to 50%. Thyroid disease is more common in geriatric patients. It may not present in the classic manner.

- Gastrointestinal bleeding most often affects patients between 60 and 90 years of age. It has a mortality rate of about 10%. Bowel obstruction generally occurs in patients with prior abdominal surgeries or hernias. It also occurs in those with colon cancer. Some geriatric patients may have problems with continence or elimination.
- Aging results in a gradual decrease in epidermal cellular turnover. It also results in loss of deep and dermal vessels. Capillary circulation leads to changes in thermal regulation and skin-related complications.
- Osteoarthritis is a common form of arthritis in geriatric patients. It results from cartilage loss and wear and tear on the joints. The loss in bone density from osteoporosis causes bones to become brittle. These bones may fracture easily.
- As persons age, they may experience problems with vision, hearing, and speech.
- Geriatric patients are at an increased risk for adverse drug reactions because of age-related changes in body makeup and drug distribution. It also is the result of metabolism and excretion. Moreover, the risk for adverse drug reactions often stems from multiple prescribed drugs. Alcohol abuse is a common problem in geriatric patients.
- Geriatric patients may develop hypothermia while indoors. This may be the result of cold surroundings or an illness that alters heat production or conservation. Hyperthermia most likely results from exposure to high temperatures that continue for several days.
- Depression is common in geriatric patients. It can result from physiologic and psychological causes. The rate of completed suicides for geriatric patients is higher than that of the general population.
- One third of traumatic deaths in persons 65 to 74 years of age result from vehicular trauma. Twenty-five percent result from falls. In those older than 80 years of age, falls account for 50% of injury-related deaths. The risk of fatality from multiple trauma is estimated to be three times greater at 70 years of age than at 20 years of age.
- Elder abuse is classified as physical abuse, psychological abuse, financial or material abuse, and neglect.

REVIEW QUESTIONS

1. An 85-year-old woman falls down an escalator at a department store. Explain how age-related changes in each of the following areas increase her risk of sustaining a traumatic injury or influence her body's response to a major injury.

   a. Respiratory system:

   ____

   ____

   b. Cardiovascular system:

   ____

   ____

   c. Renal system:

   ____

   ____

   d. Musculoskeletal system:

   ____

   ____

   e. Thermoregulation:

   ____

   ____

2. A 70-year-old man fell to the kitchen floor. He says he is just fine. His daughter states that he has a history of diabetes, a heart attack, heart failure, and lung disease. His home medications include Lanoxin, insulin, furosemide, Slow-K, and a number of vitamins and laxatives. He is on oxygen at 2 L/min by nasal cannula.

    a. What factors will make it difficult to assess and determine the nature of his acute problem?

____

____

____

____

    b. List eight possible causes of his fall.

a. __________	**e.** __________
b. __________	**f.** __________
c. __________	**g.** __________
d. __________	**h.** __________

Questions 3 to 5 pertain to the following case study:

A 70-year-old man calls you to his home complaining of dyspnea and weakness. He has no underlying pulmonary problems. His ECG is shown in Fig. 49-1.

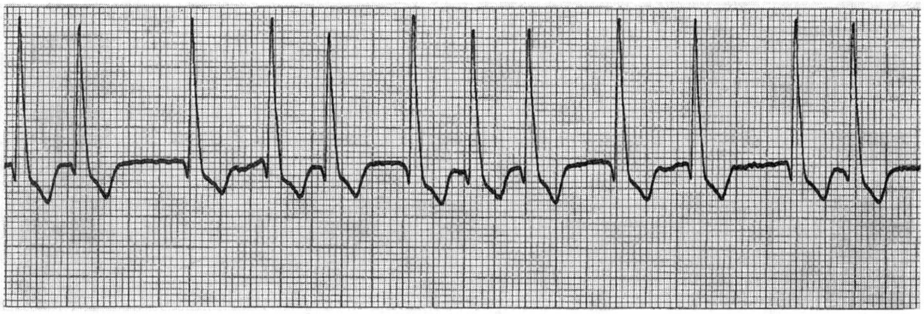

Figure 49-1

3. Why should you assess the appropriate history and physical examination for myocardial infarction and pulmonary embolism on this patient?

____

4. What is your interpretation of the ECG rhythm?

____

5. List two complications associated with this dysrhythmia.

    a. ____

    b. ____

679

6. A 76-year-old woman complains of diffuse abdominal pain. Identify four conditions that can cause this symptom.

a. ____

b. ____

c. ____

d. ____

7. Briefly describe the following characteristics of delirium:

a. Onset:

____

b. Duration:

____

c. Metabolic causes:

____

8. List four reversible causes of dementia.

a. ___________________________ **c.** ___________________________

b. ___________________________ **d.** ___________________________

Questions 9 to 11 pertain to the following case study:

An 80-year-old man experiences a syncopal episode in church. He is conscious but pale and diaphoretic. His blood pressure is 80/50 mm Hg. His ECG is shown in Fig. 49-2.

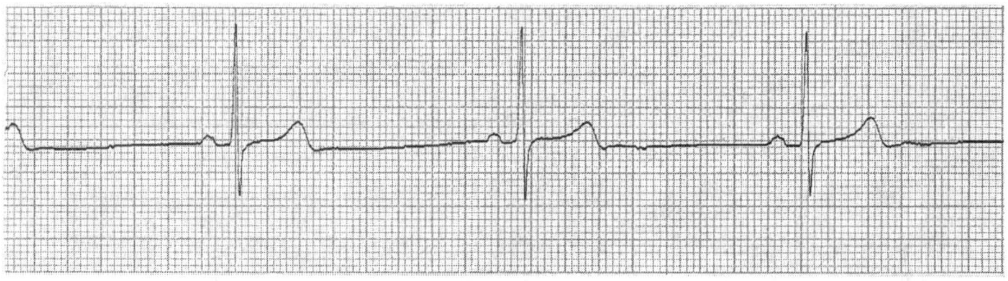

Figure 49-2

9. What is your interpretation of the rhythm?

____

10. a. State the dose and route of administration of the drug used to treat this rhythm.

____

b. What other intervention should be considered if drug therapy is unsuccessful?

____

11. List two possible causes of the signs and symptoms this patient is experiencing.

a. ____

b. ____

Questions 12 to 15 pertain to the following case study:

A 69-year-old woman complains of dyspnea and chills. She has been ill with a mild cough and weakness for approximately 1 week. Her skin is cold and clammy. Vital signs are BP, 108/70 mm Hg; P, 135/min; and R, 30/min. Breath sounds in the right base are diminished with scattered crackles. Her ECG is shown in Fig. 49-3.

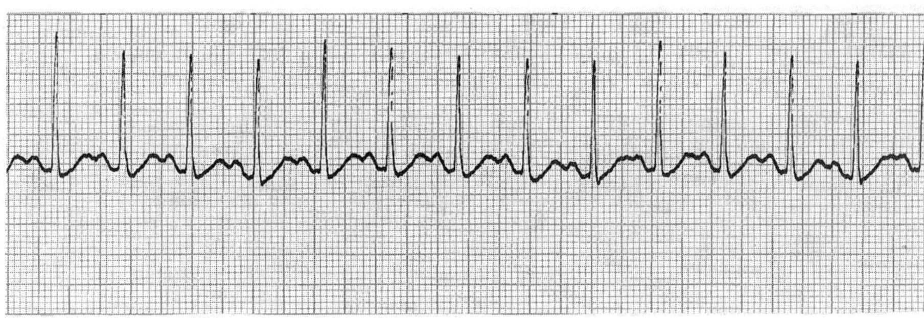

Figure 49-3

12. Identify the rhythm.

____

13. What illness do you suspect?

____

14. Should you use synchronized cardioversion or adenosine to treat her? Explain your answer.

____

15. What other interventions are indicated for this patient?

____

____

16. An 76-year-old man with a history of chronic lung disease is being transferred to another hospital. Oxygen is being supplied by Venturi mask at 24%. His vital signs are within normal limits. His ECG tracing is shown in Fig. 49-4.

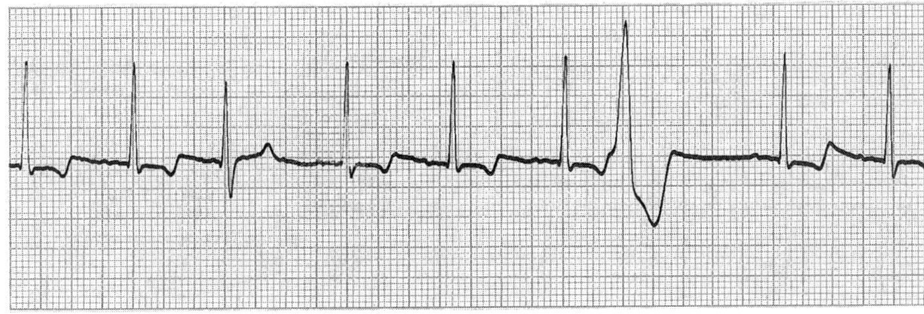

Figure 49-4

a. Identify the rhythm strip.

____

b. What interventions are indicated with this rhythm?

____

c. For what signs and symptoms of acute decompensation of COPD will you observe?

____

17. An 82-year-old woman who had a syncopal episode is now awake and has the following vital signs: BP, 108/70 mm Hg; P, 50/min; and R, 18/min and unlabored. Her lungs are clear. The ECG is shown in Fig. 49-5.

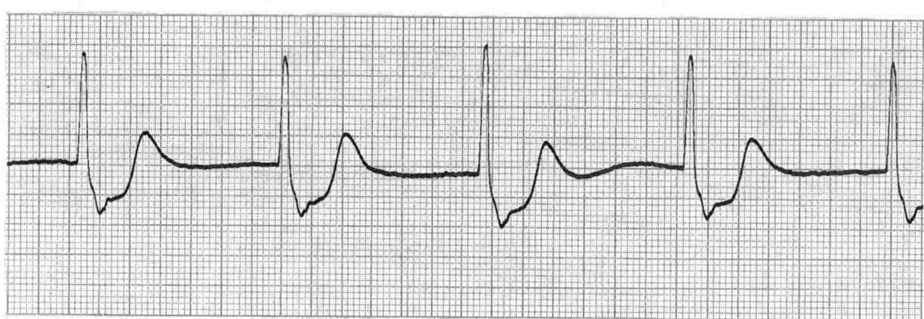

Figure 49-5

a. Identify the rhythm strip.

____

b. After oxygen has been administered and intravenous therapy started, what interventions should be performed en route to the medical center?

____

c. What age-related changes predispose this patient to developing this rhythm?

____

Questions 18 to 21 refer to the following case study:

The family of a 72-year-old man states that he suddenly became confused and disoriented to time and place over the past few hours. His vital signs are BP, 168/110 mm Hg; P, 100/min; and R, 20/min. His ECG is shown in Fig. 49-6.

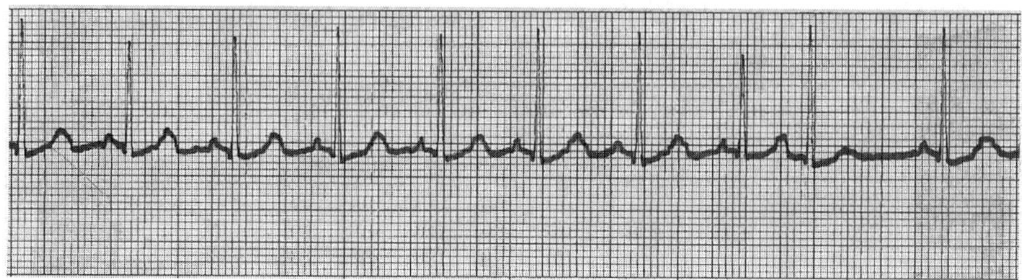

Figure 49-6

18. Is he likely experiencing dementia or delirium?

____

19. Identify the rhythm strip.

____

20. Are his symptoms related to his ECG tracing? Explain your answer.

____

21. List two factors that could cause this change in behavior.

a. ____

b. ____

Questions 22 and 23 refer to the following case study:

An 80-year-old woman complains of dizziness and shortness of breath. Her vital signs are BP, 82/50 mm Hg; P, 50/min; and R, 24/min. Her ECG tracing is shown in Fig. 49-7.

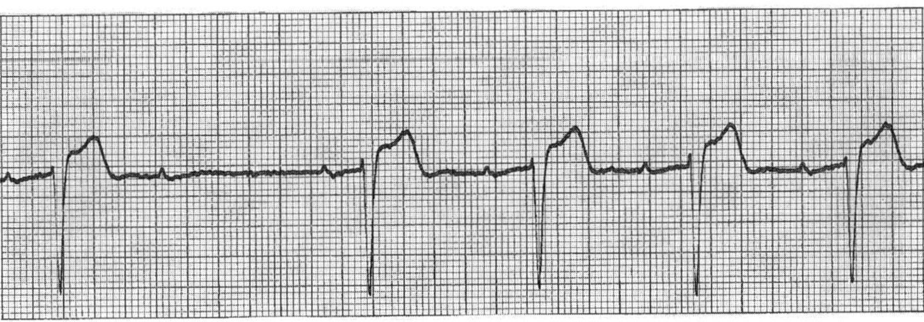

Figure 49-7

22. Identify the rhythm strip.

____

23. a. What illness may be causing her signs and symptoms?

____

b. List prehospital interventions that you will consider for this patient.

____

24. A 94-year-old woman who was found in her apartment is confused and difficult to arouse. You note that it feels very cold inside, and her temperature is 95°F (35°C). List at least nine reasons (physiologic, social, or medical) why she is at risk for hypothermia.

____

____

____

25. Adverse drug reactions are common in older adults. For each of the following drugs or drug groups, list two signs or symptoms associated with overdose or adverse effects.

a. Anticoagulants:

____

____

b. Diuretics:

____

____

c. Digitalis:

____

____

d. Tricyclic antidepressants:

____

____

e. Sedative–hypnotic drugs:

____

____

f. Propranolol:

____

____

g. Theophylline:

____

____

h. Quinidine:

____

____

Questions 26 to 29 refer to the following case study:

You are on the scene of a single-car accident in which a compact car struck a bridge abutment at high speed. The driver, an anxious 75-year-old man, complains of mild abdominal discomfort. Vital signs are BP, 90/70 mm Hg; P, 70/min; and R, 24/min and somewhat labored. His skin is pale and clammy, and his nailbeds are dusky.

26. What vital sign assessment does not fit with this man's clinical picture?

---

27. What aspect of his history may explain this discrepancy?

---

28. Because he has just mild abdominal pain, should you be concerned?

---

29. What prehospital treatment should be given after the cervical spine has been appropriately immobilized?

---

30. A 94-year-old man appears dehydrated and very dirty. You note large ecchymotic areas on his back and hips. The daughter, who lives with him, says his bruises were caused by a fall.

    a. If you suspect elder abuse, what should you do?

---

    b. Does the caregiver have any characteristics of an elder abuser?

STUDENT SELF-ASSESSMENT

31. What can alterations in lung and chest wall compliance in the older adult cause to decrease?
    a. Alveolar diameter   **c.** Total lung capacity
    b. Residual volume   **d.** Vital capacity

32. What is the medical term for humpback posture that develops as a result of osteoporosis?
    a. Kyphosis   **c.** Osteoarthritis
    b. Lordosis   **d.** Scoliosis

33. An elderly man has paroxysmal nocturnal dyspnea. Crackles and wheezes are auscultated. He had an MI 3 years ago. Vital signs are BP, 170/94 mm Hg; P, 124/min; R, 28/min; and SaO_2, 90% on room air. You administer oxygen. What drug is indicated next?
    a. Albuterol   **c.** Epinephrine
    b. Furosemide   **d.** Nitroglycerin

34. An elderly patient is on bed rest after treatment for metastatic breast cancer.. She suddenly develops dyspnea and tachycardia. Which is a likely cause of her symptoms?
    a. Chronic obstructive pulmonary disease
    b. Emphysema
    c. Lung cancer
    d. Pulmonary embolus

35. Which is a possible cause of dementia?
    a. Alzheimer disease
    b. Epilepsy
    c. Hyperglycemia
    d. Pneumonia

36. Which illness causes trembling; a rigid posture; slow movement; and shuffling, unbalanced walking?
    a. Alzheimer disease
    b. Delirium
    c. Dementia
    d. Parkinson disease

37. Which is a critical prehospital intervention for an unconscious patient with diabetes who has hyperglycemic hyperosmolar nonketotic coma?
    a. Dextrose
    b. Glucagon
    c. IV fluids
    d. Sodium bicarbonate

38. Which consequence of thyroid dysfunction that might lead to a call for EMS?
    a. Altered mental status
    b. Bradycardia
    c. Diarrhea
    d. Weight gain

39. Your elderly male patient is unable to urinate. What condition should you inquire about specifically when obtaining his history?
    a. Constipation
    b. Epididymitis
    c. Kidney stones
    d. Prostate enlargement

40. What causes pressure ulcers?
    a. Burns
    b. Tissue hypoxia
    c. Infection
    d. Tears of the tissue

41. Which eye condition causes damage to the optic nerve and can result in blindness if untreated?
    a. Cataracts
    b. Conjunctivitis
    c. Corneal abrasion
    d. Glaucoma

42. A patient is being treated for Parkinson disease. What sign, if present, might you attribute to drug toxicity?
    a. Altered vision
    b. Hypokalemia
    c. Paresthesias
    d. Tardive dyskinesia

43. Which medication increases the elderly patient's risk of hyperthermia?
    a. Amitriptyline
    b. Aspirin
    c. Cimetidine (Tagamet)
    d. Coumadin

44. What is a physiologic cause of depression in an elderly patient?
    a. Hyperglycemia
    b. Hypertension
    c. Hyponatremia
    d. Hypothermia

45. What is the most common psychiatric disorder in older adults?
    a. Bipolar disorder
    b. Depression
    c. Hysteria
    d. Schizophrenia

46. Why might the symptoms of increased intracranial pressure be delayed in an older patient?
    a. Altered blood–brain barrier
    b. Cerebral atrophy
    c. Decreased cerebral blood flow
    d. Fragile bridging veins

686

47. Which bone is most often fractured in falls by older adults?

    a. Ankle   **c.** Hip

    b. Clavicle   **d.** Wrist

48. Which home medication increases the older person's risk of falling?

    a. Alprazolam   **c.** Hydrochlorothiazide

    b. Digoxin   **d.** Dipyridamole

WRAP IT UP

Your partner groans as your dispatcher sends you to a familiar address for a "person down with possible forcible entry." The 80-year-old patient is well known because of her frequent 9-1-1 calls to "assist the invalid" when she misses her walker and slides to the floor. Since her stroke 3 months ago, she calls 9-1-1 several times a week despite attempts to identify appropriate social services. Her home is locked, and you can see that she is sitting on the floor, but she oddly won't acknowledge the knocking on the window. The fire captain quickly breaks out a pane of glass on a rear door and unlocks it, permitting you to enter her steamy home. "Mabel, what's going on today?" you call out. As you approach her, you recognize that something is wrong; instead of her typical crooked smile, she is staring blankly ahead, showing no sign she recognizes you. Her skin color isn't right either; she looks pale and sweaty, and her usually neatly coifed hair is disheveled and dirty. As you grasp her wrist, you feel her rapid, irregular pulse and note that her breathing is labored and fast. Her oxygen saturation is only 89%, much lower than her normal reading, and you can hear some basilar crackles in her lungs. A quick scan of her body reveals no obvious injuries. "Mabel, what's wrong? Are you in pain? Did you fall?" you ask. She looks blankly at you, and the usually polite and articulate woman mumbles some obscenities and pushes you away. You administer oxygen and assess her vital signs, which are BP, 102/60 mm Hg; P, 124/min; and R, 24/min. Her pupils are 3 mm, equal, and reactive to light. By then your partner has the cot at her side, and you guide her onto it and secure the straps. In the ambulance, her ECG shows atrial fibrillation, and a blood sugar reading of 78 mg/dL is obtained as you start her IV. As you look through her sack of familiar medicines (furosemide, Plavix, aspirin, Glucotrol, Lipitor, Lanoxin, Paxil), you realize that some of them are empty, and based on the date they were prescribed, they should not be. Her Sao$_2$ is improving on oxygen, and her vital signs are unchanged, but she is still muttering obscenities. You look more carefully head to toe to see if you've missed something on your initial exam, but you find nothing additional. As you sit writing your report at the hospital, you recall your last visit, 3 days ago, and try to think of anything unusual that may have occurred, but nothing seemed out of place.

1. Based on the information given, list five chronic problems this patient is likely to have.

    a. ____

    b. ____

    c. ____

    d. ____

    e. ____

2. Place a ✓ beside some possible causes for this patient's altered level of consciousness.

    a. _______ Delirium   **f.** _______ Hypoxia

    b. _______ Dementia   **g.** _______ Hypoglycemia

    c. _______ Head injury   **h.** _______ Overdose

    d. _______ Hyperthermia   **i.** _______ Sepsis

    e. _______ Depression   **j.** _______ Stroke

3. **a.** Would this patient be a candidate for fibrinolytic therapy if an acute stroke were diagnosed? Yes/No
   b. Explain your answer:

____

____

4. Which of the patient's social or medical conditions would not put her at high risk for complications related to her diabetes?
   a. Aspirin use
   b. Decreased ability to care for herself
   c. Living alone
   d. Other illnesses

5. If you think she has taken an overdose, what problems should you anticipate during transport based on your knowledge of her prescription drugs.

CHAPTER 49 ANSWERS

REVIEW QUESTIONS

1. a. Because the baseline Pao_2 is lower, the body is less able to compensate if chest trauma is sustained or if the patient is hypoxic because of trauma (e.g., inhalation injury). The chest wall is less elastic and more susceptible to injury.
   b. Myocardial contusion can cause pump failure stemming from poor cardiac reserve. A decreased ability to increase the heart rate can result in a decreased ability to compensate for shock, and dysrhythmias can cause syncope and precipitate a fall.
   c. Renal blood flow is decreased; therefore, a sudden traumatic event that causes shock and hypoperfusion to the kidneys can precipitate the onset of renal failure; decreased renal function can make an older adult more susceptible to toxic drug effects, leading to CNS depression, disturbances in balance, hypotension, and dysrhythmias, all of which can increase the risk of falls.
   d. Kyphosis may alter balance and predispose a person to falls, and osteoporosis increases the incidence of fractures after falls.
   e. Advancing age can result in decreased peripheral vasoconstriction, a lowered metabolic rate, and poor peripheral circulation and can impair the body's ability to regulate temperature effectively, especially during stressful events such as traumatic injury. Hypothermia may occur rapidly.
   (Objective 1)

2. a. His multiple illnesses and drugs make it difficult to assess for new onset of signs or symptoms. Diabetes: Impairs pain perception and retards healing. Heart attack and heart failure: Cardiac output may be impaired from chronic conditions, and dysrhythmias may be chronic. Lung disease: Patient's baseline must be determined. Cyanosis, increased respiratory rate, and abnormal lung sounds may be chronic. Lanoxin: Therapeutic effects slow heart rate; the patient may not become tachycardic in response to trauma, and toxic effects may cause dysrhythmias. Insulin: Excessive amounts may cause hypoglycemia and produce central nervous system impairment. Furosemide: Diuretics may cause an electrolyte imbalance that can affect muscle strength and may precipitate dysrhythmias that can cause syncope and falls. His baseline SaO_2 may be lower than normal.
   (Objective 2)

   b. Dysrhythmias, visual impairment, neurologic disabilities, arthritis, changes in gait, postural hypotension, syncope, cerebrovascular accident or transient ischemic attack, medications, slippery surfaces, loose rugs, objects on floors, poor lighting, pets, low beds or toilet seats, defective walking equipment, and lack of handrails on stairs
   (Objective 8)

3. In an older adult, dyspnea and weakness may be the only presenting history for myocardial infarction. Carefully obtain a patient history; perform a physical examination, including a 12-lead ECG; and treat with a high index of suspicion for myocardial infarction (these signs and symptoms also accompany pulmonary embolus).
   (Objective 3)

4. Atrial fibrillation
(Objective 3)

5. Cerebrovascular accident and pulmonary embolism
(Objective 3)

6. Cholecystitis, colonic diverticular disease, appendicitis, aortic abdominal aneurysm, mesenteric artery occlusion, and mesenteric vein thrombosis
(Objective 2)

7. a. Rapid
b. Variable: It is usually self-limited and can be corrected quickly when the cause is identified.
c. Electrolyte imbalance, hypoglycemia, hyperglycemia, acid–base imbalance, hypoxia, vital organ failure, and Wernicke encephalopathy
(Objective 3)

8. Hypothyroidism, Cushing syndrome, vitamin deficiencies, and hydrocephalus
(Objective 3)

9. Sinus bradycardia, rate 30 beats/min
(Objective 3)

10. a. Atropine 0.5 mg IV
(Objective 3)

b. Transcutaneous pacing
(Objective 3)

11. Acute myocardial infarction, drug toxicity, or vagal response
(Objective 3)

12. Sinus tachycardia
(Objective 3)

13. Bacterial pneumonia or pulmonary embolus
(Objective 3)

14. No to both; you must treat the patient and her underlying problem.
(Objective 3)

15. Administer high-flow oxygen via a non-rebreather mask, initiate intravenous therapy, and monitor the patient's response and vital signs closely en route.
(Objective 3)

16. a. Normal sinus rhythm with a premature atrial contraction and a premature ventricular contraction
b. Continue to monitor the patient and the electrocardiographic rhythm.
c. Assess for limited airflow, increased work of breathing, dyspnea, hypoxemia, or hemodynamic compromise. Measure for excessive increases in $EtCO_2$ if available.
(Objective 3)

17. a. Junctional rhythm
b. Observe the patient for any signs of hemodynamic compromise related to the slow rhythm (monitor vital signs and electrocardiogram). Consider drug administration or pacing if unstable.
c. Functional cells are lost in the sinoatrial and atrioventricular nodes during aging, which contributes to dysrhythmias.
(Objectives 2, 3)

18. Delirium (sudden onset)
(Objective 3)

19. Normal sinus rhythm with a premature atrial contraction
(Objective 3)

20. There is no reason for this ECG to cause these symptoms.
(Objective 3)

21. Intoxication or poisoning, withdrawal from drugs, metabolic disturbances, infectious processes, CNS trauma, and stroke
(Objective 3)

22. Second-degree heart block Mobitz type II
(Objective 3)

23. a. Myocardial infarction is the most likely cause.
(Objective 3)

b. Administer high-concentration oxygen. Continue assessment to include breath sounds and observe for signs of congestive heart failure; perform a head-to-toe survey. Initiate IV therapy at a TKO rate. Prepare to apply transcutaneous pacing. Consult with medical direction regarding administration of sedation (with caution because of dyspnea and hypotension). Provide rapid transport for definitive cardiac care. Perform a 12-lead ECG if available.
(Objective 3)

24. Decreased ability to sense changes in ambient temperature, less total body water to store heat, reduced likelihood of becoming tachycardic to compensate for cold stress, decreased ability to shiver, inability to pay utilities for heat, insufficient insulation, malnutrition, arthritis, drug overdose, hepatic failure, hypoglycemia, infection, Parkinson disease, stroke, thyroid disease, and uremia
(Objective 6)

25. a. Bleeding problems, increased hemorrhage from trauma, multiple contusions, and allergic   reactions
b. Electrolyte abnormalities (sodium and potassium) and dehydration
c. Influenza-like symptoms, multiple dysrhythmias, and bradycardia
d. Dry mouth, tachycardia, ventricular dysrhythmias, seizures, and impaired level of consciousness
e. Impaired perception (increased risk of falls) and decreased level of consciousness with respiratory depression
f. Decreased heart rate (excessive), bronchoconstriction, and mood alteration
g. Tachycardia, dysrhythmias, and CNS stimulation
h. Dysrhythmias and clotting abnormalities
(Objective 5)

26. His heart rate is slow relative to the rest of his clinical picture (everything else indicates impending shock or hypoxia).
(Objective 8)

27. He may have a pacemaker or may be taking medications (e.g., digitalis or beta blockers) that prevent his heart rate from becoming tachycardic in response to a decrease in cardiac output.
(Objective 8)

28. Yes, abdominal injuries are frequently lethal in older adults. His perception of pain may be impaired, and this situation could deteriorate quickly, especially with signs of shock.
(Objective 8)

29. Ensure a patent airway; deliver high-flow oxygen by non-rebreather mask; apply pneumatic antishock garments (if indicated by local protocol); en route to a trauma center, start two large-bore intravenous lines and administer small fluid challenges in consultation with medical direction; frequently monitor vital signs and lung sounds (for increased rales [crackles]) to make sure the patient is not developing a volume overload.
(Objective 8)

30. a. Follow local protocols and report to appropriate authority (e.g., local law enforcement, abuse hotline, medical direction) as indicated; report findings to receiving hospital and document findings thoroughly on prehospital run report.
b. Yes, the daughter lives with her parent.
(Objective 9)

STUDENT SELF-ASSESSMENT

31. d. Total lung capacity remains unchanged because the loss of chest wall compliance balances the weakened respiratory muscles. The residual volume increases as a result of variable increases in alveolar diameter and the tendency for distal airways to collapse on expiration.
(Objective 1)

690

32. a. Lordosis is the normal S curve of the spine. Osteolysis is degeneration of bone. Scoliosis is lateral curvature of the spine, usually found in childhood.
(Objective 3)

33. d. The patient has no history of COPD. His history and clinical presentation point to left-sided heart failure. Nitroglycerin would be the drug of choice.
(Objective 3)

34. d. Pulmonary embolus is a higher risk in patients with cancer and in bedridden patients. It should be suspected when there is sudden onset of dyspnea.
(Objective 3)

35. a. The other conditions may cause delirium.
(Objective 3)

36. d. These signs can be reduced or eliminated with drug therapy.
(Objective 3)

37. c. This condition results from excessive glucose in the blood and causes serious dehydration; IV fluids are indicated in the prehospital setting to treat the severe dehydration. Sodium bicarbonate may be indicated after arterial blood gas analysis or if the patient experiences cardiac arrest.
(Objective 3)

38. a. Thyroid dysfunction may also cause tachydysrhythmias, constipation, weight loss, anemia, or musculoskeletal complaints.
(Objective 3)

39. d. Prostate enlargement is a cause of dysuria commonly found in this age group.
(Objective 3)

40. b. The ulcers often become infected because of the poor blood supply to the area.
(Objective 3)

41. d. Cataracts are a loss in transparency of the lens of the eye. Conjunctivitis is an inflammation of the conjunctiva of the eye. Corneal abrasion is a scraping-off of the outer layer of the cornea.
(Objective 4)

42. d. Some of the older drugs prescribed for patients with Parkinson disease may produce this reaction.
(Objective 5)

43. a. Cyclic antidepressants, antidysrhythmics, and beta-blockers may increase the risk of hyperthermia.
(Objective 6)

44. c. This may result from diuretic or other drug therapy and can have a very slow onset.
(Objective 7)

45. b. It may be caused by physiological or psychological factors.
(Objective 7)

46. b. The venous blood of a subdural hematoma takes longer to fill the larger space between the skull and the brain.
(Objective 8)

47. c
(Objective 8)

48. a. Sedative–hypnotic drugs put older patients at greater risk for falls.
(Objective 8)

WRAP IT UP

1. Stroke (in history and Coumadin); congestive heart failure (Lanoxin, furosemide); atrial fibrillation (Lanoxin); type 2 diabetes (Glucotrol); high cholesterol (Lipitor); depression or anxiety (Paxil)
(Objectives 2, 3)

2. a (sudden onset of confusion); c (altered level of consciousness); d (house is hot); e (age and Paxil); f (Sao_2 and crackles); h (missing pills); i (elders are at high risk; crackles in lungs); j (prior stroke, atrial fibrillation)
(Objective 3)

3. a. No
   b. Unknown time of onset of symptoms (must be less than 3 hours)
   (Objective 2)

4. a. All of the other factors listed increase her risk of having poorly controlled diabetes.
   (Objective 3)

5. Possibility for bleeding (Coumadin, aspirin); acidosis (aspirin); hypoglycemia (Glucotrol); bradycardia or dysrhythmias (Lanoxin); depressed respirations (Paxil)
   (Objective 2)

50 Abuse and Neglect

Chapter 50, pages 1415-1428, in *Mosby's Paramedic Textbook,* ed. 4.

OBJECTIVES

Upon completion of this chapter, the paramedic student will be able to do the following:

1. Define *battering*.
2. Describe the characteristics of abusive relationships.
3. Outline findings that indicate a battered patient.
4. Describe prehospital considerations when responding to and caring for battered patients.
5. Identify types of elder abuse.
6. Discuss legal considerations related to all forms of abuse.
7. Describe characteristics of abused children and their abusers.
8. Outline the physical examination of the abused child.
9. Describe the characteristics of sexual assault.
10. Outline prehospital patient care considerations for the patient who has been sexually assaulted.

SUMMARY

- Battering is the establishment of control and fear in a relationship through violence and other forms of abuse.
- Domestic violence follows a cycle of three phases. Phase one involves arguing and verbal abuse. Phase two progresses to physical and sexual abuse. Phase three consists of denial and apologies. Certain personality traits may predispose a person to abusive relationships.
- The paramedic may have a hard time identifying the battered patient. Injuries from domestic violence often involve contusions and lacerations of the face, neck, head, breast, and abdomen.
- The paramedic must ensure scene and personal safety in domestic violence events. The paramedic should manage physical injuries according to standard protocols. The paramedic should direct special attention toward the emotional needs of the victim as well. Assault is a crime. The perpetrator is often released soon after arrest. This is a dangerous time for the victim.
- Elder abuse is classified into four categories: physical abuse, psychological abuse, financial or material abuse, and neglect.
- All 50 states have elder abuse statutes. Reporting of suspected elder abuse also is mandatory under law in most states.
- Most child abusers are the child's parents (77%). Eleven percent are other relatives of the victim. Abused children often exhibit behavior that provides key clues about abuse and neglect. The paramedic should observe carefully the child younger than 6 years of age who is passive or the child older than 6 years of age who is aggressive.
- If the child volunteers the history of the event without hesitation and matches the history that the parent provides (and the history is suitable for the injury), child abuse is unlikely.
- Injuries may include soft tissue injuries, fractures, head injuries, and abdominal injuries.
- Sexual assault generally refers to any genital, anal, oral, or manual penetration of the victim's body by way of force and without the victim's consent.
- After managing all threats to life, the paramedic should provide emotional support to the victim. The paramedic should deliver care in a way that preserves evidence.

Questions 1 to 5 pertain to the following case study:

You are called to a private residence by a woman who says her husband "beat her up." When you arrive, you hear loud shouting coming from the house.

1. What measures should be taken before entering the home?

____

____

2. When you begin your examination, what measures should you take to enhance safety and allow for a better history and examination?

____

____

    The patient's vital signs are stable. She has several bruises around her face, but she is alert and oriented and does not want further care. You contact medical direction, and despite both your and their recommendations, the patient refuses transport.

3. What reasons might someone have for staying with an abusive partner?

____

____

4. If you tell her to move out immediately, would that be the safest course of action without planning on her part? Why or why not?

____

____

5. What advice and resources can you offer her before you leave the scene?

____

____

Questions 6 to 8 refer to the following case study:

You are dispatched to a residence in a middle-class neighborhood for an "accidental injury." An 80-year-old widow has a tender, swollen, ecchymotic left upper arm. She is awake and alert but very withdrawn. You note multiple other bruises on both arms and her back that are yellow, brown, and green. Her 60-year-old daughter lives with her and says that her mother tripped and fell. When you ask the patient to confirm this, she nods slowly; when you ask about the old bruises, she just shrugs. She has a history of heart disease, emphysema, and type 2 diabetes. Her vital signs are normal.

6. What characteristics typical of an "average" victim of elder abuse does this woman have?

____

7. What physical findings suggest possible abuse?

____

8. What action should you take if you suspect abuse on this call?

____

____

Questions 9 to 12 refer to the following case study:

You are dispatched to an address in your district that is well known to you and your partner. Both the woman that lives at this address and her boyfriend are heavy drinkers, and you have responded to multiple calls at their home. When you arrive, you find a 2-year-old girl with bilateral circumferential second-degree burns to her feet, lower legs, and buttocks. The mother says that when she was filling the tub to bathe the child after she dirtied her pants, the child stepped into the tub and got burned. You take the child to the ambulance and notice that she does not cry for her mother to be with her. She shudders when you touch her and jumps every time someone approaches.

9. What characteristics of an abusive family situation are present in this situation?

____

____

10. What specific characteristics of the injuries increase your suspicion of possible abuse?

____

____

11. How does the child's behavior suggest the possibility of an abusive family situation?

____

____

12. What are your legal responsibilities with regard to this situation?

____

____

13. List five measures to help preserve evidence on a sexual assault call.

    a. ____

    b. ____

    c. ____

    d. ____

    e. ____

14. List at least four injuries that may accompany sexual assault.

    a. ____

    b. ____

    c. ____

    d. ____

15. What term describes establishing control and fear in a relationship through violence and other forms of abuse ?
   a. Assault
   b. Battering
   c. Intimidation
   d. Terrorism

16. What typically occurs in the third phase of the domestic violence cycle?
   a. An argument occurs.
   b. Threats of violence.
   c. Physical or sexual abuse occurs.
   d. The abuser apologizes.

17. What does the victim of domestic violence often fear most?
   a. That her children will be harmed or taken away.
   b. That she will be humiliated in front of their friends.
   c. That she will not be able to achieve financial independence.
   d. That the abuser will hurt himself if the victim leaves.

18. Which characteristic may an abuser or victim of domestic violence have?
   a. Alcohol or drug dependence
   b. Dislike of discipline
   c. Fear of love and affection
   d. Rigid personal boundaries

19. Which of the following injury patterns is most suggestive of domestic abuse?
   a. Contusions of the breast
   b. Fracture of the ankle
   c. Laceration of the finger
   d. Scald burn of the hand

20. How should you treat a patient who you suspect was injured in a domestic violence situation?
   a. Ask the police to speak to her partner so you can examine her privately.
   b. Don't pry if she doesn't volunteer any information about abuse.
   c. If she won't talk, ask her, "You've been abused, haven't you?"
   d. Force her to go to the hospital even if she doesn't want to.

21. Which is an example of psychological abuse of an elder?
   a. Sexual molestation
   b. Theft of property
   c. Verbal threats
   d. Withholding food

22. What action should the paramedic take if elder abuse is suspected?
   a. Confront the suspected abuser about the abusive behavior and threaten to report it.
   b. Report your suspicions to medical direction and the appropriate state agency.
   c. Discuss the patient's rights and ways to follow up with authorities.
   d. Wait to see whether it happens again before you take action so you can be sure.

23. Which of the following descriptions is most characteristic of a child abuser?
   a. 20-year-old mother
   b. 45-year-old female neighbor
   c. 50-year-old father
   d. 70-year-old uncle

24. What is usually helpful to determine if a child's injury is accidental or inflicted by an adult?
   a. Assessing the family for the characteristics of abusers
   b. Checking with the police to see whether a record of abuse exists
   c. Matching the description of the event to the injury
   d. Performing a careful, detailed physical examination

25. Which statements about sexual assault is true?
   a. All victims of sexual assault are women.
   b. Rape is motivated by sexual desire.
   c. Threats of harm or use of weapons during the attack are rare.
   d. Victims often know their attackers.

26. What statement by the paramedic may be most helpful to a child who has been sexually assaulted?
   a. "Don't worry about anything; you are OK."
   b. "They'll probably get the person who did this."
   c. "You didn't do anything wrong; this wasn't your fault."
   d. "You're really lucky; it could have been a lot worse."

WRAP IT UP

You are dispatched to a large, elegant home for a "maternity case." The dispatcher notes that the caller requests no lights and sirens and that the crew use a rear entrance. The patient's husband meets you; you recognize him, from his frequent television commercials, as a prominent injury claims attorney. He tells you that his wife is in labor. The patient is crying and telling you, "It's too early." She has two other children, has miscarried several times, and is at 30 weeks' gestation. She says her contractions began an hour ago, are very painful, and are coming every 3 minutes. You note her skin is pale. Her vital signs are BP, 80/50 mm Hg; P, 132/min; and R, 28/min. The Sao$_2$ does not register. When you drape the patient and examine her perineum during a contraction to determine if she is crowning, you are alarmed to see that her undergarments are soaked with dark red blood, much different from the mucousy bloody show you've seen in the past. Your partner is unable to find fetal heart tones on the Doppler. The patient grimaces in pain when the Doppler is pressed against her abdomen, where you note an ecchymotic area lateral to her umbilicus. When you ask the patient if she has any risk factors for abruption, toxemia, high blood pressure, or trauma, she glances nervously at her husband but denies all. He quickly interrupts and says, "Well, she did fall down a couple of steps this morning." As you administer oxygen, she whispers to you that her husband punched her in the abdomen during an argument earlier today. As you quickly secure the patient to your cot and raise her legs, you explain to her that her pain and blood pressure concern you, so you will be starting an IV and transporting her to the closest hospital with high-risk OB services. The husband is crying and telling her that he loves her as you wheel her out the door. The patient appears embarrassed and tells you, "I should have left him years ago, but I know he'll take the other kids. He's really a good person, but he just has a bad temper. It's all my fault." You start an IV line en route and deliver her to the labor and delivery unit, where a team is waiting with four units of blood to rush her for an emergency C-section based on your report. Subsequently, you learn that the patient survived but her baby did not. Her husband plea bargained, so you are thankful you did not have to testify at trial.

1. Which is true about battered women?
   a. City dwellers are at higher risk of abuse.
   b. Domestic abuse calls pose little threat to rescuers.
   c. About 15% to 25% of pregnant women are battered.
   d. Wife batterers do not usually abuse their children.

2. What clues to abuse did you note before the patient told you she had been assaulted?

____

____

3. Which action or actions could have increased the potential for violence directed at the EMS crew?

____

____

____

4. Put a ✓ beside interventions related to this patient's abuse that would have been appropriate for you to provide during transport.
   a. _______ Listen with a nonjudgmental attitude
   b. _______ Encourage the patient to get control of life
   c. _______ Provide access to community resources
   d. _______ Provide a written list of community resources for the patient
   e. _______ Confirm that she is not at fault her
   f. _______ Treat her in a sensitive manner

REVIEW QUESTIONS

1. Request and await police to help assess and maintain scene safety. Domestic violence calls are very dangerous. (Objective 4)

2. Move the patient to the ambulance as soon as possible. Do not ask about the violence until you have the patient alone. Have the police remain with the alleged abuser while you perform your examination. (Objective 4)

3. The patient may fear for her own safety or the safety of her children if she leaves. A victim often believes that the offender's behavior will change. She may not have the money or emotional support to help her leave. She may believe that she is the cause of the behavior or that abuse is a normal part of marriage. (Objective 2)

4. Often the perpetrator is released from jail within several hours. A woman who leaves is 75% more likely to be killed by her partner. A woman who leaves should be directed to community support agencies that can maximize her safety. Sometimes it is more prudent for her to stay and carefully plan a safe departure than to leave suddenly. (Objective 4)

5. Accept her decision and support her by confirming that she is not at fault and doesn't deserve to be abused. Give her written information (preferably on something small enough to hide) about community agencies that can provide financial, emotional, safety-related, and legal resources to assist her. Help her prepare a quick way out. Identify safety precautions for her. (Objective 4)

6. The victim is a widow who is older than 75 years of age. She has multiple chronic health problems and lives with her adult child. (Objective 7)

7. The patient seems hesitant to confirm the source of the injury and has aging bruises. (Objective 5)

8. If you suspect abuse, you should report your suspicions to medical direction and call the agency mandated by law to report suspected elder abuse. (Objective 6)

9. This child is with a parent, and alcohol abuse is evident, which greatly increases the risk of physical abuse. You also have received many calls to this home. (Objective 7)

10. The burns involve both extremities and the buttocks and are circumferential, indicating that the child was probably forcibly held in the hot water. (Objective 8)

11. The child does not mind separation from the parents, appears fearful, and does not like to be touched. (Objective 7)

12. This case should be reported to the appropriate state agency for child abuse on arrival at the hospital (refer to local reporting protocols). Document in detail your observations and quote any significant remarks by the adults. (Objective 7)

13. a. Take steps to preserve evidence.
    b. Do not allow the patient to urinate, defecate, douche, or bathe.
    c. Do not remove evidence from areas of sexual contact.
    d. Notify law enforcement immediately.
    e. Maintain a chain of evidence with clothing and other items.
    (Objective 10)

14. a. Abrasions or bruises on the upper limb, head, and neck
   b. Forcible signs of restraint
   c. Petechiae of the face and conjunctiva
   d. Broken teeth, swollen jaw or cheekbone, or eye injuries
   e. Muscle soreness or stiffness of the shoulder, neck, knee, hip, or back
   (Objective 9)

15. b. Battering may include physical abuse (assault) or psychological abuse such as intimidation, isolation, or threats to control another person.
   (Objective 1)

16. d. This is known as the honeymoon phase.
   (Objective 2)

17. a. Usually all these fears exist, but children most often are the most compelling reason for the victim to stay.
   (Objective 2)

18. a. Abusers may believe that abuse is a form of discipline. Abusers or victims often have an intense need for love and affection and are unable to set personal boundaries.
   (Objective 2)

19. a. Abusive injuries are more commonly found on the face, head, neck, breasts, and abdomen.
   (Objective 3)

20. a. The partner may be reluctant to leave the victim alone and may need to be distracted for you to be able to conduct an effective history. If the victim does not volunteer information, you could say something nonthreatening, such as, "I'm concerned for you because I've seen these types of injuries in people who have been hit by others." Do not intimidate or accuse the victim. You cannot insist on transport if the adult patient is competent.
   (Objective 4)

21. c. Sexual molestation is physical abuse, theft is financial or material abuse, and withholding food is neglect.
   (Objective 5)

22. b. Report it to the authorities so they will have complete information if a pattern of abuse exists.
   (Objective 6)

23. a. Most perpetrators are a parent, female, and younger than 40 years of age.
   (Objective 7)

24. c. If the child volunteers the same story as the parents without prompting and the story is consistent with the injuries you see, abuse is not likely. You probably will not have time in the field to assess the family or check police records.
   (Objective 8)

25. d. About 49,000 men report sexual assault each year. Rape is a crime of violence, not a sexual act. Threats of harm or the use of weapons for intimidation are common.
   (Objective 9)

26. c. Abused children should understand that the assault was not their fault and that they won't be punished. False reassurances serve no purpose.
   (Objective 10)

1. c. Abuse is also common in rural and suburban areas. Domestic violence calls pose a high risk of violence toward police and EMS. More than half of wife batterers also abuse their children.
   (Objective 2)

2. The request to respond on the quiet; the obvious trauma to the abdomen (characteristic of abuse); a pregnant patient with possible abruption (trauma is a possible cause); the changing story (no mention of trauma initially); and the high incidence of abuse during pregnancy
   (Objective 3)

3. Confronting or questioning the husband about the abuse
   (Objective 4)

4. a, e, f. The patient is experiencing a life-threatening injury, and the other interventions would not be appropriate at this time. A detailed report to hospital staff members, who can refer her to the appropriate social services after her recovery, would also be indicated.
   (Objective 4)

700

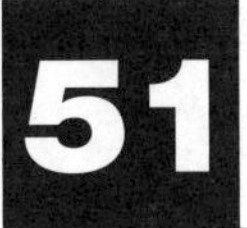 **Patients with Special Challenges**

Chapter 51, pages 1429-1444, in *Mosby's Paramedic Textbook,* ed. 4.

OBJECTIVES

Upon completion of this chapter, the paramedic student will be able to do the following:

1. Identify considerations in prehospital management related to physical challenges such as hearing, visual, and speech impairments; obesity; and paraplegia or quadriplegia.
2. Identify considerations in prehospital management of patients who have mental illness, are developmentally disabled, or are emotionally or mentally impaired.
3. Describe special considerations for prehospital management of patients with selected pathological challenges.
4. Outline considerations in management of culturally diverse patients.
5. Describe special considerations in the prehospital management of terminally ill patients.
6. Identify special considerations in management of patients with communicable diseases.
7. Describe special considerations in the prehospital management of patients with financial challenges.

SUMMARY

- Certain accommodations may be needed for a hearing impaired patient. These include helping with a patient's hearing aid, providing paper and pen to aid in communication, speaking softly into the patient's ear, and speaking in clear view of the patient.
- When caring for the visually impaired patient, the paramedic should help the patient use his or her glasses or other visual aids. The paramedic also should describe all procedures before performing them.
- Allow extra time for the history of a patient with a speech impairment. If appropriate, provide aids such as a pen and paper to assist in communication.
- When caring for an obese patient, use the properly sized diagnostic devices. Also, secure extra personnel if needed to move the patient for transport.
- When transporting patients with paraplegia or quadriplegia, extra personnel may be needed to move special equipment.
- After rapport and trust have been established with a patient who has a mental illness, the paramedic should proceed with care in the standard manner.
- When caring for a patient with developmental delays, the paramedic should allow enough time to obtain a history, perform an assessment, deliver care, and prepare for transport.
- The challenge in assessing patients with emotional impairments is distinguishing between symptoms produced by stress and those caused by serious medical illness.
- Pathological conditions may call for special assessment and management skills. The paramedic should ask about current medications and the patient's normal level of functioning.
- *Diversity* refers to differences of any kind. These include race, class, religion, gender, sexual preference, personal habitat, and physical ability. Good health care depends on sensitivity toward these differences.
- Often, calls involving the care of a terminally ill patient will be emotionally charged. They require a great deal of empathy and compassion for the patient and his or her loved ones.
- Some infectious diseases will take a toll on the emotional well-being of affected patients, their families, and loved ones. Paramedics should be sensitive to the psychological needs of the patient and his or her family.
- Financial challenges can deprive a patient of basic health care services. These patients may be reluctant to seek care for illness or injury.

Match the pathological condition in column II with the appropriate description in column I. Use each condition only once.

Column I

1. _______ Nonprogressive disorders of movement and posture

2. _______ Inherited disorder that causes slow muscle deterioration

3. _______ Congenital defect that exposes part of the spinal cord

4. _______ Autoimmune disorder that weakens the muscles of the head and extremities

5. _______ Inflammation of the joints

6. _______ Inherited disease of the lungs and digestive tract

7. _______ Autoimmune disease that affects the CNS

Column II

a. Arthritis
b. Cerebral palsy
c. Cystic fibrosis
d. Multiple sclerosis
e. Muscular dystrophy
f. Myasthenia gravis
g. Poliomyelitis
h. Spina bifida

For the patient situations in questions 8 to 20, identify which of the following prehospital considerations may be necessary to accommodate the patient's special needs. More than one answer may be required.

a. Provide communication aids.

b. Allow additional time for history and management.

c. Obtain detailed information about the preexisting condition.

d. Determine baseline level of functioning.

e. Obtain additional resources and manpower to prepare for transport.

8. _______ The patient had a stroke 6 months ago, has weakness on the right side, and speaks slowly and with a stutter. He called you today complaining of inability to urinate.

9. _______ Your patient complains of crushing chest pain. He weighs approximately 475 lb (215 kg).

10. _______ You are transferring a patient with quadriplegia who is in halo traction.

11. _______ A man with schizophrenia has difficulty breathing related to asthma.

12. _______ A 12-year-old girl with Down syndrome has extreme weakness after chemotherapy for leukemia.

13. _______ A moderately retarded man lacerated his finger at his job in the cafeteria.

14. _______ A patient with severe arthritis was involved in a motor vehicle crash.

15. _______ A 14-year-old patient with quadriplegic spastic paralysis and mental retardation caused by cerebral palsy is febrile and congested.

16. _______ A child with cystic fibrosis has vomiting and diarrhea.

17. _______ A 43-year-old woman with multiple sclerosis complains of severe vertigo.

18. _______ An 8-year-old boy with Duchenne muscular dystrophy says he can't breathe.

19. _______ A 45-year-old patient who sustained a head injury 5 years ago is confused and pale.

20. _______ A 65-year-old man tells you he is being treated for tuberculosis.

21. Which accommodation might be helpful to many patients with hearing impairment?
 a. No accommodation is necessary.
 b. Speaking very loudly into the patient's ear
 c. Speaking very slowly with very exaggerated lip movements
 d. Writing key questions or instructions on a piece of paper

22. How is obesity defined?
 a. A person who is impaired as a result of excessive weight
 b. A person who weighs 20% or more than the maximum desirable weight relative to height
 c. A person who weighs 50 lb (23 kg) more than the average weight for someone of that age
 d. A person who weighs more than 250 lb (114 kg)

23. During the initial examination of a patient with a mental illness, what is your priority?
 a. To determine whether the patient is aware of the mental illness
 b. To determine whether the patient is dangerous
 c. To determine the patient's specific form of mental illness
 d. To determine the type of medications the patient is taking

24. What challenge is posed by caring for a patient who is emotionally impaired?
 a. Determining whether symptoms are produced by stress or medical illness
 b. Determining whether the patient is lying or telling the truth
 c. Obtaining an accurate medical history from caregivers
 d. Winning the patient's trust so you can perform the examination

25. A patient with severe arthritis of the spine falls down some steps. What is likely to be the most significant challenge in caring for this patient?
 a. Communicating so you can understand the patient
 b. Determining whether the patient has any serious injuries
 c. Obtaining a reliable patient history and medication list
 d. Securing the patient to a spine board to minimize pain

26. Which term describes involuntary writhing movements found in patients with cerebral palsy?
 a. Ataxia
 b. Athetosis
 c. Diplegia
 d. Mucoviscidosis

27. During transport of a patient with severe cystic fibrosis, you should anticipate the need for which of the following?
 a. Antidysrhythmic treatment
 b. Blood glucose monitoring
 c. Nitrous oxide inhalation
 d. Suctioning

28. Which of the following is true about cultural diversity in prehospital patient care?
 a. All generations in a culture share the same beliefs.
 b. Personal prejudices and belief systems should not interfere with patient care.
 c. People must accept your explanation of the causes of their illnesses.
 d. You should agree with every aspect of a patient's cultural beliefs.

29. What is a primary consideration during transport of a terminally ill patient?
 a. The family should be encouraged to deal with the imminent death.
 b. Talking to the family may interfere with their grieving process.
 c. Comfort is usually the priority of care.
 d. Rapid transport is essential for definitive care.

30. How can you show respect for the dignity of a patient with AIDS during transport?
 a. Don't discuss the patient's disease process.
 b. To keep the patient from feeling ashamed, don't use BSI.
 c. Encourage the patient to express feelings related to the disease.
 d. Respecting the patient's dignity should not be a primary concern during prehospital care.

31. What statement may be helpful when transporting a patient who has serious financial concerns?
 a. "Don't worry; the ambulance bill won't come for a couple of months."
 b. "I don't see why you're worried. You're sick now—worry about the money later."
 c. "I'll ask the nurse to contact social services to see whether there is a program to help you."
 d. "We have people who never pay a dime for our service, and they abuse us all the time."

  Chapter **51** **Patients with Special Challenges**

You could have predicted it—a light, drizzly rain always causes multiple "fender benders" at this very busy corner. As you approach the scene, you can see that a van has struck the rear of a large dump truck. There is almost no visible damage to the truck, but the van has considerable front-end damage. The van's driver, a woman in her thirties, is crying and calling out to her rear-seat passenger, a 13-year-old boy who was thrown out of his wheelchair, which had been secured in the specialized van. He is crying, making a high-pitched, moaning sound. As you approach him, the driver, his mother, tells you that his name is Michael, he has cerebral palsy with diplegic spasticity, and he is blind and has mental retardation. She tries to calm him, but his persistent cries pierce the environment, making it difficult to concentrate and impossible to hear anything on your assessment. He is recumbent with his arms and legs drawn toward his chest in a fetal-like position. "Michael," you say loudly as you grasp one wrist and place the other hand on his shoulder, "I'm here to help you." His pulse is rapid, his breathing is normal, and his skin is warm and dry. He has a laceration on the left temporal area of his head but no other visible soft tissue injury or any evidence of other injury. Vital signs are BP, 96 mm Hg by palpation; P, 120/min; R, 20/min; and Sao_2, 97%. His pupils are 3 mm, equal, round, and react to light. By now your partner has evaluated the mother; she appears uninjured and refuses any care. You ask her to help you to calm her son. She rubs his back while singing a familiar song into his ear, and his moaning begins to slow. After realizing that standard spinal immobilization would be impossible because of the rigid spasticity of the boy's limbs, you and your partner determine that applying a cervical collar and a half spine board device will provide stabilization of the spine. Medical direction concurs. In simple language, you explain each step of the process, which his mother relays to him. Although his agitation increases, it is manageable. After the immobilization is applied, you position him on the stretcher in a semi-sitting position with blankets and pillows supporting his legs. You allow his mother to sit seat belted beside him, where she soothes him. She tells you his behavior is appropriate. He is treated in the ED and released several hours later.

1. What difficulties were posed by the assessment of this patient?

   ____

2. Why is it appropriate to have the parent remain with the child in this situation?

   ____

3. What does diplegic spasticity mean?
   a. It affects both arms and legs.
   b. It is intermittent.
   c. It affects both limbs on one side of the body.
   d. It causes involuntary writhing movements.

   ____

4. Explain why it would be appropriate to deviate from standard spinal immobilization protocol in this situation.

   ____

   ____

CHAPTER 51 ANSWERS

REVIEW QUESTIONS

1. b

2. e

3. h

4. f

5. a

6. c

7. d
(Questions 1–7, Objective 3)

8. a, b, c, d
(Objective 1)

9. c, e
(Objective 1)

10. b, c, d, e
(Objective 1)

11. c, d
(Objective 2)

12. b, c, d
(Objective 2)

13. b, d
(Objective 2)

14. b, c, e (possibly)
(Objective 3)

15. c, d, e
(Objective 3)

16. c, d
(Objective 3)

17. c, d
(Objective 3)

18. c, d
(Objective 3)

19. c, d
(Objective 3)

20. c
(Objective 6)

STUDENT SELF-ASSESSMENT

21. d. Speak in low tones into the patient's ear if residual hearing exists. Otherwise, if the patient reads lips, speak at a regular speed in view of the patient.
(Objective 1)

22. b
(Objective 1)

23. b. The safety of the patient, crew, and bystanders should always be prioritized.
(Objective 2)

24. a. Anxiety can produce a host of symptoms that mimic serious medical illness.
(Objective 2)

25. d. The arthritic pain and deformity can make spinal immobilization challenging.
(Objective 3)

26. b. Ataxia is a loss of coordination and balance. Diplegic cerebral palsy affects all four limbs, the legs more
severely than the arms. Mucoviscidosis is cystic fibrosis.
(Objective 3)

27. d. These patients often have excessive secretions, and the paramedic should anticipate the need for suctioning.
(Objective 3)

28. b. Individual beliefs exist even within specific cultures. People may choose to have their own beliefs about the
cause of their illness despite your explanations. You need not agree with all aspects of a patient's cultural
beliefs, but you should not let your opinion interfere with patient care or interaction.
(Objective 4)

29. c. Some families will not be fully prepared for the death regardless of the length of illness. The paramedic should
support the patient and family with honest and empathetic care. Talking to the patient and family should be
encouraged if the patient's condition permits.
(Objective 5)

30. c. There is no reason not to mention the disease to the patient, but the condition should remain confidential with
regard to others. Use BSI as you would for any other patient care situation. The dignity of each patient is an
important part of prehospital patient care delivery.
(Objective 6)

31. c. The patient may worry about receiving poor credit ratings, adding to a mounting debt, and being a deadbeat.
Offer constructive suggestions related to their financial concerns rather than empty statements.
(Objective 7)

WRAP IT UP

1. He is unable to communicate effectively, he is blind and so is probably terrified because he has no idea what
happened to him, and he is mentally retarded.
(Objective 2)

2. The mother knows how to communicate with her child, can calm him, and can tell medical providers what
behaviors are normal or abnormal for her son.
(Objective 1)

3. a. All four limbs are affected, the legs more than the arms. Athetosis describes writhing movements.
(Objective 3)

4. Positioning this patient supine on a long spine board would be impossible. Adaptations in care should take into
consideration the physical needs of the patient and the potential for injury. Consultation with medical direction can
be helpful.
(Objective 3)

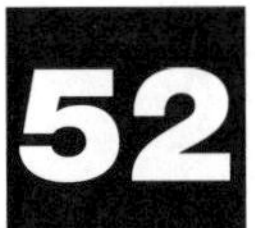# Acute Interventions for Home Care

READING ASSIGNMENT

Chapter 52, pages 1445-1464, in *Mosby's Paramedic Textbook,* ed. 4.

OBJECTIVES

Upon completion of this chapter, the paramedic student will be able to do the following:

1. Discuss general issues related to the home health care patient.
2. Outline general principles of assessment and management of the home health care patient.
3. Describe medical equipment, assessment, and management of the home health care patient with inadequate respiratory support.
4. Identify assessment findings and acute interventions for problems related to vascular access devices in the home health care setting.
5. Describe medical equipment, assessment, and management of the patient with a gastrointestinal or genitourinary crisis in the home health care setting.
6. Identify key assessments and principles of wound care management in the home health care patient.
7. Outline maternal and child problems that may be encountered early in the postpartum period in the home health care setting.
8. Describe medical therapy associated with hospice and comfort care in the home health care setting.

SUMMARY

- About 25% of home health care patients have heart and circulatory diseases as their primary diagnosis. Other common diagnoses of home health care patients include cancer, diabetes, and hypertension. Typical emergency medical services calls to a home health care setting may include respiratory failure, cardiac decompensation, septic complications, equipment malfunction, and other medical problems.
- After arrival at the scene of a home health care patient, the scene size-up should include standard precautions, elements of scene safety, and environmental setting. The initial assessment should focus on illness or injury that poses a threat to life. The paramedic should take appropriate measures as indicated.
- Patients with diseases of the respiratory system being cared for at home are at increased risk for airway infections. In addition, the progression of their illnesses may lead to difficulty breathing, making current support equipment inadequate.
- Assessment findings that may require acute interventions in patients with ventricular assist devices include infection, hemorrhage, hemodynamic compromise from circulatory overload or embolus, obstruction of the vascular device, and catheter damage with leakage of medication.
- Patients with diseases of the digestive or genitourinary system may have medical devices such as urinary catheters or urostomies, indwelling nutritional support devices (e.g., percutaneous endoscopic gastrostomy tube or gastrostomy tube), colostomies, and nasogastric tubes. Acute interventions required for these patients can result from urinary tract infection, urosepsis, urinary retention, and problems with gastric emptying or feeding.
- Home health care patients with acute infections have an increased the death rate from sepsis and severe peripheral infections. Many also have a decreased ability to perceive pain or perform self-care.
- Maternal and child conditions that one may encounter in the home health care setting during the postpartum period include postpartum hemorrhage, infection, pulmonary embolism, postpartum depression, septicemia in the newborn, infantile apnea, and failure to thrive.
- Hospice services include supportive social, emotional, and spiritual services for terminally ill patients. They also provide support for a patient's family. Palliative care is directed mainly at providing relief to a terminally ill person. This is done this through symptom and pain management.

Questions 1 to 4 refer to the following case study:

A 32-year-old patient complains of difficulty breathing. You find him at home with a tracheostomy and on a ventilator. The low pressure alarm is sounding.

1. What signs and symptoms might the patient have if he were hypoxic?

____

2. What should your first action be?

____

____

3. What will you check on the ventilator to assess the problem?

____

____

4. How can you calm the patient before reconnecting him to the ventilator?

____

____

____

Questions 5 to 7 refer to the following case study:

An elderly patient has a home IV infusion. You are called to treat her for difficulty breathing. She has a history of multiple myeloma. Her husband thinks the pump hasn't been working correctly and too much fluid has run in.

5. What specifically would you assess to check for fluid overload?

____

The patient has crackles in the bases of both lungs, and her neck veins are distended. Her vital signs are 160/84 mm Hg; P, 100/min; and R, 24/min. Her Sao_2 is 93% on room air.

6. What interventions should you perform in cooperation with medical direction?

____

____

7. Should you transport the patient for evaluation by a physician?

____

Questions 8 to 13 pertain to the following case study:

You are called to a home for an "assist invalid" call. An elderly woman greets you, and after you help her husband to bed (he couldn't get off the commode), she asks you to check his arm. He burned it 4 days ago. When you remove the dressing, you note a green wound bed surrounded by black tissue. The drainage is green and foul smelling.

8. What does the appearance of this wound suggest?

____

9. How would it look if it were healing normally?

____

10. What should you look for in the surrounding skin?

____

The skin around the wound is reddened and warm to the touch.

11. What does this assessment suggest?

____

12. What systemic assessment should you perform on this patient?

____

The patient's vital signs are BP, 150/80 mm Hg; P, 110/min; and R, 16/min. His skin feels hot to the touch. The rest of the exam is normal.

13. What action should you take?

____

Questions 14 to 17 refer to the following case study:

You respond to a call for "baby not breathing." You find a woman sobbing while holding her 4-day-old infant in her arms. The baby is awake, lying quietly in her mother's arms. The parents state that they had just put her down for a nap when they noticed that she wasn't breathing and her color looked "bad." They state that the episode lasted about 15 to 20 seconds.

14. What assessments should you perform?

____

____

The baby's examination looks normal. While you are on the phone with medical direction, your partner shouts at you. She states that the baby stopped breathing for almost 20 seconds and was very pale, and her heart rate dropped to 80 beats/min on the monitor. Now she is breathing normally.

15. What are some possible causes of infantile apnea?

____

____

16. What interventions should you perform?

____

____

17. What equipment should you prepare and keep easily accessible during transport?

____

____

18. What was the historical focus of home health care?
   a. To reduce the incidence of infection
   b. To care for rural patients
   c. To provide wider physician care
   d. To provide preventive care

19. What do home health care services in the United States commonly include?
   a. Diagnostic radiology
   b. Minor surgical procedures
   c. IV antibiotic therapy
   d. Physician visits for acute illness

20. The Haddon matrix states that any injury or disease can be broken down into three components. Which of the following shows the correct three?
   a. Agent, host, and environment
   b. Agent, host, and mechanical force
   c. Patient, host, and environment
   d. Agent, disease, and environment

21. What type of infection control standards should be practiced in the home health setting?
   a. No precautions are needed.
   b. Use precautions only for HIV patients.
   c. Wear reusable rubber gloves.
   d. Observe universal precautions.

22. Assessment of the milieu in home care includes evaluation to ensure which of the following?
   a. Infectious waste is disposed of properly.
   b. Dogs and other pets are contained.
   c. No hazards are present in the home.
   d. The home has heat, water, and electricity.

23. On arrival at a call in which home care is provided, your priority (after making sure the scene is safe) is to assess for which of the following?
   a. Abusive caregivers
   b. Equipment failure
   c. Life-threatening illness or injury
   d. Medical device malfunction

24. Which of the following systems will not work during a power failure?
   a. Demand valve
   b. Liquid oxygen
   c. Oxygen concentrators
   d. Oxygen cylinders

25. You are called because the high pressure alarm keeps sounding on a home care ventilator. What might this indicate?
   a. Cuff leak
   b. Disconnected tubing
   c. Insufficient oxygen
   d. Water in tubing

26. Which of the following is a peripheral vascular access device?
  a. Groshong   **c.** Intracath
  b. Hickman   **d.** MediPort

27. Which complication of peripheral vascular access devices is associated with the risk of sepsis?
  a. Circulatory overload   **c.** Hemorrhage
  b. Embolus   **d.** Phlebitis

28. Which is a sign of air embolus that may occur if air enters a vascular access device?
  a. Distended neck veins   **c.** Hypotension
  b. Fever   **d.** Pulmonary congestion

29. What is used to flush a peripheral vascular device?
  a. Aspirin   **c.** Heparin
  b. Coumadin   **d.** Normal saline

30. What complication can result from infection associated with a urinary catheter?
  a. Kidney stones   **c.** Sepsis
  b. Prostatic hypertrophy   **d.** Urinary retention

31. Which complication of tube feedings can cause serious skin breakdown and fluid and electrolyte imbalances?
  a. Bowel obstruction   **c.** Diarrhea
  b. Choking   **d.** Irritable bowel syndrome

32. How can you reduce the risk of infection when transporting a patient with a urinary catheter?
  a. Cap the catheter during transport and reattach the bag on arrival.
  b. Flush the catheter with normal saline to clear any bacteria.
  c. Keep the catheter bag lower than the level of the urethra.
  d. Administer a prophylactic dose of antibiotic.

33. Which of the following enhances wound repair?
  a. Environmental contamination   **c.** Moisture
  b. Eschar   **d.** Necrotic tissue

34. Your patient delivered a baby 3 days ago. She is complaining of severe abdominal pain, weakness, and shaking chills. What postpartum complication should be anticipated?
  a. Appendicitis   **c.** Hemorrhage
  b. Endometritis   **d.** Pulmonary embolism

35. You are called to the home of a woman who appears to have signs and symptoms of postpartum depression. Your priority should be to assess for which of the following?
  a. Depressive psychosis   **c.** Severe sleep disturbances
  b. Forgetfulness or memory loss   **d.** The well-being of the baby

36. A mother calls you to evaluate her 11-day-old infant. She says she has been nursing him, but he "doesn't seem right." He is difficult to awaken and pale, and he has dry mucous membranes and a sunken fontanelle. She thinks he hasn't wet a diaper in about 18 hours. What do you suspect?
  a. Apnea   **c.** Jaundice
  b. Dehydration   **d.** Sepsis

37. Which term describes abnormal infant growth and development caused by maternal deprivation or malnutrition?
  a. Cerebral palsy   **c.** Failure to thrive
  b. Cystic fibrosis   **d.** Muscular dystrophy

      Chapter **52**   **Acute Interventions for Home Care**

38. What is the primary goal of palliative care?
   a. To make sure that optimal nutritional requirements are met
   b. To help families accept the reality of impending death
   c. To improve the quality of a person's life as death approaches
   d. To provide complete relief of any pain or discomfort

WRAP IT UP

When you enter the neat, single-story home, you find a 35-year-old man sitting upright in a wheelchair using a ventilator. With great difficulty, he tells you that he has high-level quadriplegia. He directs you to papers that describe his medical history. He has a ventilator, a G tube, a urinary catheter, and several splints on his extremities. He has an oral antibiotic that was prescribed today. He says he is "sick; just doesn't feel well," and his doctor would like him transported to the ED for evaluation. His vital signs are T, 102.6°F (38.8°C) axilla; BP, 90/68 mm Hg; and P, 128/min. His ventilator is set at a rate of 12 with a tidal volume of 500 mL on room air; his Sao_2 is 90%. You can hear wheezes in his lungs, so you connect some oxygen to the ventilator. The urine in his catheter bag is a milky color. The rest of his exam is unremarkable. It takes a few moments for you and your partner to plan how to effectively move him to the cot without disturbing the ventilator. You make sure the G tube is clamped securely and move the urinary catheter so you won't pull on it. The patient says he can breathe spontaneously for several minutes on his own, so you momentarily disconnect him as you perform the lift. In the ambulance, you administer a bronchodilator updraft treatment while your partner starts an IV and delivers a 200-mL normal saline bolus. Reassessment in a few minutes shows that his vital signs are now BP, 100/70 mm Hg; P, 120/min; and Sao_2, 97%.

1. Why is it important to review the medical papers of the home care patient?

2. Put a ✓ beside the type(s) of home care services this patient is likely to need on an ongoing basis.

   a. ______ Cardiopulmonary care   **e.** ______ Hospice care

   b. ______ Dermatological or wound care   **f.** ______ Orthopedic care

   c. ______ Catheter management   **g.** ______ Pain management

   d. ______ Gastroenterologic care   **h.** ______ Rehabilitative care

3. What complications requiring emergency care could occur based on this patient's use of a

   a. Ventilator:____________________________________

   b. Gtube:____________________________________

   c. Foley catheter:______________________________

4. If you could not transport the patient with his ventilator, what should you do?

CHAPTER 52 ANSWERS

REVIEW QUESTIONS

1. A hypoxic patient may be restless, confused, tachycardic, hypertensive, dyspneic, or cyanotic or may have a headache. When you monitor the patient, you may find a low Sao_2 or cardiac dysrhythmias. (Objective 3)

2. If he appears to be in distress, immediately begin ventilation with a bag-valve device and 100% O_2. Then you can evaluate the equipment problem. Determine the need for suctioning.
(Objective 3)

3. Check the ventilator for disconnected tubing or power cords; check the settings; make sure the tracheostomy tube is in the proper place and the balloon is adequately inflated.
(Objective 3)

4. Reassure the patient that the problem has been fixed, perhaps showing him how you fixed it. Tell him you will remain with him for several minutes after you reconnect him to the ventilator to make sure that everything continues to work properly.
(Objective 3)

5. Assess the patient's level of consciousness and level of distress; respiratory rate and lung sounds; the neck for signs of JVD; skin color, temperature, and moisture; and vital signs.
(Objective 4)

6. Slow the infusion to a keep-open rate, provide high-concentration oxygen, elevate the patient's head, maintain body warmth, monitor vital signs, and reassess. If her condition does not improve, consider the need for a diuretic.
(Objective 4)

7. The need to transport depends on the patient's response to your interventions, other anticipated complications based on the contents of the infusion, and the patient's wishes with regard to transport. The decision should be made in consultation with medical direction.
(Objective 4)

8. The wound has many signs of infection and necrosis.
(Objective 6)

9. A properly healing wound has a pink or red wound bed, clear or serosanguineous drainage, and no odor.
(Objective 6)

10. The surrounding skin should be assessed for color, warmth, and swelling.
(Objective 6)

11. The redness and warmth of the surrounding skin suggest infection.
(Objective 6)

12. A full assessment is necessary. Specifically, vital signs, including temperature and lung sounds, should be evaluated.
(Objective 6)

13. His physical examination suggests systemic infection. You should administer high-concentration oxygen, start IV fluids, assess his temperature, and transport him.
(Objective 6)

14. A full assessment is indicated, including initial assessment, vital signs, blood glucose, and ECG and oxygen saturation monitoring.
(Objective 7)

15. Infantile apnea may be caused by hypoglycemia, hypocalcemia, hypothermia, sepsis, pneumonia, meningitis, CNS hemorrhage, hypoxic injury, seizures, respiratory distress, hyaline membrane disease, and obstruction.
(Objective 7)

16. Keep the baby warm; administer dextrose if the glucose level is low; administer high-concentration oxygen by mask or blow-by; start an IV line (in consultation with medical direction); continually monitor breathing, color, oxygen saturation, and ECG; transport. (Objective 7)

17. Make sure that resuscitation equipment is within easy reach. Open the appropriate size bag-mask for the child and connect it so that it is easily accessible should another apneic episode occur. (Objective 7)

STUDENT SELF-ASSESSMENT

18. d. The growing population of immigrants in large cities stimulated the growth of nurse-provided home care for the poor. (Objective 1)

19. c. The home health field may continue to expand, perhaps offering these services in the future. (Objective 1)

20. a. These factors occur in three phases: preinjury, injury, and postinjury. (Objective 1)

21. d. The same precautions should be used as in the hospital setting. (Objective 1)

22. d. Environmental assessments include infectious waste, pets, and hazards. (Objective 2)

23. c. Life threats should be identified before further assessment is done. (Objective 2)

24. c. The patient should keep an oxygen cylinder on hand in case this happens. (Objective 3)

25. d. Cuff leakage and disconnected tubing trigger a low pressure alarm. The oxygen alarm sounds if the oxygen supply is inadequate. (Objective 3)

26. c. The rest are central venous access devices. (Objective 4)

27. d. Although a site infection is not an immediate life threat, it can cause sepsis and possibly death if it spreads and becomes systemic. (Objective 4)

28. c. Fever is a sign of infection. Distended neck veins and pulmonary congestion are signs of fluid overload. Other signs and symptoms of embolus include cyanosis; a weak, rapid pulse; and loss of consciousness. (Objective 4)

29. c (Objective 4)

30. c. Urosepsis is managed with antibiotic therapy. (Objective 5)

31. c. Excessive diarrhea can cause skin to break down rapidly, as well as dehydration and electrolyte imbalances. A change in the volume or type of tube feeding may remedy the problem.
(Objective 5)

32. c. Urine from the bag and tubing can contain bacteria and should not be allowed to flow back into the bladder.
(Objective 5)

33. c. An adequate blood supply and sufficient oxygen and nutrition are also essential.
(Objective 6)

34. c. Fever and abdominal pain are the most common signs and symptoms of postpartum hemorrhage.
(Objective 7)

35. d. Some women with this condition fantasize about harming their babies. All of the other symptoms should be assessed after the physical well-being of the mother and baby have been ensured.
(Objective 7)

36. b. Further evaluation is necessary, but the patient's clinical presentation suggests severe dehydration, which requires immediate fluid resuscitation and rapid transport.
(Objective 7)

37. c. This condition can also be caused by chromosomal abnormalities and major organ system defects.
(Objective 7)

38. c. Palliative care customizes treatment for patients and their families, providing pain and symptom management if needed and mental and spiritual guidance with the goal of improving quality of life.
(Objective 8)

WRAP IT UP

1. To determine his normal state of functioning, other medical conditions, home medications, any special instructions regarding care, legal papers, including advanced directives, normal vital signs, and private physician and hospital of choice
(Objective 2)

2. a, b, c, d, h
(Objective 1)

3. a. The ventilator could fail as a result of power loss, kinks or water in the tubing, or excessive secretions. Patients can develop pneumothorax or experience anxiety attacks if they feel as if they are not being ventilated. Oxygen supply (if present) can fail.
b. G tube: Aspiration and severe diarrhea can occur.
c. A urinary catheter can become infected, resulting in sepsis. It can cause urethral trauma if pulled out forcefully with the balloon inflated, and the patient can develop serious signs and symptoms if the catheter is removed and urinary retention occurs.
(Objectives 3, 5)

4. Ventilate the patient with a bag-mask device or place on an automatic transport ventilator adjusted closely to the settings the patient was on at home.
(Objective 3)

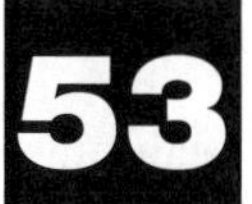 **Ground and Air Ambulance Operations**

Chapter 53, pages 1466-1476, in *Mosby's Paramedic Textbook,* ed 4.

OBJECTIVES

Upon completion of this chapter, the paramedic student will be able to do the following:

1. List standards that govern ambulance performance and specifications.
2. Discuss the tracking of equipment, supplies, and maintenance on an ambulance.
3. Outline the considerations for appropriate stationing of ambulances.
4. Describe measures that can influence safe operation of an ambulance.
5. Identify aeromedical crew members and training.
6. Describe the appropriate use of aeromedical services in the prehospital setting.

SUMMARY

- The federal KKK A-1822 standards provide the foundation of uniformity for the design of ambulance vehicles.
- Completing an equipment and supply checklist at the start of every work shift is important. It is essential for safety, patient care, and risk management. It also helps to ensure proper handling and safekeeping of scheduled medications.
- The methods for estimating ambulance service needs and placement in a community have changed. Compliance in providing emergency medical services within time frames that meet national standards is the method that now is commonly used.
- Factors that influence safe ambulance operation include proper use of escorts, environmental conditions, proper use of warning devices, proceeding safely through intersections, parking at the emergency scene, and operating with due regard for the safety of all others.
- The staffing of air ambulances includes a pilot and various health care professionals. These individuals undergo specialized training in flight physiology and the use of special medical equipment and procedures.
- When paramedics request aeromedical service, the flight crew should be advised of the type of emergency response, the number of patients, and the location of the landing zone and any prominent landmarks and hazards. Paramedics should always follow strict safety measures during helicopter landings. This helps to prevent injury to air medical crews, ground crews, the patient, and bystanders.

REVIEW QUESTIONS

1. Cite the standard that defines ambulance design or performance.

   ____

2. List three types of prehospital care supplies that should be routinely checked on an ambulance.

   a. ____

   b. ____

   c. ____

3. What would be a consequence of the following supply or equipment problems?

   a. The batteries aren't charged on the portable suction unit, and your patient is trapped in a car with a mouth full of blood and vomit.

   ____

   b. The defibrillator doesn't work, and the patient is in ventricular fibrillation.

   ____

   c. You run out of strips to check blood glucose levels on a call with an elderly man who has an altered level of consciousness and no available history.

   ____

   d. Someone forgot to replace the OB (delivery) kit after the last delivery.

   ____

   e. You run out of oxygen while on a call for pulmonary edema.

   ____

4. EMS and community planners must consider a number of factors when determining ambulance placement to provide acceptable availability and response times. List four of these factors.

   a. ____

   b. ____

   c. ____

   d. ____

5. Explain how you can reduce the risk of vehicle accidents in each of the following situations:

   a. You are being followed by a police escort.

   ____

   b. It's 0500, and driving conditions include a light rain and heavy fog.

   ____

   c. The lights and sirens are on, and you are preparing to proceed through a red light at an intersection.

   ____

Questions 6 to 10 refer to the following case study:

You respond to a rollover MVC with a patient ejected at 0800. On arrival, you find a 4-year-old girl who was thrown 20 feet from the vehicle. She is unconscious; has rapid, shallow respirations; and shows signs of shock. The nearest hospital is 40 minutes away; a pediatric trauma center is 45 minutes away by ground or 20 minutes by air. Air medical ETA to your location would be 10 minutes.

6. Give two reasons why this is an appropriate situation for use of air medical transport.

   a. ____

   b. ____

7. What information should you give the dispatcher when you call to activate the air medical transport?

   ____

   ____

   ____

8. Describe landing zone selection and preparation for this air medical response.

   ____

   ____

   The crash occurred across from a baseball diamond that is easily accessible, and the LZ is set up there.

9. What patient management procedures should be performed before the helicopter arrives?

   ____

   ____

10. List three safety measures that should be taken as you approach the helicopter to load the patient when it lands.

    a. ____

    b. ____

    c. ____

STUDENT SELF-ASSESSMENT

11. Which of the following is true of the KKK A-1822 standards?
    a. They contradict the AMD 001-009 performance standards.
    b. They designate design standards for types I, II, and III ambulances.
    c. They define performance specifications for air ambulances.
    d. They outline ambulance driving standards and qualifications.

12. Why are routine ambulance equipment checks essential?
    a. So that accurate patient billing and reimbursement can occur in a timely manner
    b. So that disciplinary action will not be necessary if an equipment failure occurs
    c. So that essential equipment is available and in working order during patient care
    d. So that state laws and regulations can be met and licensure can be maintained

13. What should determine emergency vehicle placement in a community?
    a. Average response times that meet national standards
    b. The number of receiving hospitals in the region
    c. The projected revenue flow from reimbursement
    d. Where the citizens would like to have ambulances

14. Which of the following help promote safety when driving an ambulance?
    a. Drive no faster than 20 miles per hour over the speed limit on routine calls.
    b. Make sure that only the driver and the patient are always restrained.
    c. Use extreme caution at intersections, especially when using lights and sirens.
    d. Use lights and sirens often so that other drivers will yield the right of way.

15. How can the paramedic promote safety when responding to a vehicle crash on the highway?
    a. Park 100 feet past the crash.
    b. Park downhill from hazardous materials.
    c. Park on the opposite side of the road.
    d. Turn off emergency lights.

16. All air medical crew members should receive specialized training in which of the following areas?
    a. Airway management techniques
    b. Flight physiology
    c. Medication administration
    d. Vascular access techniques

17. Which of the following situations would justify the use of air medical transport by an advanced life support unit with an ETA of 40 minutes?
    a. Possible fractured tibia with good pulses
    b. Possible aneurysm with absent pedal pulses
    c. Home delivery with both patients stable
    d. Asthma patient with P, 100/min; R, 20/min

18. Which of the following safety measures should be used when approaching the helicopter to load patients?
    a. Approach the aircraft as soon as it lands.
    b. At least six people should help load the aircraft.
    c. Long objects should be carried vertically to maintain control.
    d. The aircraft should be approached from the front.

WRAP IT UP

"C-crew," your partner mutters as you begin your morning ambulance check. It's frustrating because things just don't seem as neat and clean as you like them, and there's always some little thing missing or out of place. You complete the equipment checklist and then go to the office to fill out a maintenance request for the broken latch on the medication drawer. Because it's the first day of the month, the sealed pediatric bag is opened and checked to make sure that none of the drugs have expired. Just as break time begins, you are dispatched to a call for an electrocution. The pumper is responding with you, so you and your partner follow it at a distance, taking care to change the siren tone as you pass motorists that have pulled to the right. At each light, you change your siren and sound the air horn, stop, and make sure all traffic has stopped before you proceed. En route, you ask dispatch to place the air medical team on standby because the burn center is an hour away. You are thankful that your new engine house is so close to the scene; it will probably save you a couple of minutes on this response.

You find that your patient touched some high-voltage wires with a tree trimmer and is critically burned, so you immediately ask that the aircraft be launched. Your captain sends two of his crew members to set up the landing zone in an adjacent parking lot while the rest of the team works to assess and treat the patient. When the flight crew lands, you give a report, explaining that intubation is impossible because the man's jaw is clenched. After assessing the patient, the air crew performs rapid-sequence induction and intubates the patient, ensuring a secure airway in flight. You help them with loading, being careful to stay to the front of the aircraft away from the tail rotor. Back at the station, you restock and document the call and then get your well-deserved cup of coffee.

1. Put a ✓ beside the items that would have consequences if you had failed to check the ambulance equipment or to maintain it properly before this call.

a. __________ Batteries dead in saturation monitor   e. __________ Traction splint unavailable

b. __________ Inability to defibrillate   f. __________ No oxygen available

c. __________ Breakdown en route to the hospital   g. __________ Appropriate drug not on the ambulance

d. __________ Drugs expired   h. __________ Ambulance tire blowout

2. What advantage of constructing a new station is described here?

____

3. List two additional safe driving considerations that were not mentioned in this case study.

____

____

4. List two advantages of aeromedical transport that were described in this situation.

____

____

CHAPTER 53 ANSWERS

REVIEW QUESTIONS

1. KKK A-1822D
   (Objective 1)

2. a. Supplies (airway, vascular access, dressings)
   b. Medications (number and expiration dates, oxygen supply)
   c. Equipment (including routine maintenance, battery loads, supplementary supplies)
   (Objective 2)

3. a. The patient may aspirate and die.
   b. You will be unable to defibrillate until another unit arrives, and the patient may deteriorate into asystole and die.
   c. You will be unable to determine whether the altered consciousness is attributable to hypoglycemia. If you administer glucose and the patient's altered level of consciousness is related to a stroke, this action may worsen his condition.
   d. You will have to search for other appropriate supplies, wasting time to care for the patient and baby. What will you use to cut the cord and then clamp it?
   e. The patient's hypoxia may worsen, resulting in death.
   (Objective 2)

4. a. National response time standards
   b. Geographical area
   c. Population and patient demand
   d. Traffic conditions

   Others include time of day and appropriate placement of vehicles.
   (Objective 3)

     Chapter **53** **Ground and Air Ambulance Operations**

5. a. Make sure that the police follow at a safe distance. Use a siren tone different from that used by the police.
   b. Slow the ambulance to a safe speed and use the low-beam lights.
   c. Remember that not all drivers will hear your sirens or see your lights. Stop and look to make sure that all traffic is stopping (make eye contact if possible). Use the yelp mode of the siren and remain vigilant as you proceed.
   (Objective 4)

6. Your patient is critical and requires specialized resources, and you are far from a hospital.
   (Objective 6)

7. Advise the flight crew that you are at an MVC with a critically ill child. Let them know the location of the landing zone and any prominent landmarks or hazards.
   (Objective 6)

8. The landing zone should be 100 × 100 feet. It should have few vertical structures and should be relatively flat and free of high grass, crops, debris, and rough terrain (check local standards for specific variations).
   (Objective 6)

9. As many patient care procedures as possible should be done, depending on the ETA of the helicopter. The airway should be secured and the patient ventilated appropriately. The patient should be secured to a long spine board with straps and cervical immobilization. Vascular access should be obtained, and other patient assessment and care should be continued (e.g., maintain warmth) until the helicopter arrives.
   (Objective 6)

10. Do not approach the aircraft unless directed to do so by the crew. Approach from the front of the aircraft and stay clear of the tail rotor. Allow a minimal number of people to help load. Secure loose objects. Walk in a crouched position. Carry objects at waist height. Depart from the front in view of the pilot. Wear eye protection.
    (Objective 6)

STUDENT SELF-ASSESSMENT

11. b. The AMD 001-009 performance standards have been incorporated into the latest KKK standards.
    (Objective 1)

12. c. Lack or failure of essential patient equipment could mean the difference between life and death.
    (Objective 2)

13. a. A number of factors will affect those times, and they can vary by time of day and other variables. This should be monitored on a continuing basis.
    (Objective 3)

14. c. Paramedics driving an ambulance should remain at or below the speed limit except in extreme circumstances. For maximal safety, the paramedic attendant should also be restrained except when patient care requires movement. Lights and sirens should be used only on emergency responses (as dictated by policy) and when a patient in critical condition is being transported.
    (Objective 4)

15. a. Ideally, the ambulance should be on the same side of the road as the crash. Emergency lights should be left on. Ambulances should be parked uphill and upwind from hazardous materials incidents.
    (Objective 4)

16. b. Some air medical services require training in specialized airway and vascular access techniques, as well as expanded medication administration knowledge. This varies by agency.
    (Objective 5)

17. b. Unless inclement weather or impassable roads prohibit transport, all the other patients could be appropriately transported by ground ALS service.
(Objective 6)

18. d. No one should approach the aircraft until a crew member signals that it is OK. A minimal number of people should approach the aircraft. No objects should be held up.
(Objective 6)

WRAP IT UP

1. a (Are replacements available on the ambulance, are the batteries fully charged on the defibrillator, and are there defibrillator pads on truck?); c (Is preventive maintenance being done?); d (What effect would giving an expired drug have?); e (How will that affect the patient's pain and further damage/bleeding?); f (What if your patient is critical?; Would you have to call another ambulance?); g (How would you explain that in court?); h (What might the consequence be?; Are you checking the tires each day and reporting wear?)
(Objective 2)

2. Reduction in response time
(Objective 3)

3. Wearing seatbelts; driving the speed limit, except as allowed by law; parking safely at the scene
(Objective 4)

4. The crew is trained and authorized to perform advanced techniques; a specialized resource center can be reached more quickly.
(Objectives 5, 6)

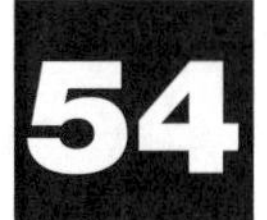 **Medical Incident Command**

Chapter 54, pages 1477-1493, in *Mosby's Paramedic Textbook,* ed. 4.

OBJECTIVES

Upon completion of this chapter, the paramedic student will be able to do the following:

1. Outline the components that define a major incident.
2. Identify the components of an effective incident command system (ICS).
3. Outline the activities of the preplanning, scene management, and postdisaster follow-up phases of an incident.
4. Identify the five major functions of the ICS.
5. List command responsibilities during a major incident response.
6. Describe the section responsibilities in the ICS.
7. Identify situations that may be classified as major incidents.
8. Describe the steps necessary to establish and operate the ICS.
9. Given a major incident, describe the groups or divisions that would need to be established and the responsibilities of each.
10. List common problems related to the ICS and to mass casualty incidents.
11. Outline the principles and technology of triage.
12. Identify resources for the management of critical incident stress.

SUMMARY

- Major incidents are events for which available resources are not adequate to manage the number of casualties or the type of emergency.
- The incident command system (ICS) organizational structure should be adaptable to any agency or to any incident requiring emergency management. The ICS also must be expandable. It must be able to expand from dealing with a nonmajor incident to a major one in a logical way.
- The five major functions of the ICS organization are command, planning, operations, logistics, and finance and administration.
- The responsibility of command should belong to one person. This should be a person who can effectively manage the emergency scene. In multiagency and multijurisdictional incidents, unified command may be used.
- The planning section should provide past, present, and future information about the incident and the status of resources. The operations section directs and coordinates all operations. It also ensures the safety of all personnel. The logistics section is responsible for providing supplies and equipment (including personnel to operate the equipment), facilities, services, food, and communications support. The finance or administration section tracks incident and reimbursement costs.
- All participating response agencies must agree to the preplan (phase 1 of the ICS). The preplan must address common goals and the specific duties of each group. Phase 2 requires the development of a strategy to manage the emergency scene. Phase 3 includes a postdisaster review of lessons learned from the incident and the determination of ways to improve.
- The need to expand the ICS at a medical incident is based on the number of casualties and the nature of the event.
- The first emergency medical services unit to arrive at the scene should make a quick and rapid assessment of the situation. Command must immediately establish radio contact with the communications center or emergency operations center. Additional units should be requested as soon as the need has been identified.
- Common divisions or groups that may need to be established include extrication and rescue, treatment, and transportation. A staging area and support branch may also be needed. The rescue and extrication group is responsible for managing trapped patients at the scene. The treatment group provides advanced care and stabilization until the patients are transported to a medical facility. The transportation group communicates with the receiving hospital, ambulances, and aeromedical services for patient transport. The staging area is used in large incidents to prevent vehicle congestion and delays in response. The rehabilitation area allows rescue personnel to receive physical and psychological rest. The support branch coordinates the gathering and distribution of equipment and supplies for all divisions and groups.

727

- Problems of mass casualty incidents and incident command systems stem from numerous issues related to communication, resource allocation, and delegation.
- Triage is a method used to categorize patients for priorities of treatment. START triage uses a 60-second assessment. It focuses on the patient's ability to walk, respiratory effort, pulses and perfusion, and neurologic status. The METTAG system is one of a number of tape, tag, and label systems used to categorize patients during triage.
- Critical incident stress debriefing is part of a critical incident stress management program. Such debriefing should be part of postdisaster standard operating procedures.

REVIEW QUESTIONS

Match the terms in column II with their definitions in column I. Use each term only once.

Column I

1. _________ Contracts agreeing to interagency exchange of resources when necessary

2. _________ Pumpers, ladder trucks, rescue trucks

3. _________ Rendezvous location for all arriving EMS, fire, and rescue equipment

4. _________ Responsible for coordination of major incident situation

Column II

a. Apparatus
b. Command
c. Command post
d. Communication center
e. Mutual aid
f. Branch
g. Staging area

Questions 5 to 13 refer to the following case study:

Dispatch radios your crew to respond to a local sports stadium for a bleacher collapse at a college football game. During your initial size-up, you determine that 50 to 100 people are injured, with a substantial number of victims still trapped under the fallen concrete seats. It is rush hour, and traffic conditions will be heavy for at least 2 more hours.

5. List three actions that should be taken by the first unit arriving at the scene.

6. a. How will command be determined?

   b. Will single or unified command be used?

7. List nine command responsibilities during this incident.

   a. ____

   b. ____

   c. ____

   d. ____

   e. ____

f. ____

g. ____

h. ____

i. ____

8. Fill in Fig. 54-1 with the appropriate positions needed in this incident command situation.

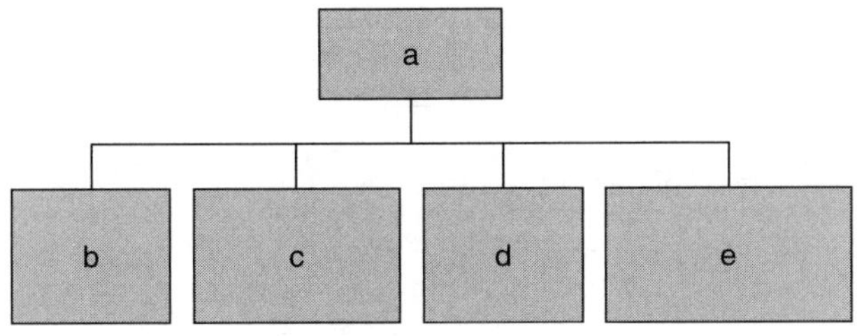

Figure 54-1

9. Briefly describe the responsibilities of each of the following sectors that command has established for this incident.

a. Support branch:

____

____

b. Staging area:

____

____

c. Extrication group:

____

____

d. Treatment group:

____

____

e. Transportation:

____

____

10. Explain how communications can be initiated in an effective manner in this situation.

____

____

____

11. a. What special resources will be needed during this incident?

____

____

    b. How will command know where to obtain those resources?

____

____

12. Triage each of the following patients injured at this scene using START triage and METTAG categories.

    a. A man walks over to you complaining of chest pain.

____

    b. A woman has a respiratory rate of 20 breaths/min and no radial pulse but a carotid pulse is present.

____

    c. A man is lying under a bleacher. His respiratory rate is 24 breaths/min, a radial pulse is present, he can't touch his nose with his index finger, and he knows his name but not the date or year.

____

    d. A woman is leaning against a bleacher unable to walk. Her respiratory rate is 16 breaths/min; a radial pulse is present; she can stick out her tongue and touch her nose with her index finger; and she knows her name, the date, and the year.

____

    e. A man has a respiratory rate of 8 breaths/min. He has no radial pulse, but a carotid pulse is present.

____

    f. A woman is trapped under a post. She is not breathing and has no pulse.

____

13. During triage, what care should be provided to the patients in question 12?

____

14. An ideal incident command system would have which of the following characteristics?
   a. It would be able to expand to a larger incident in a logical manner.
   b. It would be used only for large or complex mass casualty situations.
   c. It would provide for just single jurisdiction involvement.
   d. It would respond to one specific incident or situation.

15. Which phase of major incident planning involves establishing an inventory of community resources needed for selected disasters?
   a. Logistics operations
   b. Postdisaster follow-up
   c. Scene management
   d. The preplan

16. What are the five major components of FEMA's ICS organization?
   a. Communications, logistics, operations, staging, support
   b. Communications, finance, staging, support, treatment
   c. Command, finance, logistics, operations, planning
   d. Command, operations, planning, transportation, treatment

17. What has the highest priority when the incident commander is considering whether to expand the ICS organization during an incident?
   a. Cost
   b. Incident stability
   c. Life safety
   d. Property conservation

18. What is the primary responsibility of the section chiefs in an MCI situation?
   a. To assume overall accountability for the MCI situation
   b. To make sure that section members are working toward a common goal
   c. To operate rescue equipment and supervise staff in the area
   d. To provide patient care and stabilization within a defined area

19. Which section has overall responsibility for the areas that provide care to medical staff?
   a. Finance
   b. Logistics
   c. Operations
   d. Planning

20. Which situation would be likely to be declared a major incident?
   a. Rural EMS service, motor vehicle collision requiring four EMS units
   b. City EMS service, train derailment, possibly four patients
   c. Rural EMS service, tractor roll-over with rescue
   d. City EMS service, two-person motor vehicle collision, no patient trapped

21. What group usually provides patient care in the ICS system?
   a. Extrication
   b. Support
   c. Treatment
   d. Triage

22. What is an appropriate role for a physician brought to the scene from a local hospital?
   a. Incident commander
   b. Extrication group resource
   c. Staging area resource
   d. Transport group resource

23. The most appropriate radio communication during a mass casualty incident would be between which of the following crew members?
   a. Command and sector officers
   b. Individuals within each unit
   c. Treatment group and hospital
   d. Public information officer and press

24. Which of the following may create a problem at an MCI?
  a. Organizing patients rapidly at a treatment area
  b. Transporting patients prematurely
  c. Performing rapid "initial" stabilization of patients
  d. Wearing identification vests

25. Patient classification during mass casualty incidents should be based on which of the following?
  a. Physiologic signs, mechanism of injury, and anatomic injury
  b. Mechanism of injury, anatomic injury, and patient age
  c. Chief complaint, physiologic signs, and anatomic injury
  d. Physiologic signs, anatomic injury, and concurrent disease

26. Your patient has a gunshot wound to the chest, is conscious, and has a respiratory rate of 36 breaths/min. Which of the following would be the appropriate triage category using the triage systems discussed in the text?
  a. Urgent, yellow
  b. Critical, red
  c. Dead/dying, black
  d. Delayed, green

27. Mental status examination during START triage should include which of the following?
  a. Asking the patient to touch his nose
  b. AVPU
  c. Glasgow Coma Scale
  d. Observing for arm drift

28. What information should be included on the patient tracking log?
  a. Patient's age
  b. Patient's injuries
  c. Patient's next of kin
  d. Patient's priority

29. What service is typically provided in a critical incident stress management program?
  a. Part of command during large-scale incidents
  b. Defusing services 2 weeks after a large-scale incident
  c. Long-term psychiatric counseling
  d. On-scene support for distressed personnel

30. What best defines a major incident that requires use of the incident command system?
  a. The specific situation is spelled out in detail in a community-wide preplan
  b. Rescuers do not have enough help or equipment to manage the scene in a timely manner
  c. Motor vehicle collision with more than two cars or more than four patients
  d. Shooting with more than one patient and unknown location of the shooter

WRAP IT UP

At 0828 on a foggy morning, a large passenger aircraft runs off runway M2R, striking the perimeter fence around the airport. Your ambulance is the first to arrive on the scene. The local fire chief is the incident commander, and he immediately delegates your supervisor to lead the EMS branch. She in turn asks that you lead the rescue and extrication group. You send your partner to do a quick size-up of the patients who are out of the aircraft. The initial assessment reveals that the pilot was found not breathing and pulseless; three crew members and three passengers are noted to have inhalation injuries and severe respiratory distress; the other 19 patients appear on initial exam to be walking and complaining of minor injuries. The next hour is frantic and chaotic at times as the patients are sorted, treated, and finally transported.

During an incident debriefing 3 days later, you review the whole situation. The incident commander shows how he laid out the groups: rescue and extrication (triage, treatment, transport), staging, and transportation. A PIO officer helped deal with the huge media presence, and a liaison officer helped to communicate with the unified command. Problems identified in the situation included difficulty with communication, a delay in getting ambulances to the scene, a traffic jam at the scene, difficulty identifying branch leaders, and failure to update the hospitals about incoming patients. Some suggestions are offered for remedying these problems, and another planning meeting is scheduled for 2 weeks later.

1. What additional support staff person should have been appointed by command in addition to the public relations

and liaison officers? ____

2. What are some possible causes of the difficulties identified in this situation, and which sectors or branches are responsible for identifying solutions?

732

Problem	Possible Causes	Sector or Branch Responsible for Solution
a. Difficulty with communication		
b. Delay in ambulance arrival		
c. Traffic jam on scene		
d. difficulty identifying command		
e. Failure to update hospitals		

3. Based on the limited information you have, how many patients would you triage as

    a. Dead or dying:____

    b. Critical:____

    c. Urgent: ____

    d. Delayed: ____

CHAPTER 54 ANSWERS

REVIEW QUESTIONS

1. e
2. a
3. g
4. b
(Questions 1–4, Objective 2)

5. A rapid scene assessment should be performed. Communication should be established with the communications center or emergency operations center (as dictated by local policy). Additional units should be requested as soon as the need has been identified.
(Objective 8)

6. a. Command is determined by the preplanned system of arriving emergency units. The person assuming command must be familiar with ICS structure and the operating procedures of responding units.
(Objective 8)

    b. It will likely be a unified command involving EMS, fire and rescue, and police. Some communities have public safety departments that incorporate all three functions. In that case, a single command will likely be used.
(Objective 5)

7. Assuming an effective command position that has a good vantage point and is away from any danger of the bleachers, some responsibilities would include transmitting initial radio reports to the communications center; evaluating the scene rapidly (visually and with reports of other first responders); developing a strategy to safely extricate, triage, treat, transport, and provide security on scene; requesting additional equipment and personnel resources and assigning command roles; assigning sectors and identifying objectives in cooperation with section chiefs; evaluating information to determine the progress of the event; sending units no longer needed back into service; terminating command at an appropriate time; and evaluating the effectiveness of operations (may be done retrospectively).
(Objective 5)

8. Incident command organizational chart completed. a. Command b. Finance c. Logistic d. Operation e. Planning
(Objective 4)

9. a. Procuring and distributing supplies (medicine, food, water, protective gear) and resources (heavy equipment, special tools)

    b. Designating and staffing a safe helicopter landing zone and designating and staffing a staging area where all arriving apparatus will report and be assigned to areas where needed

c. Triaging victims and moving them to a designated treatment area, securing necessary experts to determine the safest extrication procedures for this structure, coordinating physical rescue operations (including direction of heavy equipment), and ensuring scene safety

d. Selecting a site close to but at a safe distance from the collapse site, categorizing patients on arrival and sending them to the appropriate segment of the treatment area or immediate or delayed zones, providing patient care and stabilization until transport can be provided, and communicating frequently with the transportation sector so that appropriate patient transfers can be facilitated

e. Coordinating patient transport with the staging area manager and treatment groups, communicating with receiving hospitals so that appropriate resources can be selected, and assigning patients to ambulances or helicopters and directing them to the appropriate facilities
(Objective 9)

10. Effective communications can be enhanced by using a common frequency (command frequency) for interdisciplinary communication when necessary; using the radio frequencies designated in the plan; using different frequencies for fire, EMS, and other support agencies; making sure that common terminology is used; ensuring clear, concise radio traffic; preparing messages before transmitting; limiting use of radios; and identifying the speaker only by sector
(Objective 8)

11. a. Air medical transport because of heavy traffic and heavy equipment needed to extricate victims from under the bleachers
(Objective 9)

b. The preplan should identify the availability and location of specialized resources that may be needed during an MCI situation.
(Objective 3)

12. a. Delayed: yellow (may be upgraded after retriage in treatment sector)
b. Critical: red
c. Critical: yellow
d. Delayed: green
e. Critical: red
f. Dead or dying: black
(Objective 11)

13. The airway may be opened if necessary and hemorrhage controlled.
(Objective 11)

STUDENT SELF-ASSESSMENT

14. a. The ICS should be adaptable to small or large situations involving one or more jurisdictions as the need arises.
(Objective 2)

15. d. Preidentification of resources ensures rapid deployment by logistics during a disaster.
(Objective 3)

16. c. Command, finance, logistics, operations, and planning (C-FLOP) are the foundations on which the ICS is built.
(Objective 4)

17. c. The priority is always the safety of the emergency responders and the public.
(Objective 5)

18. b. The incident commander has overall responsibility. The section chiefs should be directing staff in their sectors, not performing physical tasks or providing patient care.
(Objective 4)

19. b. The rehab branch falls under the command of the logistics section.
(Objective 4)

20. a. In most urban EMS systems, this type of patient situation would not overwhelm the system, requiring a mass casualty plan.
(Objective 7)

21. c. In triage, patients are sorted, airways are opened, and hemorrhage is controlled.
(Objective 9)

22. b. Physicians are probably not appropriately trained for command. Their services may be more useful in assisting with triage and providing emergency surgery to facilitate extrication (all extrication sector responsibilities). A physician may also be assigned to the treatment sector.
(Objective 4)

23. a. As much verbal communication as possible should take place during the mass casualty incident to permit essential communication on the airwaves.
(Objective 8)

24. b
(Objective 10)

25. d. Abnormal vital signs, obvious anatomic injury, and other obvious preexisting illnesses and injuries should be considered when triaging patients.
(Objective 11)

26. b. A respiratory rate over 30 breaths/min indicates critical status in the START triage method. This patient obviously has a serious anatomic injury and abnormal physiologic signs, indicating that urgent care is necessary.
(Objective 11)

27. a. The patient should also be asked to state his name and the current date, including the year.
(Objective 11)

28. d. Patient identification, transporting unit, and hospital destination should also be noted.
(Objective 11)

29. d. The services provided depend on the local CISM team. Defusing is provided immediately after an incident.
(Objective 12)

30. b. Although c and d would merit the use of the ICS, b is the broadest definition.
(Objective 1)

WRAP IT UP

1. There should always be a safety officer.
(Objective 2)

2.

Problem	Possible Causes	Sector or Branch Responsible for Solution
a. Difficulty with communication	Failure to designate specific channels in preplan or early in the incident Excessive talking on the radio; failure to use face-to-face communication	Incident Command Sector officers
b. Delay in ambulance arrival	Possible failure to request resources early Possible failure to adequately control the perimeter and access roads	Incident command
c. Traffic jam on scene	Failure to designate staging area early Failure to designate areas spread apart (e.g., transportation, staging, command)	Law enforcement Incident command
d. Difficulty identifying command	Possible failure to declare who is in command on the radio Failure to wear identification vests or to mark the command area adequately	Incident command
e. Failure to update hospitals	Failure to give hospitals a brief report when wounded are leaving	Transportation group leader

(Objective 10)

3. a. 1
b. 3
c. 0
d. 19
(Objective 11)

 Rescue Awareness and Operations

READING ASSIGNMENT

Chapter 55, pages 1494-1514 in *Mosby's Paramedic Textbook,* ed. 4.

OBJECTIVES

Upon completion of this chapter, the paramedic student will be able to do the following:

1. Describe factors that must be considered to ensure appropriate timing of medical and mechanical skills during a rescue.
2. Outline each phase of a rescue operation.
3. Identify the appropriate personal protective equipment for rescue operations.
4. Describe important considerations for emergency medical services (EMS) crews in a surface water rescue.
5. Discuss important considerations for EMS crews in rescues associated with hazardous atmospheres, including confined spaces and trench or cave-in situations.
6. Describe hazards that may be present during an EMS rescue operation on a highway.
7. Describe important considerations for EMS crews in a rescue involving hazardous terrain.
8. Outline special considerations for prehospital assessment and management during a rescue operation.

SUMMARY

- Rescue is a patient-driven event. It calls for specialized medical and mechanical skills. The right amount of each must be applied at the right time. The main role of the paramedic in rescues is to have the proper training and the appropriate personal protective equipment (PPE). These allow safe access to the patient and the provision of treatment at the site and throughout the incident.
- The seven phases of a rescue operation are arrival and scene size-up, hazard control, gaining access to the patient, medical treatment, disentanglement, patient packaging, and transportation.
- The standards for protective clothing and personal protection equipment established by the National Fire Protection Association and Occupational Safety and Health Administration have been adopted by many fire and emergency medical services (EMS) agencies. The appropriate PPE depends on the level of rescuer involvement and the nature of the incident.
- Water rescue should never be attempted by a single rescuer or by one who is untrained.
- Water hazards include obstructions to flow and foot or extremity pins that can trap victims and drag them under water. Some factors that contribute to flat water drowning are alcohol or other drug use. Also, cool water temperatures contribute to such drownings.
- Hazardous atmospheres are environments with low oxygen. These environments can occur in confined spaces. The six major hazards associated with confined spaces are oxygen-deficient atmospheres, chemical or toxic exposure and explosion, engulfment, machinery entrapment, electricity, and structural concerns.
- Traffic flow is the biggest hazard in EMS highway operations. Other scene hazards associated with highway operations include fuel or fire hazards, electrical power, unstable vehicles, airbags and supplemental restraint systems, and hazardous cargoes.
- Hazardous terrain can create major difficulties during rescue events. Three common classifications of hazardous terrain are low-angle terrain, high-angle terrain, and flat terrain with obstructions.

Questions 1 and 2 refer to the following case study:

A woman who is kayaking on a winter day is swept under the ice. You can see her about 3 feet (1 meter) from the edge of the ice, where the water is rolling up over a large rock. Her team is frantically screaming at you to do something.

1. What hazards do you face if you enter the water to attempt a rescue?

Additional equipment is requested, and a cut is made in the ice to retrieve the woman. However, she does not survive the 90-minute submersion.

2. What services of the local CISM team might your crew need after this incident?

Questions 3 to 8 refer to the following case study:

A partygoer falls into an open sewer standpipe. You estimate that he is approximately 30 feet down the 48-inch pipe. Bystanders report that he was talking to them when they arrived, but you hear him moaning only occasionally at this time.

3. What additional assistance will you request?

4. What potential injuries should you worry about in this patient?

5. Why must the rescue team test the air quality at several levels in the pipe?

6. Why might the rescuer who enters the pipe wear an SABA instead of an SCBA during this rescue?

7. What can cause problems when using an SABA?

8. Aside from a confined-space rescue, what other hazardous rescue situation exists here?

Questions 9 to 18 refer to the following case study:

You are called to the scene of a motor vehicle collision at a busy urban shopping center. On arrival, you find that a large sedan has hit the side of a compact car, wedging it between the sedan and a storefront. A large crowd of spectators has gathered and is impeding your access to the patient. You note a trickle of gasoline coming from one of the vehicles. No other equipment or law enforcement personnel have been dispatched.

9. What should you be looking for as you do your scene size-up?

____

10. What information or assistance did you receive on your response?

____

____

11. What steps should you take to gain control of the crowd?

____

____

____

One patient was pulled from the sedan by bystanders before your arrival. He is pale and complains of abdominal pain. Your partner begins care. A second patient in the compact car is unconscious. He is trapped and inaccessible.

12. List the additional equipment and other resources you should request at this time.

____

13. What hazards have you identified that should be reported to incoming crews?

____

14. What actions can be taken to reduce the risks associated with the hazards you identified?

____

____

A rescue truck arrives, and the crew breaks a window in the compact car, providing limited access to the patient while rescue operations proceed.

15. What can you do for your patient at this time?

____

16. How can you ensure patient safety during the rescue?

____

____

Chapter **55** **Rescue Awareness and Operations**

A brief primary survey reveals an unconscious patient with gurgling respirations and a strong radial pulse of 70 beats/min. You observe a large ecchymotic area on the temporal region of the patient's head.

17. You have limited time and access to the patient. What are your priorities of care?

____

____

18. Describe the disentanglement, packaging, and removal segments of the rescue operation and your responsibilities to the patient during these phases.

____

____

____

____

19. At the scene of an accident in which an energized wire is in contact with an involved automobile, what safety measures should be taken for:

a. Rescuers:

____

____

b. People trapped in the involved automobile:

____

____

20. Give two examples of equipment that may be used to disentangle a person who is trapped inside a vehicle.

a. ____

b. ____

STUDENT SELF-ASSESSMENT

21. Aside from ensuring safety, the rescue operations should be guided by which of the following?
   a. Performance of techniques in the standardized manner
   b. The desire of the rescue team to complete the task
   c. The medical and physical needs of the patient
   d. The number of bystanders observing the scene

22. What is the responsibility of the paramedic in any rescue situation?
   a. To coordinate overall scene safety
   b. To direct scene and tactical operations
   c. To know when it is safe to attempt rescue
   d. To operate all rescue and extrication equipment

23. Whose safety is the first priority at the scene of any rescue?
   a. Bystanders   **c.** Injured
   b. Crew   **d.** Trapped

740

24. When does scene size-up begin on a call for rescue?
   a. On arrival to the scene
   b. When specialized teams arrive
   c. When the call is received
   d. When the patient is visible

25. Which is true regarding medical treatment during a rescue situation for a safely accessible patient?
   a. All standardized procedures should be followed.
   b. Medical treatment should be directed by the rescue commander.
   c. No treatment should be attempted until the patient has been freed.
   d. Rapid assessment and basic stabilization should be attempted.

26. What routine safety measures should be used to protect the patient during a vehicle rescue that does not involve fire or hazardous materials?
   a. Blanket
   b. Air bags
   c. Surgical mask
   d. An SCBA

27. According to NFPA and OSHA standards, EMS rescue personnel should have access to which of the following personal protective equipment?
   a. Ear plugs
   b. Protective helmet
   c. Firefighting turnout gear
   d. Leather boots

28. Which is true when responding to a rescue in swift water?
   a. A foot trapped in water should be freed the opposite way it went in.
   b. Do not walk through fast-moving water that is over knee deep.
   c. Flat water does not create any serious hazard.
   d. High dams create more dangerous situations than low dams.

29. What factors contribute to drowning?
   a. Cool water temperature
   b. Advanced patient age
   c. PFDs worn properly
   d. Swimming after eating

30. What factor would be an acceptable reason not to resuscitate a person who has drowned?
   a. More than 5 minutes of submersion was documented by witnesses.
   b. Evidence of activation of the mammalian diving reflex exists.
   c. The patient is cold, and temperature can't be detected on a regular thermometer.
   d. Rigor mortis or dependent lividity is present.

31. What is the first measure that should be used to attempt rescue for a person in the water?
   a. Go
   b. Reach
   c. Row
   d. Throw

32. Which of the following oxygen levels is considered hazardous?
   a. Over 19.5%
   b. Over 22%
   c. Over 21%
   d. Under 21%

33. Which is a clue to help identify an oxygen-limiting silo?
   a. An audible tone will sound.
   b. The color is usually blue.
   c. The placard states this information.
   d. The smell will be sweet.

34. You arrive at the scene of a trench collapse. When should you enter the trench to rescue the patient without specialized rescue equipment?
   a. The patient is unconscious.
   b. The patient is completely covered.
   c. The trench is less than waist deep.
   d. The trench is more than 3 feet wide.

35. Which of the following techniques may be used to increase safety at the scene of a vehicle accident with a gasoline leak at night?
  a. Put flares adjacent to the involved vehicles to alert motorists.
  b. Stage all apparatus on the highway and not on side roads.
  c. Use all warning lights and headlights to increase visibility.
  d. Wear high-visibility clothing, such as ANSI 2 vests.

36. What should the paramedic do to reduce the risk of fire at the scene of a motor vehicle collision?
  a. Disconnect the battery cable.
  b. Douse the vehicle with foam.
  c. Place a tarp over the spilled fuel.
  d. Turn off the automobile ignition.

37. Which type of extinguisher can be used to suppress a combustible metal fire?
  a. Class A
  b. Class B
  c. Class C
  d. Class D

38. What type of equipment is helpful for vehicle stabilization during rescue?
  a. Chain saws
  b. Cribbing
  c. Hurst tools
  d. Pry bars

39. You respond to a vehicle crash involving an undeployed air bag. What measure may create a hazard for rescuers?
  a. Using tools that generate sparks
  b. Cutting the steering column to disable the system
  c. Disconnecting or cutting both battery cables
  d. Cutting into the air bag module

40. What is the primary risk associated with hazardous terrain rescue?
  a. Avalanche of debris
  b. Dropping the patient
  c. Injury from falls
  d. Injury from projectiles

41. Which term describes rescue on steep terrain that can be walked on without use of the hands?
  a. Graded terrain rescue
  b. High-angle rescue
  c. Low-angle rescue
  d. Rescue on flat terrain with obstructions

42. Which of the following factors that can interfere with a paramedic's ability to adequately assess and treat a patient is unique to a rescue situation?
  a. Cumbersome personal protective equipment
  b. Lack of cooperation among your team members
  c. Hostile, uncommunicative patient
  d. Unstable vital signs and neurologic status

43. Which is a complication of crush syndrome?
  a. Hypertension
  b. Metabolic alkalosis
  c. Myoglobinemia
  d. Sepsis

44. You are trying to free a driver involved in a head-on crash who is seriously injured. The car shows major front-end damage; also, the passenger air bag has deployed, but the driver-side air bag has not. How will this affect your approach to the rescue?
  a. When the ignition is off, the bag will not open unless there is a fire.
  b. It will not affect your approach to this patient.
  c. You will put a board between the patient and the unopened bag.
  d. You will keep at least 10 inches or more away from the path of the bag.

742

You sense panic as you pull up to the scene of a mine explosion. Six men were down in the narrow shaft when a rumbling noise was heard, and then a plume of dark smoke slowly wound out of the mine. The incident commander and mine supervisor are reviewing the situation, trying to determine the best approach. An alternate shaft is available, but there is a fear of secondary danger. One garbled radio transmission from below indicates that there are survivors, but several are trapped under the rubble. It is determined that you and your partner will go in first because of your advanced, confined-space rescue training. The two of you don SABA and rappelling harness and are lowered slowly down the secondary shaft. At the bottom, water is slowly creeping up the walls of the enclosure. Your lamps provide a glimpse of some movement through the haze, and you carefully move along the side of the wall, taking care not to catch your air hoses on the protruding rocks. When you reach the miners, two are dead, three are in good condition, and one is entangled in some twisted rebar. Over the next 4 hours, first the three men in good condition are lifted up the narrow shaft in a rescue harness; then the rebar is cut, the fourth miner is removed from the wreckage, his wounds are treated, and he is pulled to the top wrapped securely in a Stokes basket. Finally, the agonizing job of respectfully packaging and lifting the bodies is undertaken.

1. Put a ✓ beside potential hazards faced by the rescuers in this situation.

    a. _________ Collapse and engulfment   **d.** _________ Hypothermia

    b. _________ Electrical   **e.** _________ Oxygen deficiency

    c. _________ Explosion   **f.** _________ Toxic gases

2. Identify steps that should be taken to minimize the risks you indicated for the trapped miners and for the rescuers.

____

____

____

3. What personal protective equipment should the rescuers be using in this situation?

____

4. Which phase of the rescue operation was it when the rescuers cut the rebar and freed the miner?
    a. Disentanglement   **c.** Hazard control
    b. Gaining access to the patient   **d.** Patient packaging

5. Which elements of low- or high-angle rescue did the rescuers need to consider during this situation?

____

____

6. Why should only specially trained rescuers be sent down the shaft on this type of call?

____

____

       Chapter **55** **Rescue Awareness and Operations**

REVIEW QUESTIONS

1. Drowning, foot or extremity entrapment, hypothermia, recirculating current
   (Objective 4)

2. Defusing immediately after the incident if the emotional impact is high, critical incident stress debriefing 24 to 72 hours after the incident, follow-up to ensure that specific crew members are recovering, and specialty debriefing for the people with the patient (if your team provides that service)
   (Objective 2)

3. Rescue truck, possibly specialized hazardous materials team, high-angle rescue specialists
   (Objective 2)

4. Asphyxiation, toxic inhalation, trauma, drowning, and exposure (depending on the time of year)
   (Objective 5)

5. Toxic gas may exist or oxygen levels may be low, and these conditions may vary at different levels in the pipe.
   (Objective 5)

6. It may be difficult to maneuver in the pipe with a standard air tank, and the time required for the rescue may exceed the tank capacity.
   (Objective 5)

7. The line may kink or tangle or the equipment may fail.
   (Objective 5)

8. High-angle rescue probably will be necessary to retrieve the patient.
   (Objective 7)

9. During arrival and scene size-up, you should look for environmental risks, the number of patients, and the need for medical care and rescue and then request additional resources.
   (Objectives 2, 6)

10. Information was limited to location and the fact that a crash had occurred. No additional equipment was dispatched (or has arrived).
    (Objective 2)

11. Immediately delegate several crowd members to move the crowd to a safe distance to allow for patient care and the arrival of additional equipment. Call for law enforcement officers to take charge of crowd control.
    (Objective 2)

12. Advanced life support ambulance, rescue truck, pumper, and law enforcement officers
    (Objective 2)

13. Hazards identified are a crowd and the gasoline spill.
    (Objective 2)

14. Make sure no one is smoking near the crash. Also, disconnect the vehicle battery cables.
    (Objective 2)

15. Begin initial patient assessment and airway management (if indicated).
    (Objective 8)

16. Protect the patient with blankets, shields, or flame-retardant coverings.
    (Objective 8)

744

17. Securing an open airway, protecting the cervical spine, and assisting ventilations with high-concentration oxygen if possible
(Objective 8)

18. Disentanglement involves removing the wreckage from the patient. Rescuers must protect the patient and maintain the airway, cervical spine immobilization, and breathing to the best of their ability. Packaging involves immobilization and removal of the patient from the scene to the emergency response vehicle. Rescuers must protect the patient's spine, splint or bandage injuries if appropriate (based on the acuteness of the patient's condition), and make sure the patient is adequately secured before removal begins. The paramedic should oversee safe transport of the patient by the rescue team to the ambulance.
(Objective 2)

19. a. Contact utility workers to move downed wires or shut off power, keep bystanders away, and secure energized wires with a dry fire hose or other appropriate means.
b. Advise occupants to stay in the car.
(Objective 6)

20. Ropes, air bags, pry bars, jacks, wedges, cutters, spreaders, and winches
(Objective 6)

STUDENT SELF-ASSESSMENT

21. c. Other than safety, the patient is the primary focus of the rescue.
(Objective 1)

22. c. Unless responding as part of a specialized fire and rescue team, the paramedic is not responsible for coordinating the rescue, serving as the safety officer, or operating equipment. Although everyone on the scene should be alert for overall safety considerations, the paramedic's responsibilities are to recognize when a rescue is safe before arrival of specialized teams and to provide patient care and monitoring during a rescue situation.
(Objective 1)

23. b. Initial efforts should ensure that the crew is uninjured so their EMS functions can be maintained.
(Objective 1)

24. c. The dispatch call can provide the first information paramedics need to size up a rescue situation and respond to it with the appropriate safety measures.
(Objective 2)

25. d. Moving all standardized equipment into the rescue area is not practical. Basic assessment and stabilization should be attempted until the patient is in the ambulance. In certain situations, when the surroundings are unsafe or the patient is inaccessible, delivery of care may not be possible.
(Objective 2)

26. a. Ear and eye protection may also be necessary. A face mask with supplemental air or oxygen would be needed only in situations in which the oxygen supply is inadequate or toxic fumes are present.
(Objective 2)

27. a. Although ear plugs are helpful during the response, they may impair communication on a rescue.
(Objective 3)

28. b. Walking in swift water could result in a foot becoming trapped, and the paramedic could be dragged under the surface.
(Objective 4)

29. a. Alcohol and drug use also contribute to drowning. Properly worn PFDs reduce the risk of drowning.
(Objective 4)

30. d. Survival after cold water drowning is difficult to predict; rigor mortis, dependent lividity, or putrefaction indicates death.
(Objective 4)

31. b. If the person is close enough, the rescuer should reach out with a long device. The next measure would be to throw a device to the person. Then, if this is unsuccessful, a boat should be taken to rescue the person. Finally, if no other option exists, a trained rescuer with appropriate PPE should enter the water in an attempt to rescue the individual.
(Objective 4)

32. b. High oxygen concentrations create a risk of rapid combustion to fuel fire or explosion. Concentrations below 19.5% are considered an atmospheric hazard.
(Objective 5)

33. b. Personnel on the scene may be helpful and may also provide that information.
(Objective 5)

34. c. Rescuer safety should be the primary concern.
(Objective 5)

35. d. Flares would be dangerous in the presence of a gasoline leak. Apparatus should be staged off the highway if possible. Placing one large apparatus in front of the scene so that safe loading can occur may be helpful. Use warning lights cautiously and make sure that headlights are not pointed at oncoming traffic.
(Objective 6)

36. d. In some cases, the battery may be left connected. The other measures would be unnecessary in the absence of flames.
(Objective 6)

37. d. Class A is used to extinguish ordinary combustibles; class B, flammable liquids; and class C, energized electrical equipment.
(Objective 6)

38. b. The other tools are used for disentanglement.
(Objective 6)

39. c. The steering column should not be cut.
(Objective 6)

40. c. Both the rescuers and patient are at risk for falls during rescue from hazardous terrain.
(Objective 7)

41. c. High angle refers to cliffs or the sides of buildings or other structures; rope or aerial apparatus is needed for such rescues. Flat terrain with obstacles may include large rocks, loose soil, and waterbeds or creeks.
(Objective 7)

42. a. Ideally, team cooperation is a standard on all scenes. Hostile or unstable patients are not unique to rescue situations.
(Objective 8)

43. c. When the muscles are crushed, they release their pigment (myoglobin), which can cause renal failure. Hypotension and metabolic acidosis may also occur.
(Objective 8)

44. d. If possible, avoid that side of the car for your safety.
(Objective 8)

746

1. a, b, c, d, e, f
(Objective 5)

2. Collapse: The incident commander should confer with the site engineer to determine the risk of further collapse.
Electrical: The incident commander and site engineer should make sure that power is disabled if the risk of
electrical injury exists.
Explosion: The cause of the initial explosion should be identified, if possible, and the risk of secondary explosion
determined. Measurements should be taken in the shaft to determine if explosive gas levels are present.
Hypothermia: The depth of the cold water and the potential for the water to rise to a dangerous level, posing the
risk of hypothermia or drowning, should be determined.
Oxygen deficiency and toxic gases: Gas levels should be monitored.
(Objective 5)

3. Helmet, light, face shield or goggles, gloves, boots with steel toe shank, Nomex jumpsuit, PFD if risk of water
rising exists
(Objective 3)

4. a. Gaining access to the patient was accomplished if the patient were accessible at first contact. Hazard control
should have started before the rescuers entered the shaft and continued until conclusion of the rescue. Packaging
covered the activities involved in securing the patient in the Stokes basket.
(Objective 2)

5. Low-angle rescue considerations would develop as the rescuers moved through the obstructions and hazards in the
shaft. High-angle rescue principles would have been applied when the rescuers were lowered into the shaft and the
miners were removed.
(Objective 7)

6. Confined space rescue is a very hazardous, specialized rescue. Attempting to enter the shaft without proper
training would be very dangerous. It would likely violate OSHA rules.
(Objective 8)

<table><tr><td>**56**</td><td># Crime Scene Awareness</td></tr></table>

READING ASSIGNMENT

Chapter 56, pages 1515-1526, in *Mosby's Paramedic Textbook,* ed. 4.

OBJECTIVES

Upon completion of this chapter, the paramedic student will be able to do the following:

1. Describe general techniques for determining whether a scene is violent and choosing the appropriate response to a violent scene.
2. Outline techniques for recognizing and responding to potentially dangerous residential calls.
3. Outline techniques for recognizing and responding to potentially dangerous calls on the highway.
4. Describe signs of danger and emergency medical services (EMS) response to violent street incidents.
5. Identify characteristics of and EMS response to situations involving gangs, clandestine drug labs, and domestic violence situations.
6. Outline general safety tactics that EMS personnel can use if they find themselves in a dangerous situation.
7. Describe special EMS considerations when providing tactical patient care.
8. Discuss EMS documentation and preservation of evidence at a crime scene.

SUMMARY

- A key point in ensuring scene safety is to identify and respond to dangers before they threaten. If the scene is known to be violent, the emergency medical services (EMS) crew should remain at a safe and out-of-sight distance from the area. They should remain at this distance until the scene has been secured.
- The paramedic should look for warning signs of violence during response to a residence. He or she should retreat from the scene if danger becomes evident.
- A response to a highway incident may present the dangers associated with traffic and extrication. However, it may present danger from violence as well. Occupants may be armed, wanted or fleeing felons, intoxicated or drugged, or violent or abusive from an altered mental state.
- The paramedic should monitor for warning signs of danger in violent street incidents. He or she should retreat from the scene if necessary.
- A gang is any group of people who take part in socially disruptive or criminal behavior. Some gangs are involved in violent criminal activities. EMS personnel often look like law enforcement officers. Thus, they should be very cautious about their personal safety when working in gang areas.
- Clandestine lab activities can produce explosive and toxic gases. Other risks include booby traps that can maim or kill an intruder as well as armed or violent occupants.
- EMS personnel who respond to a scene of domestic violence should be aware that acts of violence may be directed toward them by the perpetrator; they should take all safety precautions.
- Tactics for safety include avoidance, tactical retreat, cover and concealment, and distraction and evasive maneuvers.
- Tactical patient care refers to care activities that occur inside the scene perimeter. This is known as the "hot zone." Providing care in this area calls for special training and authorization; body armor and a tactical uniform; compact and functional equipment; and in some operations, personal defensive weapons.
- The paramedic's observations at a crime scene are important. They should be carefully documented. Evidence should be protected while caring for the patient. This can be done by not unnecessarily disturbing the scene or destroying evidence.

Questions 1 and 2 apply to the following case study:

You are responding to a routine call in a residential neighborhood.

1. When should your scene size-up begin?

\
\

2. List six warning signs of danger that you should look for on this call.

a. ____

b. ____

c. ____

d. ____

e. ____

f. ____

3. List strategies to increase safety as you approach each of the following:

a. A darkened residence:

\
\

b. A vehicle stopped on the side of the highway:

\
\
\

4. For each of the situations below, indicate which of the following tactics would best increase your safety and describe how you would use it.

a. Avoidance   c. Cover and concealment

b. Tactical retreat   d. Distraction and evasive maneuvers

a. You respond to a school shooting. En route, you determine that several shots fired in a school classroom have been reported; however, there is no confirmation that the perpetrator has been apprehended.

\
\

b. You are providing care to an injured fan at a large soccer match when irate fans begin to hurl bottles at you and your partner.

\
\

c. You are on bike patrol at a community picnic. You respond to a call for a "person injured." You find a teenager dressed in known gang attire who was punched in the face. As you begin your care, you hear the sound of gunfire nearby.

\
\

750

d. During assessment of a patient with an altered level of consciousness in the living room of a small home, his behavior escalates suddenly, and he starts yelling and threatening to hurt you as he lunges toward you.

____

____

5. List six types of physical evidence that may be found at a crime scene.

a. ____

b. ____

c. ____

d. ____

e. ____

f. ____

6. When should assessment of the potential for violence at the scene begin?
a. If the patient threatens the crew   **c.** When the patient is encountered
b. On arrival at the scene   **d.** En route to the call

7. What may indicate that the residence you are about to enter is potentially dangerous?
a. Darkened residence   **c.** No car in the driveway
b. History of multiple calls   **d.** Person waving you in

8. Which represents the safest approach to a single vehicle stopped on the highway?
a. Approach from the passenger side of the vehicle
b. Simultaneous approach by both crew members
c. Ambulance lights turned off to eliminate glare
d. Walking between the ambulance and the other vehicle

9. Which of the following is most likely to protect the paramedic from danger during a violent street scene?
a. Allow police to control the scene and proceed as usual.
b. Attempt to disperse the crowd while providing care.
c. Retreat immediately from the scene with the patient.
d. There is no danger; crowds will not attack paramedics.

10. How can you learn about gang-related activity in your EMS response area?
a. CDC data   **c.** Census data
b. School officials   **d.** All of the above

11. Why is a response to a methamphetamine drug lab risky?
a. The lab may be booby trapped to harm intruders.
b. Cyanide gas is often present during production.
c. Production involves cryogenics and can cause frostbite.
d. Infectious agents may be in the environment.

12. Which of the following is most suspicious for domestic violence?
a. Darkened rooms   **c.** Inaccurate medical history
b. Excessive nervous talking   **d.** Inconsistent injuries

13. Which of the following is the safest EMS safety strategy in a dangerous situation?
    a. Avoidance
    b. Contact
    c. Negotiation
    d. Use of weapons

14. Which is an appropriate location for cover during gunfire?
    a. Bushes
    b. Car door
    c. Large tree
    d. Wooden sign

15. Which of the following provides a clue that a patient may become violent?
    a. Crossed legs
    b. Hands on hips
    c. Quiet dialogue
    d. Verbal abuse

16. Which is true regarding body armor?
    a. They protect the entire torso.
    b. An ice pick may pass through it.
    c. It stops high-velocity rifle bullets.
    d. Shot gun pellets easily penetrate it.

17. Which of the following does tactical paramedic training usually include?
    a. HAZMAT decontamination
    b. Advanced hazard assessment
    c. Radiographic interpretation
    d. Suturing and advanced wound care

18. Which of the following is an appropriate way to approach a crime scene?
    a. Document any suspicions you may have.
    b. Follow the same path to and from the victim.
    c. Move visible evidence so police can find it.
    d. Save patient items in a plastic bag.

WRAP IT UP

As you respond to a call for a suicidal patient, dispatch notifies you that this address is flagged because the occupant is heavily armed and has shown violent behavior in the past. The dispatcher notifies you that the police are en route. The 9-1-1 call was placed by the patient's girlfriend, who said that he was threatening to "blow his brains out." You stage a block away from the home, out of sight of the scene, until dispatch notifies you, "The scene is safe; you may proceed in." You enter the darkened house and find your patient, a very tall, muscular man in his sixties. He is a retired police officer and has many weapons, which are evident to you. You hear loud barking from behind a closed bedroom door. Police tell you that a German shepherd that had been trained as an attack dog was secured in that room. As you begin to question the patient, he somehow escapes the grip of the police and grabs a gun. You and your partner quickly flee the house and run behind the ambulance engine block, where you seek cover. A prolonged standoff with the police ensues until finally the tactical police squad throws a stun grenade into the home, subduing the patient, and the incident is over.

1. What is the rationale for staging a block away from this scene?

2. Aside from known information about previous violent episodes, what are some other situational clues that this may be a violent scene?

3. Put a ✓ beside the safety tactics that were used at this scene.

    a. _______ Avoidance

    b. _______ Cover and concealment

    c. _______ Distraction and evasive maneuvers

    d. _______ Tactical retreat

4. If you were to hide behind the ambulance box, which of the following would be true?
   a. It would provide cover.
   b. It would protect you from gunfire.
   c. It would provide protection from any potential danger.
   d. It would provide temporary concealment.

5. a. Is this a crime scene? Yes/No

   b. If you answered yes, what additional responsibilities do you have on the call?

____

____

CHAPTER 56 ANSWERS

REVIEW QUESTIONS

1. Scene size-up for danger should begin during response and be based on dispatch information, knowledge of the area, and physical assessment of the scene during the approach.
(Objective 1)

2. a. Past history of problems or violence
   b. Known drug or gang area
   c. Loud noises indicating violent activity
   d. Presence of alcohol or drug use
   e. Presence of dangerous pets
   f. Unusual silence or darkened residence
(Objective 2)

3. a. Avoid use of lights and sirens as you get close, use unconventional pathways to approach the house, avoid positioning yourself between the ambulance lights and the residence, listen for signs of danger before entry, and stand on the doorknob side of the entry door.
(Objective 2)

   b. One crew member should approach the car while the other remains in the ambulance, ambulance lights should be used to light the vehicle, the approach should be made from the passenger side, and the paramedic should not walk between the ambulance and the other vehicle. Observe for unusual activity in the rear seat and do not move forward from post C if a threat is suspected. If any warning signs of danger are noted, retreat until law enforcement secures the scene.

   (Objective 3)

4. a. Avoidance should be used. The EMS crew should stage their ambulance at a safe distance until law enforcement officers indicate that the scene is safe enough to proceed.
   b. Tactical retreat should be used, and cover should be sought. The paramedics should immediately retreat to a safe area of cover for protection against the projectiles and the possibility of further crowd violence.
   c. Cover and concealment should immediately be sought. Seek cover behind a solid object that will not allow penetration of a bullet. If possible conceal yourself from the perpetrator until the scene is safe or retreat can be done safely.
   d. Distraction and evasive maneuvers may be attempted during retreat. Try to move something between you and the patient to slow an attack as you quickly retreat.
   (Objective 6)

5. a. Fingerprints
   b. Footprints
   c. Blood or other body fluids
   d. Hair
   e. Carpet fibers
   f. Clothing fibers
   (Objective 8)

6. d. Locations of unsafe scenes may be known, as may the presence of crowds, intoxicated people on the scene, violence on the scene, or weapons.
(Objective 1)

7. a. Other indications of a potentially dangerous residence are a history of violence, known drug or gang area, loud noises, witnessing acts of violence, alcohol or drug use, and dangerous pets.
(Objective 2)

8. a. Lights should be left on, and only one crew member should approach, leaving the second crew member to call for help if needed.
(Objective 3)

9. c. Police may lose control of the scene, which would put you, your partner, and the patient in danger. Leave the scene as quickly as possible. Angry people may direct violence at uniformed paramedics.
(Objective 4)

10. b. Gang-related activity varies by region. Police and other social service agencies may provide you with information that can alert you to danger related to gang activities.
(Objective 5)

11. a. This process can produce hazardous gases, explosive forces, or fires as well as threats from violence.
(Objective 5)

12. d. Injuries that aren't consistent with the history or mechanism of injury should be viewed with suspicion. An inaccurate medical history may reflect poor patient knowledge. Excessive nervous talking may be related to many factors.
(Objective 5)

13. a. Avoidance requires alertness to detect and avoid dangerous situations.
(Objective 6)

14. c. The other choices provide concealment but can easily be penetrated by a bullet and therefore should not be used for cover.
(Objective 6)

15. d. The boxer stance and clenched fists are also signs of increasing aggression.
(Objective 6)

16. b. High-velocity rifle bullets or thin- or dual-edged weapons, such as ice picks, may penetrate body armor.
(Objective 7)

17. b. Other areas of training include hostage survival, care under fire, weapons and ballistics, medical threat assessment, forensic medicine, assessment under special situations, safe searches, dental injury management, medical issues related to drug lab raids, and rescue and extraction.
(Objective 7)

18. b. Document only objective findings; try not to disturb any evidence; save patient items in a paper bag.
(Objective 8)

1. If the patient is violent, he may come after the EMS crew, injuring or killing crew members or taking a hostage. (Objectives 1, 2)

2. The house is dark, the patient has numerous visible weapons, and a dangerous pet is on the premises. (Objective 2)

3. a (staging); b (behind ambulance); d (running from the house) (Objective 6)

4. d. It would temporarily hide you from the perpetrator, but it does not afford complete protection from gunfire. (Objective 6)

5. Yes. Objective observations should be carefully worded. Any significant statements from the patient should be recorded in quotes. (Objective 8)

 **Hazardous Materials Awareness**

READING ASSIGNMENT

Chapter 57, pages 1527-1548, in *Mosby's Paramedic Textbook,* ed. 4.

OBJECTIVES

Upon completion of this chapter, the paramedic student will be able to do the following:

1. Define hazardous materials terminology.
2. Identify legislation about hazardous materials that influences emergency health care workers.
3. Describe resources to assist in identification and management of hazardous materials incidents.
4. Identify the protective clothing and equipment needed to respond to selected hazardous materials incidents.
5. Describe the pathophysiology, signs, and symptoms of internal damage caused by exposure to selected hazardous materials.
6. Identify the pathophysiology, signs and symptoms, and prehospital management of selected hazardous materials that produce external damage.
7. Outline the prehospital response to a hazardous materials emergency.
8. Describe medical monitoring and rehabilitation of rescue workers who respond to a hazardous materials emergency.
9. Describe emergency decontamination and management of patients who have been contaminated by hazardous materials.
10. Outline the eight steps to decontaminate rescue personnel and equipment at a hazardous materials incident.

SUMMARY

- A hazardous material is any substance or material that is capable of posing an unreasonable risk to health, safety, and property.
- The Superfund Amendments and Reauthorization Act of 1986 established requirements for federal, state, and local governments and industry regarding emergency planning and the reporting of hazardous materials-related incidents. In 1989, the Occupational Safety and Health Administration and the Environmental Protection Agency published rules to govern training requirements, emergency plans, medical checkups, and other safety precautions for workers at uncontrolled hazardous waste sites and those responding to hazardous chemical spills. In addition, the National Fire Protection Association has published standards that address competencies for emergency medical services workers at hazmat scenes.
- There are two methods used to identify hazardous materials. One is informal product identification. (This includes visual, olfactory, and verbal clues.) The other is formal product identification. (This includes, for example, placards and shipping papers.) Resources for hazardous materials reference include the *North American Emergency Response Guidebook*, regional poison control centers, CHEMTREC, CHEMTEL, and CAMEO.
- It is crucial that anyone dealing with hazardous materials use proper protection. This includes using the proper respiratory devices. It also includes wearing protective clothing. This clothing is made of a variety of materials and is designed for certain chemical exposures. Thus, the manufacturer's guidelines must be followed.
- Hazardous materials may enter the body through inhalation, ingestion, injection, and absorption. Internal damage to the human body from hazardous materials exposure may involve the respiratory tract, central nervous system, or other internal organs. Chemicals producing internal damage include irritants, asphyxiants, nerve poisons, anesthetics, narcotics, hepatotoxins, cardiotoxins, nephrotoxins, neurotoxins, and carcinogens.
- Exposure to hazardous materials may result in burns. It also may result in severe tissue damage.
- The first agency to arrive at the scene of a hazardous materials incident must detect and identify the materials involved, assess the risk of exposure to rescue personnel and others, consider the potential risk of fire or explosion, gather information from onsite personnel or other sources, and confine and control the incident.
- A hazmat medical monitoring program may include medical examination for members of hazmat response teams, providing medical care, record keeping, and periodic evaluation of the surveillance program.

- The primary goals of decontamination are to reduce the patient's dosage of material, decrease the threat of secondary contamination, and reduce the risk of rescuer injury.
- Rescuers should follow strict protocols for proper decontamination of themselves, their clothing, and any contaminated equipment.

REVIEW QUESTIONS

Match the HAZMAT terms in column II with the appropriate definition in column I. Use each term only once.

Column I

1. _________ Weight of pure vapor compared with the weight of an equal volume of dry air

2. _________ Dose of chemical that will kill 50% of animals

3. _________ Exposure limit of 15 minutes

4. _________ Gas or vapor concentration that will burn or explode with ignition source

5. _________ Safe exposure for a 40-hour work week

6. _________ Minimum temperature to ignite gas without spark or flame

7. _________ Atmosphere that causes immediate harm

8. _________ Vapor's ability to mix with water

9. _________ Maximum concentration not to be exceeded even for a moment

10. _________ Temperature at which liquid produces enough vapor to ignite and flash over but not continue to burn without more heat

Column II

a. Flammable or exposure limits
b. Flash point
c. IDLH
d. Ignition temperature
e. LD50
f. PEL
g. TLV-C
h. TLV-STEL
i. Vapor density
j. Vapor pressure
k. Vapor solubility

Match each of the hazardous chemicals in column I with all the terms in column II that describe the chemical's associated health hazards. Answers may be used more than once.

Column I

11. _________ Arsenic

12. _________ Halogenated hydrocarbons

13. _________ Hydrochloric acid

14. _________ Hydrogen cyanide

15. _________ Lead

16. _________ Malathion

17. _________ Mercury

Column II

a. Asphyxiant
b. Anesthetic
c. Carcinogen
d. Cardiotoxin
e. Hemotoxin
f. Hepatotoxin
g. Irritant
h. Nephrotoxin
i. Nerve poison
j. Neurotoxin

18. Briefly describe each of the five categories of emergency response personnel who may respond to a hazardous materials situation:

   a. First responder—awareness:

____

____

b. First responder—operations:

____

____

c. Hazardous materials technician:

____

____

d. Hazardous materials specialist:

____

____

e. On-scene incident commander:

____

____

19. You arrive on the scene of a motor vehicle collision involving an overturned tanker truck. A cloud of white vapor is escaping from a relief valve on top of the truck. Describe the formal and informal means of identifying hazardous materials that may be involved in this situation.

a. Formal:

____

____

b. Informal:

____

20. After a hazardous material has been identified, what other resources can help the emergency response crew to determine the dangers and management of the scene?

____

21. Describe the protective clothing needed in the following hazardous materials response situations:

a. The hazardous materials crew provides emergency care to a seriously injured worker who is lying in an area contaminated with a liquid acidic chemical. No contaminated gas is present from the spill.

____

____

759

b. Your fire rescue team must enter a burning building to extricate trapped victims. No known hazardous materials are reported on the scene.

c. An equipment malfunction inside a chemical manufacturing plant has resulted in the release of toxic gases. Hazardous materials specialists must enter to attempt to locate a victim known to be just inside the hot zone.

22. Describe the health problems that can be encountered when an individual is exposed to the following agents:

a. Irritants:

b. Asphyxiants:

c. Nerve poisons, anesthetics, and narcotics:

d. Hepatotoxins:

e. Cardiotoxins:

f. Neurotoxins:

g. Hemotoxins:

h. Carcinogens:

23. You respond to the scene of a fire in which hazardous materials of unknown origin are involved. Describe signs and symptoms shown by scene workers that may cause you to suspect exposure to hazardous materials.

24. Your crew arrives at an industrial chemical manufacturing plant where a worker has sustained a splash exposure of a corrosive chemical to the eyes. Describe patient management in this situation.

760

25. Label Fig. 57-1 and briefly describe each of the three safety zones for a hazardous materials situation that have been established by hazardous materials specialists.

A. ____

B. ____

C. ____

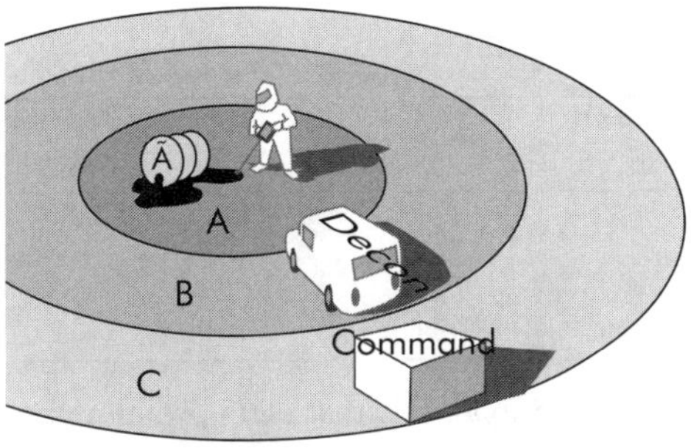

Figure 57-1

Questions 26 to 28 refer to the following case study:

You are the first team dispatched to the scene of a train derailment where three victims remain trapped. The bystanders who called in the incident report that several of the involved train cars have placards indicating the presence of hazardous materials.

26. What actions should you take during your initial response to this situation?

____

____

____

____

____

27. Describe special considerations in the prehospital management of contaminated patients.

____

____

____

____

28. The incident commander at this scene delegates your EMS crew to establish a medical monitoring station. Describe the responsibilities of this role.

____

____

____

29. What measures should rescuers follow as they leave the hot zone of a HAZMAT scene?

____

____

STUDENT SELF-ASSESSMENT

30. What term is used for substances and materials that can pose an unreasonable risk to health, safety, and property?
 a. External hazards
 b. Hazardous materials
 c. Immediately dangerous to life and health
 d. Internal hazards

31. What term describes the legislation, enacted in 1986, that established requirements for federal, state, and local governments and industry regarding emergency planning and the reporting of hazardous materials?
 a. Hazardous Materials Control Act
 b. Occupational Health and Safety Law
 c. Ryan White Law
 d. Superfund Amendments and Reauthorization Act

32. According to the HAZWOPER rules, the five categories of individuals who may respond to an emergency involving hazardous materials include
 a. CERT teams
 b. DOT officials
 c. Hazardous material specialist
 d. Rescue operation technician

33. Which of the following is a formal means of identifying hazardous products?
 a. Container characteristics
 b. Incident location
 c. Patient signs and symptoms
 d. United Nations labeling system

34. On what type of hazardous materials location will you find Material Safety Data Sheets?
 a. Airplane
 b. Train
 c. Tanker truck
 d. Hospital

35. Which is a general sign or symptom of inhalation exposure to a hazardous material?
 a. Hemiplegia
 b. Hematemesis
 c. Seizure
 d. Urticaria

36. External exposure to corrosive chemicals generally causes which of the following?
 a. Acidosis
 b. Burns
 c. Coughing
 d. Systemic effects

37. Which long-term sign or symptom would be most indicative of hazmat exposure to a hepatoxin?
 a. Confusion and lightheadedness
 b. Shortness of breath and coughing
 c. Tingling of the extremities
 d. Jaundice and vomiting

762

38. How should rescuers approach the scene of a hazardous materials incident?

    a. Downhill and downwind   **c.** Uphill and downwind

    b. Downhill and upwind   **d.** Uphill and upwind

39. Which of the following is included in the "pre-suit" medical monitoring of an individual who will be entering a hazardous materials situation?

    a. End-tidal CO_2 **c.** Blood glucose

    b. Reflexes   **d.** Weight

40. General recommendations for emergency management of contaminated patients include:

    a. Emergency patient care overrides all safety considerations.

    b. All patients in the cold zone are considered contaminated.

    c. Intravenous therapy should be initiated on patients in the hot zone.

    d. The patient's clothing should be completely cut off.

41. Which of the following is an appropriate step in the decontamination of a rescuer leaving a HAZMAT site?

    a. Shave all body hair.

    b. Shake clothing vigorously before reapplying.

    c. Take the HAZMAT suit to the ambulance to be used later.

    d. Shower and wash with soap.

WRAP IT UP

The crash seems minor; a car struck the rear of a delivery truck, causing it to topple over onto its side. All of the occupants of both vehicles are out and moving around, but as approach, you note tears streaming down their faces, and a man is standing next to the truck coughing vigorously. "Stop," you tell your driver, "let's park upwind aways." You pick up the microphone for the loud speaker. "Move away from the truck," you command, instructing the group to follow your ambulance to a higher location, several hundred feet away from the truck. You contact dispatch to ask for fire department and HAZMAT team response. You notice a faint ammonia smell that is becoming weaker as you move away from the scene, and you pull out your binoculars to get a better look at the scene. No placards are visible, and you do not see any liquid pools around either vehicle.

When the truck driver and the two occupants of the car get to the ambulance, they report a very strong smell of ammonia and severe burning of their eyes, noses, and throats, as well as difficulty breathing. They say that they didn't see anything spilled or any gas cloud. You immediately administer oxygen, and when you listen to their lungs, you hear diffuse wheezes. The patients are tachycardic and tachypneic but have normal blood pressure. You remove the patients' clothing outside the ambulance. You begin treatment with a bronchodilator and place a nasal cannula over their eyes to begin continuous irrigation with normal saline. You ask the truck driver about his cargo and request his shipping papers, but he is evasive; he gets up and tries to run from the scene, but the police tackle and subdue him, confiscating a handgun from his pocket. HAZMAT teams arrive, establish zones around the contaminated area, and find a variety of hazardous chemicals in the back of the truck, which turns out to be a mobile methamphetamine lab. Apparently, an ammonia tank ruptured in the collision, releasing the irritant gas and exposing your patients.

1. What methods of identification of the hazardous materials did the first rescuers attempt to use in this situation?

    a. Informal:

    b. Formal:

        Chapter **57** **Hazardous Materials Awareness**

2. What additional resources were contacted immediately to assist with the incident?

3. Put a ✓ beside the signs or symptoms of hazardous materials exposure that were observed in these patients.

a. _______ Confusion, dizziness		**g.** _______ Numbness	
b. _______ Chest tightness		**h.** _______ Loss of coordination	
c. _______ Double vision		**i.** _______ Nausea, vomiting	
d. _______ Changes in skin color		**j.** _______ Drooling, rhinorrhea	
e. _______ Coughing		**k.** _______ Tearing	
f. _______ Difficulty breathing		**l.** _______ Unconsciousness	

4. Why was gross water decontamination done even though the situation involved a gas exposure?

____

____

5. Could the ambulance crew be charged with abandonment for pulling past the scene of an emergency? Explain your answer.

____

____

6. Describe the zones that the HAZMAT team established around the scene.

____

____

CHAPTER 57 ANSWERS

REVIEW QUESTIONS

1. i

2. e

3. h

4. a

5. f

6. d

7. c

8. k

764

9. g

10. b
(Questions 1–10, Objective 1)

11. j, e

12. f, d

13. g

14. a

15. j, e

16. i

17. h, j, e
(Questions 11–17, Objective 5)

18.

Category	Description
a. First responder–awareness	May witness or discover hazardous materials release but job does not include emergency response duties pertaining to hazardous materials
b. First responder–operations	Responds to hazardous materials release to protect nearby people, property, or the environment without trying to stop the release
c. Hazardous material technician	Responds to hazardous materials situations to stop the release
d. Hazardous materials specialist	Has direct or specific knowledge of various hazardous substances and provides support to hazardous materials technicians
e. On-scene incident commander	Trained to assume control of a hazardous materials event

(Objective 2)

19. a. Placards on trucks, shipping papers, and Material Safety Data Sheets
b. Visual indicators (vapor), container characteristics, company name on truck, and smell
(Objective 3)

20. Hazardous materials texts, poison control centers, CHEMTREC, federal agencies, commercial agencies, subject experts, site coordinators, and regional, state, and local agencies
(Objective 3)

21. a. Chemical splash protective clothing to protect the skin and eyes from direct chemical contact
b. Structural firefighting clothing, including helmet, positive-pressure self-contained breathing apparatus, turnout coat and pants, gloves and boots, and a protective hood of fire-resistant material
c. Vapor-protective clothing (suit with a self-contained breathing apparatus worn inside or outside the suit or a supplied-air breathing apparatus with emergency escape capabilities)
(Objective 4)

22. a. Irritants damage the upper and lower respiratory tracts and irritate the eyes.

b. Asphyxiants deprive the body tissues of oxygen.

c. Nerve gases, anesthetics, and narcotics act on the nervous system, causing disruption of cardiorespiratory function.

d. Hepatotoxins destroy the liver's ability to function in a normal capacity.

e. Cardiotoxins may induce myocardial ischemia and cardiac dysrhythmias.

f. Neurotoxins may cause cerebral hypoxia or neurologic or behavioral disruption.

g. Hemotoxins cause destruction of red blood cells, resulting in hemolytic anemia.

h. Carcinogens are cancer-causing agents.

(Objective 5)

23. Confusion, anxiety, dizziness, visual disturbances, changes in skin color, shortness of breath or burning of the upper airway, tingling or numbness of extremities, loss of coordination, seizures, nausea and vomiting, abdominal cramps, diarrhea, and unconsciousness

(Objective 5)

24. Don protective gear; remove contact lenses; and flush with copious amounts of water, normal saline, or lactated Ringer solution.

(Objective 6)

25. A. The hot zone is the area that includes the hazardous material and any associated wastes. Only specially trained and clothed personnel may enter this area.

B. The warm zone is the area that can become contaminated if the hot zone is unstable. Decontamination and patient care activities take place here.

C. The cold zone is the area around the warm zone. Minimal protective clothing is required. The command post and other support agencies are located here.

(Objective 7)

26. En route to the emergency scene, the EMS crew should attempt to identify the hazardous material and obtain preliminary information about the potential hazards and recommended safety equipment, initial first aid, and a safe distance factor for response to the area. Medical control should be notified so that appropriate measures can be taken at the hospital for potential victims. If the involved substance is identified, the dispatching agency should contact the appropriate authorities and other experts (e.g., CHEMTREC) to get additional information and support. The scene should be approached from uphill and upwind, and the EMS crew should call for additional help as needed. The arriving crew should be alert to any fire hazards and leakage of gas or liquid from the involved cars and remain clear of all vapors and spills.

(Objective 7)

27. Nonambulatory patients should be removed from the hot zone by trained personnel who have adequate protective clothing. All patients in the hot zone should be considered contaminated. Patient care in the hot zone should consist only of airway and breathing management, spinal immobilization, and control of hemorrhage. Intravenous lines should be avoided unless absolutely necessary to prevent internal introduction of contaminants. Decontamination should be attempted only with adequate protection of the rescue workers; often, removal of the victim's clothing removes most of the contaminant, with the remainder being washed with copious amounts of water and mild detergent soap. All contaminated clothing from the patient and rescuers should be left in the decontamination area. Further patient care should be provided in the support area before transport. The patient should be wrapped tightly in blankets.

(Objective 9)

28. Pre-suit examination: Assess baseline vital signs and instruct rescuers about possible symptoms to anticipate if contamination or exposure occurs. Postentry examination: Assess vital signs and monitor rescuer for signs or symptoms of exposure or heat-related illness.

(Objective 8)

29. Outer gloves and boots should be removed and placed in a receptacle. Remove contaminated breathing apparatus. Remove protective clothing and assess the need to remove outer clothing (based on type of chemical). Shower and wash twice. Put on clean clothing. Obtain medical evaluation.

(Objective 8)

766

30. b. Whereas external hazards are materials that produce external damage, internal hazards cause internal damage. Not all HAZMAT substances are IDLH.
(Objective 1)

31. d. The Ryan White law pertains to exposure to infectious diseases.
(Objective 2)

32. c. The categories are first responder–awareness, first responder–operations, hazardous materials technician, hazardous materials specialist, and on-scene incident commander.
(Objective 2)

33. d. All other responses are informal means of recognizing and identifying hazardous materials.
(Objective 3)

34. d. Information regarding hazardous materials in the workplace is found in MSDS.
(Objective 3)

35. c. The others would not usually be associated with this type of exposure.
(Objective 5)

36. b. The other signs described are systemic effects, which are not the most common findings in external exposure to corrosive chemicals.
(Objective 6)

37. d. A high index of suspicion for rescuer exposure should always be maintained.
(Objective 5)

38. d. This ensures that hazardous gases and liquids are moving away from the ambulance.
(Objective 7)

39. d. In addition, a full set of vital signs, including temperature, should be assessed.
(Objective 8)

40. d. Safety overrides all considerations.
(Objective 10)

41. d. Shaving may permit internal entry of chemicals. Clothing should be left at the exit point and appropriately cleaned or discarded.
(Objective 9)

WRAP IT UP

1. a. Observation of the patient's signs and symptoms; smell
b. Checking for placards, shipping papers
(Objective 3)

2. Fire department, HAZMAT team
(Objective 7)

3. e, f, k
(Objectives 5, 6)

4. To remove any chemical irritant present on the skin or clothes and to prevent subsequent off-gassing of chemicals
(Objective 9)

5. The first priority in an incident, especially a HAZMAT incident, is scene safety. Pulling onto the scene would have been dangerous, so no abandonment claim could be made.
(Objective 7)

6. Hot (contamination) zone: Area where actual contaminant is located; only personnel in appropriate PPE are allowed entry.
Warm (control) zone: Surrounds hot zone and is the location of decontamination
Cold (safe) zone: Normal operations
(Objective 7)

58 Bioterrorism and Weapons of Mass Destruction

READING ASSIGNMENT

Chapter 58, pages 1549-1566, in *Mosby's Paramedic Textbook,* ed. 4.

OBJECTIVES

Upon completion of this chapter, the paramedic student will be able to do the following:

1. List five types of weapons of mass destruction (WMD).
2. Identify actions, signs and symptoms, methods of distribution, and management of biologic WMD.
3. Identify actions, signs and symptoms, methods of distribution, and management of chemical WMD.
4. Identify actions, signs and symptoms, methods of distribution, and management of nuclear WMD.
5. Identify measures to be taken by paramedics who respond to incidents with suspected WMD involvement.

SUMMARY

- The five categories of weapons of mass destruction (WMD) are biologic, nuclear, incendiary, chemical, and explosive.
- Biologic agents include anthrax, botulism, plague, ricin, tularemia, and smallpox.
- Person-to-person spread is possible in patients who are infected with plague or smallpox.
- Nerve agents include Sarin, Soman, Tabun, and VX. Exposure causes a cholinergic overdrive. The antidote for nerve agent exposure is atropine and pralidoxime chloride.
- Poisonous gases such as chlorine and phosgene cause severe respiratory problems. They also can cause skin and eye injury. Move exposed patients to safety, remove their clothing, and treat their symptoms.
- Dirty bombs could cause heat damage and radiation sickness, severe burns, and cancer.
- Emergency responders at a WMD incident should recognize hazmat incidents, know protocols to detect WMD, use personal protective equipment, know crime-scene procedures, know how to activate more resources, and implement incident operations.

REVIEW QUESTIONS

Match the terms in column II with the description in column I. A term may be used more than once.

Column I	Column II
1. ________ Illness caused by bacteria found in rodents	**a.** Anthrax
2. ________ Nerve agent that has a camphorlike odor	**b.** Chlorine
3. ________ Thick, odorless liquid used as a nerve agent	**c.** Phosgene
4. ________ Gray, poisonous gas that smells like mown hay	**d.** Plague
5. ________ Odorless nerve agent	**e.** Ricin
6. ________ Bacterial disease spread by rodent fleas	**f.** Sarin
7. ________ Poisonous cytotoxin from a plant	**g.** Soman
8. ________ Nerve agent that has a fruity odor	**h.** Tabun
	i. Tularemia
	j. VX

9. Supply the words that form the following acronym for weapons of mass destruction.

B ____

N ____

I ____

C ____

E ____

Match the categories in column II with the characteristics of biological agents in column I. Each category may be used more than once.

Column I

10. _______ Emerging pathogen

11. _______ Q fever

12. _______ Second highest priority agents

13. _______ Nipah virus

14. _______ National security risk

15. _______ Anthrax

Column II

a. Category A
b. Category B
c. Category C

16. Provide the missing information for each of the following biological weapons of mass destruction.

Agent	Signs and Symptoms	Outcomes	Treatment
a. Anthrax			
b.	Fever, fainting, shortness of breath, cough, bloody sputum, GI symptoms		
c.		35% mortality from septicemia	
d. Botulism			
e.			Antibiotics, supportive treatment; vaccine under study
f. Ricin			
g.		DIC, respiratory failure, death (5%)	

17. You are called to investigate multiple reports of difficulty breathing at the airport. When you arrive, approximately 30 people rush toward the ambulance with tears streaming down their faces. They report a sudden onset of difficulty breathing, blurred vision, headache, and weakness. Most were in the baggage pickup area when their symptoms began. You note that they are sweating profusely, some are faint, and they have fasciculations.

a. List four agents that can cause this clinical presentation.

____

b. What precautions should you take before transport of these patients?

____

____

____

c. List three drugs that may be indicated in the management of these patients.

____

____

____

18. Your patients were working at an immigration center when they smelled an odor they described as "like fresh cut hay." They then developed severe dyspnea, a burning sensation in the chest, and a nonproductive cough.

a. What WMD agent do you suspect?

____

b. What interventions would you perform?

____

____

____

19. List three factors that would affect the degree of contamination from a dirty bomb.

a. ____

b. ____

c. ____

20. Describe three special considerations for a paramedic responding to a WMD incident.

a. ____

b. ____

c. ____

21. People in your community are becoming very ill with rashes and severe respiratory symptoms. Many have died, and new cases are spreading among people who appear to have had contact with the first group. What WMD infectious agent may be involved?

a. Anthrax   **c.** Smallpox
b. Plague   **d.** Tularemia

22. According to the CDC categorization of biologic agents, which category includes agents that cause moderate morbidity and low mortality and includes Q fever?

a. Category A   **c.** Category C
b. Category B   **d.** Category D

23. Which WMD exposure route has the potential for the greatest number of casualties?

a. Aerosol   **c.** Liquid ingestion
b. Direct contact   **d.** Solid ingestion

24. Which of the following is true about anthrax infection?

a. All those who come in contact with the infected patient should be quarantined.
b. It can cause severe respiratory distress and sepsis in later stages.
c. Treatment with antibiotics is not indicated and is ineffective.
d. Vaccination is routinely recommended for health care workers.

25. A large number of patients who ate at the salad bar of a local restaurant are complaining of nausea, blurred vision, and dry mouth. Several have difficulty swallowing and complain that they are having trouble breathing. Which of the following may be associated with this presentation?

a. Botulism   **c.** Soman
b. Ricin   **d.** Tularemia

26. Which of the following WMD agents can be spread from person to person?

a. Botulism   **c.** Ricin
b. Plague   **d.** Tularemia

27. You are caring for a patient suspected to have smallpox. What personal protective measure is indicated?

a. Have hazmat perform a full decontamination before care
b. None unless you are performing invasive procedures
c. Respiratory and contact protection
d. Normal universal precautions

28. A large number of patients at a court house have excessive tearing, salivation, severe dyspnea with wheezing, weakness, drooling, and hypotension. After HAZMAT teams have decontaminated the patients and while oxygen is administered, which treatments should you give next to improve their condition?

a. Albuterol, fluid bolus   **c.** Atropine, fluid bolus
b. Albuterol, atropine   **d.** Atropine, pralidoxime chloride

29. A tanker transporting chlorine has collided with a van carrying six occupants. A slow gas leak is streaming from the side of the truck. All of those involved in the accident are ambulatory but complaining of severe burning of the eyes, coughing, and difficulty breathing. You have staged away from the incident. After calling for appropriate additional resources, what should your immediate priorities be for these patients?

a. Administer oxygen and an antidote.
b. Have them remain in place until the HAZMAT team arrives.
c. Instruct them to move upwind to higher ground.
d. Take oxygen and albuterol to the patients to begin care.

30. According to the Office for Domestic Preparedness, what are the responsibilities of EMS providers in preparing for and responding to incidents of terrorism involving WMD agents?
   a. Contain hazardous materials.
   b. Detect and identify agents used as WMDs.
   c. Implement incident operations.
   d. Protect the crime scene perimeter.

WRAP IT UP

As you pull up on the scene, you see more than 100 people streaming from a church where your dispatcher tells you there have been multiple calls for difficulty breathing. People noticed a faint "fruity" odor when the minister lit the incense oil pots, and watering eyes, drooling, sweating, and coughing quickly developed. You call for an MCI response and a HAZMAT team. Several people have fallen to the ground, and you note a child having a grand mal seizure on the grass. Other people are running from the scene to their cars. The incident commander and HAZMAT team arrive, and a decision is quickly made that a vaporized nerve agent has been used. Therefore, the patients' clothing is removed and gross decontamination performed before treatment and transport to eliminate any possibility of off-gassing. You and your partner are in charge of the triage division and direct next-arriving crews to initiate START triage. The supply branch is in charge of locating and procuring MARK-I kits deployed in the city and having them sent to the treatment division. After disrobing and undergoing gross decontamination, patients are moved to the treatment division, where antidote administration and supportive care begin until appropriate transport can be arranged. It is 2 hours before the 97th patient is transported to the hospital, leaving only seven who were tagged unsalvageable to be transported to the county medical examiner's office and the police and HAZMAT teams to finish up their work.

1. Which nerve agent has the characteristics described in this scenario?

____

2. Put a ✓ beside the signs or symptoms that a patient exposed to a nerve agent may experience (even if not described in the above scenario).

a. ______ Blurred vision		**h.** ______ Hypotension
b. ______ Bradycardia		**i.** ______ Renal failure
c. ______ Cardiac arrest		**j.** ______ Seizures
d. ______ Drooling		**k.** ______ Sweating
e. ______ Dry skin		**l.** ______ Watery eyes
f. ______ Headache		**m.** ______ Wheezing
g. ______ Hypertension		**n.** ______ Loss of consciousness

3. What drugs does the MARK-I kit contain?

4. What additional interventions are needed for patients poisoned by a nerve agent?

773

REVIEW QUESTIONS

1. d, i
   (Objective 2)

2. b
   (Objective 3)

3. j
   (Objective 3)

4. c
   (Objective 3)

5. f
   (Objective 3)

6. d
   (Objective 2)

7. e
   (Objective 2)

8. h
   (Objective 3)

9. B—biological; N—nuclear; I—incendiary; C—chemical; E—explosives
   (Objective 1)

10. c

11. b

12. b

13. c

14. a

15. a
    (Questions 10–15, Objective 2)

16.

Agent	Signs and Symptoms	Outcomes	Treatment
a. Anthrax	Itching, papular lesion that becomes vesicular, black eschar; signs and symptoms resembling those of a cold followed by respiratory distress and sepsis	High mortality rate if untreated	Antibiotics, vaccines (controversial)
b. Plague (*Yersinia pestis*)	Fever, fainting, shortness of breath, cough, bloody sputum, GI symptoms	Septic shock; high mortality rate	Antibiotics, postexposure drug therapy, isolation
c. Smallpox (variola virus)	High fever, fatigue, headache and backache; within 2 to 3 days, rash and skin lesions that crust and scar; joint deformities, blindness	35% mortality rate from septicemia	Vaccine, antivirals (experimental), supportive care isolation
d. Botulism	Nausea, dry mouth, blurred vision, dysphagia, fatigue, dyspnea	Recovery may occur with weeks supportive care	Antitoxin, mechanical ventilation
e. Tularemia	Fever, HA, chills, malaise, GI illness, DIC, ARF; death possible	Severe incapacitation; low death rate	Antibiotics, supportive treatment; vaccine under study
f. Ricin	Severe respiratory symptoms within 8 hours; respiratory failure in 36 to 72 hours; severe GI symptoms; vascular collapse; seizures	Respiratory failure, shock, death	No antidote; only supportive care possible; avoid exposure, eliminate toxin, and decontaminate
g. Tularemia	Fever, chills, general malaise, GI illness	DIC, respiratory failure, death (5%)	Antibiotics, supportive care; vaccine under review

(Objective 2)

17. a. Sarin, soman, tabun, VX
   b. Secondary exposure is possible from off-gassing of clothes; clothing should be removed before transport.
   c. Atropine, pralidoxime chloride, and diazepam or lorazepam are indicated for the management of nerve agent poisoning.
   (Objective 3)

18. a. Phosgene gas; **b.** decontamination if needed, supportive care with oxygen and management of symptoms
   (Objective 3)

19. The size of the explosive, the amount and type of radioactive material used, and the weather (Objective 4)

20. Danger to EMS crews from secondary devices or armed resistance; crowd control and public panic situations; the need to preserve the crime scene
   (Objective 6)

STUDENT SELF-ASSESSMENT

21. c. Smallpox is spread easily from person to person, causes a progressive rash, and has a high mortality rate in unvaccinated individuals.
   (Objective 2)

22. b. Category A agents (which include anthrax) have high morbidity and mortality rates; category C agents (which include Nipah virus) are emerging pathogens. There is no category D.
   (Objective 2)

     Chapter **58** **Bioterrorism and Weapons of Mass Destruction**

23. a. Aerosolized agents can be distributed easily over a wide area, exposing large numbers of victims in a short time.
(Objective 2)

24. b. Person-to-person contact does not transmit the infection. Antibiotics should be given as soon as possible to minimize the risk of death. Vaccination is recommended only for military personnel and for researchers who work with anthrax.
(Objective 2)

25. a. Ricin produces pulmonary symptoms, soman is a nerve agent, and tularemia does not typically cause blurred vision or dysphagia.
(Objective 2)

26. b. Botulism and tularemia are not known to spread from person to person. Ricin is not an infectious agent.
(Objective 2)

27. c. Smallpox can be spread by inhalation or by contact with clothing or lesions.
(Objective 3)

28. d. Atropine and pralidoxime chloride (PAM) are direct antidotes to nerve agents and should be given immediately to reverse the effect of the nerve poisons.
(Objective 3)

29. Any attempt to move to the contaminated area without appropriate PPE would be dangerous. Supportive care can begin after patients are in a safe area and their clothing has been removed.
(Objective 3)

30. c. HAZMAT teams are typically responsible for containing the hazardous material and identifying specific agents using special monitoring devices. Police should control the perimeter of the crime scene.
(Objective 4)

WRAP IT UP

1. Tabun; it has a fruity odor, vaporizes when heated, causes symptoms within seconds of exposure to the vapor, and produces the signs and symptoms described.
(Objective 3)

2. a, b, c, d, f, h, i, j, k, l, m
(Objective 3)

3. Atropine and pralidoxime chloride
(Objective 3)

4. IV fluids, oxygen, and diazepam or lorazepam for seizures
(Objective 3)

59 Putting It All Together: Assessment-Based Management

READING ASSIGNMENT

Chapter 59, pages 1567-1573, in *Mosby's Paramedic Textbook,* ed. 4.

OBJECTIVES

Upon completion of this chapter, the paramedic student will be able to do the following:

1. Discuss how assessment-based management contributes to effective patient and scene assessment.
2. Describe factors that affect assessment and decision making in the prehospital setting.
3. Outline effective techniques for scene and patient assessment and choreography.
4. Identify essential take-in equipment for general and selected patient situations.
5. Outline strategies for patient approach that promote an effective patient encounter.
6. Describe techniques to permit efficient and accurate presentation of the patient.

SUMMARY

- Assessment-based management "puts it all together." This means that the paramedic gathers, evaluates, and synthesizes information. The paramedic makes proper decisions based on the information. Then the paramedic takes the appropriate actions required for the patient's care.
- Factors that can affect the quality of assessment and decision making include the paramedic's attitude, the patient's willingness to cooperate, distracting injuries, labeling and tunnel vision, the environment, patient compliance, and considerations of personnel availability.
- Promoting a coherent assessment is the goal. Thus members of the response team should have a preplan for determining roles and responsibilities.
- The paramedic crew should always be prepared for the worst event. They should carry essential equipment to manage every aspect of patient care.
- A calm and orderly manner is essential for the paramedic. This is especially the case when approaching a patient. During the initial assessment, the paramedic must look actively for problems that pose a threat to life.
- Presenting the patient in the course of prehospital and hospital care is twofold. *Presentation* refers to the skills of effective communication. *Presentation* also refers to the effective transfer of patient information.

REVIEW QUESTIONS

For questions 1 to 5, what is your field impression based on the patterns described in each of the following scenarios (knowing that further assessment is necessary to confirm each)? Describe the key differences in each pair that distinguish the patterns.

1. **a.** A 24-year-old patient with a history of diabetes is found confused and diaphoretic with weakness on the right side.

b. An 80-year-old patient with a history of hypertension is found confused and diaphoretic with weakness on the right side.

c. Key differences in patterns:

2. a. A 20-year-old woman whose last menstrual period was 8 weeks ago has severe right lower quadrant abdominal pain and signs of shock.

____

b. A 12-year-old boy has severe right lower quadrant abdominal pain, fever, and vomiting.

____

c. Key differences in patterns:

____

3. a. A 38-year-old man has severe left lower back pain that radiates down into his testicle, and he has hematuria.

____

b. A 70-year-old man had a sudden onset of lower back pain described as "ripping." He is pale, wants to have a bowel movement, and has a cool left foot.

____

c. Key differences in patterns:

____

4. a. A healthy 4-month-old infant is found pulseless, with rigor mortis, and in bed with no obvious signs of trauma.

____

b. A healthy 16-year-old patient is found pulseless, with rigor mortis, and in bed with no obvious signs of trauma.

____

c. Key differences in patterns:

____

5. a. A 70-year-old man complains of crushing substernal chest pain. He is diaphoretic and having multifocal premature ventricular contractions. His history includes hypertension, smoking, and diabetes.

____

b. A 25-year-old woman complains of crushing substernal chest pain. She is diaphoretic and having multifocal premature ventricular contractions. Her chest struck the steering wheel in a motor vehicle crash 10 minutes ago.

____

c. Key differences in patterns:

____

778

Questions 6 and 7 refer to the following case study:

Your patient is an alcoholic who calls often for minor problems. She curses at you for taking so long to respond and then says she fell out of bed yesterday, hit her head, and now has a headache. You note a large bruise on the temporal area of her head but no other injuries. Her speech is slurred, and she has a staggering gait. Her vital signs are BP 160/100 mm Hg, P, 64/min, and R 16/min. You advise her that she will be okay, and she declines transport. The next day, she is found unconscious and is diagnosed with a large subdural hematoma that resulted in her death.

6. List factors that may have contributed to your decision in this case.

____

____

7. Why is this patient at increased risk for intracerebral bleeding?

____

Questions 8 to 12 refer to the following case study:

You are dispatched for a stabbing. A 17-year-old boy was stabbed at a street party. It is dark, and the police are trying to control a large, loud, belligerent crowd that has gathered at the scene. Your patient says he cannot breathe, and when you pull his shirt off, you note a stab wound above the right nipple. Breath sounds are equal. You apply an occlusive dressing, and you elect to move the patient to the ambulance for further assessment and care.

8. During the initial contact with this patient, what are the responsibilities for each of the following team members?

    a. Team leader:

____

    b. Patient care person (as described in this textbook):

____

____

9. Should you carry your drug box with you on a call like this? Why?

____

10. Explain why the contemplative or the resuscitative approach would be appropriate for this call.

____

____

When you get in the ambulance, you talk to the patient, assess his airway and breathing, and apply oxygen. Your partner begins transport. As you begin to initiate an IV, you note blood dripping off the side of the ambulance cot. You cut the patient's clothing off and find a wound in the groin spurting blood.

11. List two factors that you think delayed detection of the patient's bleeding.

    a. ____

    b. ____

12. What pertinent positives should be included in your patient care report?

____

779

        Chapter **59** **Putting It All Together: Assessment-Based Management**

13. Which term describes the process of gathering, evaluating, and synthesizing information; making appropriate decisions based on available information; and taking the appropriate actions required for patient care?
  a. Assessment-based management
  b. Primary assessment
  c. Patient reassessment
  d. Patient-focused care

14. What should your field impression be based on?
  a. Information gathered before any physical examination
  b. Advice of medical direction and perception of the call
  c. The paramedic's "gut instinct" and pattern recognition
  d. The patient's chief complaint and assessment of the problem

15. What should you rule out if you encounter an uncooperative patient?
  a. Chest pain or dyspnea
  b. Hypoxia or hypoglycemia
  c. Neuromuscular disorder
  d. Personality disorder

16. Why is it important to predesignate roles for emergency medical services calls?
  a. To identify who is at fault if a problem occurs on a call
  b. To allow all paramedics to perform the skills at which they excel
  c. To ensure appropriate skills acquisition
  d. To promote coherent, efficient patient care delivery

17. What is the advantage of taking notes while obtaining the patient history?
  a. To obtain adequate billing information
  b. To provide evidence that may be used in court
  c. To prevent the need for repetitive questioning of the patient
  d. To reassure the patient that you are listening

18. In which situation would the contemplative approach to patient care be appropriate?
  a. A large bleeding laceration
  b. Cramping abdominal pain
  c. Decreased level of consciousness
  d. Dyspnea and diaphoresis

19. A 24-year-old woman is hyperventilating. What is the last condition to rule out when performing your history and physical exam?
  a. Anxiety attack
  b. Asthma
  c. Diabetic ketoacidosis
  d. Pulmonary embolus

20. A patient is seriously injured after a fall. What is a serious consequence of inadequately presenting your patient during your report to the hospital?
  a. Appropriate resources may not be ready.
  b. The nursing staff will be angry with you.
  c. The patient may misunderstand you.
  d. You may have an increased time out of service.

21. Which of the following is a characteristic of an effective patient presentation?
  a. Every assessment finding is described.
  b. It should last no longer than 5 minutes.
  c. It should include the name of the patient and the doctor.
  d. It should follow a standard format and be concise.

Your partner groans as you pull up to the three-story apartment building where you are responding for a "person passed out." You know the address, you know the patient, and you know that this is probably no emergency because you have been here many times for minor complaints of headache, constipation, and blood pressure checks. "What should we bring?" he asks wearily. "Let's bring it all," you say, grabbing the monitor, airway bag, and jump kit even though you realize it is probably just an exercise in weight lifting. You enter the apartment, and your patient, a 70-year-old man, is lying on the sofa. When you ask what is going on, he tells you he must have pulled something in his back, it has been bothering him all day, and then he "fell out" and when he woke up, he called 911. "Tell me about your pain," you inquire, as vital signs are taken and his medicines (labetalol, hydrochlorothiazide, potassium, aspirin) are recorded. "Well, it's in my back, and it's real bad, kind of like I tore something in there, and it goes down in my leg," he says, grimacing suddenly as he relates his story. You notice his skin is cool; his lips and nailbeds are pale; and when you grab his wrist, his heart rate, while not rapid, is weak. His vital signs are BP 104/64 mm Hg, P 68/min, R 20/min, and SaO_2 93%. "That pressure's a bit low for you," your partner tells the patient as he opens a nasal cannula and places it on his face. On the physical exam, you note a tender pulsatile mass above his umbilicus to the right of the midline. Femoral pulses are weak, and you cannot feel any pulses in his cool, pale feet. You establish a line and send your partner and the police officer to retrieve the stretcher from the ambulance. Your patient is monitored, packaged, and transported to the hospital after you call report. Based on your notification, the ED resuscitation room is set up, and the patient is quickly diagnosed with abdominal aortic aneurysm. He is in surgery by the time you complete your report and is hospitalized for several weeks because of renal complications.

1. What findings fit the "pattern" of abdominal aortic aneurysm in this case study?

   ____

2. How would your impression of the situation have changed if the following were true?
   a. The patient was 17 years old, had no medical history (no daily medications), and was unknown to the paramedics
   b. The patient did not have a pulsating mass
   c. You found a heart rhythm disturbance before you palpated his abdomen

3. **a.** Which vital sign assessment did not fit the "pattern?"

   b. What could explain this altered vital sign?

4. Which factor had the potential to have a negative impact on your assessment of this patient?

   a. Distracting environment
   b. Labeling and tunnel vision
   c. Personnel considerations
   d. Uncooperative patient

5. Place a check mark beside the team leader responsibilities that you observed on this call.

   a. __________ Accompanies patient to hospital   e. __________ Presents the patient

   b. __________ Establishes dialogue with patient   f. __________ Completes documentation

   c. __________ Obtains history   g. __________ Team leadership

   d. __________ Performs physical exam

   Chapter **59**   **Putting It All Together: Assessment-Based Management**

CHAPTER 59 ANSWERS

REVIEW QUESTIONS

1. a. Hypoglycemia (further assessment to rule out stroke would also be needed)
   b. Stroke
   c. Age (stroke is more common in elderly adults) and history (the patient in a. had a history of diabetes, and the patient in b. had a history of hypertension)
   (Objective 1)

2. a. Ectopic pregnancy
   b. Appendicitis
   c. Sex (the boy in b. would not have gynecologic complaints), age (appendicitis is common in this age group), and clinical signs (shock in ectopic pregnancy versus fever in appendicitis)
   (Objective 1)

3. a. Nephrolithiasis (kidney stone)
   b. Abdominal aortic aneurysm
   c. Age (aneurysms are more common in men 60 to 70 years of age), clinical signs or symptoms (hematuria is common in kidney stones; urge to defecate, cool extremities, and signs of shock are consistent with aneurysms)
   (Objective 1)

4. a. Sudden infant death syndrome or child abuse
   b. Drug or alcohol toxicity or suicide
   c. Age (sudden infant death syndrome and abuse are more common in infants; suicide and drug abuse and overdose are more common in teens)
   (Objective 1)

5. a. Myocardial infarction
   b. Myocardial contusion
   c. Age (myocardial infarction is more common in older patients; history of a. is consistent with risk factors of myocardial infarction; mechanism of injury in b. is consistent with myocardial injury)
   (Objective 1)

6. Your attitude, the patient's willingness to cooperate, and labeling or tunnel vision (the expectation that her signs and symptoms were related to alcohol intoxication) may have contributed to your decision.
   (Objective 2)

7. Chronic alcoholism can impair the clotting mechanisms, putting the patient at risk for bleeding. Poor coordination caused by intoxication increases the risk of injury (falls) in patients with alcoholism.
   (Objective 2)

8. a. The team leader establishes contact and begins dialogue with the patient, obtains the history, and performs the physical examination.
   b. The patient care person provides scene cover (watches the crowd), gathers scene information (size and type of weapon), obtains vital signs, and performs skills.
   (Objective 3)

9. When moving into a volatile situation such as this one, you should take the minimum amount of equipment; the drug box would not be indicated based on the dispatch information. (This may vary by agency based on the size and contents of the drug box.)
   (Objective 4)

10. The resuscitative approach is necessary because a life threat exists.
    (Objective 5)

11. a. The presence of distracting injuries (the chest wound)
   b. The environment (dangerous and dark)
   (Objective 2)

12. The patient is conscious, and breath sounds are present and equal bilaterally.
   (Objective 6)

13. a. Initial assessment and ongoing assessment are components of assessment-based management.
   (Objective 1)

14. c. The field impression is based on a careful history, physical examination, and then analysis and evaluation based
   on the paramedic's knowledge and past experiences.
   (Objective 2)

15. b. Alcohol or drug intoxication, hypovolemia, and head injury or concussion are other physiological problems that
   may cause a patient to be uncooperative.
   (Objective 3)

16. d. This becomes especially important when multiple units respond to a scene.
   (Objective 4)

17. c. Taking notes keeps you from forgetting critical information that will be necessary when you complete your
   patient care report later.
   (Objective 5)

18. b. The contemplative approach is appropriate only when immediate intervention to manage a life threat is not
   needed.
   (Objective 5)

19. a. All of the other conditions represent life-threatening problems associated with hyperventilation; therefore, your
   examination should be tailored to rule out those problems first.
   (Objective 5)

20. a. An inadequate or inaccurate report can result in delayed patient care related to room or resource (medical staff,
   equipment) unavailability.
   (Objective 6)

21. d. Ideally, the report should be concise, follow a standard format, and include pertinent positives and negatives.
   The patient's name should not be included if radio communication is used.
   (Objective 6)

WRAP IT UP

1. Patient age, history of hypertension (from medications), description and location of pain, pulsatile mass, location
   of mass, diminished pulses in extremities, hypotension, syncopal episode
   (Objective 1)

2. a. An aneurysm would be unlikely (but not impossible) in someone that age and with no previous history. The
   patient would still need similar interventions and urgent transport because of the physical findings (cool skin,
   weak pulse, low SaO_2 for age).
   b. The treatment and impression should not change. A pulsatile mass is not always palpable.
   c. The history and description of the pain should still lead you to suspect aneurysm.
   (Objective 2)

     Chapter **59**   **Putting It All Together: Assessment-Based Management**

3. a. Tachycardia would have been expected.
   b. Patient was taking a beta-blocker, which will not permit the heart to speed up effectively to compensate for shock.
   (Objective 2)

4. b. Having been to many "false alarms," it would be possible to discount the patient's complaints and, if a comprehensive exam was not done, to miss this critical condition.
   (Objective 2)

5. a, b, c, d, e, f, g
   (Objective 3)

Emergency Drug Index

1. List the actions, indications, and side effects of steroids.

____

____

2. For each of the following two drugs, list the time of onset, duration, and dose:
  a. Methylprednisolone:

____

  b. Dexamethasone:

____

Fill in the blank for each of the scenarios in questions 3 to 28 and complete the corresponding flashcard (after the electrocardiogram flashcards at the end of this workbook) with the appropriate drug information, including trade name, class, description, indications, contraindications, adverse reactions, onset, duration, dose (adult and pediatric, if appropriate), and special considerations. Verify your drug choice before completing the flashcard by looking at the generic drug name on the back.

3. Your patient has urticaria and severe itching resulting from an allergic reaction. His vital signs are stable, and no wheezes are audible on auscultation of his lungs. You administer ___________________. (Complete Flashcard 23.)

4. After defibrillating a patient in ventricular fibrillation cardiac arrest and continuing CPR, you wish to give a potent vasoconstrictor with a long duration of action. What do you administer? ___________________. (Complete Flashcard 24.)

5. Your crew is unable to initiate an intravenous line on an unconscious diabetic patient who is known to be hypoglycemic. Transport time is 45 minutes. The drug of choice to increase the blood glucose level is ___________________. (Complete Flashcard 25.)

6. A 35-year-old with an injured ankle is very nauseated. What antiemetic can you administer that will dissolve on the tongue? ___________________ (Complete Flashcard 26)

7. Your patient is in stable ventricular tachycardia. List an antidysrhythmic drug you may administer that can also be used to treat some narrow QRS tachycardias. ___________________. (Complete Flashcard 27.)

8. A 65-year-old woman complains of dyspnea and chest pain radiating down her left arm. Her blood pressure is 110/70 mm Hg. The initial drug of choice to relieve her pain is ___________________. (Complete Flashcard 28.)

9. A 42-year-old patient has a pounding sensation in her chest. Her ECG rhythm is ventricular tachycardia. The patient's blood pressure is normal, she has no chest pain, and the rest of the history and physical examination is unremarkable. If amiodarone is not available, which antidysrhythmic is indicated? ___________________. (Complete Flashcard 29.)

10. Your 30-year-old patient fell and has obvious deformity of the right wrist with significant pain. What nonnarcotic analgesic can you give him intramuscularly or intravenously? ___________________ (Complete Flashcard 30.)

11. You are called to an outpatient surgery center to evaluate a nurse who is unconscious. Coworkers confide that they have suspected drug abuse for some time, and there is an empty fentanyl (Sublimaze) Tubex in her pocket. Her pupils are pinpoint, and her respirations are 12 breaths/min and shallow. What drug is indicated first? ___________________ (Complete Flashcard 31.)

12. You perform transcutaneous pacing on a conscious patient. He complains of severe discomfort related to the procedure. BP is 110/70 mm Hg. What short-acting IV medicine can you administer to reduce anxiety, relax skeletal muscles, and provide amnesia? _____________________ (Complete Flashcard 32.)

13. An 88-year-old woman fainted. The patient has sinus bradycardia at a rate of 40/min and has a blood pressure of 80 mm Hg systolic by palpation. What drug is indicated? _____________________ (Complete Flashcard 33.)

14. An initial electrical countershock and good CPR do not successfully convert your cardiac arrest patient from ventricular fibrillation. An adrenergic drug that should be repeated every 3 to 5 minutes is _____________________. (Complete Flashcard 34.)

15. A 32-year-old patient fell and has an apparent dislocation of the left shoulder, which is very painful. Medical direction wishes to administer a short-acting analgesic. What self-administered analgesic is indicated? _____________________ (Complete Flashcard 35.)

16. A 73-year-old woman who is in cardiac arrest. Tricyclic antidepressant overdose is suspected. What electrolyte may be considered during resuscitation? _____________________ (Complete Flashcard 36.)

17. The police call you to evaluate an unconscious person. The patient is a known alcoholic, and friends say that he has not eaten for several days. He has a blood glucose level of 40 mg/dL (reference range, 80–120 mg/dL). No drug use is suspected. The two drugs indicated for this patient are _____________________ and _____________________. (Complete Flashcards 37 and 38.)

18. A 32-year-old woman is experiencing repetitive grand mal seizures. She is known to have epilepsy, and she has not taken any phenytoin (Dilantin) for 2 days. What is your drug of choice under these circumstances? (You do not have lorazepam or midazolam.) _____________________ (Complete Flashcard 39.)

19. A 24-year-old man is known to have asthma, and he is acutely dyspneic. Inspiratory and expiratory wheezes are audible, and the patient's HR is 100 beats/min. What drug would you administer by inhalation? _____________________ (Complete Flashcard 40.)

20. A 56-year-old woman has severe crushing substernal chest pain. What antiplatelet drug should you administer? _____________________ (Complete Flashcard 41.)

21. A 32-year-old woman has a sudden onset of palpitations. The electrocardiogram reveals a rapid supraventricular tachycardia. Which drug is indicated first? _____________________ (Complete Flashcard 42.)

22. A mechanic's arm is trapped in the landing gear of a small aircraft. Extrication time is lengthy, and the patient is in extreme distress because of pain. Vital signs are stable, and no other injuries are noted. List two narcotic analgesics that may be administered to this patient. _____________________ and _____________________ (Complete Flashcards 43 and 44.)

23. A 67-year-old patient has a headache resulting from his elevated blood pressure, which is now 230/160 mm Hg. He is awake and cooperative. After you consult with medical direction, which alpha- and beta-adrenergic blocker drug may improve this situation by lowering the blood pressure? _____________________ (Complete Flashcard 45.)

24. A 21-year-old took an SSRI overdose of an antidepressant 10 minutes ago and is awake and alert. What drug may be used to prevent absorption of this drug? _____________________ (Complete Flashcard 46.)

25. Your patient is 8 months pregnant and has been diagnosed with preeclampsia. Coworkers found her having a grand mal seizure in the restroom. The patient appears to be in a postictal state. Blood pressure is 160/116 mm Hg. What drug may be given for her seizure activity? _____________________ (Complete Flashcard 47.)

26. An 86-year-old patient from a nursing home has the following vital signs: blood pressure, 80/50 mm Hg; pulse, 124 beats/min; and respirations, 24 breaths/min. The urine in her urinary catheter bag is milky green and foul smelling. What is the drug of choice to treat her hypotension after fluid resuscitation in this situation? _____________________ (Complete Flashcard 48.)

27. A 35-year-old patient has the following vital signs: blood pressure, 130/90 mm Hg; pulse, 160 beats/min; and respirations, 24 breaths/min. The electrocardiogram monitor shows atrial fibrillation with a rapid ventricular response. She has mild signs of congestive heart failure, but all other physical findings are negative. What class IV antidysrhythmic drug is indicated? _____________________ (Complete Flashcard 49.)

28. A 72-year-old patient has severe dyspnea that began suddenly during the night. She is in obvious distress. Lung sounds reveal rales and wheezes throughout, and she has a cough that produces frothy, pink sputum. Vital signs are blood pressure, 170/108 mm Hg; pulse, 132 beats/min; and respirations, 32 breaths/min. Identify the diuretic medical direction may order after CPAP and nitroglycerin are administered. _________________ (Complete Flashcard 50.)

29. You have just delivered a healthy baby boy followed minutes later by a complete placenta. Despite vigorous massage, the patient's uterus is very soft, and she is experiencing profuse vaginal bleeding. What can you administer to help control this bleeding? _________________ (Complete Flashcard 51.)

30. You wish to intubate a combative trauma patient. Which short-acting drug can help facilitate this process? _________________

Complete the remaining flashcards with drugs not included in the previous questions that are administered within your emergency medical services system.

STUDENT SELF-ASSESSMENT

31. When is the use of dopamine most clearly indicated?
- **a.** Blood pressure 70/50 mm Hg
- **b.** Cardiogenic shock
- **c.** Unresponsive patient
- **d.** Internal bleeding

32. Which drug is indicated for a 72-year-old with a history of severe COPD and a possible hip fracture whose vital signs are stable?
- **a.** Fentanyl 2 mcg/kg IV
- **b.** Morphine 8 mg IV
- **c.** Nitrous oxide/oxygen inhaled
- **d.** None of the above

33. For what condition should you administer epinephrine 1:1000 intramuscularly?
- **a.** Anaphylaxis
- **b.** Hypovolemic shock
- **c.** Pulseless electrical activity
- **d.** Ventricular fibrillation

34. Which drug is recommended to control atrial fibrillation with a rate of 170 beats/min when the patient has Wolff-Parkinson-White syndrome?
- **a.** Adenosine
- **b.** Amiodarone
- **c.** Atenolol
- **d.** Diltiazem

35. Which is true regarding use of atropine?
- **a.** It can be given intranasal.
- **b.** It inhibits vagal stimulation.
- **c.** It should be given in asystole.
- **d.** It is an antidote for verapamil.

36. Which is true of oral administration of ondansetron?
- **a.** Allow the tablet to dissolve on the tongue.
- **b.** It is not effective and not indicated in the field.
- **c.** Have the patient swallow with liquid that contains sugar.
- **d.** It is safe to administer in a patient with jaundice.

37. A 68-year-old man has chest pain. His 12-lead electrocardiogram shows ST segment elevation in leads II, III, and aV_F. His breath sounds are clear. His vital signs are blood pressure is 86/50 mm Hg, pulse is 64 beats/min, respirations are 20 breaths/min. Which drug is indicated?
- **a.** Aspirin
- **b.** Morphine
- **c.** Nitroglycerin
- **d.** Metoprolol

38. A patient is in ventricular fibrillation. Which sympathomimetic is indicated during her care?
- **a.** Epinephrine
- **b.** Amiodarone
- **c.** Magnesium sulfate
- **d.** Vasopressin

39. Which of the following drugs does **not** cause bronchodilation?
- **a.** Albuterol
- **b.** Epinephrine
- **c.** Diphenhydramine
- **d.** Isoproterenol

40. Verapamil is contraindicated for which patient situation?
- **a.** Complaining of palpitations
- **b.** Hypotensive
- **c.** Tachycardic
- **d.** Younger than age 45 years

41. Which drug is self-administered by mask for relief of pain?
- **a.** Fentanyl
- **b.** Morphine sulfate
- **c.** Nitroglycerin
- **d.** Nitrous oxide and oxygen

42. Which drug is indicated to treat stable narrow QRS complex atrial fibrillation at a rate of 152 beats/min?
- **a.** Adenosine
- **b.** Diltiazem
- **c.** Lidocaine
- **d.** Magnesium

Emergency Drug Index

43. Which drug inhibits platelet aggregation?
   a. Aspirin
   b. Reteplase
   c. Streptokinase
   d. Tissue plasminogen activator
44. What drug is indicated to prevent Wernicke-Korsakoff syndrome?
   a. Glucagon
   b. Naloxone
   c. Methylprednisolone
   d. Thiamine
45. When is mannitol indicated?
   a. Congestive heart failure
   b. Acute cerebral edema
   c. Cor pulmonale
   d. Shock
46. Which drug is indicated to treat status epilepticus, anxiety, and skeletal muscle spasms?
   a. Diazepam
   b. Morphine
   c. Naloxone
   d. Phenytoin
47. Which drug is indicated for management of postpartum bleeding?
   a. Dopamine
   b. Insulin
   c. Magnesium sulfate
   d. Oxytocin
48. When is diphenhydramine contraindicated?
   a. Anaphylactic shock
   b. Acute asthma attack
   c. Allergic reactions
   d. Patients who are nauseated
49. For which toxic ingestion is charcoal administered?
   a. Cyanide
   b. Ethanol
   c. Lithium
   d. Strattera
50. Which drug will naloxone antagonize?
   a. Diazepam
   b. Methamphetamine
   c. OxyContin
   d. Phenobarbital
51. Which medication may cause respiratory depression?
   a. Atropine
   b. Dexamethasone
   c. Magnesium sulfate
   d. Sodium bicarbonate
52. A patient has monomorphic ventricular tachycardia at 160 beats/min (normal Q-T interval). Her blood pressure is 100 mm Hg, she has crackles in both lung bases. Which drug is preferred to manage this rhythm?
   a. Amiodarone
   b. Magnesium sulfate
   c. Metoprolol
   d. Lidocaine
53. Which side effect may occur after nitroglycerin ingestion?
   a. Headache
   b. Hypertension
   c. Urticaria
   d. Priapism
54. Which drug exerts a positive chronotropic effect?
   a. Adenosine
   b. Epinephrine
   c. Labetalol
   d. Digoxin
55. What condition may furosemide worsen?
   a. Hypertension
   b. Cor pulmonale
   c. Pneumonia
   d. Pulmonary edema
56. Which calcium channel blocker slows conduction and heart rate in atrial flutter?
   a. Adenosine
   b. Albuterol
   c. Dobutamine
   d. Diltiazem
57. Which drug has the highest priority for administration in pulmonary edema?
   a. Aspirin
   b. Furosemide
   c. Morphine
   d. Nitroglycerin
58. What vital sign alteration should be expected after administering metoprolol?
   a. Hypertension
   b. Rising temperature
   c. Bronchodilation
   d. Decreased heart rate
59. A 35-year-old man is psychotic and violent. Which drug is indicated?
   a. Haloperidol
   b. Hydroxyzine
   c. Etomidate
   d. Midazolam
60. What is a desired action of methylprednisolone?
   a. Nausea reduction
   b. Enhanced heart contraction
   c. Reduced inflammation
   d. Pain relief

1. Actions: suppress acute or chronic inflammation and potentiate relaxation of vascular smooth muscle by beta-adrenergic agonist. Indications: anaphylaxis, asthma, shock, and spinal cord injury. Adverse reactions: hypertension, sodium and water retention, hypokalemia, hypocalcemia, alkalosis, and headache

2. a. Onset: 1 to 2 hours. Duration: 8 to 24 hours. Dose: 40 to 125 mg IV (in spinal cord injury medical control may order higher doses)
   b. Onset: 4 to 8 hours. Duration: 24 to 72 hours. Dose: 4 to 24 mg IV

3. Diphenhydramine (Benadryl). Class: antihistamine. Description: Prevents histamine from reaching H_1 receptor sites. Indications: allergic reactions, anaphylaxis, and acute extrapyramidal reactions. Contraindications: patients taking non-selective monoamine oxidase inhibitors, hypersensitivity, narrow-angle glaucoma, newborns, and nursing mothers. Adverse reactions: drowsiness, sedation, disturbed coordination, hypotension, palpitations, tachycardia or bradycardia, thickening of bronchial secretions, and dry mouth and throat. Onset: maximal effects in 1 to 3 hours. Duration: 6 to 12 hours. Dose: adult—10 to 50 mg deep IM or slow IV injection; pediatric—1.25 mg/kg/dose in divided doses IV or IM. Special considerations: pregnancy Category C.

4. Vasopressin (Pitressin). Class: antidiuretic hormone. Description: stimulates smooth muscles; in high doses is a nonadrenergic peripheral vasoconstrictor. Indications: adult cardiac arrest to replace the first or second dose of epinephrine; vasodilatory shock. Contraindications: responsive patients with coronary artery disease. Adverse reactions: ischemic chest pain, abdominal distress, sweating, nausea, vomiting, tremors. Onset: immediate. Duration: variable. Dose: adult cardiac arrest—40 units IV or IO 1 time; pediatric—0.4 to 1 unit/kg IV or IO (maximum, 40 units). Special considerations: Drug may cause cardiac ischemia and angina.

5. Glucagon. Class: pancreatic hormone and antihypoglycemic agent. Description: Stimulates glycogenolysis; positive inotropic effect on the heart. Indications: treatment of hypoglycemia if glucose administration not possible; calcium channel blocker or beta-blocker toxicity. Contraindications: hypersensitivity to proteins. Adverse reactions: tachycardia, hypotension, nausea, vomiting, and urticaria. Onset: within 1 minute. Duration: 60 to 90 minutes. Dose: adult—0.5 to 1.0 mg IM; children weighing more than 20 kg—0.5 to 1.0 mg IM. Calcium channel blocker or beta-blocker toxicity, adult 3 to 10 mg slow over 3 to 5 minutes. Special considerations: not first-line choice for hypoglycemia; may potentiate the effects of oral anticoagulants.

6. a. Ondansetron (Zofran). Class: antiemetic. Description: Selective serotonin blocking antiemetic. Indications: nausea and vomiting. Contraindications: hypersensitivity, liver disease, GI obstruction. Onset within 30 min. Duration: 3 to 6 hours. Dose: IV up to 4 mg over 30 sec; deep IM 4 mg; oral film 4 mg. Special considerations: pregnancy Category B; allow tablet to dissolve on tongue.

7. Amiodarone (Cordarone). Class: Class III antidysrhythmic. Description: prolongs action potential and refractory period; alpha-adrenoreceptor and calcium channel blocker. Indications: treatment and prophylaxis of frequently recurring ventricular fibrillation and unstable ventricular tachycardia. Contraindications: pulmonary congestion, cardiogenic shock, second- or third-degree heart block (if no pacemaker) sensitivity to amiodarone or iodine. Adverse reactions: hypotension, bradycardia, headache, dizziness, atrioventricular conduction abnormalities, flushing, abnormal salivation, pain at IV site, liver function abnormalities, congestive heart failure, abnormal thyroid function. Onset: within minutes. Duration: variable. Dose: adult cardiac arrest—300 mg IV push; supplemental bolus for cardiac arrest—150 mg IV push in 3 to 5 minutes. Wide complex tachycardias—150 mg IV over 10 min; may repeat in 10 min if needed. Follow with 1 mg/min infusion for 6 hours; then 0.5 mg/min infusion for 18 hr.

8. Nitroglycerin (Nitrostat). Class: vasodilator. Description: dilates peripheral venous and arteriolar blood vessels; reduces cardiac workload and oxygen demand. Indications: ischemic chest pain, acute myocardial infarction, hypertensive emergencies, congestive heart failure. Contraindications: volume depletion, hypersensitivity, systolic blood pressure below 90 mm Hg or above 30 mm Hg below baseline; if heart rate is below 50 beats/min or above 100 beats/min (in the absence of heart failure), head injury, right ventricular infarction; cerebral hemorrhage; recent use of tadalafil, vardenafil, or sildenafil. Adverse reactions: headache, postural syncope, reflex tachycardia, hypotension, nausea, vomiting, flushing, diaphoresis. Onset: 1 to 3 minutes. Duration: 30 to 60 minutes. Dose: tablet—0.4 mg sublingually; may repeat in 5 minutes twice; metered spray—0.4 mg/spray, one to two sublingual sprays; that may be repeated in 5 minutes to a maximum of 3 sprays in 15 minutes; infusion begins at a rate of 10 mcg/min, increased to desired effect (ceiling dose, 200 mcg/min). Special considerations: keep in an airtight container protected from light; older adults have an increased risk of hypotension. Administer with caution if at all to patients with inferior wall MI and suspected to have RV infarct.

9. Lidocaine (Xylocaine). Class: Class I-B antidysrhythmic, local anesthetic. Description: Suppresses premature ventricular contractions and raises ventricular fibrillation threshold. Indications: ventricular fibrillation, ventricular tachycardia, significant ventricular ectopy in the presence of myocardial ischemia or infarction; wide-complex tachycardia of unknown origin. Contraindications: hypersensitivity, Stokes-Adams syndrome, and second- or third-degree heart block in the absence of an artificial pacemaker. Adverse reactions: lightheadedness, confusion, blurred vision, hypotension, cardiovascular collapse, bradycardia, and central nervous system depression and

789

Emergency Drug Index

seizures with high doses. Onset: 30 to 90 seconds. Duration: 10 to 20 minutes. Dose: adult—administration IV or via endotracheal bolus (at 2–2.5 times IV dose) followed by a continuous infusion; for ventricular fibrillation, 1.0 to 1.5 mg/kg IV repeated at 0.5 to 0.75 mg/kg in 3 to 5 minutes to a total loading dose of 3 mg/kg; for ventricular ectopy or stable ventricular tachycardia, 0.5 to 0.75 mg/kg (≤1 to 1.5 mg/kg IV may be used) repeated in 5 to 10 minutes at 0.5 to 0.75 mg/kg to a total dose of 3 mg/kg; given via infusion—maintenance infusion at 1 to 4 mg/ min; pediatric—1 mg/kg/dose IV or IO; Infusion—20 to 50 mcg/kg/min. Special considerations: short half-life; treat bradycardia with premature ventricular contractions with atropine first; high doses can result in coma or death; decrease dose in elderly adults. Avoid lidocaine in reperfusion dysrhythmias after thrombolytic therapy; use caution in patients with hepatic disease, heart failure, marked hypoxia, severe respiratory depression, hypovolemia, or shock.

10. Ketorolac tromethamine (Toradol). Class: nonsteroidal antiinflammatory. Description: antiinflammatory drug that exhibits peripherally acting nonnarcotic analgesic activity by inhibiting prostaglandin synthesis. Indications: moderate to severe pain. Contraindications: hypersensitivity, allergies to aspirin or other nonsteroidal antiinflammatory drugs, bleeding disorders, renal failure, active peptic ulcer disease. Adverse reactions: anaphylaxis, edema, sedation, bleeding disorders, rash, nausea, headache. Onset: within 10 minutes. Duration: 6 to 8 hours. Dose: adult—60 mg IM or 30 mg IM (patients >65 years); 30 mg IV; one half dose (15 mg) for patients older than 65 years old and those with renal impairment or weight less than 50 kg. Special considerations: pregnancy Category C safety.

11. Naloxone (Narcan). Class: synthetic opioid antagonist. Description: a competitive narcotic antagonist reverses overdoses caused by narcotics and synthetic narcotic agents. Indications: complete or partial reversal of central nervous system depression and respiratory depression resulting from opioids, including narcotic agonists, narcotic agonist/antagonists, and others; decreased level of consciousness, coma of unknown origin. Contraindications: hypersensitivity and caution with narcotic-dependent patients, who may experience withdrawal syndrome; avoid use in meperidine-induced seizures. Adverse reactions: tachycardia, hypertension, dysrhythmias, nausea, vomiting, blurred vision, withdrawal, and diaphoresis. Onset: within 2 minutes. Duration: 30 to 60 minutes. Dose: adult—0.4 mg IV use higher doses (up to 2 mg) for complete narcotic reversal (can administer 6–10 mg over 10 min.) or 0.4 to 0.8 mg IM or subcutaneously. May be repeated in 5-minute intervals to a maximum of 10 mg; children—0.1 mg/kg/dose IV, IM, or subcutaneously or via endotracheal administration (diluted). Special considerations: seizures have been reported; drug may not reverse hypotension and may cause withdrawal syndrome; use smaller doses if patient is a suspected narcotic addict. Naloxone has shorter duration than some narcotics; monitor patient carefully after administration. Intranasal use has been cited in literature.

12. Midazolam hydrochloride (Versed). Class: short-acting benzodiazepine. Description: benzodiazepine that may be administered for conscious sedation to relieve apprehension or impair memory before tracheal intubation or cardioversion. Indications: premedication for trachea intubation or cardioversion. Seizures in children. Contraindications: hypersensitivity; glaucoma; shock; coma; alcohol intoxication (relative); depressed vital signs; concomitant use of barbiturates, alcohol, narcotics, or other central nervous system depressants. Adverse reactions: respiratory depression, hiccups, cough, oversedation, pain at injection site, nausea and vomiting, headache, blurred vision, fluctuations in vital signs, hypotension, and respiratory arrest. Onset: 1 to 3 minutes. Duration: 2 to 6 hours, dose dependent. Dose: adult—1 to 2.5 mg slow IV (over 2–3 minutes); repeat as needed in small increments (total maximum dose not to exceed 0.1 mg/kg); elderly adults—0.5 mg slow IV (maximum of 1.5 mg in a 2-minute period); pediatric—loading dose 0.05 to 0.2 mg/kg followed by continued infusion at 1 to 2 mcg/kg/ min. Seizures in children: 0.1 to 0.15 mg/kg (maximum dose, 5 mg) IV slow over 1 to 2 minutes or IM. Special considerations: pregnancy Category D; continuously monitor respiratory and cardiac function; have resuscitation equipment and medication readily at hand; never administer medication as an intravenous bolus.

13. Atropine sulfate (atropine and others). Class: anticholinergic agent. Description: inhibits the action of acetylcholine at postganglionic parasympathetic receptor sites; blocks vagus nerve and increases heart rate and enhances atrioventricular conduction. Indications: hemodynamically significant bradycardia and organophosphate or nerve gas poisoning. Contraindications: tachycardia, hypersensitivity, unstable cardiovascular status in acute hemorrhage and myocardial ischemia, narrow-angle glaucoma, obstructive disease of the gastrointestinal tract, obstructive uropathy, and thyrotoxicosis. Adverse reactions: tachycardia; paradoxical bradycardia when pushed slowly or when used at doses less than 0.5 mg; palpitations; dysrhythmias; headache; dizziness; anticholinergic effects (dry mouth, nose, skin, photophobia, blurred vision, urine retention); nausea; vomiting; flushed, hot, dry skin; and allergic reactions. Onset: rapid. Duration: 2 to 6 hours. Dose: bradydysrhythmias: adult—0.5 mg IV every 3 to 5 minutes as needed (maximum total dose, 3 mg); pediatric—0.02 mg/kg/dose IV or IO (minimum dose, 0.1 mg; maximum single dose, 0.5 mg; may repeat dose once). Anticholinesterase poisoning: adult—1 to 2 mg IV every 5 to 15 minutes until atropine effects observed; pediatric (<12 years)—0.02 to 0.05 mg/kg/dose IV or IO, repeated as needed every 20 to 30 minutes until muscarinic effect is observed; pediatric (>12 years) 2 mg IV or IO; then 1 to 2 mg IV or IO every 20 to 30 minutes until muscarinic symptoms reverse. Special considerations: pregnancy Category C. Causes pupil dilation. Avoid use in hypothermic bradycardia.

14. Epinephrine (Adrenalin). Class: sympathomimetic. Description: stimulates alpha- and beta-receptors; causes bronchodilation and, when administered via rapid intravenous injection, causes rapid increases in systolic pressure, ventricular contractility, and heart rate; causes vasoconstriction of the arterioles of the skin, mucosa, and splanchnic areas; and antagonizes the effects of histamine. Indications: bronchial asthma, acute allergic reactions, cardiac arrest symptomatic bradycardia. Contraindications: hypersensitivity, hypovolemic shock, coronary insufficiency (should be used with caution). Adverse reactions: headache, restlessness, weakness, dysrhythmias, hypertension, nausea, vomiting, tremors, dyspnea, precipitation of angina pectoris and tachycardia. Onset: 5 to 10 minutes (subcutaneously), 1 to 2 minutes (IV). Duration: 5 to 10 minutes. Dose: cardiac arrest: adult—1 mg IV push repeated every 3 to 5 minutes; pediatric—0.01 mg/kg 1:10,000 IV or IO or via endotracheal administration (diluted to 3–5 mL). Bradycardia refractory to other interventions: adult—2 to 10 mcg/min; pediatric—IV/IO 0.01 mg/kg/0.1 mL/kg of 1:10,000 standard concentration) infusion at 0.1 to 1 mcg/kg/min. Anaphylactic reaction or bronchoconstriction: adult—mild to moderate: 0.3 to 0.5 mL (1:1000), IM for anaphylaxis; severe: 0.1 mg (1 mL of 1:10,000) slow IV injection; pediatric—0.01 mg/kg IM (1:1000), maximum of 0.3 mL. Special considerations: syncope has been reported after administration in children; it may increase myocardial oxygen demand. Do not administer 1:1000 epinephrine IV bolus.

15. Nitrous oxide:oxygen (50:50; Nitronox). Class: Self-administered gaseous analgesic and anesthetic. Description: depresses the central nervous system and causes anesthesia. Indications: moderate to severe pain. Contraindications: impaired level of consciousness, head injury, chest trauma (pneumothorax), inability to comply with instructions, decompression sickness, undiagnosed abdominal pain, bowel obstruction, hypotension, shock, and chronic obstructive pulmonary disease. Adverse reactions: dizziness, apnea, cyanosis, nausea, vomiting, and malignant hyperthermia. Onset: 2 to 5 minutes. Duration: 2 to 5 minutes. Dose: adult—invert cylinder several times before use and instruct the patient to inhale deeply through the mask or mouthpiece, which the patient must hold; pediatric—same. Special considerations: The drug increases the incidence of spontaneous abortion; it diffuses into gas-filled pockets trapped in the patient (e.g., pneumothorax, intestinal obstruction) and may cause rupture; nitrous oxide is a nonexplosive gas.

16. Sodium bicarbonate. Class: buffer, alkalinizing agent, electrolyte supplement. Description: reacts with hydrogen ions to form water and carbon dioxide to buffer metabolic acidosis. Indications: known preexisting metabolic acidosis, hyperkalemia, tricyclic antidepressant overdose, and alkalinization for treatment of specific intoxications. Contraindications: patients with chloride loss from vomiting or gastrointestinal suction, respiratory alkalosis, pulmonary edema, hypernatremia, hypokalemia, hypocalcemia, and abdominal pain of unknown origin. Adverse reactions: metabolic alkalosis, hypoxia, rise in intracellular PCO_2 and increased tissue acidosis, hypernatremia, seizures, and tissue sloughing at injection site. Onset: 2 to 10 minutes. Duration: 30 to 60 minutes. Dose: urgent forms of metabolic acidosis: adult—1 mEq/kg IV; pediatric—same as adult; infuse slowly. Special considerations: if possible, arterial blood gas analysis should guide administration of this drug; it may increase edematous or sodium-retaining states; it initially may worsen cellular acidosis or hyperkalemia; it may worsen congestive heart failure. Precipitates when infused with calcium chloride; inactivated epinephrine when given in the same infusion.

17. a. Thiamine (Betaxin). Class: vitamin (B_1). Description: vitamin necessary for carbohydrate metabolism. Indications: coma of unknown origin (with administration of dextrose 50% or naloxone), delirium tremens, beriberi, and Wernicke's encephalopathy. Contraindications: none significant. Adverse reactions: hypotension (from rapid injection or a large dose), anxiety, diaphoresis, nausea, vomiting, and allergic reaction (rare). Onset: rapid. Duration: depends on degree of deficiency. Dose: adult—100 mg slow IV or IM. Special considerations: anaphylactic reactions have been reported.

b. Dextrose 50%. Class: carbohydrate and hypertonic solution. Description: the principal carbohydrate used in the body. Indications: hypoglycemia, altered level of consciousness, coma of unknown cause, seizure of unknown cause. Contraindications: intracranial hemorrhage, increased intracranial pressure, or suspected stroke in the absence of hypoglycemia. Adverse reactions: warmth, pain, burning from medication infusion, hyperglycemia, thrombophlebitis. Onset: less than 1 minute. Duration: depends on degree of hypoglycemia. Dose: adult—12.5 to 25 g slow IV or IO (may repeat once); pediatric—0.5 to 1 g/kg/dose IV or IO (maximum recommended concentration, 25%); 2 to 4 mL/kg 25%; 5 to 10 mL/kg 10%. Special considerations: blood glucose analysis should be performed before administration, if possible; extravasation may cause tissue necrosis; it may sometimes precipitate severe neurologic symptoms (Wernicke's encephalopathy) in patients with thiamine depletion, such as people with alcoholism; high-risk groups should receive thiamine.

18. Diazepam (Valium and others). Class: benzodiazepine. Description: raises seizure threshold in the cerebral cortex and acts on the limbic, thalamic, and hypothalamic regions of the brain to potentiate the effects of inhibitory neurotransmitters. Indications: acute anxiety states, acute alcohol withdrawal, muscle relaxation, seizure activity, and premedication to countershock or transcutaneous pacing. Contraindications: hypersensitivity, substance abuse (use with caution), coma, shock, central nervous system depression after head injury, respiratory depression. Adverse reactions: hypotension, reflex tachycardia, respiratory depression, ataxia, dizziness, drowsiness, blurred vision, psychomotor impairment, confusion, and nausea. Onset: 1 to 5 minutes (IV); 15 to 30 minutes (IM).

Duration: 15 minutes to 1 hour (IV), 15 minutes to 1 hour (IM). Dose: Seizure activity: adult—5 mg IV over 2 minutes (may give up to 10 mg for most adults); pediatric—infants 30 days to 5 years: 0.2 to 0.5 mg slow IV or IO every 2 to 5 minutes (maximum, 5 mg); children older than 5 years: 1 mg every 2 to 5 minutes to maximum 10 mg slow IV. Premedication for cardioversion: adult—5 to 15 mg IV 5 to 10 minutes before procedure. Special considerations: diazepam may cause local venous irritation; dose should be reduced by 50% in older adults; resuscitation equipment should be readily available; anticonvulsant effect has a short duration.

19. Albuterol (Proventil, Ventolin). Class: sympathomimetic bronchodilator. Description: a beta2-specific sympathomimetic stimulant that relaxes bronchiolar smooth muscle and peripheral vasculature. Indications: relief of bronchospasm in patients with reversible obstructive airway disease; anaphylaxis; hyperkalemia. Contraindications: hypersensitivity, cardiac dysrhythmias associated with tachycardia. Adverse reactions: restlessness, apprehension, tremors, dizziness, palpitations, increased blood pressure, and dysrhythmias. Onset: 5 to 8 minutes via inhalation. Duration: 2 to 6 hours via inhalation. Dose: bronchial asthma: adults—via metered-dose inhaler, 1 to 2 inhalations (90–180 mcg) every 4 to 6 hours (5 minutes between inhalations); via inhalation, 2.5 mg (0.5 mL of 0.5% solution) diluted to 3 mL with 0.9% NaCl administered over 5 to 15 minutes; pediatric—via solution, 0.01 to 0.03 mL (0.05–0.15 mg) per kilogram per dose to a maximum of 0.5 mL/dose diluted in 2 mL of 0.9% normal saline (may be repeated every 20 minutes). Special considerations: sympathomimetics may exacerbate adverse cardiac effects; drug may potentiate hypokalemia; it may precipitate angina pectoris and dysrhythmias; it should be used with caution with patients with diabetes mellitus, hyperthyroidism, prostatic hypertrophy, cardiovascular disorder, or seizure disorder; it should be administered only by inhalation in prehospital care.

20. Aspirin (ASA, Bayer, Ecotrin, St. Joseph, others). Class: analgesic, antiinflammatory, antiplatelet, antipyretic. Description: drug that blocks pain impulses in the central nervous system, dilates peripheral vessels, and decreases platelet aggregation. Indications: mild to moderate pain or fever; prevention of platelet aggregation in ischemia and thromboembolism; unstable angina; prevention of myocardial infarction or reinfarction. Contraindications: hypersensitivity to salicylates; gastrointestinal bleeding; active ulcer disease; hemorrhagic stroke; bleeding disorders; children with flu-like symptoms. Adverse reactions: stomach irritation, heartburn or indigestion, nausea or vomiting, allergic reaction. Onset: 15 to 30 minutes. Duration: 4 to 6 hours. Dose: adult—mild pain or fever: 325 to 650 mg PO q4h; myocardial infarction—160 to 325 mg PO (chew).

21. Adenosine (Adenocard). Class: endogenous nucleotide, miscellaneous antidysrhythmic agent. Description: slows tachycardia associated with the atrioventricular node via modulation of the autonomic nervous system without causing negative inotropic effects and acts directly on sinus pacemaker cells and vagal nerve terminals to decrease chronotropic and dromotropic activity. Indications: treatment of paroxysmal supraventricular tachycardia. Contraindications: second- or third-degree atrioventricular block, sick sinus syndrome, and hypersensitivity to adenosine; drug-induced tachycardia. Adverse reactions: facial flushing, lightheadedness, paresthesia, headache, diaphoresis, palpitations, chest pain, hypotension, dyspnea, nausea, metallic taste. Transient sinus bradycardia, sinus pause, bradyasystole ventricular ectopy. Onset: immediate. Duration: 10 seconds. Dose: adult—initial, 6 mg over 1 to 3 seconds, if no response in 1 to 2 minutes, administration of 12 mg over 1 to 3 seconds; pediatric—0.1 mg/kg rapid IV or IO; (maximum single dose, 6 mg); second dose, 0.2 mg/kg IV or IO followed with 5 to 10 mL NS flush. Special considerations: methylxanthines antagonize the action of adenosine; dipyridamole potentiates the effect of adenosine; carbamazepine may potentiate the atrioventricular-nodal blocking effect of adenosine; adenosine may produce bronchoconstriction in patients with asthma or bronchopulmonary disease; asystole (≤15 seconds) followed by normal sinus rhythm is common after administration.

22. a. Morphine sulfate (Astramorph/PF and others). Class: opioid analgesic. Description: increases peripheral venous capacitance and decreases venous return; promotes analgesia, euphoria, and respiratory and physical depression; decreases myocardial oxygen demand; a Schedule II drug. Indications: chest pain associated with acute coronary syndrome, moderate to severe acute or chronic pain, and pulmonary edema. Contraindications: hypersensitivity to narcotics, hypovolemia, hypotension, head injury, and patients who have taken monoamine oxidase inhibitors within 14 days; increased intracranial pressure; and severe respiratory depression. Use with caution in right ventricular infarction. Adverse reactions: hypotension, tachycardia, bradycardia, palpitations, syncope, facial flushing, respiratory depression, euphoria, bronchospasm, dry mouth, and allergic reaction. Onset: 1 to 2 minutes. Duration: 2 to 7 hours. Dose: adult—STEMI: 2 to 4 mg IV; may give additional doses of 2 to 8 mg IV at 5- to 15-minute intervals; UA/NSTEMI: 1 to 5 mg IV if symptoms are not relieved by nitrates. Pain: 2 to 4 mg slow IV over1 to 5 min.; pediatric—0.1 to 0.2 mg/kg/dose IV (maximum, 15-mg total dose). Special considerations: narcotics rapidly cross the placenta; drug should be used with caution with older adults, patients with asthma, and patients susceptible to central nervous system depression; naloxone should be readily available; drug may worsen bradycardia or heart block in inferior myocardial infarction (vagotonic effect).

    b. Fentanyl (Sublimaze). Class: opioid analgesic. Description: an opioid agonist that produces analgesia. Indications: moderate to severe pain. Contraindications: hypersensitivity to opiates, respiratory depression, hypotension, head injury, cardiac dysrhythmias, myasthenia gravis. Adverse reactions: respiratory depression, bradaycardia, hypotension, nausea, and vomiting, chest muscle rigidity. Onset: 1 to 2 minutes (intravenously).

792

Duration: 1/2 to 1 hour. Dose: adult—0.05 to 0.1 mg slow IV over 1 to 2 min every 1-2 hr,; pediatric—1 to 2 mcg/kg/dose (rarely used prehospital). Special considerations: Drug should be used with caution in elderly patients and in those with severe respiratory disorders, seizure disorders, cardiac disorders or pregnancy; nalaxone should be readily available.

23. Metoprolol (Lopressor). Class: Beta-adrenergic blocker. Description: beta-receptor blocker used to control ventricular response during supraventricular dysrhythmias (second-line). Indications: MI and unstable angina; adjunct with fibrinolytic thereapy. Slow ventricular rate in supraventricular dysrhythmias. Contraindications: bronchial asthma (relative), uncompensated congestive heart failure, second- and third-degree heart block, bradycardia, cardiogenic shock, BP <100 mm Hg, PR interval >.24 sec. Adverse reactions: hypotension, bradycardia, AV condution delays, palpitations, nausea and vomiting. Onset: 1 to 2 minutes. Duration: 3 to 4 hours. Dose: adult—5 mg slow intravenous bolus over 5 minutes; additional injections at 5-minute intervals as needed (maximum 15 mg). Special considerations: pregnancy safety category C; monitor blood pressure, pulse, electrocardiogram continuously; observe for signs of congestive heart failure, bradycardia, bronchospasm; concurrent administration with IV calcium channel blockers can cause severe hypotension.

24. Activated charcoal (Actidose-Aqua, Liqui-Char). Class: adsorbent, antidote. Description: drug that binds and adsorbs ingested toxins. Indications: many oral poisonings and medication overdoses. Contraindications: corrosives, caustics, and petroleum distillates. Adverse reactions: nausea (indirectly), vomiting, and constipation. Onset: immediate. Duration: continual in gastrointestinal tract. Dose: prepared in a slurry and administered by mouth or slowly by gastric tube; adult—30 to 100 g; pediatric—15 to 30 g; infant younger than 1 year—1 g/kg. Special considerations: drug does not adsorb all drugs and toxic substances (e.g., phenobarbital, aspirin, cyanide, lithium, iron, lead, and arsenic).

25. Magnesium sulfate. Class: electrolyte, anticonvulsant. Description: drug that reduces striated muscle contractions and blocks peripheral neuromuscular transmission by reducing acetylcholine release at the myoneural junction. Indications: seizures resulting from eclampsia, torsades de pointes, refractory ventricular fibrillation, with suspected hypomagnesemia status asthmaticus. Contraindications: heart block or myocardial damage. Adverse reactions: diaphoresis, facial flushing, hypotension, depressed reflexes, hypothermia, reduced heart rate, circulatory collapse, diarrhea, and respiratory depression. Onset: (IV) immediate. Duration: 30 minutes. Dose: seizures associated with pregnancy: 1 to 4 g (8–32 mEq) IV; maximum dose of 30–40 g per day. Pulseless arrest (torsades de pointes or hypomagnesemic state): adult—1 to 2 g in 10 mL of D5W IV over 5 to 20 minutes; pediatric—25 to 50 mg/kg over 10 to 20 minutes. Special considerations: other central nervous system depressants may enhance central nervous system depressant effects; drug should not be administered in the 2 hours before delivery; calcium gluconate or calcium chloride should be available as antagonist; drug may be needed for up to 48 hours after delivery; use with caution in patients with renal failure.

26. Dopamine (Intropin). Class: sympathomimetic. Description: drug that acts on alpha$_1$- and beta-adrenergic receptors, increasing systemic vascular resistance and exerting a positive inotropic effect on the heart. Indications: hemodynamically significant hypotension in the absence of hypovolemia. Contraindications: tachydysrhythmias, ventricular fibrillation, and patients with pheochromocytoma. Adverse reactions: dose-related tachycardias, hypertension, and increased myocardial oxygen demand. Onset: 2 to 4 minutes. Duration: 10 to 15 minutes. Dose: adult—dosage range of 2 to 20 mcg/kg/min recommended; pediatric—2 to 20 mcg/kg/min; IV or IO titrated to patient response (not to exceed 20 mcg/kg/min). Special considerations: Drug should be infused through a large, stable vein to avoid extravasation injury; patients should be monitored for signs of compromised circulation; infusion pump is recommended.

27. Verapamil (Isoptin). Class: calcium channel blocker (class IV antidysrhythmic). Description: antidysrhythmic, antianginal, antihypertensive; inhibits the movement of calcium ions across cell membranes, decreases atrial automaticity, reduces atrioventricular conduction velocity, prolongs the atrioventricular nodal refractory period, decreases myocardial contractility, reduces vascular smooth muscle tone, and dilates coronary arteries and arterioles. Indications: paroxysmal supraventricular tachycardia (unresponsive to vagal maneuvers or adenosine), atrial flutter with rapid ventricular response, and atrial fibrillation with a rapid ventricular response; unstable angina. Contraindications: hypersensitivity, sick sinus syndrome (unless the patient has a pacemaker), second- or third-degree heart block, hypotension, cardiogenic shock, severe congestive heart failure, Wolff-Parkinson-White syndrome with atrial fibrillation or flutter, patients receiving intravenously administered beta-blockers, wide-complex tachycardias. Adverse reactions: dizziness, headache, nausea, vomiting, hypotension, bradycardia, complete atrioventricular block, and peripheral edema. Onset: 1 to 5 minutes. Duration: 30 to 60 minutes. Dose: adult—2.5 to 5.0 mg IV bolus over 2 minutes; repeat with 5 to 10 mg in 15 to 30 minutes, as necessary (maximum, 30 mg). Alternative dosing: 5 mg IV over 2 minutes every 15 minutes to a maximum dose of 30 mg. Special considerations: vital signs should be monitored closely; be prepared to resuscitate the patient; atrioventricular block or asystole may occur because of slowed atrioventricular conduction; decrease dose when administering to elderly or borderline hypotensive patients.

28. Furosemide (Lasix). Class: loop diuretic. Description: drug that inhibits reabsorption of sodium and chloride in the proximal tubule and loop of Henle; IV doses can increase venous capacitance and decrease preload. Indications:

Emergency Drug Index

pulmonary edema associated with congestive heart failure, and hepatic or renal disease. Contraindications: anuria, hypokalemia, hypersensitivity; states of severe electrolyte depletion; dehydration; known allergy to sulfonamides. Adverse reactions: hypotension, electrocardiogram changes, dry mouth, hypocalcemia, hypochloremia, hypokalemia, hyponatremia, and hyperglycemia; may cause hearing loss if the infusion of large doses is too rapid. Onset: vascular effects within 5 minutes IV; diuresis, 15 to 20 minutes. Duration: 2 hours. Dose: adult—0.5 to 1.0 mg/kg slow IV injection; if no response, double dose to 2 mg/kg slow over 2 minutes; pediatric—1 mg/kg/dose. Special considerations: Drug has been known to cause fetal abnormalities; it should be protected from light.

29. Oxytocin (Pitocin). Class: pituitary hormone. Description: drug that indirectly stimulates uterine smooth muscle contractions, which transiently reduce uterine blood flow and stimulates the mammary gland to increase lactation. Indications: postpartum hemorrhage after infant and placental delivery; induces labor at term (not a prehospital indication). Contraindications: presence of a second fetus; hypertonic or hyperactive uterus fetal distress. Adverse reactions: tachycardia, hypertension, dysrhythmias, angina pectoris, anxiety, seizure, nausea, vomiting, allergic reaction, and uterine rupture (excessive dose). Onset: IV—immediate; IM—3 to 5 minutes. Duration: IV—20 minutes; IM—30 to 60 minutes. Dose: IM—3 to 10 units after delivery of the placenta; IV—mix 10 to 40 units in 1000 mL normal saline or lactated Ringer solution and infuse at 10 to 40 milliunits/min, titrated to the severity of bleeding and uterine response. Special considerations: vasopressors may potentiate hypertension; vital signs and uterine tone should be monitored closely. Administer in prehospital setting after all fetuses delivered.

30. Etomidate (Amidate). Class: nonbarbiturate hypnotic, anesthetic. Description: acts at reticular activating system to produce anesthesia. Short-acting agent used for conscious sedation. Contraindications: hypersensitivity; labor and delivery. Adverse reactions: nausea and vomiting, dysrhythmias, dyspnea, hypotension, hypertension, involuntary muscle movement, pain at injection site. Onset: IV within 30 sec. Duration: 3 to 5 min. Dose: adult: 0.2 to 0.4 mg/kg IV over 30 to 60 seconds. Pediatric (older than 10 years of age): 0.2 to 0.4 mg/kg for rapid sequence intubation (RSI). Special considerations: regnancy Category C; can suppress adrenal secretion of steroids.

31. b. Dopamine is used to increase stroke volume.
32. d. Nitrous oxide is contraindicated in severe COPD. Fentanyl should be used with caution, if at all in older adults with severe respiratory disease.
33. a. Epinephrine 1:10,000 IV is indicated for all other conditions listed.
34. b. Adenosine, beta-blockers (atenolol), and calcium blockers (diltiazem) are not recommended to control rate in atrial fibrillation or flutter in the presence of Wolff-Parkinson-White syndrome.
35. b. It blocks parasympathetic stimulation. It is not indicated in asystole.
36. a. Do not administer to patients with liver disease.
37. a. Aspirin should be administered. The blood pressure is too low to administer the other drugs.
38. a. All of the other drugs are not sympathomimetic.
39. c. All others are beta-agonists.
40. b. Verapamil vasodilates and further decreases blood pressure.
41. d. Morphine and fentanyl is given IV or IM. Nitroglycerin is given by infusion, SL tablet, or spray for chest pain.
42. b.
43. a. The of the other drugs listed increase the plasmin in the blood, which causes degradation of fibrin threads and fibrinogen.
44. d. Naloxone is administered to reverse potential narcotic intoxication. Thiamine promotes uptake of glucose in the brain and prevents the development of Wernicke's encephalopathy when glucose is administered.
45. b. It is an osmotic diuretic and pulls excess fluid from the brain, temporarily decreasing intracranial pressure.
46. a.
47. d. Oxytocin should be administered only after delivery of all of the babies.
48. b. Benadryl causes thickening of the bronchial secretions and exacerbates an asthma attack.
49. d. It is contraindicated with the other ingestions listed.
50. c. It is not effective against barbiturates, stimulants, or benzodiazepines.
51. c. It also may cause hypotension.
52. a. Magnesium would be given if the Q-T interval were prolonged. Beta-blockers would be an option for polymorphic ventricular tachycardia. Lidocaine can be used if amiodarone is not available.
53. a. Hypotension and burning under the tongue are also often encountered.
54. b. Digoxin has positive inotropic but not chronotropic effects.
55. c. Furosemide decreases intravascular volume and may thicken secretions in pneumonia.
56. d. Adenosine is not a calcium channel blocker and is not used to treat atrial flutter.
57. d. Nitroglycerin is the only class I recommended drug.
58. d. Beta-blockers decrease heart rate and contractility. They may cause bronchoconstriction.
59. a. Haloperidol (Haldol) is a major tranquilizer.
60. c. It is a steroid antiinflammatory agent.

Illustration Credits and Acknowledgments

Figs. 10-1, 10-4, 10-5, 10-10, 10-11, 10-13, 10-14, 10-16, 10-17 and 10-18 Thibodeau GA: *Structure & function of the body,* ed 9, St Louis, 1992, Mosby.

Figs. 10-6, 10-8 Seeley R, Stephens T, Tate P: *Anatomy & physiology,* ed 2, St Louis, 1992, Mosby.

Fig. 10-15 Seeley R: *Anatomy & physiology,* ed 2, St Louis, 1992, Mosby (Sims/Illustrator Jody L. Fulks).

Figs. 22-1, 22-3 Cotton S: *Mosby's paramedic study guide,* St Louis, 1989, Mosby.

Figs. 22-4, 22-12 Huszar R: *Basic dysrhythmias,* ed 2, St Louis, 1994, Mosby.

The following ECG strips and drug flashcards are included to make the task of studying easier. The cards should be completed in accordance with the questions in Chapter 22. However, they are not designed to be used in just those areas.

Challenge yourself and use the drug cards:

- With a fellow student as flashcards to study
- To review drugs in subsequent chapters
- In the cardiovascular section to enhance your instructor's lecture
- While on clinical sites as an easy reference
- Before final examinations as a quick, portable review

The ECG cards may be helpful:

- During ECG study, group them according to their similarities, and later, as you master them, mix them up and identify each one
- To make up scenarios in study groups
- When practicing for cardiac algorithm practicals
- To bring along during hospital and field clinicals as an easy reference

Be creative and invent your own uses for these flashcards. They are here so you can improve your knowledge and enhance success in study.

● FLASHCARD 1

Fig. 22-8

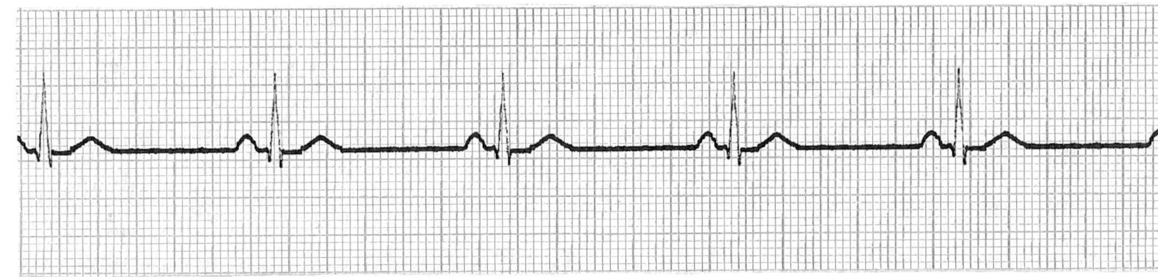

43.

QRS:_________________________ P wave: _________________________________

Rate: _________________________ Rhythm:__________________ PRI: _________________

Interpretation: ___**Sinus bradycardia**_______________________________

Distinguishing features: ____

Treatment: ____

● FLASHCARD 2

Fig. 22-9

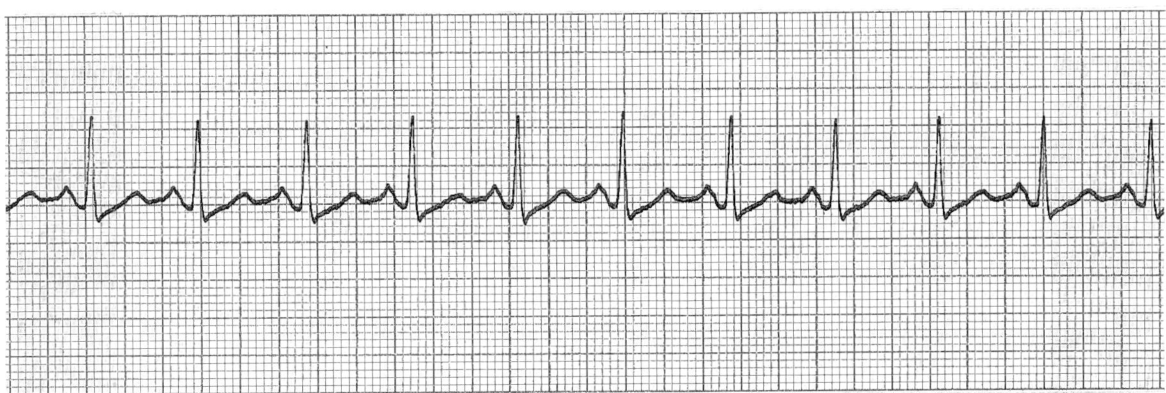

● FLASHCARD 3

Fig. 22-10

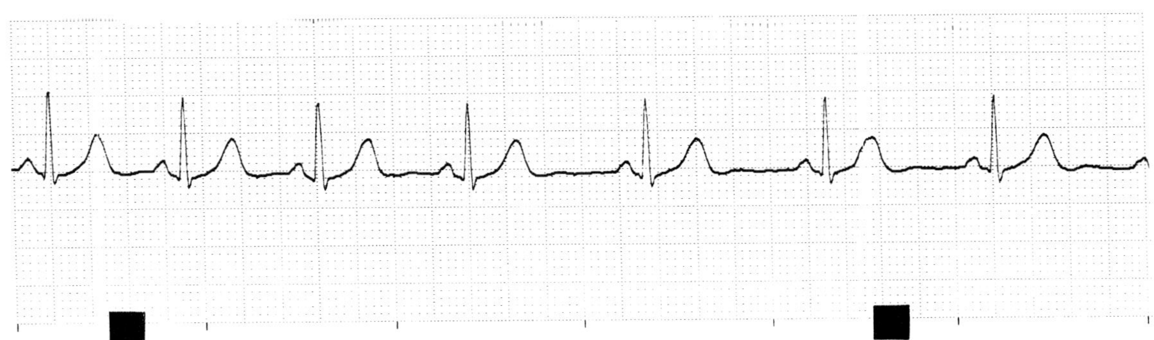

● FLASHCARD 4

Fig. 22-11

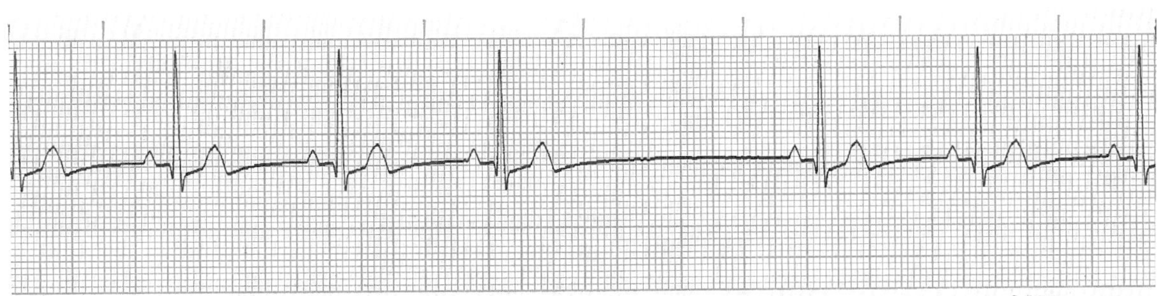

44.

QRS:_______________________________ P wave: _______________________________________

Rate: _______________________________ Rhythm:_______________________ PRI: _______________________

Interpretation:____**Sinus tachycardia**____

Distinguishing features: ____

Treatment: ____

____

45.

QRS:_______________________________ P wave: _______________________________________

Rate: _______________________________ Rhythm:_______________________ PRI: _______________________

Interpretation:____**Sinus dysrhythmia**____

Distinguishing features: ____

Treatment: ____

____

46.

QRS:_______________________________ P wave: _______________________________________

Rate: _______________________________ Rhythm:_______________________ PRI: _______________________

Interpretation:____**Sinus arrest**____

Distinguishing features: ____

Treatment: ____

____

Fig. 22-12

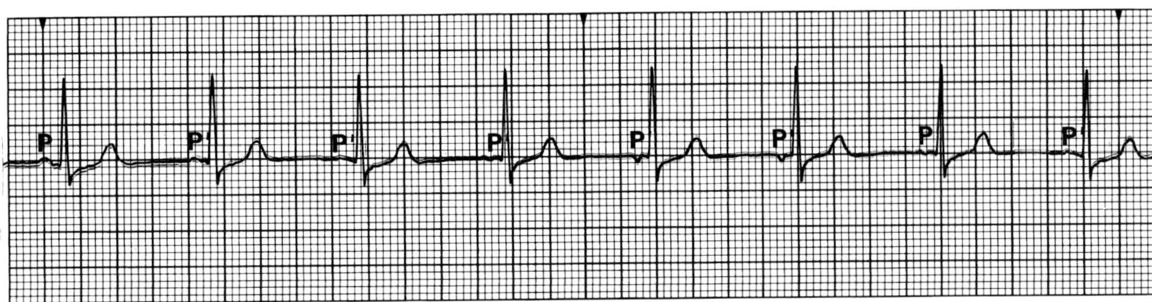

Fig. 22-13

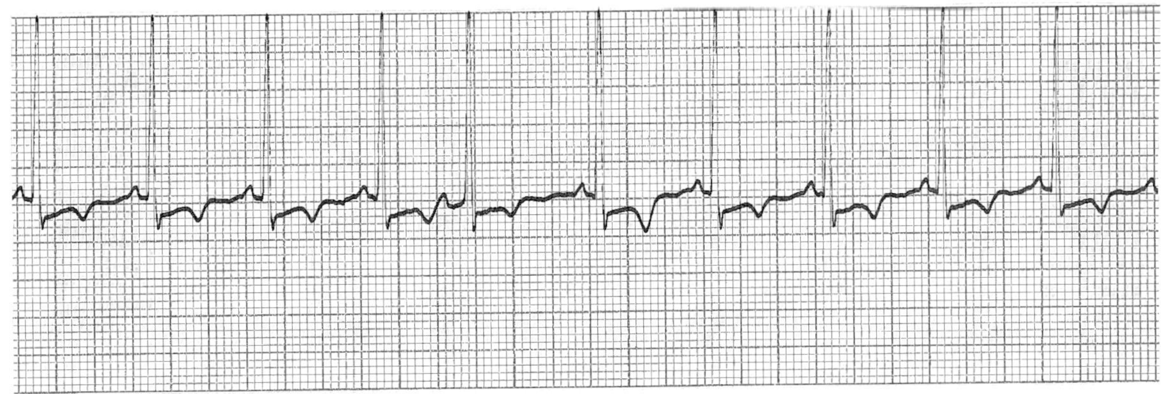

Fig. 22-14

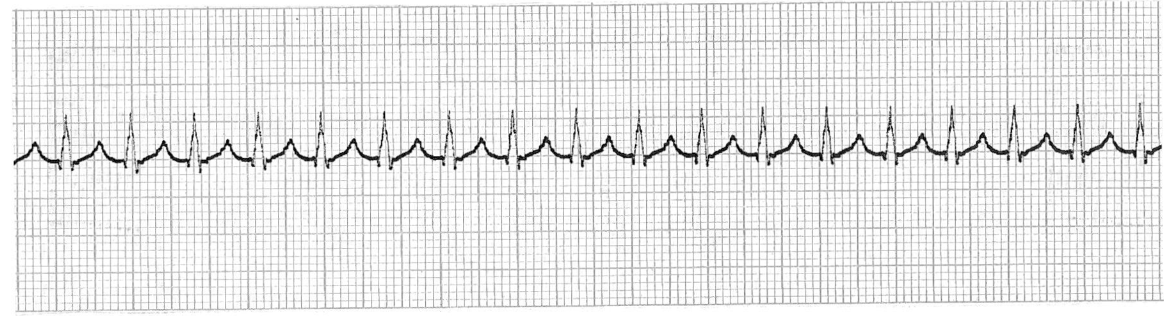

50.

QRS:_________________________________ P wave: ____

Rate: _________________________________ Rhythm:_____________________________ PRI: _________________________________

Interpretation:_____**Wandering atrial pacemaker**_______________________________________

Distinguishing features: ____

Treatment: ____

____

51.

QRS:_________________________________ P wave: ____

Rate: _________________________________ Rhythm:_____________________________ PRI: _________________________________

Interpretation:_____**Premature atrial contraction**_______________________________________

Distinguishing features: ____

Treatment: ____

____

52.

QRS:_________________________________ P wave: ____

Rate: _________________________________ Rhythm:_____________________________ PRI: _________________________________

Interpretation:_____**Supraventricular tachycardia**_______________________________________

Distinguishing features: ____

Treatment: ____

____

● FLASHCARD 8

Fig. 22-15

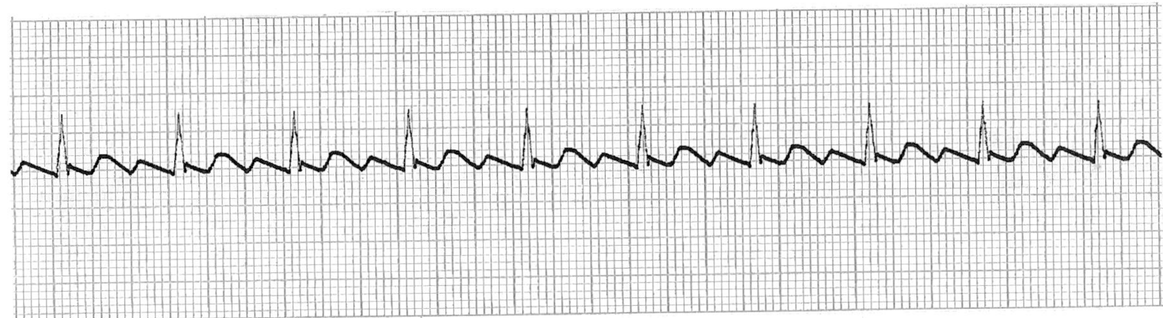

● FLASHCARD 9

Fig. 22-16

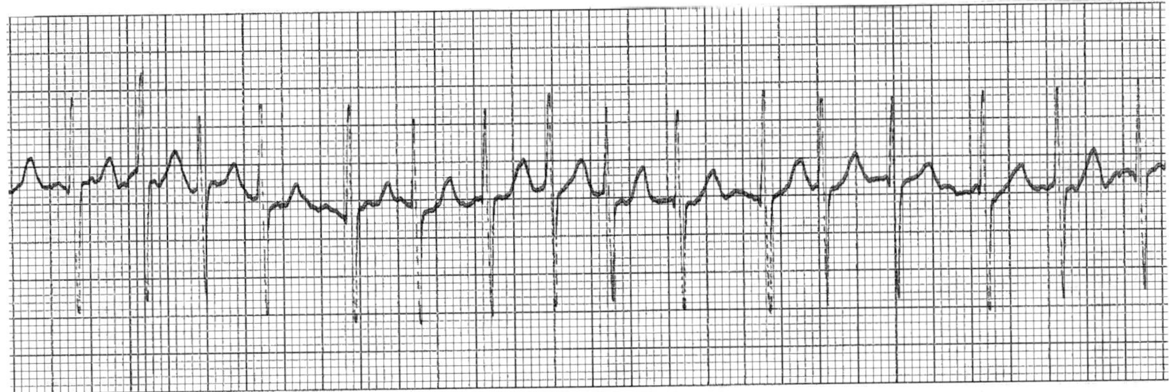

● FLASHCARD 10

Fig. 22-17

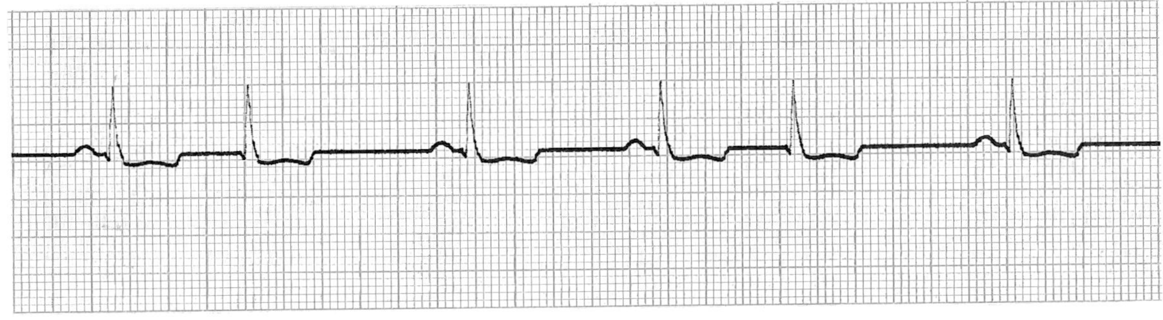

53.

QRS:_______________________ P wave: _______________________

Rate: _______________________ Rhythm:_______________________ PRI: _______________________

Interpretation:___**Atrial flutter with 3:1 conduction**_______________________

Distinguishing features: _______________________

Treatment: _______________________

____

54.

QRS:_______________________ P wave: _______________________

Rate: _______________________ Rhythm:_______________________ PRI: _______________________

Interpretation:___**Atrial fibrillation**_______________________

Distinguishing features: _______________________

Treatment: _______________________

____

57.

QRS:_______________________ P wave: _______________________

Rate: _______________________ Rhythm:_______________________ PRI: _______________________

Interpretation:___**Sinus rhythm (borderline bradycardia) with two premature junctional contractions**_______________________

Distinguishing features: _______________________

Treatment: _______________________

● **FLASHCARD 11**

Fig. 22-18

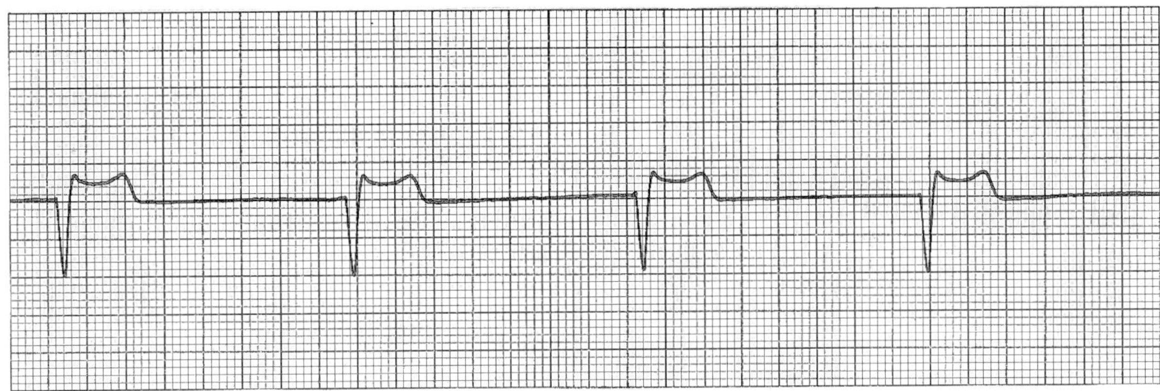

● **FLASHCARD 12**

Fig. 22-19

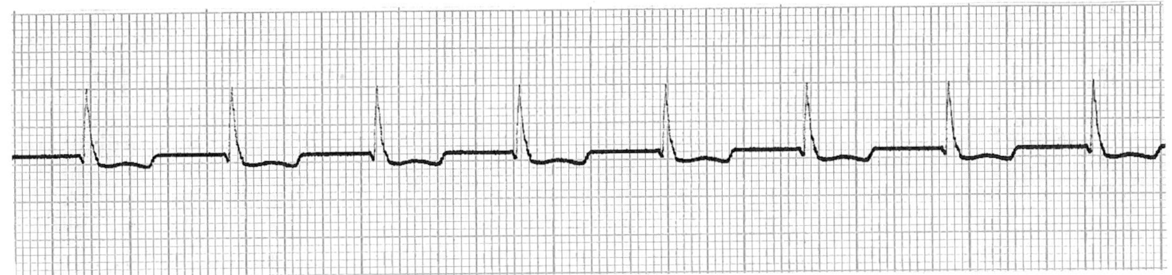

● **FLASHCARD 13**

Fig. 22-20

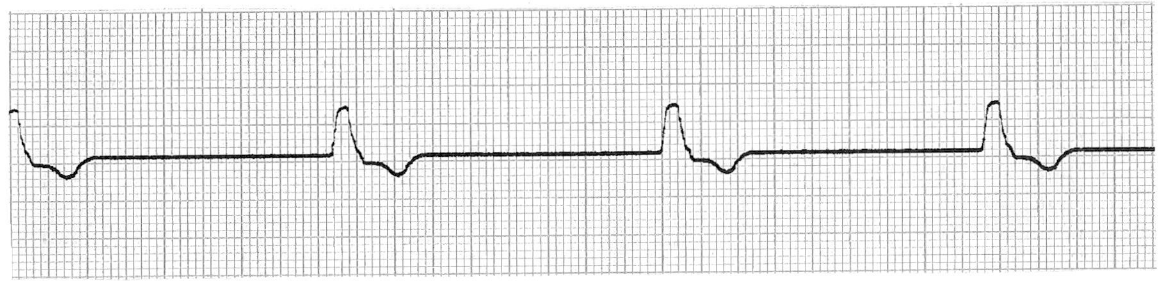

58.

QRS:_____________________ P wave: ________________________

Rate: __________________ Rhythm:________________ PRI: ___________________

Interpretation:___**Junctional escape rhythm**________________________

Distinguishing features: ________________________________

Treatment: ____________________________________

____

59.

QRS:_____________________ P wave: ________________________

Rate: __________________ Rhythm:________________ PRI: ___________________

Interpretation:___**Accelerated junctional rhythm**___________________

Distinguishing features: ________________________________

Treatment: ____________________________________

____

63.

QRS:_____________________ P wave: ________________________

Rate: __________________ Rhythm:________________ PRI: ___________________

Interpretation:___**Ventricular escape rhythm**___________________

Distinguishing features: ________________________________

Treatment: ____________________________________

____

● FLASHCARD 14

Fig. 22-21

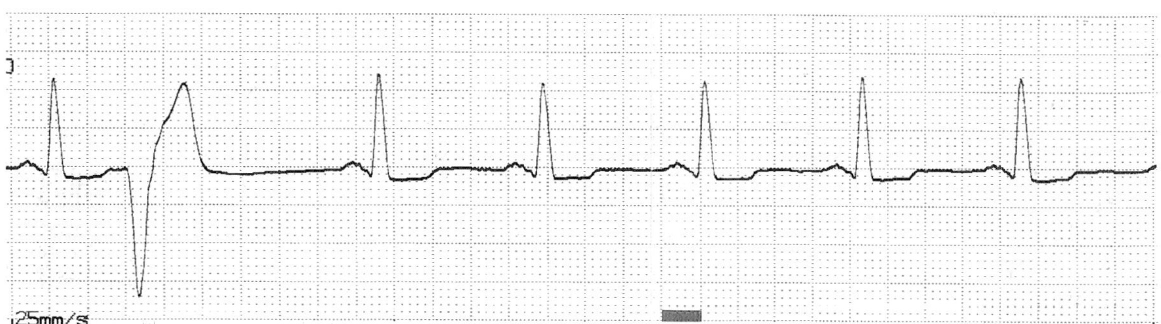

● FLASHCARD 15

Fig. 22-22

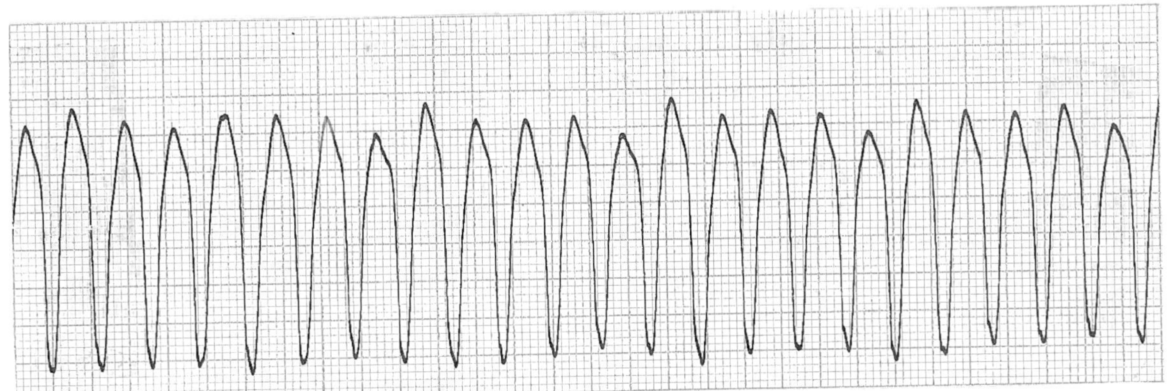

● FLASHCARD 16

Fig. 22-23

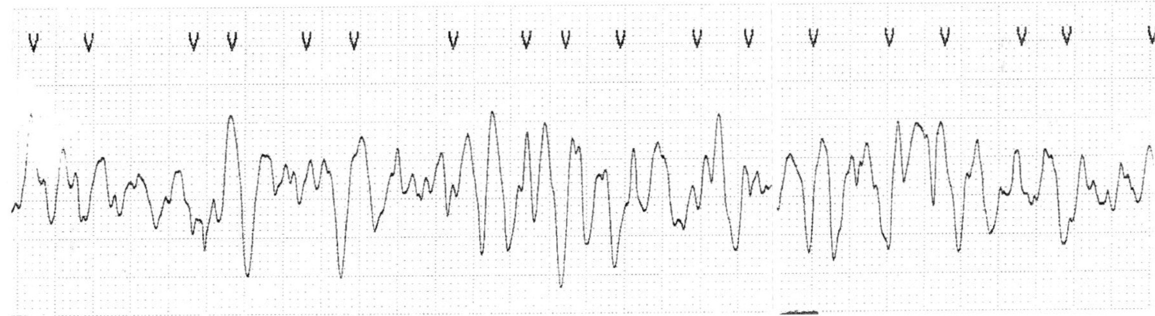

64.

QRS:___________________________ P wave: ___________________________________

Rate: _________________________ Rhythm:___________________ PRI: _________________________

Interpretation:____**Normal sinus rhythm with one premature ventricular contraction**___________

Distinguishing features: ____

Treatment: ____

____

65.

QRS:___________________________ P wave: ___________________________________

Rate: _________________________ Rhythm:___________________ PRI: _________________________

Interpretation:____**Monomorphic ventricular tachycardia**___________________________________

Distinguishing features: ____

Treatment: ____

____

66.

QRS:___________________________ P wave: ___________________________________

Rate: _________________________ Rhythm:___________________ PRI: _________________________

Interpretation:____**Ventricular fibrillation**____

Distinguishing features: ____

Treatment: ____

____

- **FLASHCARD 17**

Fig. 22-24

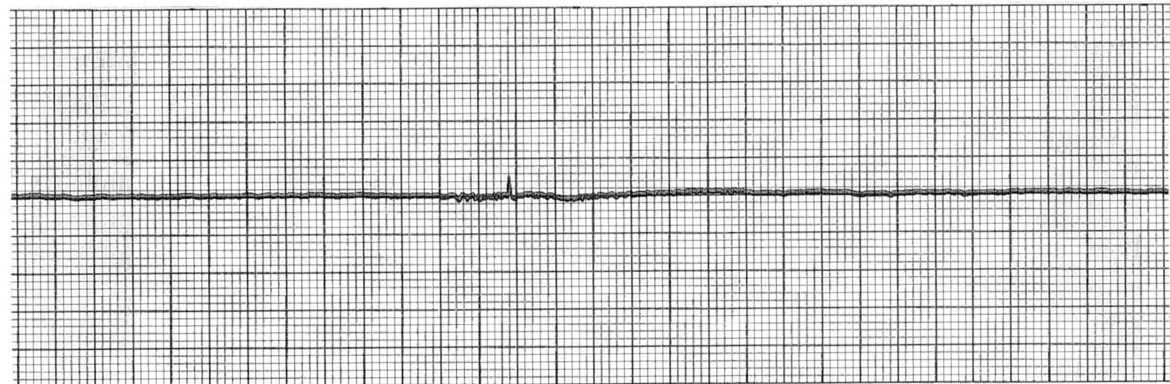

- **FLASHCARD 18**

Fig. 22-25

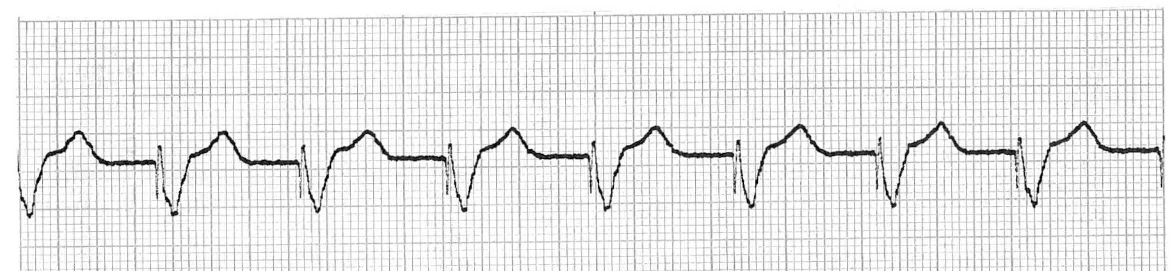

- **FLASHCARD 19**

Fig. 22-26

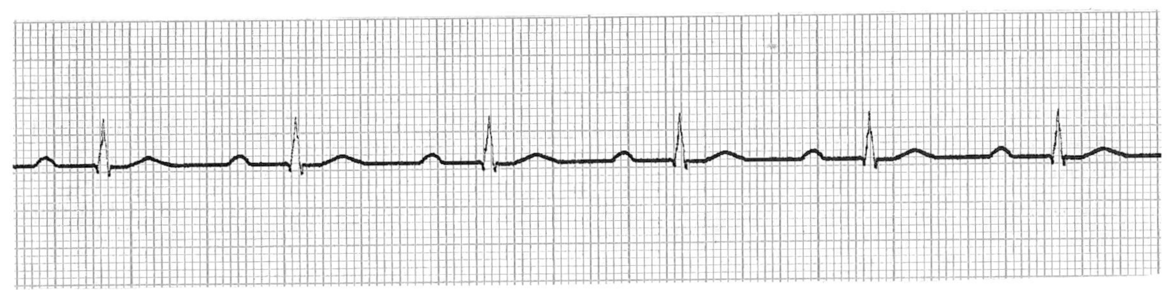

67.

QRS:_______________________________ P wave: _______________________________________

Rate: _______________________________ Rhythm:_____________________ PRI: _______________________

Interpretation:_____**Asystole**____

Distinguishing features: ____

Treatment: ____

____

68.

QRS:_______________________________ P wave: _______________________________________

Rate: _______________________________ Rhythm:_____________________ PRI: _______________________

Interpretation:_____**Ventricular paced rhythm**____

Distinguishing features: ____

Treatment: ____

____

71.

QRS:_______________________________ P wave: _______________________________________

Rate: _______________________________ Rhythm:_____________________ PRI: _______________________

Interpretation:_____**Sinus rhythm with first-degree atrioventricular block**__________________

Distinguishing features: ____

Treatment: ____

● FLASHCARD 20

Fig. 22-27

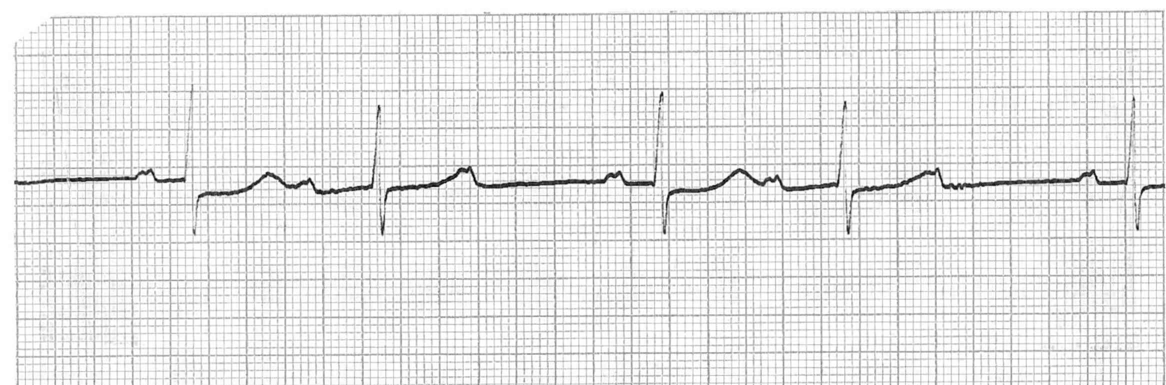

● FLASHCARD 21

Fig. 22-28

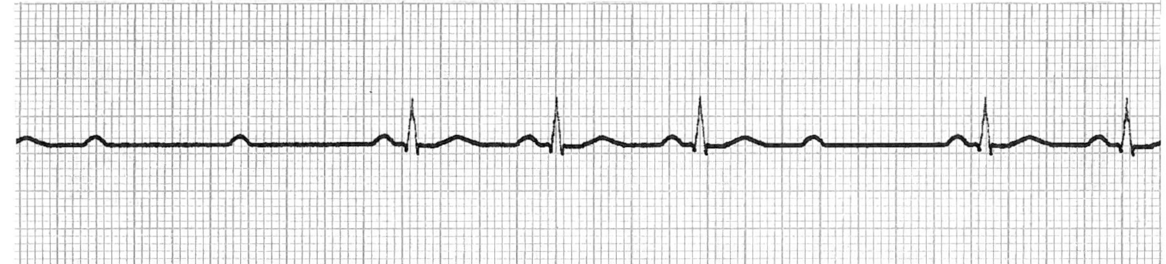

● FLASHCARD 22

Fig. 22-29

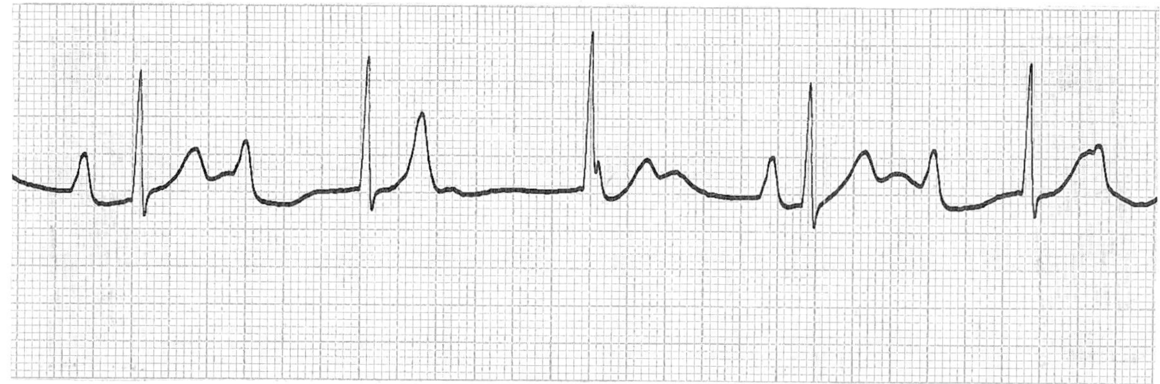

72.

QRS:_______________________ P wave: _______________________

Rate: _______________________ Rhythm:_______________________ PRI: _______________________

Interpretation:_____**Second-degree atrioventricular block (Mobitz type I or Wenckebach)**_______

Distinguishing features: _______________________

Treatment: _______________________

____

73.

QRS:_______________________ P wave: _______________________

Rate: _______________________ Rhythm:_______________________ PRI: _______________________

Interpretation:_____**Second-degree atrioventricular block (Mobitz type II)**_______

Distinguishing features: _______________________

Treatment: _______________________

____

74.

QRS:_______________________ P wave: _______________________

Rate: _______________________ Rhythm:_______________________ PRI: _______________________

Interpretation:_____**Third-degree (complete) atrioventricular block**_______

Distinguishing features: _______________________

Treatment: _______________________

____

● FLASHCARD 24	**● FLASHCARD 23**

● FLASHCARD 24

Question 4

Trade Name: _______________________________

Class: ___________________________________

Descriptions: ______________________________

____

Indications: _______________________________

____

Contraindications: __________________________

____

Adverse Reactions: _________________________

____

Onset: ___________________________________

Duration _________________________________

Dosage: __________________________________

____

____

____

Special Considerations: ______________________

____

____

● FLASHCARD 23

Question 3

Trade Name: _______________________________

Class: ___________________________________

Descriptions: ______________________________

____

Indications: _______________________________

____

Contraindications: __________________________

____

Adverse Reactions: _________________________

____

Onset: ___________________________________

Duration _________________________________

Dosage: __________________________________

____

____

____

Special Considerations: ______________________

____

____

● FLASHCARD 26

Question 6a

Trade Name: __________ N/A ________________

Class: ___________________________________

Descriptions: ______________________________

____

Indications: _______________________________

____

Contraindications: __________________________

Adverse Reactions: _________________________

____

Onset: ___________________________________

Duration _________________________________

Dosage: __________________________________

____

____

Special Considerations: ______________________

____

● FLASHCARD 25

Question 5

Trade Name: _______________________________

Class: ___________________________________

Descriptions: ______________________________

____

Indications: _______________________________

____

Contraindications: __________________________

____

Adverse Reactions: _________________________

____

Onset: ___________________________________

Duration _________________________________

Dosage: __________________________________

____

____

Special Considerations: ______________________

____

diphenhydramine

vasopressin

glucagon

procainamide

● FLASHCARD 28

Question 7

Trade Name: _______________________

Class: _______________________

Descriptions: _______________________

Indications: _______________________

Contraindications: _______________________

Adverse Reactions: _______________________

Onset: _______________________

Duration _______________________

Dosage: _______________________

Special Considerations: _______________________

● FLASHCARD 27

Question 6b

Trade Name: _______________________

Class: _______________________

Descriptions: _______________________

Indications: _______________________

Contraindications: _______________________

Adverse Reactions: _______________________

Onset: _______________________

Duration _______________________

Dosage: _______________________

Special Considerations: _______________________

● FLASHCARD 30

Question 9

Trade Name: _______________________

Class: _______________________

Descriptions: _______________________

Indications: _______________________

Contraindications: _______________________

Adverse Reactions: _______________________

Onset: _______________________

Duration _______________________

Dosage: _______________________

Special Considerations: _______________________

● FLASHCARD 29

Question 8

Trade Name: _______________________

Class: _______________________

Descriptions: _______________________

Indications: _______________________

Contraindications: _______________________

Adverse Reactions: _______________________

Onset: _______________________

Duration _______________________

Dosage: _______________________

Special Considerations: _______________________

amiodarone

nitroglycerin

lidocaine

ketorolac
tromethamine

● FLASHCARD 32

Question 11

Trade Name: _______________________________

Class: ____________________________________

Descriptions: ______________________________

____

Indications: _______________________________

____

Contraindications: __________________________

____

Adverse Reactions:__________________________

____

Onset: ___________________________________

Duration ________________________________

Dosage:__________________________________

____

____

____

Special Considerations: ______________________

____

____

● FLASHCARD 31

Question 10

Trade Name: _______________________________

Class: ____________________________________

Descriptions: ______________________________

____

Indications: _______________________________

____

Contraindications: __________________________

____

Adverse Reactions:__________________________

____

Onset: ___________________________________

Duration ________________________________

Dosage:__________________________________

____

____

____

Special Considerations: ______________________

____

____

● FLASHCARD 34

Question 13

Trade Name: _______________________________

Class: ____________________________________

Descriptions: ______________________________

____

Indications: _______________________________

____

Contraindications: __________________________

____

Adverse Reactions:__________________________

____

Onset: ___________________________________

Duration ________________________________

Dosage:__________________________________

____

Special Considerations: ______________________

____

● FLASHCARD 33

Question 12

Trade Name: _______________________________

Class: ____________________________________

Descriptions: ______________________________

____

Indications: _______________________________

____

Contraindications: __________________________

____

Adverse Reactions:__________________________

____

Onset: ___________________________________

Duration ________________________________

Dosage:__________________________________

____

____

____

Special Considerations: ______________________

____

____

naloxone

midazolam
hydrochloride

atropine sulfate

epinephrine

● FLASHCARD 36

Question 15

Trade Name: _________________ N/A _________________

Class: _______________________________________

Descriptions: _________________________________

____

Indications: __________________________________

____

Contraindications: _____________________________

____

Adverse Reactions:_____________________________

____

Onset: ______________________________________

Duration ____________________________________

Dosage:_____________________________________

____

____

____

Special Considerations: _________________________

____

____

● FLASHCARD 35

Question 14

Trade Name: __________________________________

Class: _______________________________________

Descriptions: _________________________________

____

Indications: __________________________________

____

Contraindications: _____________________________

____

Adverse Reactions:_____________________________

____

Onset: ______________________________________

Duration ____________________________________

Dosage:_____________________________________

____

____

____

Special Considerations: _________________________

____

____

● FLASHCARD 38

Question 16b

Trade Name: _________________ N/A _________________

Class: _______________________________________

Descriptions: _________________________________

____

Indications: __________________________________

____

Contraindications: _____________________________

____

Adverse Reactions:_____________________________

____

Onset: ______________________________________

Duration ____________________________________

Dosage:_____________________________________

____

____

Special Considerations: _________________________

____

____

● FLASHCARD 37

Question 16a

Trade Name: __________________________________

Class: _______________________________________

Descriptions: _________________________________

____

Indications: __________________________________

____

Contraindications: _____________________________

____

Adverse Reactions:_____________________________

____

Onset: ______________________________________

Duration ____________________________________

Dosage:_____________________________________

____

____

Special Considerations: _________________________

____

____

nitrous oxide

sodium bicarbonate

thiamine

dextrose 50%

● FLASHCARD 40

Question 18

Trade Name: _______________________________

Class: _______________________________

Descriptions: _______________________________

Indications: _______________________________

Contraindications: _______________________________

Adverse Reactions: _______________________________

Onset: _______________________________

Duration _______________________________

Dosage: _______________________________

Special Considerations: _______________________________

● FLASHCARD 39

Question 17

Trade Name: _______________________________

Class: _______________________________

Descriptions: _______________________________

Indications: _______________________________

Contraindications: _______________________________

Adverse Reactions: _______________________________

Onset: _______________________________

Duration _______________________________

Dosage: _______________________________

Special Considerations: _______________________________

● FLASHCARD 42

Question 20

Trade Name: _______________________________

Class: _______________________________

Descriptions: _______________________________

Indications: _______________________________

Contraindications: _______________________________

Adverse Reactions: _______________________________

Onset: _______________________________

Duration _______________________________

Dosage: _______________________________

Special Considerations: _______________________________

● FLASHCARD 41

Question 19

Trade Name: _______________________________

Class: _______________________________

Descriptions: _______________________________

Indications: _______________________________

Contraindications: _______________________________

Adverse Reactions: _______________________________

Onset: _______________________________

Duration _______________________________

Dosage: _______________________________

Special Considerations: _______________________________

diazepam

albuterol

aspirin

adenosine

● FLASHCARD 44

Question 21b

Trade Name: _______________________________

Class: _______________________________

Descriptions: _______________________________

____

Indications: _______________________________

____

Contraindications: _______________________________

____

Adverse Reactions: _______________________________

____

Onset: _______________________________

Duration _______________________________

Dosage: _______________________________

____

____

____

Special Considerations: _______________________________

____

____

● FLASHCARD 43

Question 21a

Trade Name: _______________________________

Class: _______________________________

Descriptions: _______________________________

____

Indications: _______________________________

____

Contraindications: _______________________________

____

Adverse Reactions: _______________________________

____

Onset: _______________________________

Duration _______________________________

Dosage: _______________________________

____

____

____

Special Considerations: _______________________________

____

____

● FLASHCARD 46

Question 23

Trade Name: _______________________________

Class: _______________________________

Descriptions: _______________________________

____

Indications: _______________________________

____

Contraindications: _______________________________

____

Adverse Reactions: _______________________________

Onset: _______________________________

Duration _______________________________

Dosage: _______________________________

____

____

Special Considerations: _______________________________

____

● FLASHCARD 45

Question 22

Trade Name: _______________________________

Class: _______________________________

Descriptions: _______________________________

____

Indications: _______________________________

____

Contraindications: _______________________________

____

Adverse Reactions: _______________________________

____

Onset: _______________________________

Duration _______________________________

Dosage: _______________________________

____

____

Special Considerations: _______________________________

____

____

morphine sulfate

meperidine

labetalol

activated charcoal

● FLASHCARD 48

Question 25

Trade Name: _______________________________

Class: _______________________________

Descriptions: _______________________________

Indications: _______________________________

Contraindications: _______________________________

Adverse Reactions: _______________________________

Onset: _______________________________

Duration _______________________________

Dosage: _______________________________

Special Considerations: _______________________________

● FLASHCARD 47

Question 24

Trade Name: _________ N/A _________

Class: _______________________________

Descriptions: _______________________________

Indications: _______________________________

Contraindications: _______________________________

Adverse Reactions: _______________________________

Onset: _______________________________

Duration _______________________________

Dosage: _______________________________

Special Considerations: _______________________________

● FLASHCARD 50

Question 27

Trade Name: _______________________________

Class: _______________________________

Descriptions: _______________________________

Indications: _______________________________

Contraindications: _______________________________

Adverse Reactions: _______________________________

Onset: _______________________________

Duration _______________________________

Dosage: _______________________________

Special Considerations: _______________________________

● FLASHCARD 49

Question 26

Trade Name: _______________________________

Class: _______________________________

Descriptions: _______________________________

Indications: _______________________________

Contraindications: _______________________________

Adverse Reactions: _______________________________

Onset: _______________________________

Duration _______________________________

Dosage: _______________________________

Special Considerations: _______________________________

magnesium sulfate

dopamine

verapamil

furosemide

oxytocin